David A. Clark '85

PHYSIOLOGY OF THE INTESTINAL CIRCULATION

Physiology of the Intestinal Circulation

Editors

A. P. Shepherd, Ph.D.
Professor of Physiology
University of Texas Health Science Center
San Antonio, Texas

D. N. Granger, Ph.D.
Professor of Physiology
College of Medicine
University of South Alabama
Mobile, Alabama

Raven Press ■ New York

Raven Press, 1140 Avenue of the Americas, New York, New York 10036

© 1984 by Raven Press Books, Ltd. All rights reserved. This book is protected by copyright. No part of it may be reproduced, stored in a retrieval system, or transmitted, in any form or by any means, electronic, mechanical, photocopying, recording, or otherwise, without the prior written permission of the publisher.

Made in the United States of America

Library of Congress Cataloging in Publication Data
Main entry under title:

Physiology of the intestinal circulation.

Includes bibliographical references and index.
1. Intestines—Blood-vessels. 2. Blood—Circulation.
I. Shepherd, A. P. (Albert P.) II. Granger, D. Neil.
[DNLM: 1. Intestines—blood supply. 2. Regional Blood
Flow. WI 400 P578]
QP156.P49   1984   599'.0132   84-9858
ISBN 0-88167-025-1

International Standard Book Number 0-88167-025-1
Library of Congress Catalog Card Number

The material contained in this volume was submitted as previously unpublished material, except in the instances in which credit has been given to the source from which some of the illustrative material was derived.

Great care has been taken to maintain the accuracy of the information contained in the volume. However, Raven Press cannot be held responsible for errors or for any consequences arising from the use of the information contained herein.

We dedicate this book with affection—

to our parents for encouraging us to get an education,

to our children
that they might do likewise,

to our families for enabling us to have scholarly pursuits,

and to all "blood and guts" physiologists that they may not only survive but prevail in an era of molecular biology.

Foreword

My interest in the circulatory system has always been centered on the basic concepts of circulatory function, especially the peculiar hemodynamic characteristics that give it a high degree of stability and the multiple control mechanisms that optimize function to the needs of the individual parts of the body. In looking at the whole circulation in this manner, I must admit to a tendency to group the intestinal circulation with other regional circulations, thus neglecting the distinctive features of this circulation in the performance of its specialized goals. Therefore, the multiple topics and depth of coverage in the chapters of this book emphasize two points: first, that a very large share of the lumped parameters that I have utilized in the consideration of the whole circulation are contributed by the intestinal circulation, and, second, that the intestinal circulation has a unique nature that makes it as worthy of study as the more widely studied regional circulations of the heart and brain.

The contents of *Physiology of the Intestinal Circulation* provide thorough sampling of worldwide research in this field. It will be of special value as a resource for investigators who themselves are working on the physiology of the intestinal circulation. The topics are organized in five major sections: (a) blood flow regulation and hemodynamics; (b) intestinal transcapillary fluid exchange; (c) mathematical models; (d) pathophysiology; and (e) pharmacology. However, embedded in these major areas are many other threads of investigation. For instance, both the metabolic and myogenic theories of autoregulation are presented along with data that led to the origin of these theories. In addition, multiple studies show the important roles of tissue metabolism, digestion of food, intestinal motility, intestinal secretion, oxygen in the arterial blood, and vascular reflexes in controlling both gross intestinal blood flow and blood flow in individual tissues of the intestines.

The physiology of intestinal fluids is discussed in detail. Consideration is given to the peculiar characteristics of capillary dynamics and capillary fluid exchange in the intestinal circulation. Also, the lymphatics, which, from a quantitative point of view, play a far greater role in the intestinal circulation than elsewhere in the body, receive just coverage.

The sections on pathophysiology and pharmacology could be classified as applied physiology of the intestinal circulation; however, in both cases, specific studies have led to important concepts that could not have been derived from experiments in normal animals. Of importance also is the section on mathematical models. The value of models is not that they provide new data but that they add tremendous depth to a research worker's thinking and analysis of his work. A mathematical analysis is "unforgiving"—it does not allow the drawing of hazy, nonquantitative conclusions. A mathematical model expresses concepts in quantitative terms; often in the past, disregarding the quantitative approach has given rise to misleading concepts. More importantly, these models lead to new experiments that can be the basis for greater depth of understanding. The mathematical models in this book provide important insights for those who study them and understand the resulting predictions.

The volume editors have been indefatigable in their study of the intestinal circulation, one emphasizing mainly the control of intestinal blood flow, and the other studying in great depth the role of the intestinal circulation in fluid exchange. A special characteristic of their work has been the introduction of multiple new experimental approaches involving new types of measuring apparatus and ingenious experimental techniques, resulting in a continuing series of significant contributions to the literature. It is fitting that Drs. Shepherd and Granger have collaborated on this most worthwhile resource book on the physiology of the intestinal circulation.

Arthur C. Guyton

Department of Physiology and Biophysics
University of Mississippi Medical Center
Jackson, Mississippi

Preface

> The local circulations are absolutely unknown. Harvey gave only the general circulations. There is a book to be written on the partial circulations.——*Claude Bernard, 1860.*

Many physiologists have taken Claude Bernard's advice and written books on various vascular beds. Books treating the coronary and cerebral circulations, in particular, are readily available to students and investigators of these areas. However, cardiovascular texts generally have treated the intestinal circulation as a stepchild, and, if addressed at all, the intestinal circulation was relegated to a miscellaneous chapter along with other visceral organs. More recently, books on the peripheral circulation occasionally have devoted a single chapter to the intestine, but such treatment today is inadequate even as a superficial summary. In the last decade, our knowledge of the intestinal circulation has burgeoned, and the community of scholars in this field, although still small, has been strengthened by talented young investigators. Therefore, we felt the time had come for a book devoted entirely to the intestinal circulation.

Claude Bernard wrote, "Science does not grow successively and regularly. It goes by bounds and revolutions." We have been privileged to participate in a decade of research in which our knowledge of the physiology of the intestinal circulation has grown rapidly. We realized that because much of the work on the intestinal circulation is recent, many of the most prominent contributors to this field were still active and could be recruited to help write this first monograph devoted completely to the physiology of the intestinal circulation. Therefore, we invited experts from around the globe to contribute chapters treating topics on which they are recognized authorities. Fortunately, few declined our invitation.

We have organized the book into five sections to facilitate the book's use as a reference:
- I. Blood Flow Regulation and Hemodynamics
- II. Intestinal Transcapillary Fluid Exchange
- III. Mathematical Models
- IV. Pathophysiology
- V. Pharmacology

Each section treats major areas of investigation of the intestinal circulation and because some areas have been more thoroughly studied than others, these sections are necessarily unequal in size. As Homer Smith observed, "the central problem of physiology is regulation within the organism." Thus, it is not surprising the bulk of the book, Section I, is devoted to the mechanisms that regulate intestinal blood flow. Here, autoregulation and the concept of local control, the sympathetic nervous system's effects on intestinal blood flow, and the potential role of gastrointestinal hormones as vasoregulators are discussed. Section I also deals with significant, often unique, aspects of the intestinal circulation, such as the response to a meal, the countercurrent exchange mechanism in the villus, and the role of the splanchnic circulation in the regulation of whole body hemodynamics and distribution of blood volume. Section II contains six chapters devoted to the transcapillary fluid exchange, since the circulation both provides the fluid for intestinal secretions and a route for the removal of absorbed water and foodstuffs. In Section III, mathematical models of tissue oxygenation, transcapillary fluid exchange, the countercurrent mechanism, and the relationship between drug absorption and intestinal blood flow are presented.

Such models, a type of systems analysis, provide a powerful means for integrating diverse experimental findings. They also force an investigator to state his assumptions explicitly and to express in rigorous form the relationships that he believes exist among the variables in his model. Like other expressions of a theory, the true test of their value is not whether they were right or wrong but whether they provide greater insight and lead to fruitful experimentation. Section IV deals with the pathophysiology of the intestinal circulation: the important role of the gut in shock, the effects of luminal obstruction on enteric perfusion, and effects of diseases such as diabetes and portal hypertension on the intestinal circulation. Finally, Section V treats the pharmacological agents that affect intestinal oxygenation and fluid exchange or that have been used to staunch gastrointestinal hemorrhage.

The chapters can be read in any sequence, but reading the book from the beginning has the advantage of first summarizing the ground to be explored. Chapter 1 provides both a conceptual overview and an historical perspective of the evolution of man's ideas about the intestinal circulation. Subsequent chapters then proceed from the normal physiological regulation of this circulation to pathophysiological derangements and therapeutic approaches to treatment.

Anyone familiar with the investigators who have made important contributions in the last decade to our understanding of the intestinal circulation will immediately realize that this book was written by experts for experts, but we have edited it with the student and novice investigator in mind. We have tried to minimize the chapter-to-chapter unevenness that a multiauthored book inevitably contains, to require that each author define his terms carefully, to avoid laboratory jargon, and to use symbols consistent with other chapters. If our editorial efforts have been successful, this book should be useful not only to seasoned investigators but also to medical and graduate students who have completed a physiology course. To these students of the intestinal circulation and to physicians and surgeons who are confronted by life-threatening diseases such as necrotizing enterocolitis, bleeding esophageal varices, and hepatic portal hypertension, we hope this book will provide knowledge and insight into the intestinal circulation.

A. P. Shepherd
D. N. Granger

San Antonio and Mobile

Acknowledgments

The editors gratefully acknowledge the assistance of Mrs. Linda Shimerda, whose meticulous attention to detail assured the successful collection of each submission and hence the successful completion of the book. The editors are also indebted to Melissa Shepherd for advice on grammar and punctuation.

Contents

Blood Flow Regulation and Hemodynamics

1. The Intestinal Circulation: A Historical Perspective   1
   D.N. Granger and A.P. Shepherd

2. Intestinal Microcirculation: Spatial Organization and Fine Structure   9
   J.R. Casley-Smith and Bren J. Gannon

3. Metabolic Regulation of the Intestinal Circulation   33
   A.P. Shepherd and D.N. Granger

4. Myogenic and Venous-Arteriolar Responses in Intestinal Circulation   49
   Paul C. Johnson

5. Neural Control and Autoregulatory Escape   61
   Clive V. Greenway

6. Control of Capacitance Vessels   73
   Carl F. Rothe

7. Countercurrent Exchange Mechanisms in the Small Intestine   83
   Mats Jodal, Ulf Haglund, and Ove Lundgren

8. Postprandial Mesenteric Hyperemia   99
   John W. Fara

9. Intestinal Blood Flow and Motility   107
   Joseph D. Fondacaro

10. Gastrointestinal Hormones and Intestinal Blood Flow   121
    C.C. Chou, M.J. Mangino, and D.R. Sawmiller

11. Physiology, Pharmacology, and Pathology of the Colonic Circulation   131
    Peter R. Kvietys and D.N. Granger

12. Tissue Oxygenation and Splanchnic Blood Flow   143
    H. Glenn Bohlen

13. Role of the Splanchnic Circulation in Reflex Control of the Cardiovascular System   153
    Loring B. Rowell and John M. Johnson

14. Cardiovascular Reflexes of Gastrointestinal Origin   165
    John C. Longhurst

15. Fetal and Neonatal Intestinal Circulations   179
    Daniel I. Edelstone and Ian R. Holzman

Intestinal Transcapillary Fluid Exchange

16. Intestinal Lymph Formation — 191
    J. A. Barrowman

17. Lymphatic Contractility — 201
    Jui S. Lee

18. Transcapillary Exchange During Intestinal Fluid Absorption — 211
    D. N. Granger, Michele Ulrich, Dale A. Parks, and Scot L. Harper

19. Capillary Fluid Exchange and Intestinal Secretion — 223
    David Mailman

20. Permeability Characteristics of Intestinal Capillaries — 233
    Michael A. Perry and D. N. Granger

21. Microvascular Pressures in the Small Intestine — 249
    H. Glenn Bohlen and Robert W. Gore

Mathematical Models

22. Microvascular Control of Intestinal Oxygenation — 261
    Harris J. Granger, Gerald A. Meininger, George E. Barnes, and Anthony H. Goodman

23. Mathematical Model of Intestinal Transcapillary Fluid and Protein Exchange — 275
    Joseph N. Benoit, Carlos A. Navia, Aubrey E. Taylor, and D. N. Granger

24. Models of the Relationship Between Drug Absorption and Intestinal Blood Flow — 289
    Dietrich Winne

Pathophysiology

25. The Small Bowel in Arterial Hypotension and Shock — 305
    Ulf Haglund, Mats Jodal, and Ove Lundgren

26. The Effects of Luminal Distension and Obstruction on the Intestinal Circulation — 321
    Ulf Öhman

27. Portal Hypertension — 335
    Charles L. Witte and Marlys H. Witte

28. Intestinal Circulation During Arterial Hypertension — 349
    Henry W. Overbeck

29. Diabetes Mellitus and the Splanchnic Vasculature — 361
    H. Glenn Bohlen

30.	The Pathophysiology of Nonocclusive Intestinal Ischemia *T.E. Bynum, Robert H. Gallavan, and Eugene D. Jacobson*	369

Pharmacology

31.	Vasopressin and Vasoconstrictor Therapy *Andres T. Blei and Roberto J. Groszmann*	377
32.	Pharmacology of Intestinal Blood Flow and Oxygen Uptake *P.D.I. Richardson*	393
33.	Pharmacology of Intestinal Transcapillary Fluid Exchange *James J. Szwed*	403

Subject Index

Contributors

George E. Barnes
Microcirculation Research Institute
and
Department of Medical Physiology
College of Medicine
Texas A & M University
College Station, Texas 77843

James A. Barrowman
Faculty of Medicine
Memorial University of Newfoundland
St. John's Newfoundland
Canada A1B 3V6

Joseph N. Benoit
Department of Physiology
College of Medicine
University of South Alabama
Mobile, Alabama 36688

Andres T. Blei
Gastroenterology Section
Department of Medicine
Lakeside VA Medical Center
Northwestern University
Chicago, Illinois 60611

H. Glenn Bohlen
Department of Physiology
Indiana University School of Medicine
635 Barnhill Drive
Indianapolis, Indiana 46223

T. E. Bynum
Division of Gastroenterology
Department of Internal Medicine
Brigham Women's Medical Center
Harvard Medical School
Boston, Massachusetts 02115

J. R. Casley-Smith
Electron Microscope Unit
University of Adelaide
G.P.O. Box 498
Adelaide, South Australia 5001
Australia

C. C. Chou
Department of Physiology
Michigan State University
East Lansing, Michigan 48824

Daniel I. Edelstone
Department of Obstetrics and Gynecology
Magee-Womens Hospital
University of Pittsburgh School of Medicine
Pittsburgh, Pennsylvania 15213

John W. Fara
Alza Corporation
950 Page Mill Road
Palo Alto, California 94304

Joseph D. Fondacaro
Gastrointestinal Pharmacology
Smith Kline and French Laboratories
Box 7929
Philadelphia, Pennsylvania 19101

Robert H. Gallavan
Department of Physiology
College of Medicine
University of Cincinnati
Cincinnati, Ohio 45267

Bren J. Gannon
Unit of Human Morphology
School of Medicine
Flinders University
Bedford Park, South Australia, 5042
Australia

Anthony H. Goodman
Microcirculation Research Institute
and
Department of Medical Physiology
College of Medicine
Texas A & M University
College Station, Texas 77843

Robert W. Gore
Department of Physiology
University of Arizona
College of Medicine
Tucson, Arizona 85724

Harris J. Granger
Microcirculation Research Institute
and
Department of Medical Physiology
College of Medicine
Texas A & M University
College Station, Texas 77843

CONTRIBUTORS

D. Neil Granger
Department of Physiology
College of Medicine
University of South Alabama
Mobile, Alabama 36688

Clive V. Greenway
Department of Pharmacology and Therapeutics
University of Manitoba
Winnipeg R3E OW3
Canada

Roberto J. Groszmann
Liver Disease Unit
Department of Medicine
West Haven VA Medical Center
Yale University
West Haven, Connecticut 06516

Ulf Haglund
Department of Surgery
Malmö General Hospital
S-214 01 Malmö
Sweden

Scot L. Harper
Department of Physiology
College of Medicine
University of South Alabama
Mobile, Alabama 36688

Ian R. Holzman
Department of Pediatrics
Magee-Womens Hospital
University of Pittsburgh School of Medicine
Pittsburgh, Pennsylvania 15213

Eugene D. Jacobson
Office of the Dean
College of Medicine
University of Cincinnati
Cincinnati, Ohio 45267

Mats Jodal
Department of Physiology
University of Göteborg
Box 33031
S-400 33 Göteborg
Sweden

Paul C. Johnson
Department of Physiology
College of Medicine
University of Arizona
Tucson, Arizona 85724

John M. Johnson
Department of Physiology
University of Texas Health Science Center at San Antonio
San Antonio, Texas 78284

Peter R. Kvietys
Department of Physiology
College of Medicine
University of South Alabama
Mobile, Alabama 36688

J. S. Lee
Department of Physiology
6-255 Millard Hall
University of Minnesota
Minneapolis, Minnesota 55455

John C. Longhurst
Cardiology Division
Department of Medicine
University of California, San Diego
La Jolla, California 92093

Ove Lundgren
Department of Physiology
University of Göteborg
Box 33031
S-400 33 Göteborg
Sweden

David Mailman
Biology Department
University of Houston
Houston, Texas 77004

M. J. Mangino
Department of Physiology
Michigan State University
East Lansing, Michigan 48824

Gerald A. Meininger
Microcirculation Research Institute
and
Department of Medical Physiology
College of Medicine
Texas A & M University
College Station, Texas 77843

Carlos A. Navia
Department of Physiology
College of Medicine
University of South Alabama
Mobile, Alabama 36688

CONTRIBUTORS

Ulf Öhman
Department of Surgery
Karolinska Sjukhuset
S-104 01 Stockholm
Sweden

Henry W. Overbeck
Department of Medicine
Cardiovascular Research and Training Center
University of Alabama
Birmingham, Alabama 35294

Dale A. Parks
Department of Physiology
College of Medicine
University of South Alabama
Mobile, Alabama 36688

Michael A. Perry
School of Physiology and Pharmacology
University of New South Wales
Kensington, N.S.W.
2033 Australia

Peter D. I. Richardson
Astra Pharmaceuticals
St. Peter's House
Bricket Road, St. Albans
Hertfordshire
England AL1 3JW

Carl F. Rothe
Department of Physiology
Indiana University Medical Center
635 Barnhill Drive
Indianapolis, Indiana 46223

Loring B. Rowell
Department of Physiology and Biophysics
School of Medicine
University of Washington
Seattle, Washington 98195

D. R. Sawmiller
Department of Physiology
Michigan State University
East Lansing, Michigan 48824

A. P. Shepherd
Department of Physiology
University of Texas Health Science Center
San Antonio, Texas 78284

James J. Szwed
Nephrology Section
Community Hospital
Indianapolis, Indiana 46219

Aubrey E. Taylor
Department of Physiology
College of Medicine
University of South Alabama
Mobile, Alabama 36688

Michele Ulrich
Department of Physiology
College of Medicine
University of South Alabama
Mobile, Alabama 36688

Dietrich Winne
Division of Molecular Pharmacology
Department of Pharmacology
University of Tübingen
D-7400 Tübingen 1
Federal Republic of Germany

Charles L. Witte
Department of Surgery
University of Arizona
College of Medicine
Tucson, Arizona 85724

Marlys H. Witte
Department of Surgery
University of Arizona
College of Medicine
Tucson, Arizona 85724

The Intestinal Circulation: A Historical Perspective

*D. Neil Granger and **A. P. Shepherd

*Department of Physiology, College of Medicine, University of South Alabama, Mobile, Alabama 36688; and **Department of Physiology, University of Texas Health Sciences Center, San Antonio, Texas 78284*

It is only fitting that this monograph begin with a historical development of the men and ideas that laid the foundation for the current concepts regarding the intestinal circulation. In addition to satisfying the natural urge to retrace our steps and bare our roots, a chronology of the growth of ideas serves to amplify the marvels of the creative process and reminds us that the advancement of knowledge is a slow and perpetual process. It is indeed a humbling experience for current practitioners of intestinal vascular physiology to recount the contributions in this area of scholars such as Aristotle, Galen, Harvey, Poiseuille, and Starling. The reason the intestinal circulation captured the imagination of these creative geniuses is an enigma in itself. However, the answer may lie in the fact that in an eviscerated animal the mesenteric vasculature is the most accessible and visible of the regional circulations.

PALEOLITHIC PERIOD TO MIDDLE AGES

The earliest known attempt to portray the intestinal vasculature can be found crudely sketched in a cave at Lascaux, France (7). The 30,000-year-old painting depicts reddish loops of intestine dangling from the belly of a bison opened by the thrust of a spear. There is evidence that Paleolithic men not only dissected animals but viewed the viscera as a manifestation of the divine.

A preoccupation with the association of visceral organs with divination led the Egyptians to bury the intestine separately in an urn located in one corner of the sarcophagus. The urn was closed by a top modeled in the likeness of the head of a jackal. Likewise, the Greeks consulted the entrails of sacrificial animals before battle or passing judgments. The existence of such notions regarding the supernatural stifled the progress of knowledge of the intestinal circulation for many centuries.

The first written description of the splanchnic circulation appear in Egyptian medical texts prior to 1600 B.C. and the published works of Diogenes in the 5th century B.C. Diogenes and Hippocrates described direct vascular connections between the veins of the forearm and the splanchnic circulation. The belief in such a vascular communication accounts for the then common practice of phlebotomy for treatment of abdominal ailments. Phlebotomy provided a direct method of removing local excesses of blood and evil humors in the abdominal viscera (7).

Aristotle (322–384 B.C.) also accepted the notion of vascular communications between veins in the arms and abdominal viscera. In the treatise, *De partibus animalium*, he described the viscera as "rivets" that serve to fasten the mesenteric blood vessels to the body. Aristotle and his contemporaries (including Galen some 600 years later) believed that blood vessels become gradually smaller and smaller until the "tubes are too fine to admit the blood." The concept that there is a continuity of the arteries and veins (via capillaries) was not proposed by Harvey and verified microscopically by Malpighi and Leeuwenhoek for another thousand years.

Greek "physiologists" ascribed a major role to the splanchnic vascular bed in "sanguification," that is, the formation of blood from food. According to the sanguification theory, food is transported by suction through the portal vein in the liver where it is converted to blood. The red color of blood was attributed to the burning effects of "fire" in the "burning hearths of the viscera." The liver was considered the site of production of blood as well as the source of all veins. Blood, after its formation in the liver, is transported to the heart via the vena cava. The arteries were considered of secondary importance to veins and were thought to contain a mixture of air (derived from the lung) and blood. The blood was thought to move bidirectionally in the vessels with a kind of tidal movement influenced by airflow in and out of the lungs.

Erasistratos (ca. 300 B.C.), a Greek anatomist and physician, was first to claim that venous blood from the intestine must subsequently flow through the liver and then to the heart, a notion that was experimentally verified by Glisson in the mid-17th century. Erasistratos also was first to propose that gastrointestinal movements intermittently compress the mesenteric veins, thereby aiding the flow of blood to the liver.

Some 500 years after Erasistratos, Galen (ca. A.D. 129–199) wrote his monumental essays on vascular anatomy and physiology. Although Galen's assessment of the gross anatomy of the splanchnic vasculature was more exact than that of his predecessors, he also became a proponent of the sanguification theory. His efforts elevated the physiology of sanguification to a new level of sophistication. For example, he proposed that the direction of portal venous flow is determined by the relative nutritional requirements of the gastrointestinal tract and liver, that is, in the fed state portal venous blood flows to the liver, whereas it flows in the opposite direction in the fasting state.

THE MODERN PERIOD

The concept that portal venous blood is derived from sanguification of food was widely accepted for approximately 1,400 years after Galen. In the 17th century, William Harvey deduced that the quantity of blood pumped by the heart far exceeded the amount of food ingested, and he concluded that portal venous blood is the same blood that entered the arteries perfusing the stomach, pancreas, and intestine. However, Harvey (28) recognized that imperceptible amounts of chyle may enter the mesenteric veins and reach the liver.

By the middle of the 17th century, the microscope had been improved sufficiently to allow Leeuwenhoek (38), a tireless microscopic observer of nature, to describe the blood and lymphatic microvessels in intestinal villi. Leeuwenhoek's drawings of the microvessels in the intestinal mucosa clearly illustrate the now-accepted hairpin arrangement of the villus circulation. He also was the first to propose that the blood capillaries and small veins are the primary conduits (rather than the lacteals) for the transport of absorbed "chyle" to the heart.

The major advances in knowledge of the intestinal circulation during the 18th century were primarily confined to improved anatomic descriptions of the vasculature (7). The development of techniques for preserving tissues and outlining the vasculature (using injections of wax or other plastic materials) led to these advances. The 18th century also witnessed what appears to be the first experiments involving artificial perfusion of the intestinal vasculature. In 1733, Stephen Hales (26) perfused the dog aorta with a column of water equal to normal aortic pressure and measured intestinal venous outflow. He observed that hot water increased, and cold water decreased, flow and concluded that agents that decrease flow do so by constricting the vasculature, whereas the opposite is true for substances that increase flow.

A century later Poiseuille (49) demonstrated that venous outflow from a segment of horse small bowel is determined exclusively by the flow and pressure in the artery perfusing the segment. Furthermore, he observed that mesenteric venous pressure is directly related to arterial pressure, and he enjoys the distinction of being the first to measure pressure in the mesenteric vein. These and other experiments by Poiseuille led to the formulation of his currently held principle of vascular hydraulics. Poi-

TABLE 1. *Milestones in research on the physiology of the intestinal circulation*

Refs.	Publ. date	Contrib.
Asellius (1)	1627	Intestinal lymphatics and implication in absorptive functions of gut
Harvey (28)	1628	Description of the splanchnic circulation, de-emphasis of importance of sanguification
Leeuwenhoek (38)	1684	Microvascular anatomy of villi
Hales (26)	1733	First perfused intestine experiment
Cumin (15)	1823	Hemorrhagic necrosis of mucosa
Poiseuille (49)	1830	Measurement of mesenteric venous pressure and description of principles of vascular hydraulics
Heller (29), Mall (41)	1872, 1888	Vascular pattern in intestine
Langley, Anderson (35)	1895	Vasodilator action of pelvic nerves in colon
Burton-Opitz (9)	1908	Measurement of portal venous flow
Brodie, Vogt (8)	1910	Increased blood flow and oxygen uptake during absorption
Hoskins, Cunning (7)	1917	Inconsistent vascular actions of epinephrine
Florey (19)	1924	Contractile nature of intestinal lacteals
Wells, Johnson (60)	1934	Influence of intestinal circulation on absorption and secretion
Königes, Otto (34)	1937	Microvascular pressure measurements in intestinal villi
Carmichael et al. (10)	1939	Cardiovascular reflex of intestinal origin
Lawson, Chumley (36)	1940	Effect of intraenteric pressure on blood flow
Grayson (23)	1950	Measurement of colonic blood flow in man
Borgstrom, Laurell (6)	1953	Role of lymphatics in fluid absorption
Keyne et al. (33)	1956	Vasoconstrictor therapy in G.I. bleeding
Lillehei (39)	1957	Role of intestine in hemorrhagic shock
Grim, Linseth (25)	1958	Microsphere technique for flow measurement
Selkurt, Johnson (53)	1958	Capacitance function of intestinal vasculature
Sidky, Bean (58)	1958	Influence of motility on blood flow
Johnson (31)	1959	Myogenic factors regulating intestinal blood flow
Mayerson et al. (44)	1960	Permeability of intestinal capillaries
Folkow et al. (20)	1964	Autoregulatory escape
Selkurt et al. (54)	1964	Intestinal reactive hyperemia
Johnson, Hanson (32)	1966	Resistance and exchange vessel response to venous hypertension
Lundgren (40)	1967	Countercurrent exchange mechanism
Reynolds et al. (50)	1967	Vascular casts of intestinal circulation
Hulten (30)	1969	Extrinsic control of colonic blood flow
Clementi, Palade (14)	1969	Ultrastructural assessment of intestinal vascular permeability
Lee (37)	1969	Micropuncture estimates of lacteal pressure
Winne (61)	1970	Kinetic analysis of influence of blood flow on intestinal absorption
Rudolph, Heymann (51)	1970	Intestinal hemodynamic changes during growth in fetus
Chiu et al. (12)	1970	Mucosal lesions in ischemic bowel
Fara et al. (17)	1972	Role of G.I. hormones in postprandial hyperemia
Greenway, Murthy (24)	1972	Validity of microsphere technique
Shepherd, Granger (56)	1973	Mathematical model of intestinal vasoregulation
Casley-Smith et al. (11)	1975	Morphometric analysis of intestinal microcirculation
Mortillaro, Taylor (45)	1976	Analysis of forces governing intestinal transcapillary fluid exchange
Nishiyama et al. (46)	1976	Role of intestinal circulation in arterial hypertension
Chou, Grassmick (13)	1978	Influence of motility on blood flow distribution
Bohlen (4)	1980	Tissue PO_2 and microvascular responses to glucose absorption
Witte et al. (62)	1981	Microvascular exchange in man normal and cirrhotic
Parks et al. (48)	1982	Role of oxygen radicals in intestinal ischemia
Shepherd, Riedel (57)	1982	Laser-Doppler method for mucosal blood flow
Blanchet, Lebrec (3) and Vorobioff, Groszmann (59)	1982, 1983	Influence of chronic portal hypertension on blood flow

seuille's invention of the mercury manometer led to subsequent measurements of arterial and portal venous pressures by Bayliss and Starling (2) and others in the latter 19th century.

With Carl Ludwig's invention of the "stromuhr" in 1868, measurements of mesenteric and portal venous blood flows became almost commonplace. Burton-Opitz (9) was first to measure flows in the splanchnic bed with the stromuhr. As a result of the advances in instrumentation and more sophisticated concepts of hemodynamics, attention could now be focused on vasoregulation. The concept of vasomotor control of the splanchnic circulation became one of the first focal points of interest. The effects of splanchnic nerve stimulation on mesenteric blood flow and portal vein pressure in experimental animals was studied by several investigators, including Mall (42) and Burton-Opitz (9). Bayliss and Starling (2) demonstrated that such stimulation decreased the volume of isolated intestinal segments and Burton-Opitz observed that mesenteric resistance was increased.

With the discovery of epinephrine by Oliver and Schafers (47) in 1894 came studies designed to assess the role of humoral factors in intestinal vasoregulation. Although Oliver and Schafers were unable to demonstrate an effect of epinephrine (adrenal extract) on the intestinal circulation, they nonetheless assumed that the concomitant rise in arterial pressure was due "very largely to contraction of arterioles in the splanchnic area." However, subsequent studies by others, including Hoskins and Cunning, and Clarke (7), revealed that epinephrine's effects on the intestinal circulation are inconsistent and that it exerts both vasoconstrictor and vasodilator effects.

The first half of the 20th century witnessed a growing interest in the interactions between intestinal function and blood flow. Brodie and Vogt (8) measured blood flow and oxygen uptake in segments of canine small intestine and observed an increase in both during absorption of dilute salt or protein solutions. The influence of motility and intraenteric pressure on intestinal blood flow was examined by Lawson and Chumley (36) in 1940. They observed that increments of intraluminal pressure less than 30 mm Hg caused a transient decrease in blood flow followed by recovery to control values. At higher pressures (up to arterial pressure), only a partial recovery was observed. Six years earlier Wells and Johnson (60) directly observed the villus circulation and measured absorption in the dog small bowel. They observed that reduced absorption or net secretion was associated with venous congestion and arteriolar dilation. Thus, by the early 1940s interactions were described between the intestine's circulation and its functions: motility, absorption, and secretion.

Other major advancements that marked this period were the studies of Florey (19) on the rhythmic contractility of intestinal lacteals and the application of the Landis micropuncture technique for direct measurements of intestinal microvascular pressures (34). Florey described the rhythmic contractions of lacteals in the guinea pig and rat, and he noted that splanchnic nerve stimulation increased lymphatic contractility whereas vagus nerve stimulation depressed contractile amplitude. Thirteen years later Koniges and Otto (34) used micropipettes to measure the hydrostatic pressure within the lacteals, arterioles, capillaries, and venules of cat intestinal villi. Although the values obtained in all vessels are somewhat higher than those reported in recent years (see Chapters 17 and 21), this study represents the first attempt to determine the microvascular pressure profile in the small bowel.

The decade of the 1950s witnessed the development of new techniques for measurement and fractionation of blood flow as well as the birth of innovative concepts regarding the physiology of intestinal vasoregulation. During this period, Grim and Lindseth (25) introduced the microsphere technique for measuring the distribution of blood flow in the various layers of the bowel wall. Their study not only provided important new data regarding the blood flow distribution but also dispelled the then common notion that major arteriovenous shunts exist within the submucosal layer.

Another major focal point of interest in the 1950s was the role of the intestine in the pathogenesis of hemorrhagic shock. Lillehei (39) observed that the mortality rate from hemorrhagic hypotension was drastically reduced (from 90% to 10%) if the intestine of the hemorrhaged animal was perfused at a normal pressure from a donor animal. This observation led to the concept that a blood-borne toxic substance, released from the ischemic bowel, is responsible for the irreversibility of hemorrhagic shock. Through the efforts of Lillehei (39), Selkurt (52), Zwiefach et al. (63), Fine (18), and others, a role for the intestine in hemorrhagic shock was clearly established.

The period between 1958 and 1966 gave rise to many new concepts regarding the role of intrinsic and extrinsic factors in the regulation of intestinal blood flow. Johnson and Hanson (31,32) and Selkurt and colleagues, (53,54) reported the first studies on pressure-flow autoregulation, reactive hyperemia, and venous pressure elevation. Such studies led to the introduction of the notion that intrinsic vascular tone, as opposed to neurogenic tone, is primarily responsible for the partially constricted state of intestinal resistance vessels. The theory of myogenic regulation was applied to the intestinal circulation as a result of these studies. Folkow and associates (16,20,21) also made many important contributions to the field during this period. The Swedish group placed considerable emphasis on the differential responses of the series and parallel coupled vascular elements in the bowel to sympathetic nerve stimulation. Folkow coined the term "autoregulatory escape" to describe the waning resistance vessel response to sympathetic stimulation, and he also was first to apply capillary filtration coefficient (K_f) and ^{86}Rb permeability-surface area product measurements as indicators of perfused capillary density in the small bowel (16,21). On the basis of data obtained using these techniques, Folkow introduced the concept of independent control of resistance and exchange vessels. The K_f measurement was subsequently used by Johnson and Hanson (32) to study the influence of myogenic factors on perfused capillary density in the small bowel. Also, quantitative analyses of the capacitance properties of the intestinal circulation revealed the importance of this vascular bed as a blood reservoir (53). As a result of the efforts of Selkurt, Johnson, and Folkow a new era in research on the intestinal circulation began in which the concept of vasoregulation encompassed the reactions of all segments of the vasculature, namely, resistance, exchange, and capacitance vessels.

Developments and concepts that mark the latter half of the 1960s include the application of the silicone rubber method for three-dimensional study of the intramural vascular supply of the gut (50), the application of electron dense tracers for ultrastructural assessment of intestinal vascular permeability (14), and the countercurrent exchange hypothesis (40). The concept that the vascular arrangement in the villi favors the shunting of highly diffusible substances between the arteries and veins at the base of the villi was introduced in 1967 by Lundgren (40). According to this hypothesis, significant concentration gradients should exist between the tip and the base of the villi for substances such as oxygen and sodium chloride. Lundgren (see Chapter 7) and others (4,5) have obtained considerable evidence that supports the hypothesis, and it has been invoked as a factor in the pathogenesis of ischemic necrosis (see Chapter 25) and other pathologic conditions.

The 1970s marked a period of rapid expansion of knowledge of all aspects of the physiology of the intestinal circulation. This can be attributed to technological and conceptual advancements, application of more analytical approaches for studying the circulation, and the ever increasing number of investigators with an interest in this area. Refinement of analytical approaches took the form of mathematical models describing intrinsic regulation of blood flow and oxygenation (56) as well as the influence of blood flow on absorption (61), and quantitative approaches for grading ischemic injury (12) and describing the ultrastructural characteristics of the microvasculature (11). Major conceptual advancements were made regarding intrinsic vasoregulatory phenomena such as the postprandial hyperemia (17). With the development of the solid state arteriovenous oxygen difference analyzer (55), the influence of blood flow on intestinal oxygenation became a popular and fruitful area of research. This period also produced a large number of reports dealing with the influence of various pharmacologic agents on intestinal blood flow. Likewise, greater attention was given to the circulatory alterations associated with various pathologic conditions. The growing interest in the intestinal circulation during this period is exemplified by the fact that 435 articles were published on this topic between 1976 and 1979, as compared with 186 articles between 1966 and 1970.

The surge of interest in the intestinal circulation continued in the period between 1980 and the present. This period witnessed the introduction of new and more sophisticated methods for studying the intestinal circulation. Microelectrodes for measurements of intestinal tissue Po_2 were first used by Bohlen (4), who demonstrated a role for tissue oxygen tension in the vascular responses elicited by glucose absorption. Also noteworthy was the first application of laser-Doppler flowmetry for continuous measurement of mucosal and muscularis blood flows in the intestine (57). Although the method has thus far undergone only preliminary testing, indications are that it may find widespread use in studies on experimental animals and man. The renewed interest in techniques for fractionating blood flow also led to studies criticizing the validity of the microsphere technique (43) and supporting an earlier study by Greenway and Murthy (24). Also, the first book devoted entirely to the techniques used to measure splanchnic (primarily intestinal) blood flow was published in 1981 (22).

The major focal point of a larger number of reports published in the first years of this decade was intestinal vascular pathophysiology. The response of the intestinal microcirculation to chronic portal hypertension was assessed both in man (62) and experimental animals (3,59). These studies revealed a paradoxical increase in intestinal blood flow and an enhancement of diffusive protein exchange across intestinal capillaries. Another disorder that received attention was ischemic bowel disease. Parks and co-workers (48) proposed that the superoxide anion, an unstable and cytotoxic form of molecular oxygen, is primarily responsible for the mucosal lesions produced by reperfusion of the ischemic small bowel and that the enzyme xanthine oxidase is the major source of the oxygen free radical.

The exchange of ideas by investigators with an interest in the intestinal circulation was greatly facilitated in the early 1980s by the formation of the Splanchnic Circulation Group. Largely through the efforts of Dr. Ching-Chung Chou, this organization was founded in 1979 to promote formal exchanges of ideas among investigators in the field. The organization sponsored workshops on methods for estimating splanchnic blood flow (University of Utah Medical Center, 1980) and circulatory regulation of intestinal oxygen delivery (American Physiological Society Meeting, 1981), and symposia on the physiology of the intestinal circulation (American Physiological Society Meeting, 1980), the contribution of the splanchnic circulation to overall cardiovascular homeostasis (Federation of American Societies of Experimental Biology, 1982), intestinal ischemia (American Gastroenterological Association, 1982), regional vascular behavior in the intestinal wall (American Physiological Society, 1982), and vasoactive agents controlling the mesenteric circulation (American Physiological Society, 1984). A biannual forum for presentation of research on the intestinal circulation was also created in 1980 by scientific sessions devoted to splanchnic circulation in the fall and spring meetings of the American Physiological Society. The impact of the Splanchnic Circulation Group's efforts to foster communication on the intestinal circulation is exemplified by the fact that at least 24 review articles dealing with this topic were published in major journals between 1980 and 1983.

EPILOG

As a result of the efforts of many scientists over the past 400 years, there is now a wealth of data in the literature on the intestinal circulation. The major objective of the chapters comprising the remainder of this monograph is to present the "state of the art" regarding the physiology of the intestinal circulation. Although it will become apparent to the reader that the level of sophistication of research in this area has made a quantum leap since the studies of Harvey, Hales and Poiseuille, we must not lose sight of the enormity of the contributions of these early physiologists, for their discoveries laid the foundation of today's concepts.

REFERENCES

1. Asellius, G. (1627): De Lactibus sive lacteis venis Quarto Vasorum Mesaraicorum genere novo invento. *Apud Jo Baptistam Bidellium*, Mediolani.
2. Bayliss, W. M. and Starling, E. H. (1894): Observations on venous pressures and their relationship to capillary pressures. *J. Physiol. (Lond.)*, 16:159.
3. Blanchet, L., and Lebrec, D. (1982): Changes in splanchnic blood flow in portal hypertensive rats. *Eur. J. Clin. Invest.*, 12:327–330.
4. Bohlen, H. G. (1980): Intestinal tissue PO_2 and microvascular responses during glucose exposure. *Am. J. Physiol.*, 238:H164–H171.
5. Bohlen, H. G. (1982): Na-induced intestinal interstitial hyperosmolality and vascular responses during absorptive hyperemia. *Am. J. Physiol.*, 242:H785–H789.
6. Borgstrom, B., and Laurell, C. B. (1953): Studies on lymph and lymph-protein during absorption of fat and saline by rats. *Acta Physiol. Scand.*, 29:264–280.
7. Bradley, S. E. (1982): The splanchnic circulation. In: *Circulation of the Blood. Men and Ideas*, edited by A. P. Fishman and D. W. Richards, pp. 607–702. American Physiological Society, Bethesda.
8. Brodie, T. G., and Vogt, H. (1910): The gaseous metabolism of the small intestine. Part 1. The gaseous exchange during the absorption of water and dilute salt solutions. *J. Physiol.*, 40:135–172.
9. Burton-Opitz, R. (1908): Ueber die Stroemung des Blutes in dem Frebiete der Pfortader. *Arch. f. ges. Physiol.*, 124:469–510.
10. Carmichael, E. A., Doupe, J., Harper, A. A., and McSwiney, B. A. (1939): Vasomotor reflexes in man following distension. *J. Physiol. (Lond.)*, 95:276–281.
11. Casley-Smith, J. R., O'Donoghue, P. J., and Crocker, K. W. J. (1975): Quantitative relationships between fenestrae in jejunal capillaries and tissue channels: proof of "tunnel capillaries." *Microvasc. Res.*, 9:78–100.
12. Chiu, C. J., McArdle, A. H., Brown, R., Scott, H. J., and Gurd, F. N. (1970): Intestinal mucosal lesions in low flow states. *Arch Surg.*, 10:478–483.
13. Chou, C. C., and Grassmick, B. (1978): Motility and blood flow distribution within the wall of the gastrointestinal tract. *Am. J. Physiol.*, 235:H34–H39.
14. Clementi, F., and Palade, G. E. (1969): Intestinal capillaries. I. Permeability to peroxidase and ferritin. *J. Cell. Biol.*, 41:33–58.
15. Cumin, W. (1823): Cases of severe burn, with dissections and remarks. *Edinburgh Med. J.*, 19:337–344.
16. Dresel, P., Folkow, B., and Wallentin, I. (1966): Rubidium[86] clearance during neurogenic redistribution of intestinal blood flow. *Acta Physiol. Scand.*, 67:173–184.
17. Fara, J. W., Rubinstein, E. H., and Sonnenschein (1972): Intestinal hormones in mesenteric vasodilation after intraduodenal agents. *Am. J. Physiol.*, 223:1058–1067.
18. Fine, J. (1954): *The Bacterial Factor in Traumatic Shock*. Charles C. Thomas, Springfield, Illinois.
19. Florey, H. W. (1927): Observations on the contractility of lacteals. *J. Physiol.*, 62:267–272.
20. Folkow, B., Lewis, D. H., Lundgren, O., Mellander, S., and Wallentin, I. The effect of graded vasoconstrictor fibre stimulation on the intestinal resistance and capacitance vessels. *Acta Physiol. Scand.*, 6:445–457.
21. Folkow, B., Lundgren, O., and Wallentin, I. (1963): Studies on the relationship between flow resistance, capillary filtration coefficient, and regional blood volume in the intestine. *Acta Physiol. Scand.*, 57:270–283.
22. Granger, D. N., and Bulkley, G. B. (1981): *Measurement of Blood Flow. Applications to the Splanchnic Circulation*. Williams and Wilkins, Baltimore.
23. Grayson, J. (1950): Vascular reactions in the human small intestine. *J. Physiol.*, 109:439.
24. Greenway, C. V., and Murthy, V. S. (1972): Effects of vasopressin and isoprenaline infusions on the distribution of blood flow in the intestine: Criteria for the validity of microsphere studies. *Br. J. Pharmacol.*, 46:177–188.
25. Grim, E., and Lindseth, E. O. (1958): Distribution of blood flow to the tissues of the small intestine of the dog. *Univ. Minn. Med. Bull.*, 30:138–145.
26. Hales, S. (1733): *Statistical Essays: Containing Haemostaticks*. Royal Society, reprinted by Hafner Publishing Co. (1964), New York.
27. Hanson, K. M., and Johnson, P. C. (1967): Pressure-flow relationships in isolated dog colon. *Am. J. Physiol.*, 212:574–578.
28. Harvey, W. (1957): *Movement of the Heart and Blood in Animals. An Anatomical Essay*. (Translated by K. J. Franklin), Blackwell, Oxford.
29. Heller, A. (1872): Über die Blugefässe des Dunndarmes. *Ber. Sachs. Ges. Wiss.*, 24:265–171.
30. Hulten, L. (1969): Extrinsic nervous control of colonic motility and blood flow. *Acta Physiol. Scand.*, 335:1–116.
31. Johnson, P. C. (1959): Myogenic nature of increase in intestinal vascular resistance with venous pressure elevation. *Circ. Res.*, 6:992.
32. Johnson, P. C., and Hanson, K. M. (1966): Capillary filtration in the small intestine of dog. *Circ. Res.*, 19:766–773.
33. Kehne, J. H., Hughes, F. A., and Gompertz, M. L. (1956): The use of surgical pituitrin in the control of esophageal varix bleeding: An experimental study and report of two cases. *Surgery*, 39:917–925.
34. Koniges, H. G., and Otto, M. (1937): Studies on the

34. filtration mechanism of the intestinal lymph and on the action acetylcholine on it and on the circulation of the intestinal villi. *Q. J. Exp. Biol.*, 26:319–329.
35. Langley, J. N., and Andersson, H. K. (1895): On the innervation of the pelvic and adjoining viscera. *J. Physiol. (Lond.)*, 18:67–105.
36. Lawson, H., and Chumley, J. (1940): The effect of distension on blood flow through the intestine. *Am. J. Physiol.*, 131:368–377.
37. Lee, J. S. (1969): A micropuncture study of water transport by dog jejunal villi *in vitro*. *Am. J. Physiol.*, 217:1528–1533.
38. Leeuwenhoek, A. V. (1684): Antomy of the slime within the guts and the use thereof. *Philos. Trans. R. Soc. Lond.*
39. Lillehei, R. C. (1957): The intestinal factor in irreversible hemorrhagic shock. *Surgery*, 42:1043–1054.
40. Lundgren, O. (1967): Blood flow distribution and countercurrent exchange in the small intestine. *Acta Physiol. Scand. (Suppl.)*, 303:1–42.
41. Mall, J. P. (1888): Die Blut- und Lymphwege in Dunndarm des Hundes. *Abh. Sachs. Ges. Wiss.*, 14:153–189.
42. Mall, F. P. (1896): The contraction of the venae portae and its influence upon the circulation. *Johns Hopkins Hosp. Rep.*, 1:111.
43. Maxwell, L. C., Shepherd, A. P., Riedel, G. L., and Morris, M. D. (1981): Effect of microsphere size on apparent intramural distribution of intestinal blood flow. *Am. J. Physiol.*, 241:H404–H414.
44. Mayerson, H. S., Wolfrom, C. E., Shirley, H. H., and Wasserman, K. (1960): Regional difference in capillary permeability. *Am. J. Physiol.*, 198:155–160.
45. Mortillaro, N. A., and Taylor, A. E. (1976): Interaction of capillary and tissue forces in the cat small intestine. *Circ. Res.*, 39:348–358.
46. Nishiyama, K., Nishiyama, A., and Frohlich, E. D. (1976): Regional blood flow in normotensive and spontaneously hypertensive rats. *Am. J. Physiol.*, 230:691–698.
47. Oliver, G., and Schafer, E. A. (1894): On the physiological action of extract of the suprarenal capsules. *J. Physiol. (Lond.)*, 16:1.
48. Parks, D. A., Bulkley, G. B., Granger, D. N., Hamilton, S. R., and McCord, J. M. (1982): Ischemic injury in the small intestine. Role of superoxide radicals. *Gastroenterology*, 82:9–15.
49. Poiseuille, J. L. M. (1830): Recherches sur les causes du mouvement du sang les veins. *J. Univ. Hebd. Med. Chir. Prat.*, 1:289.
50. Reynolds, D. G., Brim, J., and Sheehy, T. W. (1967): The vascular architecture of the small intestinal mucosa. *Anat. Rec.*, 159:211–218.
51. Rudolph, A. M., and Heymann, M. A. (1970): Circulatory changes during growth in the fetal lamb. *Circ. Res.*, 26:289–299.
52. Selkurt, E. E. (1958): Intestinal ischemic shock and the role of the liver. *Am. J. Physiol.*, 197:281–285.
53. Selkurt, E. E., and Johnson, P. C. (1958): Effect of acute elevation of portal venous pressure on mesenteric blood volume, interstitial fluid volume and hemodynamics. *Circ. Res.*, 6:592–599.
54. Selkurt, E. E., Rothe, C. F., and Richardson, D. (1964): Characteristics of reactive hyperemia in the canine intestine. *Circ. Res.*, 15:532–544.
55. Shepherd, A. P., and Burgar, C. G. (1977): A solid state arteriovenous oxygen difference analyzer for flowing whole blood. *Am. J. Physiol.*, 232:H437–H440.
56. Shepherd, A. P., and Granger, H. J. (1973): Autoregulatory escape in the gut: A systems analysis. *Gastroenterology*, 65:77–91.
57. Shepherd, A. P., and Riedel, G. L. (1982): Continuous measurement of intestinal mucosal blood flow by laser-Doppler flowmetry. *Am. J. Physiol.*, 242:G668–G672.
58. Sidky, M., and Bean, J. W. (1958): Influence of rhythmic and tonic contraction of intestinal muscle on blood flow and blood reservoir capacity in dog intestine. *Am. J. Physiol.*, 193:386–392.
59. Vorobioff, J., Bredfeldt, J. E., and Groszmann, R. J. (1983): Hyperdynamic circulation in portal-hypertensive rat model: A primary factor for maintenance of chronic portal hypertension. *Am. J. Physiol.*, 244:G52–G57.
60. Wells, H. S., and Johnson, R. G. (1934): The intestinal villi and their circulation in relation to absorption and secretion of fluid. *Am. J. Physiol.*, 109:387–402.
61. Winne, D. (1970): Formal kinetics of water and solute absorption with regard to intestinal blood flow. *J. Theor. Biol.*, 27:1–18.
62. Witte, M. H., Witte, C. L., and Dumont, A. E. (1981): Estimates of net transcapillary water and protein flux in the liver and intestine of patients with portal hypertension from hepatic cirrhosis. *Gastroenterology*, 80:265–273.
63. Zwiefach, B. W., Gordon, H. A., Wagner, M., and Rayniers, J. A. (1958): Irreversible hemorrhagic shock in germ-free rats. *J. Exp. Med.*, 107:437–450.

Intestinal Microcirculation: Spatial Organization and Fine Structure

*J. R. Casley-Smith and **Bren J. Gannon

*Electron Microscope Unit, University of Adelaide, Adelaide, South Australia 5001, Australia; and
**Human Morphology Department, School of Medicine, The Flinders University of South Australia, Bedford Park, South Australia, 5042, Australia

The microcirculation of the alimentary tract is crucial not only for the nutritive maintenance of the alimentary tract itself but also for its vital functions of secretion and absorption, since the circulation is the ultimate source of the secreted digestive juices and the recipient of absorbed digesta. This chapter reviews the spatial organization and fine structure of the intestinal microcirculation and includes some functional considerations based on structural observation. We will principally consider the small intestine, especially its mucosal microcirculation, as this is the best known; knowledge of colonic microcirculation, as of the esophagus, remains scanty (3). The gastric microcirculation will not be considered here; interested readers should consult recent articles (8,47,48). In considering the microcirculation of the intestine, we will include the small exchange vessels of the blood circulation (capillaries and postcapillary venules), the tissue channels of the interstitium, and the initial lymphatics, all of which function in an interrelated manner in all organs (19).

EXTRAMURAL VESSELS OF THE INTESTINE

Blood supply to the small and large intestines is almost entirely by the superior (anterior) and inferior (posterior) mesenteric arteries, both direct branches of the aorta, with the division in supply between the two vessels being approximately two-thirds of the way across the transverse colon to the left in man (106). The exceptions are the proximal part of the small bowel, the duodenum, which receives partial supply from the pancreatico-duodenal vessels (derived ultimately from the coeliac axis) and the distal rectum, which is supplied via rectal arteries that arise from the internal iliacs.

The venous drainage of both small and large intestines is via the portal vein to the liver, where the blood is distributed to a second microcirculatory bed, before return to right heart. Thus, unlike most microvascular beds in the body, that of the intestine is the first of two microcirculatory beds in series. Consequently, venous pressures in the intestine need to be higher than in other beds. Venous drainage of the distal rectum, however, is via the internal iliac veins directly to the systemic circulation and thus bypasses the hepatic microcirculatory bed.

The major vessels pass to and from the intestine usually within the thin sheet of the mesentery, except where the gut is retroperitoneal (e.g., ascending and descending colons in man); there the extramural vessels are also retroperitoneal. Within the mesentery, the large vessels branch, and both arterial and venous vessels self-anastomose, so that both systems show multiple arcades at the mesenteric margin of the intestine. At this point, numerous vessels penetrate the muscularis externa to join the submucosal vascular plexuses.

Within the mesentery, the arterial vessels give off small feeder vessels to the essentially planar microvascular network of the mesentery itself (45,52). This circulation may be important not only to the fat storage and mobilization that occur in the mesentery but also for the overall fluid balance of the peritoneal cavity, given the large surface area of the mesentery that is exposed to peritoneal fluid.

In addition to major blood vessels, the mesentery also carries the main intestinal lymph drainage vessels. These lymph vessels exhibit rhythmic contractile activity (at least in some species), thus assisting the flow of their contained fluid, often rich in chylomicra, to the cysterna chyli. The latter is located retroperitoneally at the root of the mesentery. Lymph drains then via the thoracic duct to the left subclavian vein, at least in man.

The arterial and venous vessels of the submucous vascular plexuses exhibit substantial amounts of medial smooth muscle; there are characteristic differences in the arrangement of and connections between adjacent smooth muscle cells between submucous arteries and veins (73), possibly reflecting changes in electrophysiology and mechanical function between arterial and venous medial smooth muscle cells.

MAJOR INTRAMURAL BLOOD VESSELS

The major arterial vessels of the intestinal wall are located principally as an arterial plexus in the deep submucosa, just subjacent to the muscularis mucosa. This plexus self-anastamoses both around the intestinal lumen from mesenteric to antimesenteric sides and also along the length of the gut in both oral and aboral directions, receiving frequent direct feeder vessels along the mesenteric margin (35,106). The submucous venous vascular plexus is similarly self-anastamotic and drained by similar or greater numbers of vessels to the extramural arcading system of mesenteric veins. The degree of self-anastamosis of these major vessel networks within the gut wall is considered important in maintaining flow during local contraction of the muscularis externa, when supply or drainage vessels penetrating the contracting visceral muscle might be occluded. Less-frequent intramural arterial anastamoses and thus the virtual supply of regions of the duodenal mucosa by end arteries, is thought to account, at least in part, for its higher susceptibility to ulceration (84).

SMALL INTRAMURAL BLOOD VESSELS

General

The capillary networks of the various layers of the intestine—muscularis externa, submucosa, and mucosa—are each supplied by frequent branches from the submucosal vascular networks of major intramural arteries and veins. These three layers have essentially discrete microvascular networks arranged in parallel with each other. Except for the microvessels of the mucosa, the capillaries are continuous and non-fenestrated (8,35).

Muscle Microvessels

The capillaries of the longitudinal and circular external muscle coats run parallel to the surrounding smooth muscle fibres (50,79,101). Their basal laminae are attached to the endomysial connective tissue matrix of the muscle layer (6) so that, on contraction, the microvascular network is distorted in concert with the contracting muscle, as occurs in other viscera (87). The supply to the muscular capillary plexus is by frequent small arterial branches from the submucous arterial plexus (5,79). The actual number of orders of branching of the vessels (5) will vary with the size of the animal. The most superficial of the muscle microvessels of the longitudinal muscle in the small intestine (and of the taenia coli and intertaenial circular muscle of the colon) are closely subjacent to the simple squamous epithelium of the serosa.

In cat, and presumably in all larger animals, the myenteric and submucous neural plexuses have their own distinct planar microvascular networks (95,96).

Submucous Microvessels

The microcirculation of the submucosa is sparse throughout the gut (8,41,48,72,79), except in the region of the duodenum that contains Brunner's glands (7); elsewhere few capillaries supply the largely connective tissue and neural elements (Meissner's Plexus) of this layer (95,96). It is convenient to consider the relatively few capillaries of the muscularis mucosa as part of this sparse submucous microvascular network. Also located at this level are the submucosal self-anastamotic plexuses of intramural distributing arteries and collecting veins (see above).

Mucosal Microvessels: Small Intestine

Mucosal Epithelial Topology

The surface of the small intestinal columnar epithelium is disturbed by two interspersed distortions (35). First, there are the villi: small, tongue- or finger-like projections of the mucosal surface into the gut lumen (35). Typically, these are about 1 mm in length and about 100 μm in thickness measured along the long axis of the gut. In some species, e.g., cat and dog, the villi are cylindrical, whereas in others, e.g., rabbit, human, and rat, the villi are broader and tongue- to leaf-like, being 0.5 to 1 mm or more in length and lying across the gut long axis (49). The second epithelial distortion is more frequent tubular down-pocketings of the epithelium between the villi: the so-called intestinal glands or crypts of Lieberkühn (35). The crypts are typically 0.8 to 1 mm deep; the base of each intestinal villus is surrounded by the openings of a number of adjacent intestinal glands, typically six to eight in rat or rabbit (46,48,50) (see also Fig. 1E). In the duodenum, however, there are in addition large numbers of branched acinar glands (Brunner's glands), which lie in the submucosa and empty into the bases of the crypts (34). Brunner's glands are arranged in a compact mass that occupies virtually all of the submucosa in the proximal duodenum in some animals, e.g., rat (7), but are more widely distributed along the duodenum as small rosettes of acini in others (e.g., guinea pig).

The microcirculation of the small intestinal mucosa supplies these various tissues. The microvascular architecture is, in large part, dictated by the complex topology of the mucosal surface, since the capillaries lie principally in the distorted surface of the lamina propria immediately subjacent to the enterocyte layer (4, 46,49–51,74,79,85,86,90).

Mucosal Microvascular Architecture: Villi

The microvascular architecture of villi has been investigated for over a century (72,94), chiefly by light microscopy of cleared tissues following intravascular injection with opaque media. Many of these earlier reports are, however, conflicting. For example, four different patterns have been described for the dog (60,72,86,94). Second, there has been an unfortunate and even continuing tendency for workers to extrapolate findings from one species to others, and particularly to man (70,79,98,101), despite the fact that interspecies differences have been well and repeatedly established (49,60,86,94,108).

Spanner (94) classified the villus microvascular architecture according to the pattern of arteriolar breakup (Fig. 1A-C) describing a "fountain" pattern where the villus arteriole passed unbranched to the villus tip, only there branching to supply the subepithelial capillary network. His "tuft" pattern described arterial breakup into capillaries at the base of the villi, with drainage of the network via a venule originating at the villus tip, and his "stepladder" pattern described arteriolar and venular vessels extending virtually to the villus tip, with multiple capillaries joining between the two, sequentially, up the villus.

The use of acrylic plastics to cast replicas of the blood space in microvascular networks and study of corroded full and partial replicas with the scanning electron microscope (75) have recently permitted the definitive description of the microvascular architecture of the intestinal mucosa in a number of species (46,49,50,51, 79,104) including man (50,51). This approach, as well as direct intravital microscopic observation of blood flow patterns (5), especially when the two techniques are combined for the same species (46,104), has permitted the patterns of microvascular flow within individual villi and adjacent intestinal glands of particular species to be firmly established (Fig. 1D,E).

Rat villi

The flattened leaf-shaped rat villus is supplied by a single arteriole that passes unbranched from the submucous arterial plexus to the tip of the villus; there it bifurcates into two marginal vessels from which frequent branches pass to the separate capillary plexuses underlying the oral and aboral faces of the villus (49,78,79,104). The capillary network of the villus is drained usually by two symmetrically placed venules that arise about 20% of villus height above the base. The villus subepithelial capillary plexus continues below this level to the base of the villus, there to be joined by capillary-size connections to the capillary rings surrounding the openings of adjacent intestinal glands (Fig. 1D,E).

Rabbit villi

The tongue-shaped rabbit villi each receive an eccentrically located arteriolar supply vessel, which passes to the tip of the villus without branching en route (46,50). Just below the tip the vessel branches into a marginal vessel that passes around the tip and into another, which passes back down the villus margin adjacent to the arteriole. These marginal vessels branch to the capillary networks on oral and aboral faces of the rabbit villus. A single venule commences close to the margin of the villus distal to the arteriole and about 25% of villus height below the tip. This venule receives virtually all its capillary tributaries at this level, so that the capillaries appear to pass to the beginning of the venule in a radial pattern (Fig. 2D). The capillaries of the lower 50% of the rabbit villus are more or less aligned parallel to the axis of the villus, connecting at one end to the venule and at the other end to the capillary rings surrounding the adjacent intestinal gland openings (Fig. 2D); some cross-connections between these capillaries of the lower villus shaft of the rabbit are also evident.

Cat villi

Cat villi (Fig. 2A) are slender and cylindrical or finger-shaped (50,94,98). A single arteriole passes to the villus tip without branching en route. At the tip, this vessel breaks up in a classic fountain pattern to supply the subepithelial plexus, which consists mainly of capillaries lying parallel to the villus axis, but with some cross-connections (50) (See Fig. 2B). Mucosal venules commence at the level of the villus base and drain both the capillary network of the villi and the capillary rings surrounding the intestinal gland openings at that level (49).

Dog villi

Canine villi (94) are stout and finger-shaped (Fig. 3A). In the villus core, an eccentrically placed arteriole passes to the tip of the villus, and an eccentric venule commences only a little below the tip (Fig. 3B,C,E). Arteriolar breakup is in a fountain pattern at the tip (Fig. 3C). However, for the distal 50% of villus height the arteriole provides a series of connections to the subepithelial capillary network, which is here principally oriented annularly around the villus; sphincter-like constrictions are commonly found in the casts at the commencement of these small

FIG. 1. Models of mucosal microcirculation of the intestine. **A:** "Fountain" pattern of villus blood. **B:** Tuft. **C:** Stepladder. All modified after Spanner (94). **D:** Combined fountain supply to tip and tuft supply at base. *(a)* Arteriole; *(v)* venule. *(Large arrows)* Principal directions of capillary flow in each pattern. (**A–D:** Reprinted from Gannon, ref. 46, with permission.) **E:** Model of mucosal microcirculatory patterns typical of human and rabbit small intestine; (modified after Frasher and Wayland, ref. 45). VA = villus arteriole, VV = villus venule. Solid arrows indicate direction of blood flow, and open arrows indicate directions of secretion of succus entericus and of absorption of intestinal fluid.

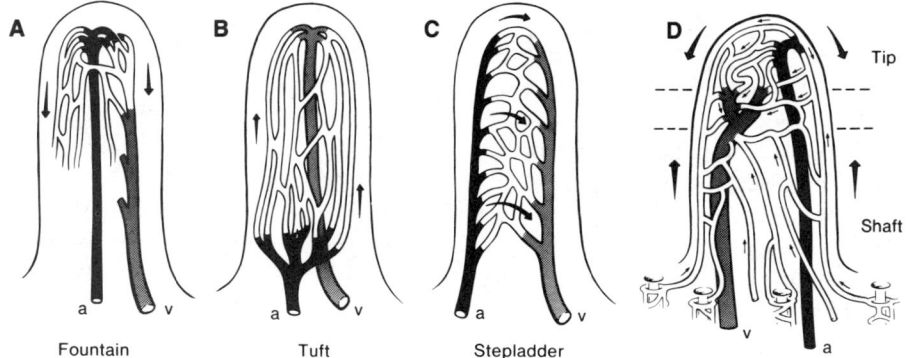

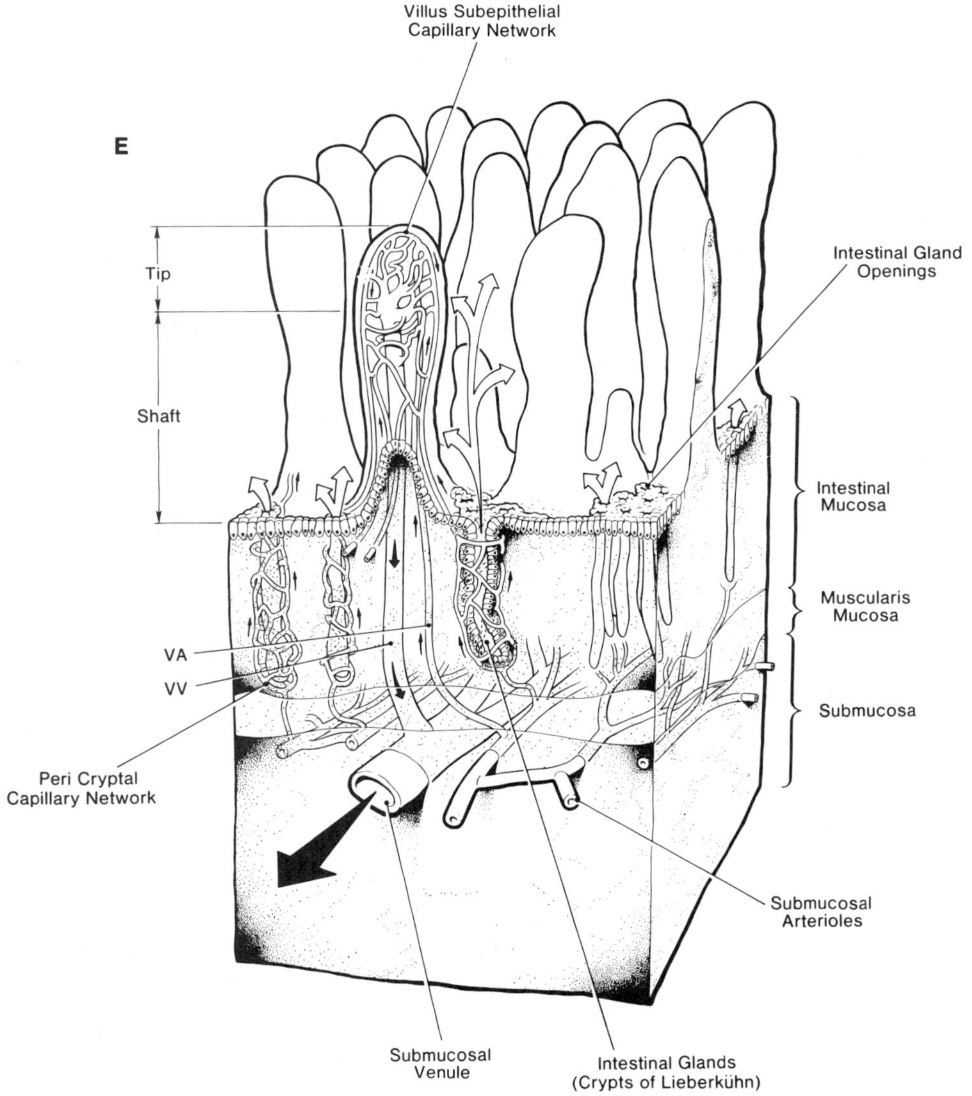

branches from the villus arteriole (49) as shown in Fig. 3E. From just below the tip region (i.e., from about 90% of villus height) down to about 50% of villus height, the villus venule also receives serial tributaries from the subepithelial capillary network (Fig. 3E). The capillary vessels in the lower ~50% of the dog villus are oriented much more parallel to the villus long axis; these vessels pass between the capillary rings surrounding the openings of the group of intestinal glands adjacent to the villus and the more annularly arranged capillaries of the upper half of the villus (Fig. 3C,D).

Human villi

There is greater variation in the shapes of adjacent villi in any single specimen from human small intestine than from the other species examined, in which intraspecies villus shape appears relatively uniform. Human villi vary in shape from short to longer finger-shaped villi, through broader tongue-shaped villi to much broader villus ridges, which appear to be the result of fusion of the lateral edges of several villi (46,49,50,51,90) (see Fig. 4A). Villus microvascular architectures reflect these variations; nevertheless, there is a constant pattern of a single eccentrically located arteriole passing to the villus tip, where it breaks up in a fountain-like pattern, and an eccentrically located venule that commences about 15% of villus height below the tip (Fig. 1E). Capillary connections to the villus venule are almost exclusively at the level of its origin. The capillaries of the lower shaft of the villus are oriented approximately parallel to the villus axis (Fig. 4B), connecting between the capillary rings surrounding adjacent intestinal gland openings and the villus venule (Fig. 4C).

Mucosal Microvascular Architecture—Crypts

The microvasculature surrounding each of the crypts consists of a tubular-shaped plexus of capillary-size vessels in the lamina propria surrounding the epithelium of each crypt (4,46,50,51,79). This capillary network is fed by direct arterial connections from the submucous vascular network (49,50,79) and perhaps partly by branches from the terminal arterioles en route to the villi, originating below the most basal (i.e., abluminal) level of the crypts (Fig. 1E). Venous drainage is into the venules that drain (and usually originate within) the villi and occurs at two principal levels. The first is by infrequent capillary-size connections from the pericryptal plexus directly to the mucosal venules efferent from the villi as the latter pass through the crypt layer (79). The second and more frequent connections are via capillary-size vessels that pass from the capillary rings surrounding the intestinal gland openings to the venules of adjacent villi. These latter capillaries form the lower portion of the villus supepithelial capillary network and join the villus venule(s) at a level characteristic of the particular species (46,49,50,51). In the rat, these capillaries efferent from the pericryptal plexus join the villus venules at ~20% of villus height above its base, in rabbit and man ~75% of villus height above the base, in the dog, ~50% of villus height above the villus base. In the cat, the venules draining the villi only originate at the very base of the villi, and the pericryptal capillaries join these at that level. Flow directions implied by these connections have been confirmed by direct *in vivo* microscopic observation (5,46) for rabbit, rat, and cat, the only species investigated to date.

FIG. 2. Scanning electron micrographs of critical point dried small intestinal villi of cat (**A**; ×165) and rabbit (**C**, ×170). Note long, slender finger shape of cat villi (**A**) and contraction of rabbit villi, as evidenced by their buckled epithelium (**C**), which also shows many small goblets of surface mucus. Scanning electron micrographs of vascular corrosion casts of cat (**B**) and rabbit (**D**). Note central arteriole *(a)* and surrounding capillaries *(c)* of cat villi, and assymmetric arteriole *(a)* and venule *(v)* of rabbit villi, capillary rings surrounding intestinal gland openings are visible between the bases of adjacent villi. (From Gannon et al., ref. 50, with permission.)

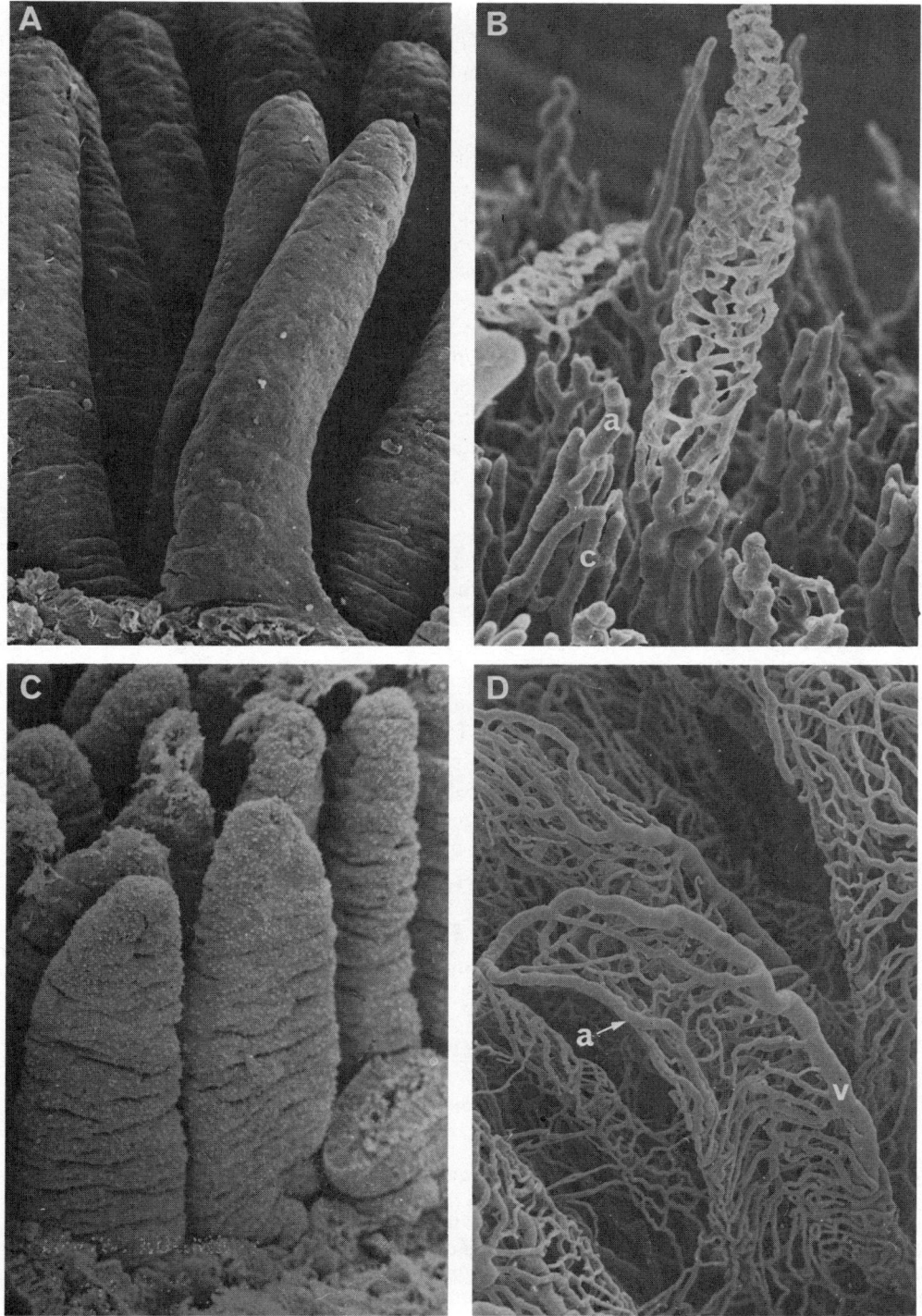

Microvascular Architecture of Duodenal Glands

The duodenal glands (Brunner's glands) are branched acinar glands that lie in the submucosa and that empty their secretions into the bases of the crypts (see above). Their specific microcirculation has not been subjected to a detailed analysis until recently (7). The arterial supply is principally to the serosal aspect of the compact mass of Brunner's glands in the rat. The gland mass is drained by several prominent venules that originate between the glands close to the crypt level and pass aborally for a substantial distance, receiving many capillary connections before draining into the submucous vascular plexus, which is located principally external to the gland mass. However, it has not been possible to define an ordered, polarized modular microvascular unit around the acini and ducts of the gland in the way this has been achieved for, for example, salivary glands (81) and for the villi and crypts of the intestine, possibly because the branching nature of the densely packed glands precludes their being arranged in an orderly, polarized fashion.

Small Intestinal Microvascular Architecture—Conclusions

As can be seen from the foregoing, classification of villi (94) as fountain, tuft, and stepladder (Fig. 1A–C) provides an inadequate description of the villus microvascular architecture of most species except the cat (which exhibits a classic fountain pattern), since most species (e.g., rat, rabbit, and man) exhibit a fountain pattern to the villus tip and a tuft pattern to the villus base (Fig. 1D). The watershed level (46) that separates these two patterns varies from quite near the villus tip (man) to quite near its base (rat). The dog shows an even more complex pattern, with a fountain pattern at the very tip, a stepladder pattern for the next approx. half the villus, and a tuft pattern for the basal half of the villus (see above). Clearly, then, villus microvascular architecture is complex, and as there are marked interspecies differences, extrapolation of microvascular architectures and of functional mechanisms dependent on such architecture (69,70) between species is of dubious validity (50,108).

For most species, the basal portion of the villus appears to receive a type of "local portal" blood supply, in that it is supplied with blood that has already perfused the pericryptal capillary network (46,49,50) as shown in Fig. 1D. Such an arrangement may be functionally significant (42,44,49), given the suggested spatial separation of transepithelial fluid movements in the intestine, secretion being reportedly from the intestinal glands (54,76,100,107), whereas absorption is apparently a function of the villi (54).

The existence or lack of arteriovenous anastamoses (AVAs) in the alimentary tract is a topic of continuing controversy (36,78,101). Despite frequent reports with earlier methods of poorer resolution, following careful scanning electron microscope analysis of corrosion casts of stomach and small intestine of several species (8,46–51,79), we consider it unlikely that connections between arterial and venous vessels with luminal diameters substantially larger than intestinal capillaries exist, at least for these regions of the alimentary tract.

Colonic Microcirculation

Microvascular architecture of the muscular and submucous layers of the colon (77) appears

FIG. 3. Micrographs of dog intestinal villi. Note stout, finger-shaped dog villi **(A)**, which contain largely annularly directed capillaries in the distal 50% of the villus (see **C–E**) but largely longitudinally oriented subepithelial capillaries for the basal 50% of the villus **(D)**. **D,E:** Micrographs of an incomplete vascular cast in which the vessels of the villus tip (~25%) were unfilled. **E:** Note asymmetrically placed arteriole *(a)* and venule *(v)*, which, near the tip, are each connected to the subcapillary network *(c)* by frequent small branches *(black arrows)*; note the sphincter-like constriction at the origin of the arteriolar to capillary connection *(white arrow)*. **B:** Note the proximity of the capillaries *(c)* to the basal lamina of the epithelium *(e)*, the arteriole *(a)* and venule *(v)* of the villus core and the large central lacteal *(c1)*.

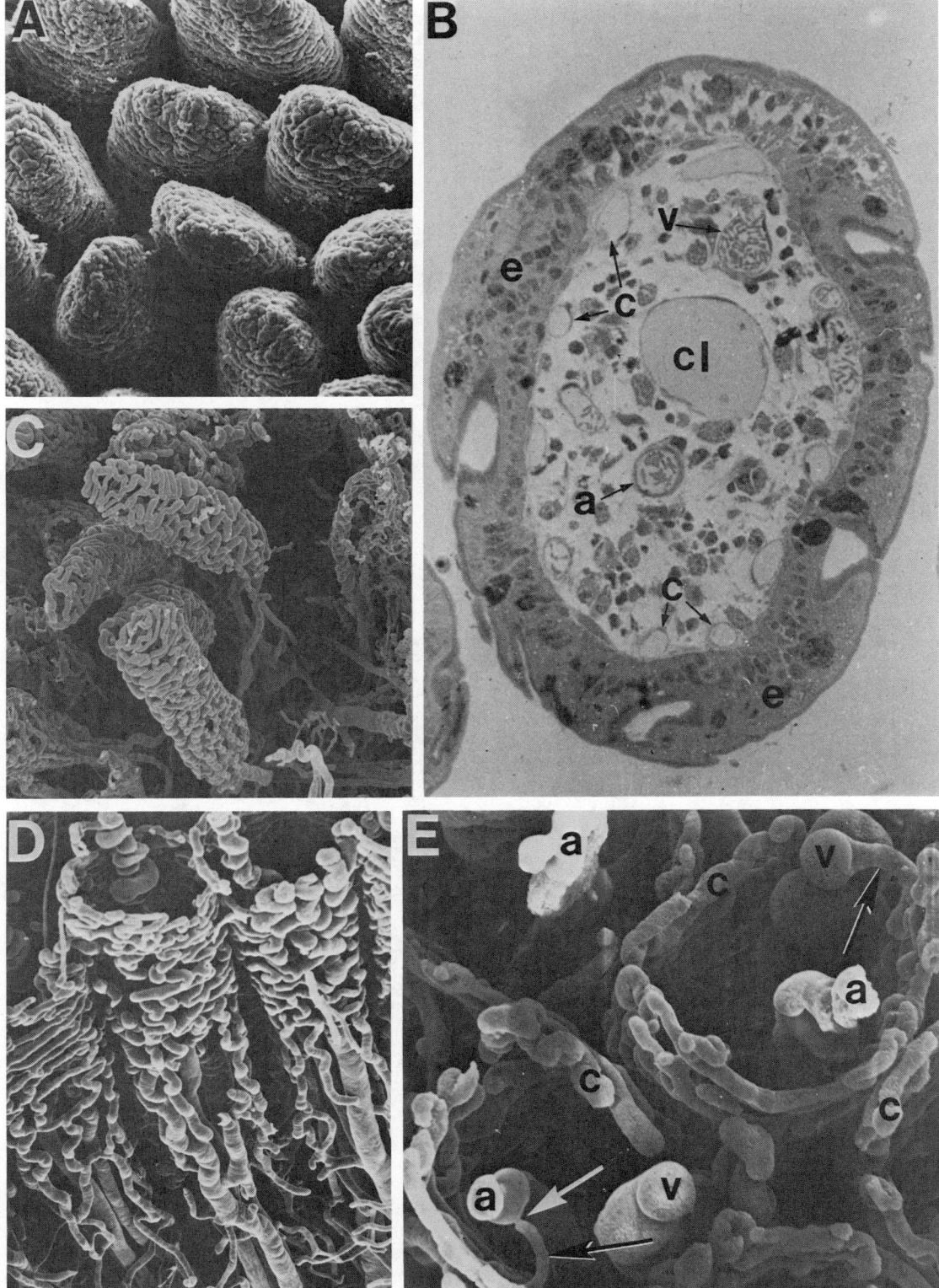

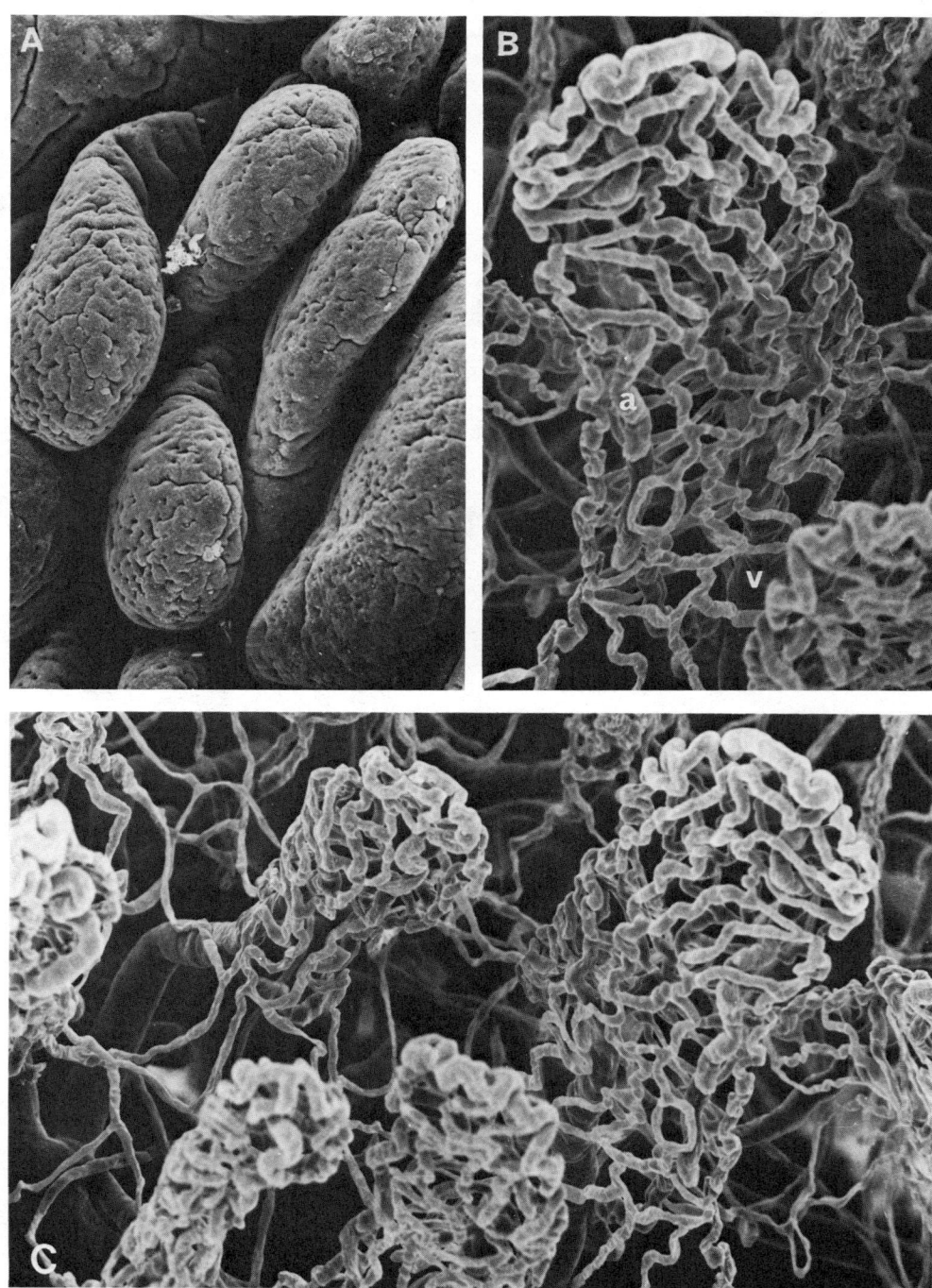

FIG. 4. Scanning electron micrographs of human villus epithelial surface **(A)** and villus vascular corrosion casts **(B,C)**. Note variation in shape of human villi **(A)**, direct arteriolar supply to the villus tip **(B,**a**)**, origin of venule high human villus **(B,**v**)**, and connection of capillaries of lower villus shaft to capillary rings surrounding openings of intervillus intestinal gland openings (c). (**A,** × 145; **B** × 185.) (Fig. 4A, B from Gannon et al., ref. 51, with permission.)

largely similar to that of the small intestine, although it has yet to be studied exhaustively (3). The mucosal microcirculation is largely that of the colonic glands, which are each surrounded by a capillary network similar to that found around the intestinal gland of the small intestine. Mucosal venules are seen by intravital microscopy to originate in the mucosa close to its luminal surface and drain the capillaries surrounding the openings of the colonic glands (B. Gannon, *unpublished observation*). Whether there are additional capillary tributaries to the mucosal venules as these pass to the submucous venous plexus remains unexplored; arterial supply to the mucosa is probably by end arterioles to the bases of the colonic glands, as for the small intestine, although this too remains to be established.

FINE STRUCTURE OF BLOOD EXCHANGE VESSELS

Capillary ultrastructure has been frequently studied (12,19,24,31,42,43,68,71,92,109). Some quantitative parameters of these vessels are shown in Table 1. Typically, the capillaries and postcapillary venules are fenestrated as in most of the viscera (Figs. 5,6). In comparison with continuous capillaries, much of their endothelium is thin (less than 100 nm deep) with many fenestrae (Fig. 5), and they contain relatively few small vesicles (92); these vessels are surrounded by a continuous basal lamina.

Cross-sectional analysis of the endothelial intercellular junctions of the mucosal blood capillaries show a similar proportion of close/tight junctions—2% (39)—as that found in continuous capillaries—6% (121). A new variety of tight junction has been found in venous capillaries of rat jejunum (97). In the villus, however, the close junctions are very unlikely to be important for the permeability of the vessels because of the large numbers of fenestrae even on the arterial limbs (24,29). Similarly, the few small vesicles are unlikely to be significant for permeability.

In the duodenum of the rat, capillary cross-sections often lack an endothelial intercellular

TABLE 1. *Some parameters of the capillaries, per 100 g of cat jejunum*[a]

Villi tips—volume 10% of total
  Capillaries
    Length: 13 km
    Surface area: 0.29 m^2
    Length of endothelial intercellular
      junctions: 29 km
  Fenestrae
    Number: 1.7×10^{12}
    Diameter: 41 nm
    Depth: 36 nm
    Numbers per cm^2 of capillary surface:
      56×10^7
Villi bases—volume 6.6% of total
  Capillaries
    Length: 5.0 km
    Surface area: 0.050 m^2
    Length of endothelial intercellular
      junctions: 9.6 km
  Fenestrae
    Number: 0.026×10^{12}
    Numbers per cm^2 of capillary surface:
      5.2×10^7
Submucosa (around crypts)—volume 21% of total
  Capillaries
    Length: 22 km
    Surface area: 0.41 m^2
    Length of endothelial intercellular
      junctions: 55 km
  Fenestrae
    Number: 0.65×10^{12}
    Diameter: 46 nm
    Depth: 37 nm
    Numbers per cm^2 of capillary surface:
      16×10^7
Muscularis externa—volume 76% of total
  Capillaries
    Length: 31 km
    Surface area: 0.5 m^2
    Length of endothelial intercellular
      junctions: 68 km
  Fenestrae
    Number: 0.04×10^{12}
    Numbers per cm^2 of capillary surface:
      0.82×10^7
cf. Dog leg muscle (per 100 g)[b]
  Capillaries
    Length: 260 km
    Surface area: 2.2 m^2
    Length of endothelial intercellular
      junctions: 450 km
  Fenestrae (not counted, but very rare)

---

[a]Adapted from reference 26, where methods of calculation are given.
[b]Adapted from reference 27, where methods of calculation are given.

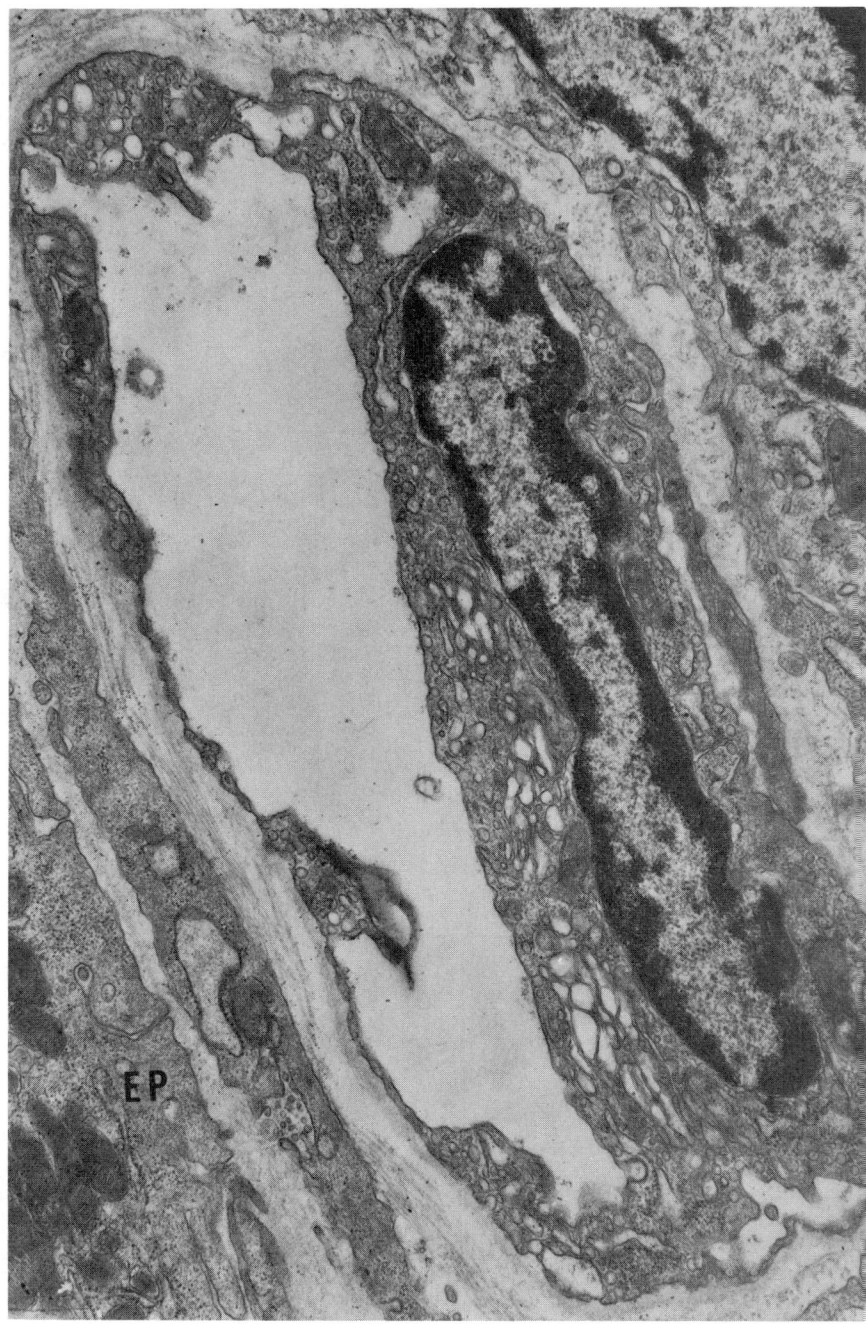

FIG. 5. A capillary on the venous side of the circulation, at the tip of a mouse villus. There are many fenestrae, especially on the side nearest the epithelium *(EP)*. ×22,000. (From Casley-Smith, ref. 12, with permission.)

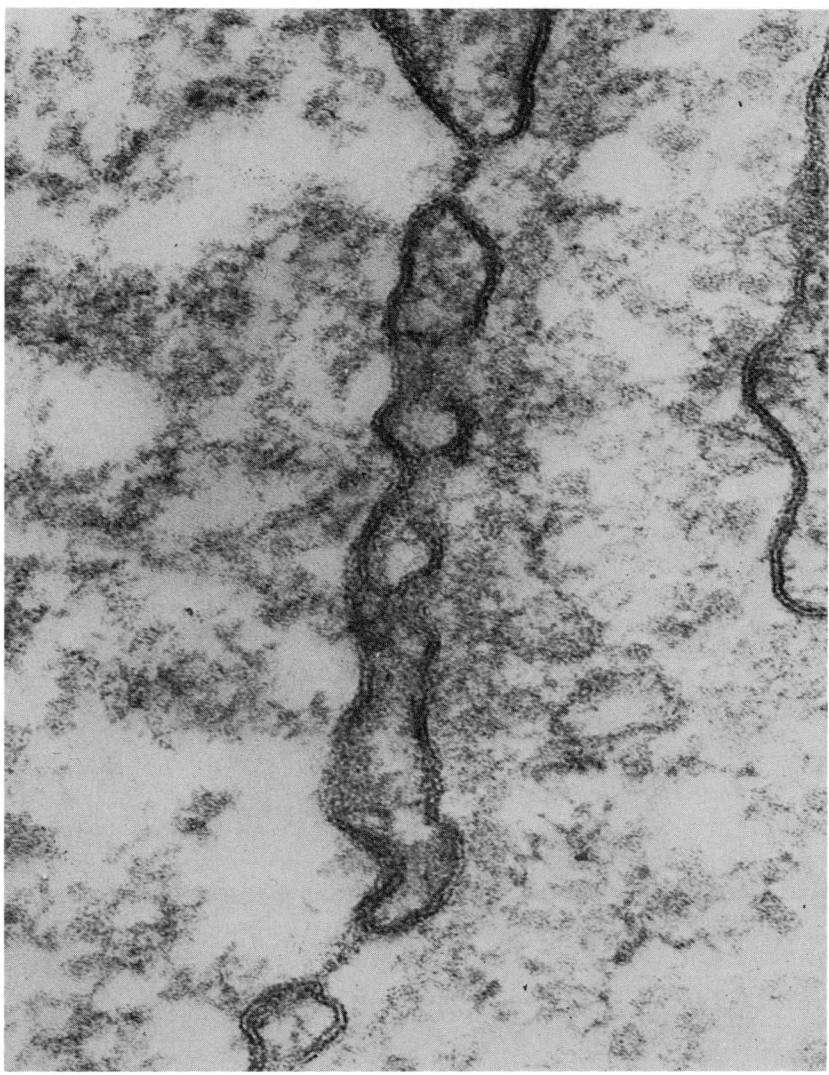

FIG. 6. As for Fig. 5, showing three fenestrae and the diaphragms × 150,000. (From Casley-Smith, ref. 12, with permission.)

junction (110). Serial sectioning proved that these were cells completely encircling the lumen and not just tangential sections. They only occur in the interconnected small capillaries, not in the main loops, and are probably a function of differing growth patterns.

The arterioles to the villi have smooth muscle in their initial segment, to the level of the tops of the crypts, but they lack smooth muscle within the villus proper (63). Microfilaments in the pericytes and endothelium, rather than muscular sphincters, may be responsible for vasoconstriction of the villous arcade vessels (63). U Uehara and co-workers *(personal communication)* have recently observed a network of microfilament containing myofibroblasts immediately subjacent to the villus epithelial basal lamina and superficial to the villus microvessel network. It is tempting to speculate that this network may have a role in the control of villus vascular perfusion and, perhaps, also in the emptying of villus interstitial compartment or the lymphatic lacteal.

The villus venules are lined by continuous epithelium and distally are surrounded by pericytes (63), which give way to muscle cells proximally.

Fenestrae: Their Fine Structure and Distribution

Fenestrae are holes (about 50 nm in diameter) passing right through endothelial cells (Figs. 5,6). They can only occur in thin endothelium, less than 100 nm, but not all thin endothelium is fenestrated. They are obviously important for exchange with the epithelium, since most of the fenestrae lie on the side of the vessel wall that faces the epithelium, whereas the nuclear region lies on the abepithelial side (Fig. 5). A similar functional polarity has been noted in many other regions in which fenestrated capillaries occur.

Fenestrae often have a diaphragm across them (Fig. 6), which may be the fused outer lamellae of the plasma membranes from the two faces of the cell. There has been much debate about whether diaphragms always exist, or whether their absence or presence is an artifact of fixation. It seems that they are real but transient structures, which are much more frequent across the fenestrae in some regions than in others (19). In mouse jejunal villi, 54% of fenestrae of the capillaries near the villus tip had diaphragms, compared with 73% near the villous base (12); in cat jejunum, these were 52% and 62%, respectively (24). EDTA destroys the diaphragms (30), as histamine may do (30), although some investigators disagree (58).

Ruthenium red easily passes from the tissues through the fenestrae and stains the endocapillary layer, which is probably composed of acidic mucopolysaccharides (68). The diaphragms of fenestrae have been shown to be anionic, more so than the plasma membrane; the membranes of vesicles are not (93).

It has been almost always reported that there are many more fenestrae at the venous end of the microcirculation than the arterial end, for example, the retia mirabile of the swim bladder and kidney, the salivary glands, the adrenal cortex, the ciliary body, the ocular muscles, the skin, and around an explanted cancer (19). The one exception to this rule is the renal glomerulus (but even this discharges into many, very fenestrated, so-called venous capillaries). This increase in total number is partly because venous vessels have greater diameters, but it also reflects a considerable increase in their numbers per unit vessel area. Arteriovenous differences have been reported for mouse (12) and cat (24) jejunal mucosa, since both these species showed many more fenestrae (per unit luminal surface area) at the villus tips than at their bases (Table 1). Rats have been reported not to show this (91). At the time of that report (91), it seemed that this arteriovenous difference was in the conventional direction, since the villus tip capillaries were then generally considered "venous." However, in the light of the more recent microvascular architectural studies, it is apparent that the rule that "most fenestrae are at the venous side of the circulation" is broken here (see above). As the arteriole goes directly to the tip of the villus in most species, it may well be that the rapid and frequent branching of the capillary plexus at the tips causes so great a drop in pressure that the capillaries soon become absorptive, even though physically close to the arterial supply; they certainly resemble venous-limb capillaries in size and in frequency of fenestrations. Alternatively, it may be that the differing numbers of fenestrae at villus tips and bases reflect the dual blood supplies to the villi (see above).

Permeability: Electron Microscope Tracers

Apart from the renal glomerulus, the fenestrae of which have long been known to be very permeable even to quite large macromolecules, it was considered for many years that the fenestrae were probably impermeable, at least to large molecules (71). We now know that they are very permeable even to ferritin molecules (11 nm) and the smaller lipoproteins (29,39,

55,91, for reviews, see 19,41,109). The effects of diaphragms are still in doubt; peroxidase appears to traverse fenestrae that always possess them. The reason for this change of opinion is of considerable interest for the light it throws on the functioning of fenestrae.

It seems very likely that the fenestrae near the arterial side of the microcirculation allow large amounts of fluid and plasma protein to enter the tissues. Although some of these will pass to the initial lymphatics, most will reenter the blood via the fenestrae on the venous side of the system. A certain amount of back-diffusion of macromolecules can occur against the bulk-flow of fluid, but this is minimal, unless the macromolecules are small, or the flow velocity is low (13,18). Since the early workers used large macromolecules injected into the blood, often at relatively low concentrations, it is not surprising that none was seen leaving the vessels. Once smaller macromolecules were used, and the concentrations greatly increased, the great permeability of the fenestrae was revealed (11,19,29,62). The microinjection of large tracers directly into the tissues also confirmed this great local flux in the intestine and renal medulla (11,64,105) and demonstrated the high permeability of the fenestrae in a number of organs (19). The endothelial intercellular junctions did not appear permeable, even to peroxidase (29,39), but this may well have been because the fenestrae were so permeable that passage via junctions was obscured.

Such structural studies and other physiological studies suggest that there is a large flux of protein (and fluid, etc.) from the arterial-limb fenestrae, most of which passes through the interstitial tissue and back to the venous-limb fenestrae, without entering the lymphatic system.

Such a large local circulation of protein makes blood-lymph studies, in regions with many fenestrated capillaries, extremely difficult to interpret. It would explain, for instance, the negative fluxes of protein (i.e., net flux towards the blood) sometimes found (56) and many other anomalous results (19, pp. 81–82). The passage of protein from the tissues to the blood in this manner has been confirmed by macrophysiological techniques in the intestine (53,67,103), particularly during the uptake of fluid, and by tracer studies (electron microscopical and macrophysiological) as mentioned earlier.

Tissue Channels

Permeating all the interstitial tissues is the continuous system of tissue channels carrying material to and from the parenchymal cells, the "ultracirculation." The presence of large interstitial fluxes of fluid from arterial to venous ends of capillaries suggests that such a system of discrete pathways within the interstitium of the intestine will be particularly well developed. These pathways or tissue channels are only beginning to be understood. They form a continuous system, throughout the body, composed of all the gaps between the cells and fibres where the ground substance is sufficiently in the sol-phase for free fluid to exist (9,20). Since one cannot fix and stain all of the constituents of the ground substance, the only way to observe the channels in the electron microscope is to attempt to adequately fill them with something identifiable. The vascular system can be perfused with methacrylate monomer, which leaks from the fenestrated capillaries of the intestine into the interstitial tissue and thus into the tissue channels and can be polymerised in them (26). After digestion of the tissue, the scanning electron microscope reveals the channels (Fig. 7). The irregular size, shape, and interconnections of the channels are well shown, as is their relative scarcity far from the vessels and their greater numbers near them.

Quantitation of channels is best performed in sections (23,26,27) by using an innocuous ion, for example, ferrocyanide, with a high charge-density (to keep it out of the gel-phase of the ground substance) and precipitating it in the channels (Fig. 8). Transmission electron microscopy and stereology can then be used. Such studies have yet to be made on intestinal tissue.

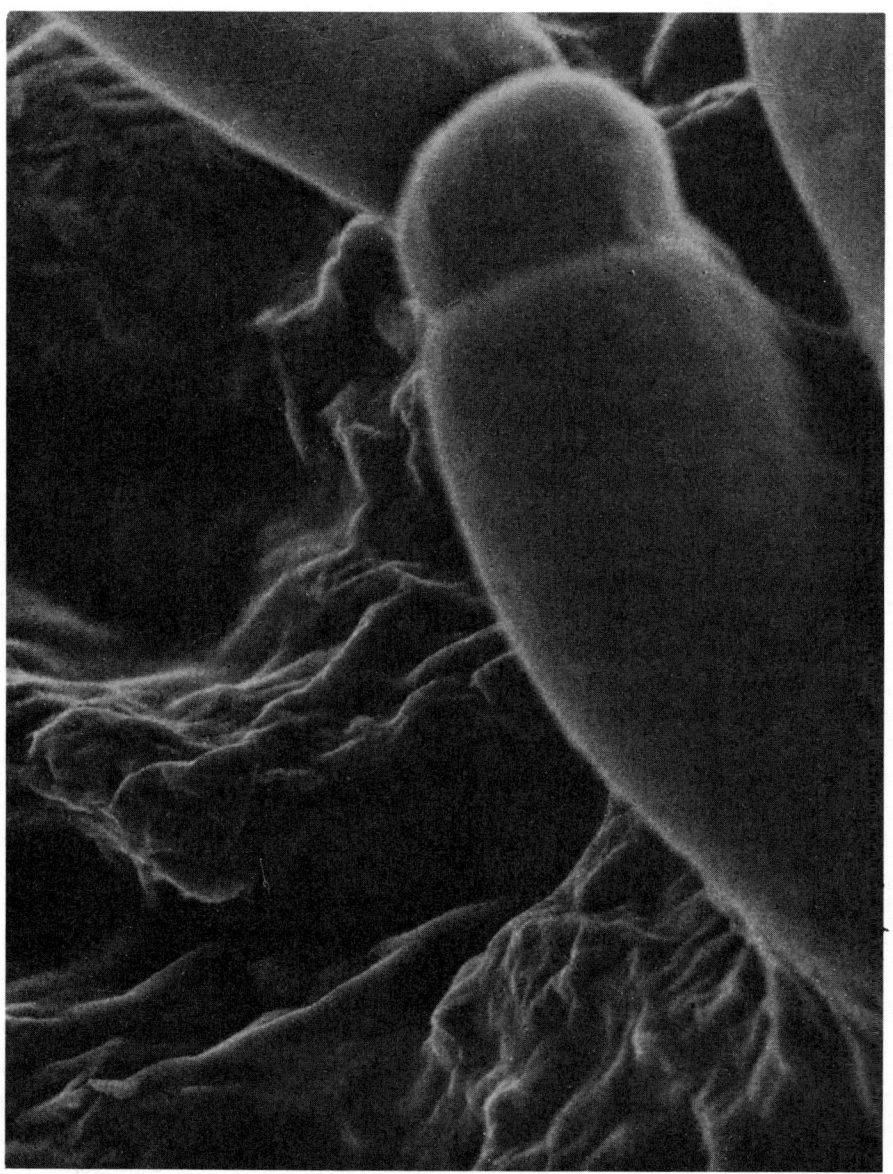

FIG. 7. Tissue channels, filled with plastic, in a rat ileal villus. Some *(top right)* pass between two blood capillaries. ×2,000. (From Casley-Smith et al., ref. 24, with permission.)

Results from normal subcutaneous tissue, brain, joint capsules, and the lining of Guyton's capsules (23,26,27) are all very similar and much the same as that calculated for cat jejunum, using the various permeability data and equations (24). The channels are normally 40 to 100 nm in diameter and there are about 0.5 to 1.5/ μm^2. Their numbers and dimensions increase markedly in edema (23) and take a long time to return to normal.

Although there is an essential randomness in the system of tissue channels (13), it seems that there is an overall directedness presumably caused by the opposing tendencies of fluid flow, which

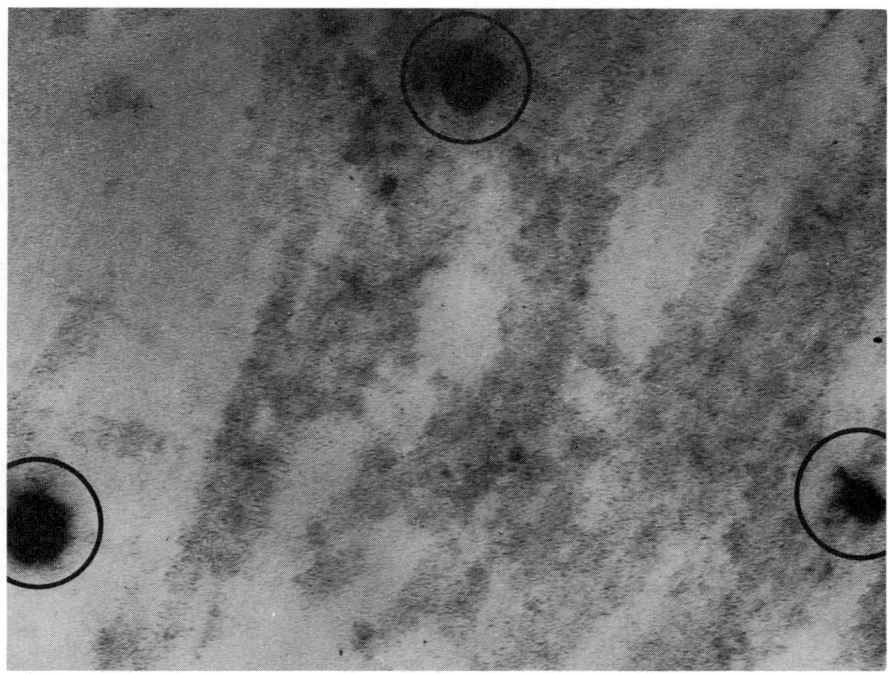

FIG. 8. Tissue channels *(circled)* contain ferri-ferrocyanide. ×80,000. (From Casley-Smith et al., ref. 24, with permission.)

will enlarge them, and the deposition of more ground substance, which will obliterate them. (19, p. 143). This presumably accounts for their alterations with time and with tissue conditions, and for their concentration generally around the venous side of the blood microcirculation. Most of them carry material from and to blood exchange-vessels, but some end at the initial lymphatics and, at times, at endothelial intercellular junctions that are either open or appear openable, as has been shown in the intestine (33).

LYMPHATIC SYSTEM

The blood exchange vessels are obviously vital to gut function; however, the lymphatics are similarly important. Functional intestinal lymphatics are important not only for the more familiar role of fat absorption and transport but also for maintenance of normal functional and indeed structural integrity of the gut itself, since their blockage causes a protein-losing enteropathy that damages gut tissues (61).

General Architecture of the Lymphatic System

Lymphatic morphology has been extensively reviewed (89,90,102,111). In the small intestine, there are initial lymphatics (lacteals) in each villus (Fig. 3B,9) with maximal diameters of 20 to 30 μm (15). In finger-like villi there is one central lacteal starting one third of the way from the tip; in leaf-like villi there are a number. In either, the total lengths of lacteals are similar (50–70 cm/cm² of gut surface); this figure is very constant wherever it has been studied (skin, muscle, diaphragm, heart, ear) (15).

Lacteals empty when the smooth muscle in the core of the villus contracts (16,102) by a longitudinal shortening in finger-like villi or by a circular constriction of the muscularis mucosa in those species with leaf-like villi. These initial lymphatics (lacteals) discharge into a submucosal plexus connected with the collecting lymphatics. Since only the villus is compressed

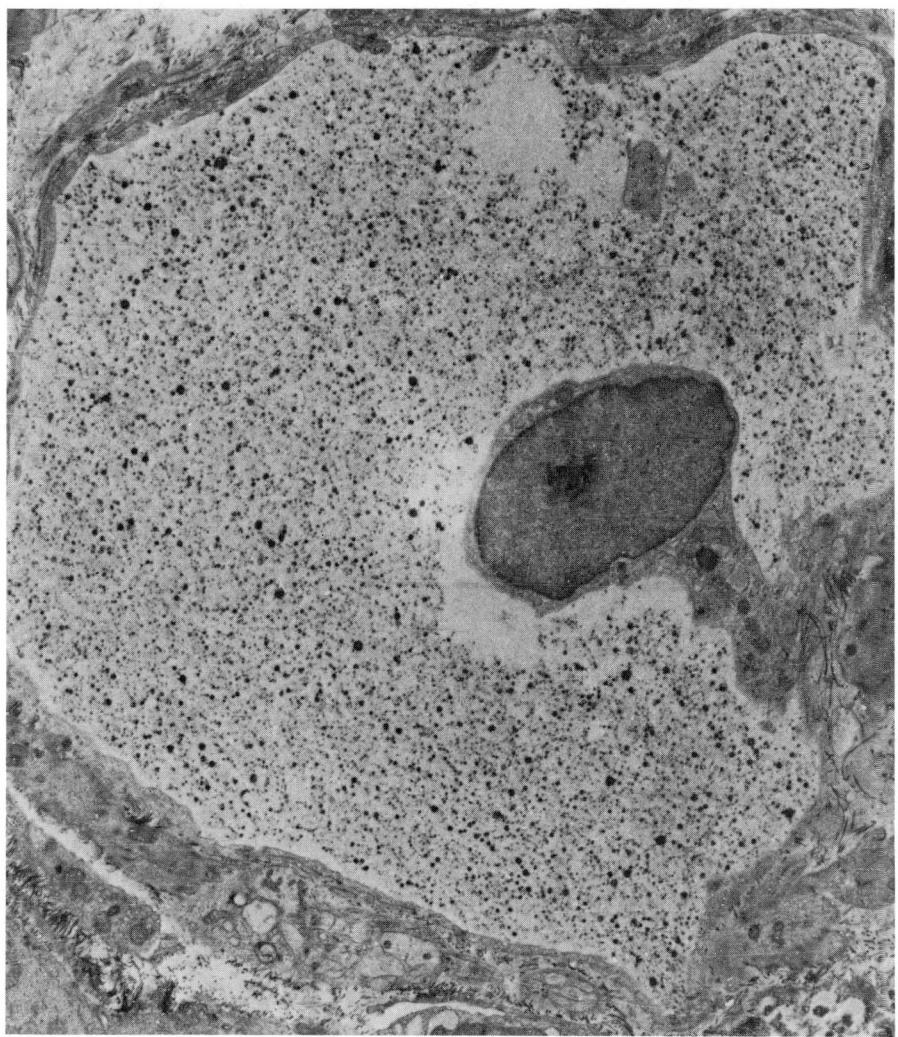

FIG. 9. Rat jejunal lacteal, containing many lipoproteins. ×5,000. (From Casley-Smith, ref. 9, with permission.)

during its emptying, there are no "adjacent collectors," that is, collecting vessels subjected to the same forces as the initial lymphatics (14). This may account for the redilution of the lymph, which had been concentrated in the initial lymphatics (14,16,25). It also accounts for the unusually high efficiency of these initial lymphatics (14–37% compared with 0.1–3% elsewhere in the body) (15). The initial lymphatics of the large intestine (99) and stomach (22,65,104) are less prominent and are further from the mucosa, a location that may reflect a reduced role for lymphatic absorption in these regions.

General Fine Structure of the Initial Lymphatics

The fine structure of intestinal lymphatics is much the same as elsewhere in the body (1,2,9,14,16,17,22,32,33,37–39,57,61,66 80,82, 83,88,99; for reviews, see 19,59,111). They are similar in size to venous capillaries (Fig. 9) but have no fenestrae, few pericytes, and tenuous basement membranes. Anchoring filaments join parts of the endothelium to the interstitial tissue, but these are much less frequent in the intestinal villi than elsewhere in the body, including the submucosal lymphatics (17,38,39). Their small vesicles (39) may be greater in frequency than those of lymphatics elsewhere or of blood capillaries (19). Lacteals also often have open endothelial intercellular junctions (Figs. 10,11).

Permeability of the Initial Lymphatics

Open junctions are characteristic of initial lymphatics. They provide the usual path into these vessels for fluid, macromolecules and particles, including chylomicra (Figs. 10,11) and lipoproteins (9,16,19,20,32,66,82,88,111). While the tissues are relaxed, the very pliable endothelial cells are pushed aside as fluid, etc., enters the vessels. Upon contraction of the surrounding muscle, the intralymphatic hydrostatic pressure rises and forces the endothelial cells against each other and the interstitial tissue, temporarily sealing the opening to macromolecules, although not to fluid. Thus the lymph becomes concentrated during this phase of the initial lymphatic cycle (14,16). Pharmacological agents have been used to make the villi stay in the relaxed or contracted state (16). They confirmed the opening of the junctions, filling of the lacteals, and dilution of the lymph during relaxation, and the reverses of these, during contraction.

Some workers, using serial sections, find no open junctions at all and consider that the visible openings are actually wide intraendothelial channels (1,2), although this would not alter the basic valve-like mechanism of lymphatic uptake. In fact, their illustrations of such channels show them adjacent to junctions, and it has often been established (e.g., 28) that open junctions usually have wide channels leading into them. These are seen as partly open junctions in most sections. Other studies of the lacteals, also with serial sections, clearly showed that there were open junctions (33).

The only quantitative study of the intestinal villi found 2.5% of the lengths of the junctions of the initial lymphatics were open (38); 10% were closed (i.e., with spaces of 4 to 6 nm between the cells), 88% were tight (i.e., with no resolvable space). Although many of the "tight" junctions could not be identified with certainty, it is likely that any open ones were identified. Some workers (19) think that so few open junctions could not account for lymphatic filling. However, a mathematical model (using these percentages) showed such numbers were quite enough to allow total filling of the initial lymphatics in a few seconds (40) because the

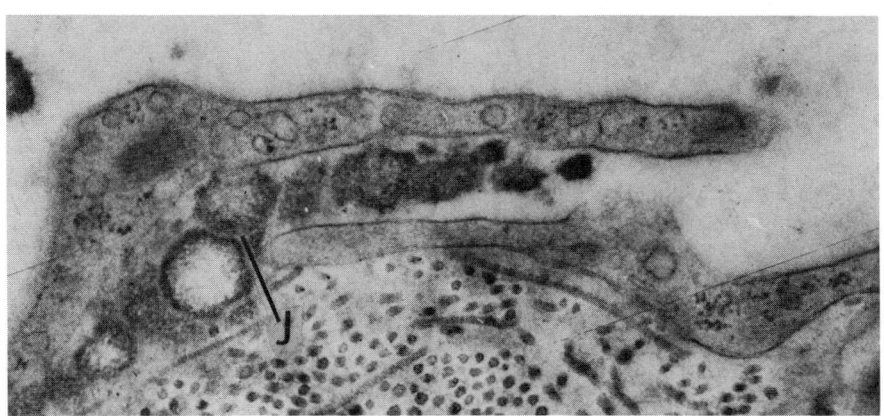

FIG. 10. Chylomicra entering a lacteal at an open junction (J). ×30,000. (From Casley-Smith, ref. 9, with permission.)

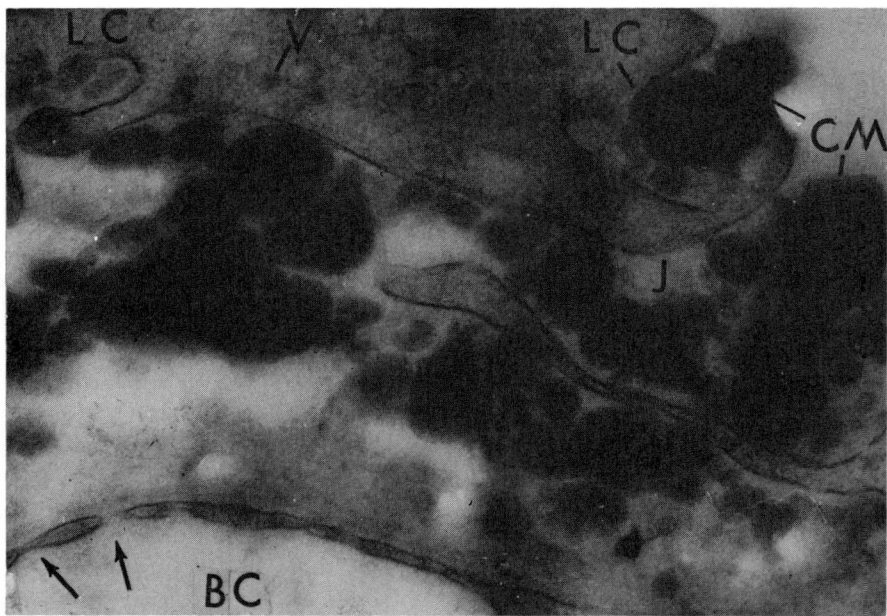

FIG. 11. Chylomicra (CM) are entering a lacteal via an open junction (J), as well as passing into the endothelium via large caveolae (LC), which become vacuoles. Small ones (probably lipoproteins) are present in vesicles (V). A blood capillary (BC) is also shown. It is evident that the chylomicra cannot enter it via its fenestrae (arrows). ×35,000. (From Casley-Smith, ref. 9, with permission.)

hydraulic conductivity of a junction varies as the cube of its width.

Chylomicra also traverse the endothelium of the initial lymphatics via large vacuoles (Fig. 11). This was suspected in the villus of the intestine (1,9,38,39), but it could not be proved, since once chylomicra emerge from the endothelium, they are free in the lumen. However, they have been observed passing, via vacuoles, from the lumen of diaphragmatic initial lymphatics into the interstitial tissue where they were trapped (10). Why should the initial lymphatics need vacuoles as well as open junctions? Possibly the vacuoles are needed during a very fatty meal. Under these conditions there will be few macromolecules, or excess fluid, in the interstitial tissue. Hence, there will be very little fluid inflow via the open junctions to carry the chylomicra into the initial lymphatics via these openings. In such circumstances, it would be very advantageous to have the second, vacuolar, path, since chylomicra are too large to enter the fenestrae of the blood vessels and must rely on the lymphatic system for transport.

REFERENCES

1. Azzali, G. (1982): Ultrastructure of small intestine submucosal and serosol-muscular lymphatic vessels. *Lymphology*, 15:106–111.
2. Azzali, G. (1982): The ultrastructural basis of lipid transport in the absorbing lymphatic vessel. *J. Submicrosc. Cytol.*, 14:45–54.
3. Baez, S. (1977): Skeletal muscle and gastrointestinal microvascular morphology. In: *Microcirculation*, edited by G. Kaley and B. M. Altura, vol. 1, pp. 69–94. University Park, Baltimore.
4. Bellamy, J. E. C., Latshaw, W. K., and Nielsen, N. O. (1983): The vascular architecture of the porcine small intestine. *Can. J. Comp. Med.*, 37:57–62.
5. Bohlen, H. G., Heinrich, H., Gore, R. W., and Johnson, P. C. (1978): Intestinal muscle and mucosal blood flow during direct sympathetic stimulation. *Am. J. Physiol.*, 235:440–445.
6. Borg, T. K., and Caulfield, J. B. (1980): Morphology of connective tissue in skeletal muscle. *Tissue Cell.*, 12:197–207.
7. Browning, J., and Gannon, B. (1984): The microvascular architecture of the rat proximal duodenum. *Biomed. Res. (submitted).*

8. Browning, J., Gannon, B. J., and O'Brien, P. (1983): The microvasculature and gastric lumenal pH of the forestomach of the rat: A comparison with the glandular stomach. *Int. J. Microcirc. Clin. Exp.*, 2:109–118.
9. Casley-Smith, J. R. (1962): The identification of chylomicra and lipoproteins in tissue sections and their passage into jejunal lacteals. *J. Cell Biol.*, 15:259–277.
10. Casley-Smith, J. R. (1964): Endothelial permeability—The passage of particles into and out of diaphragmatic lymphatics. *Q. J. Exp. Physiol.*, 49:365–383.
11. Casley-Smith, J. R. (1970): The functioning of endothelial fenestrae on the arterial and venous limb of capillaries, as indicated by the differing directions of passage of proteins. *Experientia*, 26:852–853.
12. Casley-Smith, J. R. (1971): Endothelial fenestrae in intestinal villi: Differences between the arterial and venous ends of the capillaries. *Microvasc. Res.*, 3:49–68.
13. Casley-Smith, J. R. (1976): Calculations relating to the passage of fluid and protein out of arterial-limb fenestrae, through basement membranes and connective tissue channels, and into venous-limb fenestrae and lymphatics. *Microvasc. Res.*, 12:13–34.
14. Casley-Smith, J. R. (1977): The concentrating of proteins in the initial lymphatics and their rediluting in the collecting lymphatics. *Folia Angiol.*, 25:81–89.
15. Casley-Smith, J. R. (1978): The efficiencies of the initial lymphatics. *Z. Lymphol. (J. Lymphol.)*, 2:24–29.
16. Casley-Smith, J. R. (1979): A fine structural study of variations in protein concentration in lacteals during compression and relaxation. *Lymphology*, 12:59–65.
17. Casley-Smith, J. R. (1980): Are the initial lymphatics normally pulled open by the anchoring filaments? *Lymphology*, 13:120–129.
18. Casley-Smith, J. R. (1981): Large colloidal osmotic pressures across large pores, and the passage of macromolecules up their own concentration gradients. *Microvasc. Res.*, 21:223–228.
19. Casley-Smith, J. R. (1983): The structure and functioning of the blood vessels, interstitial tissues, and lymphatics. In: *Lymphangiology*, edited by M. Földi and J. R. Casley-Smith, pp. 27–164. Schattauer, Stuttgart, New York.
20. Casley-Smith, J. R. (1982): Mechanisms in the formation of lymph. In: *International Review of Physiology, Cardiovascular Physiology IV*, edited by A. C. Guyton and J. E. Hall, vol. 26, pp. 148–187. University Park Press, Baltimore.
21. Casley-Smith, J. R., Green, H. S., Harris, J. L., and Wadey, P. J. (1975): The quantitative morphology of skeletal muscle capillaries in relation to permeability. *Microvasc. Res.*, 10:43–64.
22. Casley-Smith, J. R., and Florey, H. W. (1961): The structure of normal small lymphatics. *Q. J. Exp. Physiol.*, 46:101–106.
23. Casley-Smith, J. R., Földi-Börcsök, E., and Földi, M. (1979): A fine structural study of the tissue channels' numbers and dimensions in normal and lymphoedematous tissues. *Z. Lymphol. (J. Lymphol.)*, 3:49–58.
24. Casley-Smith, J. R., O'Donoghue, P. J., and Crocker, K. W. J. (1975): Quantitative relationships between fenestrae in jejunal capillaries and tissue channels: Proof of "Tunnel capillaries". *Microvasc. Res.*, 9:78–100.
25. Casley-Smith, J. R., and Sims, M. A. (1976): Protein concentrations in the regions with fenestrated and continuous blood capillaries and in initial and collecting lymphatics. *Microvasc. Res.*, 12:245–257.
26. Casley-Smith, J. R., and Vincent, A. H. (1978): The quantitative morphology of interstitial tissue channels in some tissues of the rat and rabbit. *Tissue Cell*, 10:571–584.
27. Casley-Smith, J. R., and Vincent, A. H. (1980): Variations in the numbers and dimensions of tissue channels after injury. *Tissue Cell*, 12:761–771.
28. Casley-Smith, J. R., and Window, J. (1976): Quantitative morphological correlations of alterations in capillary permeability, following histamine and moderate burning, in the mouse diaphragm; the effect of benzopyrones. *Microvasc. Res.*, 11:279–305.
29. Clementi, F., and Palade, G. E. (1969): Intestinal capillaries. I. Permeability to peroxidase and ferritin. *J. Cell Biol.*, 41:33–58.
30. Clementi, F., and Palade, G. E. (1969): Intestinal capillaries. II. Structural effects of EDTA and histamine. *J. Cell Biol.*, 42:706–714.
31. Cliff, W. J. (1976): *Blood Vessels*. Cambridge University Press, Cambridge.
32. Collan, Y., and Kalima, T. V. (1970): The lymphatic pump of the intestinal villus of the rat. *Scand. J. Gastroenterol.*, 5:187–196.
33. Collan, Y., and Kalima, T. V. (1974): Topographical relations of lymphatic endothelium and initial lymphatics of the villus. *Lymphology*, 7:175–184.
34. Cooke, A. R. (1976): The glands of Brunner. In: *Handbook of Physiology: Section 6, Alimentary Canal; Vol. 2, Secretion.* edited by C. F. Code, pp. 1087–1095. American Physiological Society, Washington, DC.
35. Copenhaver, W. M., Kelly, D. E., and Wood, R. L. (1978): *Bailey's Textbook of Histology*, 17th ed., pp. 455–551. Williams & Wilkins, Baltimore.
36. Dinda, P. K., Buell, M. G., DaCosta, L. R., and Beck, I. T. (1983): Simultaneous estimation of arteriolar, capillary, and shunt blood flow of the gut mucosa. *Am. J. Physiol.*, 245:G29–G37.
37. Dobbins, W. O. (1966): The intestinal mucosal lymphatic in man. *Gastroenterology*, 51:994–1003.
38. Dobbins, W. O. (1971): Intestinal mucosal lacteal in transport of macromolecules and chylomicrons. *Am. J. Clin. Nutr.*, 24:77–90.
39. Dobbins, W. O., and Rollins, E. L. (1970): Intestinal mucosal lymphatic permeability: An electron microscopic study of endothelial vesicles and cell junctions. *J. Ultrastruct. Res.*, 33:29–59.
40. Elhay, S., and Casley-Smith, J. R. (1976): Mathematical model of the initial lymphatics. *Microvasc. Res.*, 12:121–140.
41. Field, J., Hurley, J. V., and McCullum, N. E. W. (1977): The mechanism of escape of plasma protein from small blood vessels in the mucosa of the small intestine of the rat. *J. Pathol.*, 121:51–62.
42. Florey, H. W. (1961): The structure of normal and

inflamed small blood vessels of the mouse and rat colon. *Q. J. Exp. Physiol.*, 46:119–122.
43. Florey, Lord. (1968): The missing link. The structure of some types of capillary. *Q. J. Exp. Physiol.*, 53:1–5.
44. Florey, H. W., Wright, R. D., and Jennings, M. A. (1941): The secretions of the intestines. *Physiol. Rev.*, 21:36–69.
45. Frasher, W. G., Jr., and Wayland, H. (1972): Repeating modular organization of the microcirculation of cat mesentery. *Microvasc. Res.*, 4:62–76.
46. Gannon, B. J. (1981): Co-existence of fountain and tuft patterns of blood supply in intestinal villi of rabbit and man. *Bibl. Anat.*, 20:130–133.
47. Gannon, B., Browning, J., and O'Brien, P. (1983): The microvascular architecture of the glandular mucosa of rat stomach. *J. Anat.*, 135:667–683.
48. Gannon, B., Browning, J., O'Brien, P., and Rogers, P. (1984): Mucosal microvascular architecture of the fundus and body of human stomach. *Gastroenterology*, 86:866–875.
49. Gannon, B., Browning, J., Rogers, P., and Harper, B. (1983): Microvascular organization in the intestine. In: *Microcirculation of the Alimentary Tract*, edited by A. Koo, S. K. Lam, and L. H. Smaje, pp. 39–52. World Scientific, Singapore.
50. Gannon, B. J., Gore, R. W., and Rogers, P. A. W. (1981): Is there an anatomical basis for a vascular countercurrent mechanism in rabbit and human intestinal villi? *Biomed. Res. (Suppl.)*, 2:235–241.
51. Gannon, B. J., Rogers, P. A. W., and O'Brien, P. E. (1980): Two capillary plexuses in human intestinal villi. *Micron*, 11:447–448.
52. Gannon, B. J., Rosenberger, S. M., Versluis, T. D., and Johnson, P. C. (1983): Autoregulatory patterns in the arteriolar network of cat mesentery. *Microvasc. Res.*, 26:1–14.
53. Granger, D. N., Perry, M. A., Kvietys, P. R., and Taylor, A. E. (1981): Interstitium-to-blood movement of macromolecules in the absorbing intestine. *Am. J. Physiol.*, 241:G31–G36.
54. Hallbäck, D. A., Jodal, M., Sjöqvist, A., and Lundgren, O. (1982): Evidence for cholera secretion emanating from the crypts. A study of villus tissue osmolality and fluid and electrolyte transport in the small intestine of the cat. *Gastroenterology*, 83:1051–1056.
55. Hampton, J. C., and Rosario, B. (1967): Passage of exogenous peroxidase from blood capillaries into intestinal epithelium. *Anat. Rec.*, 159:159–169.
56. Hargens, A. R., and Zweifach, B. W. (1976): Transport between blood and peripheral lymph in intestine. *Microvasc. Res.*, 11:89–101.
57. Horstmann, E., and Breucker, H. (1972): Über die Lymphkapillaren in den Darmzotten von Meerschweinchen und Affe. *Z. Zellforsch. Mikrosk. Anat.*, 133:551–557.
58. Hurley, J. V., and McQueen, A. (1971): The response of the fenestrated vessels of the small intestine of rats to application of mustard oil. *J. Pathol.*, 105:21–29.
59. Huth, F. (1983): Special pathology of the lymphovascular system. In: *Lymphangiology*, ed. M. Földi and J. R. Casley-Smith, pp. 377–474, Schattauer, Stuttgart, New York.

60. Jacobson, L. F., and Noer, R. J. (1952): The vascular pattern of the intestinal villi in various laboratory animals and man. *Anat. Rec.*, 114:85–93.
61. Kalima, T. (1971): The structure and function of intestinal lymphatics and the influence of impaired lymph flow on the ileum of rats. *Scand. J. Gastroenterol. (Suppl.)*, 16(10):9–87.
62. Karnovsky, M. J. (1968): The ultrastructural basis of transcapillary exchanges. *J. Gen. Physiol.*, 52:64s–95s.
63. Knoblauch, M., Vogt, C., Hollinger, C., Neff, M., and Metry, J. M. (1981): The influence of hormones on the microcirculation of a single jejunal rat villus, with evidence for microfilament-mediated vasoconstriction. *Microvasc. Res.*, 22:232.
64. Kraehenbuhl, J. P., Gloor, E., and Blanc, B. (1967): Résorption intestinale de la ferritine chez deux espéces animales aux possibilités d'absorption protéique néontale différentes. *Z. Zellforsch.*, 76:170–186.
65. Kvietys, P. R., Wilborn, W. H., and Granger, D. N. (1981): Effects of net transmucosal volume flux on lymph flow in the canine colon. *Gastroenterology*, 81:1080–1090.
66. Ladman, A. J., Padykula, H. A., and Strauss, E. W. (1963): Morphological study of fat transport in the normal human jejunum. *Am. J. Anat.*, 112:389–419.
67. Leonard, J. I., and Abbrecht, P. H. (1973): Dynamics of plasma-interstitial fluid distribution following intravenous infusion in dog. *Circ. Res.*, 33:735–748.
68. Luft, J. H. (1973): Capillary permeability. I. Structural consideration. In: *The Inflammatory Process*, 2nd ed., edited by B. W. Zweifach, L. Grant, and R. T. McCluskey, vol. 2, pp. 47–94. Academic Press, New York and London.
69. Lundgren, O. (1967): Blood flow distribution and countercurrent exchange in the small intestine. *Acta Physiol. Scand. (Suppl.)*, 303:1–42.
70. Lundgren, O. (1978): The alimentary canal. In: *Peripheral Circulation*, edited by P. C. Johnson, pp. 225–283. Wiley, New York.
71. Majno, G. (1965): Ultrastructure of the vascular membrane. In: *Handbook of Physiology, Circulation II*, edited by W. F. Hamilton and P. Dow, pp. 2293–2375, Waverly Press, Baltimore.
72. Mall, F. P. (1888): Die Blut- und Lymphwege in Dünndarm des Hundes. *Abh. Sachs. Ges. Wiss.*, 14:153–189.
73. Miller, B. G., Woods, R. I., Bohlen, H. G., and Evan, A. P. (1982): A new morphological procedure for viewing microvessels. *Anat. Rec.*, 203:493–503.
74. Mohiuddin, A. (1965): Blood and lymph vessels in the jejunal villi of the white rat. *Anat. Rec.*, 156:83–90.
75. Murkami, T. (1971): Application of the scanning electron microscope to the study of the fine distribution of the blood vessels. *Arch. Histol. Jpn.*, 32:445–454.
76. Nasset, E. S., and Ju, J. S. (1973): Micropipet collection of succus entericus at crypt ostia of guinea-pig jejunum. *Digestion*, 9:205–211.
77. Nopanitaya, W., Aghajanian, J. G., and Gray, L. D. (1979): An improved plastic mixture for corrosion casting of the gastrointestinal microvascular system. *Scanning Electron Microscopy*, III:751–756.

78. Nylander, G., and Olerud, S. (1961): The vascular pattern of an isolated jejunal loop: A microangiographic study in the rat. *Acta Chir. Scand.*, 121:39–46.
79. Ohashi, Y., Kita, S., and Murakami, T. (1976): Microcirculation of the rat small intestine as studied by the injection replica scanning electron microscope method. *Arch. Histol. Jpn.*, 39:271–282.
80. Ohshima, Y. (1977): Electron microscopic study of the intestinal absorption of medium and long chain triglycerides in rat. *Arch. Histol. Jpn.*, 40:153–169.
81. Ohtani, O., Ohtsuka, A., Lipsett, J., and Gannon, B. (1983): The microvasculature of rat salivary glands. A scanning electron microscopic study. *Acta Anat.*, 115:345–356.
82. Palay, S. L., and Karlin, L. J. (1959): An electron microscopic study of the intestinal villus. *J. Biophys. Biochem. Cytol.*, 5:373–384.
83. Papp, M., Rohlich, P., Rusznyak, I., and Törö, I. (1962): An electron microscopic study of the central lacteal in the intestinal villus of the cat. *Z. Zellforsch. Mikrosk. Anat.*, 57:475–486.
84. Piasecki, C. (1977): Role of ischaemia in the initiation of peptic ulcer. *Ann. R. Coll. Surg. Engl.*, 59:476–478.
85. Reynolds, D. G., Brim, J., and Sheehy, T. W. (1967): The vascular architecture of the small intestine mucosa of the monkey (Macaca mulatta). *Anat. Rec.*, 159:211–218.
86. Reynolds, D. G., and Swan, K. G. (1972): Intestinal microvascular architecture in endotoxic shock. *Gastroenterology*, 63:601–609.
87. Rogers, P. A. W., and Gannon, B. J. (1983): The microvascular cast as a three-dimensional tissue skeleton: Visualization of rapid morphological changes in tissues of the rat uterus. *J. Microsc.*, 131:241–247.
88. Rubin, C. E. (1966): Electron microscopic studies of triglyceride absorption in man. *Gastroenterology*, 50:65–77.
89. Rusznyak, I., Földi, M., and Szabo, G. (1967): *Lymphatics and Lymph Circulation*, 2nd ed., Pergamon Press, London.
90. Sessions, J. T., Viegas de Andrade, S. R., and Kokas, E. (1968): Intestinal villi. *Prog. Gastroenterol.*, 1:248–260.
91. Simionescu, M., Simionescu, N., and Palade, G. E. (1972): Permeability of intestinal capillaries. *J. Cell Biol.*, 53:365–392.
92. Simionescu, M., Simionescu, N., and Palade, G. E. (1974): Morphometric data on the endothelium of blood capillaries. *J. Cell Biol.*, 60:128–152.
93. Simionescu, N., Simionescu, M., and Palade, G. E. (1981): Differentiated microdomains on the luminal surface of the capillary endothelium. I. Preferential distribution of anionic sites. *J. Cell Biol.*, 90:605–613.
94. Spanner, R. (1932): Neue Befunde über die Blutwege der Darmwand und ihre funktionelle. *Bedeutung. Morph. Jahrbuch*, 69:394–454.
95. Stach, W. (1978): Die Vaskularisation des Plexus submucous externus (Schabadasch) und des Plexus submucous internus (Meissner) im Dünndarm von Schwein und Katze. *Acta Anat.*, 101:170–178.
96. Stach, W., Hung, N., and Schoof, S. (1977): Zur Gefäßversorsung des plexus myentericus (Auerbach) im Dickdarm der Katze. *Z. Mikrosc.—Anat. Forsch., Leipzig.*, 91:S22–30.
97. Staehelin, L. A. (1975): A new occludens-like junction linking endothelial cells of small capillaries of rat jejunum. *J. Cell Sci.*, 18:545–551.
98. Svanvik, J. (1973): Mucosal blood circulation and influence on passive absorption in small intestine. *Acta Physiol. Scand. (Suppl.)*, 385:1–44.
99. Takada, M., Torisawa, K., Takada, T., Takada, K., and Saeki, S. (1970): Observations on lymphatic vessels in subserosa of rabbit large intestine: the internal pressure and structure. *Acta Anat. Nippon.*, 45:305–310.
100. Trier, J. S. (1964): Studies on small intestinal crypt epithelium. II. Evidence for and mechanisms of secretory activity by undifferentiated crypt cells of the human small intestine. *Gastroenterology*, 47:480–495.
101. Vajda, J., Raposa, T., and Herpai, Z. (1968): Structural bases of blood flow regulation in the small intestine. *Acta Morphol. Acad. Sci. Hung.*, 16:331–340.
102. Verzar, F., and McDougall, E. J. (1936): *Absorption from the Intestine*. Longmanns, London.
103. Vogel, G., Martensen, I., and Hinghofer-Szalkay, H. (1982): The influence of absorption/enterosorption and partial occlusion of the portal vein on the quantity and composition of intestinal lymph. *Lymphology*, 15:43–50.
104. Vogt, C., Métry, J. P., Holliger, C., Anliker, M., and Knoblauch, M. (1981): The microcirculatory system of the jejunal villus of the rat. Correlation of intravital microscopy, injection casts and electron microscopy. *Bibl. Anat.*, 20:69–70.
105. Warshaw, A. L., Walker, W. A., Cornell, R., and Isselbacher, K. J. (1971): Small intestinal permeability to macromolecules. *Lab. Invest.*, 25-675–684.
106. Warwick, R., and Williams, P. L. (1973): Gray's Anatomy. 35th ed., Longman, Edinburgh.
107. Welsh, M. J., Smith, P. L., Fromm, M., and Frizzell (1982): Crypts are the site of intestinal fluid and electrolyte secretion. *Science*, 218:1219–1221.
108. Winne, D. (1975): The influence of villous counter current exchange on intestinal absorption. *J. Theor. Biol.*, 53:145–176.
109. Wolff, J. R. (1977): Ultrastructure of the terminal vascular bed as related to function. In: *Microcirculation*, edited by G. Kaley and B. M. Altura, vol. 1, pp. 95–130. University Park Press, Baltimore.
110. Wolff, J. R., Moritz, A., and Güldner, F.-H. (1972): "Seamless" endothelia in fenestrated capillaries of duodenal villi (rat). *Angiologica*, 9:11–14.
111. Yoffey, J. M., and Courtice, F. C. (1970): *Lymphatics, Lymph and Lymphomyeloid Complex*. Academic Press, New York and London.

Metabolic Regulation of the Intestinal Circulation

*A. P. Shepherd and **D. Neil Granger

*Department of Physiology, University of Texas Health Science Center, San Antonio, Texas 78284; and **Department of Physiology, College of Medicine, University of South Alabama, Mobile, Alabama 36688

The concept that mechanisms within an organ control its perfusion is over a century old. In 1877 Gaskell (8), working in Ludwig's laboratory, suggested that the exercise hyperemia of skeletal muscle was due to vasodilator metabolites. The teleological appeal of this concept is that each organ could adjust its perfusion for optimal function, whereas nervous mechanisms could temporarily override local control to regulate arterial pressure reflexly and thus assure survival of the organism. In the first half of this century little progress was achieved in applying this concept to the intestinal circulation; however, in the 1950s and 1960s pressure versus flow relationships began to be reported showing the presence (6,20–23,58) or absence (17) of local control in the gut.

These early studies (17,20–23) indicated that the intestine did not autoregulate its blood flow as vigorously as some organs such as the kidney, that experimental conditions affected the probability of successfully demonstrating local control, that autoregulatory phenomena were indeed due to mechanisms intrinsic to the gut, since they persisted in spite of acute or chronic denervation, and that the two most viable theories to explain the evidence indicative of local control were the myogenic and metabolic theories.

The myogenic theory (7) primarily attempts to explain the relative constancy of blood flow in the face of perfusion pressure changes. It is based on the premise that, in response to an increase in passive stretch, vascular smooth muscle can actively contract. Thus, increased perfusion pressure, although followed by a transient rise in blood flow, would evoke an active vasoconstriction through increased transmural pressure. Hence, blood flow would be brought back down toward control. By contrast, the metabolic theory explains the return of blood flow back to control by the washout of vasodilator metabolites. At this writing, the best evidence indicates that both types of mechanisms participate in the local control of the intestinal circulation. In fact, a dual or unified theory that encompasses both the metabolic and myogenic mechanisms has been proposed (7,23). In this chapter, we discuss the evidence that a metabolic mechanism is responsible for intestinal "autoregulation," whereas the myogenic reactivity of intestinal vessels and the interaction between the myogenic and metabolic mechanisms are discussed in Chapter 4.

METABOLIC MODEL OF LOCAL CONTROL

The metabolic model of local circulatory contol that has stimulated significant research in the last 10 years is depicted in Fig. 1 (15,16,48). In this model, the oxygen flux to the parenchymal cells of the intestine is proposed to be the regulated variable. As Fig. 1 shows, two discrete microvascular mechanisms are available to regulate the delivery of oxygen to intestinal tissue: (a) arterioles regulate blood flow and thus determine the convective flux of oxygen into the intestinal capillary beds and (b) precapillary sphincters determine the number of capillaries perfused at a given instant. The number of perfused capillaries, in turn, sets two important diffusion parameters—capillary surface area and capillary-to-cell diffusion distance (27). Thus, the precapillary sphincters regulate the diffusive flux of oxygen into the tissue. A detailed de-

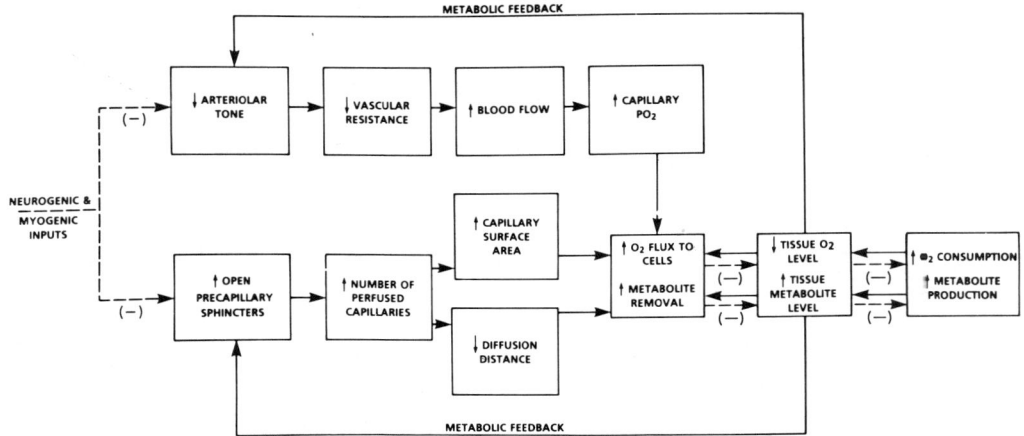

FIG. 1. Two-component metabolic model of local control. Tissue oxygenation is regulated by metabolic feedback to resistance vessels and precapillary sphincters. Feedback signals could be either a vasodilator metabolite or interstitial hypoxia. Sympathetic nervous stimulation and the myogenic reactivity of microvessels can superimpose their effects on the metabolic control system because they also affect resistance and exchange vessels. (From Shepherd, ref. 47, with permission.)

scription of this type of model is given in Chapter 22. The model was constructed on the premise that in response to inadequate tissue oxygenation parenchymal cells produce a feedback signal to dilate resistance vessels and open precapillary sphincters. Therefore, the two vascular responses to inadequate oxygenation are increased blood flow and increased perfused capillary density. Augmented blood flow increases or maintains capillary PO_2, whereas the diffusive flux of oxygen into the tissue is a function of both the capillary-to-cell PO_2 difference and the perfused capillary density. Hence, in response to transient inadequate oxygenation, the two vascular responses restore the tissue oxygen level toward its normal value.

As Fig. 1 illustrates, two different types of feedback signals could possibly work in this scheme. One possibility is that the PO_2 of interstitial fluid influences the tone of both resistance vessels and precapillary sphincters. A second possibility, however, is that parenchymal cells produce a vasodilator metabolite. Figure 1 also shows that a myogenic mechanism could be superimposed on the metabolic feedback system. For example, increased venous pressure could cause the constriction of both resistance vessels and precapillary sphincters and thus induce vascular reactions opposite to those exerted by metabolic feedback. Such myogenic-metabolic interactions are discussed in Chapter 4. Finally, neurogenic inputs such as sympathetic stimulation could also compete with metabolic feedback at the two vascular effectors (see Chapter 5).

A computer model (48) based on this two-component model of the microvascular control of tissue oxygenation provided a theoretical framework for many of the experiments on local control that were carried out in the last decade. These experiments have preceded in several stages. The first phase was to determine if resistance and exchange vessels in the gut behaved qualitatively as the metabolic model predicted during various experimental perturbations. The second phase was to quantitate the ability of resistance vessels to autoregulate flow during perfusion pressure changes and to determine the relative contributions of blood flow and capillary density to oxygen homeostasis. Indeed, a major prediction of this model was that the autoregulation of blood flow in response to perfusion pressure manipulations would be enhanced if the oxygen availability-to-demand ratio was lowered in any way. Finally, attempts have been made to identify the specific substances that could act as the metabolic feedback signal in the intestinal circulation.

Because capillary recruitment is a major component of the proposed microvascular mechanism for controlling intestinal oxygenation, it is appropriate to review briefly two methods for detecting changes in the density of the perfused capillary bed. In fact, most of the evidence favoring capillary recruitment in perfused organ studies have been obtained using either the transcapillary extraction of diffusible indicators such as ^{86}Rb from which the surface area-product (PS) of the capillary bed is computed or the water flux from capillary to tissue from which the capillary filtration coefficient (K_f) is obtained. K_f is a measurement of the hydraulic conductivity of the capillary bed. Although the measurement can be made in a variety of ways, the most common approach is to produce a known increment in capillary hydrostatic pressure by elevating venous pressure in an isolated intestinal loop. The rate of transcapillary fluid filtration is then determined by recording the subsequent change in volume or weight of the tissue. Differences in the value of K_f between control and experimental conditions indicate a change in capillary surface area, permeability, or both. Likewise, measurements of the capillary exchange capacity (PS) reflect the inseparable product of capillary surface area and permeability. Fortunately, many perturbations that cause changes in PS and K_f do not change permeability. Therefore, changes in PS and K_f generally indicate that the effective capillary density has changed. Both of these methods have been discussed in detail elsewhere (38,45).

In the following sections, we discuss the major experimental perturbations that have been employed to delineate the metabolic mechanisms regulating intestinal blood flow.

ARTERIAL HYPOXIA

Because the metabolic theory predicts that any reduction in the oxygen availability-to-demand ratio should elicit vasodilation and capillary recruitment, arterial hypoxia has been used to study the ability of the intestine to maintain tissue oxygenation. Two studies pertinent to the metabolic model have examined the effect of arterial hypoxia in the gut. Svanvik and colleagues (57), studying feline intestine perfused at constant arterial pressure, found blood flow increased 48% when the inspired P_{O_2} was reduced to 55 mm Hg. Capillary filtration coefficients increased 60%. These findings agree qualitatively with the metabolic model and with the later report of Shepherd (41), who found in canine intestine that an arterial P_{O_2} of 46 mm Hg increased blood flow 46% during constant pressure perfusion. The same level of arterial hypoxia increased the capillary exchange capacity (PS for ^{86}Rb) 60% above control during constant flow perfusion. Thus, both of these studies indicate that resistance and exchange vessels responded to arterial hypoxia as predicted by the metabolic model. Both the vasodilation and the apparent capillary recruitment should tend to maintain tissue oxygenation despite the reduced oxygen supply. As Fig. 1 shows, if the resistance feedback loop is defeated by perfusing the intestine at constant flow, the feedback loop regulating capillary density is still free to operate. Thus, isolated gut loops maintained their oxygenation within 48% of control when perfused at constant flow. However, when both blood flow and capillary density were free to increase, oxygen uptake remained within 26% of control despite the hypoxia (41). Skeletal muscle apparently maintains its oxygen consumption within 15% of control at comparable hypoxic levels (16). Thus, the intestine appears to be slightly less effective than skeletal muscle in regulating its oxygenation during arterial hypoxia. The nearly fivefold greater oxygen demands of the intestine may partly explain this difference.

Three major observations made during arterial hypoxia support the metabolic theory: vasodilation, increased PS and K_f, and the tendency of oxygen uptake to remain relatively constant. However, several problems remain to be resolved and new uncertainties have recently been uncovered. For example, the complete relationship between arterial P_{O_2} and capillary exchange capacity is still unknown; neither has the dependence of oxygen uptake on arterial P_{O_2} been completely characterized by lowering arterial P_{O_2} continuously. Also, increases in oxygen extraction can result either from capillary recruitment or from an increase in the capillary-to-cell P_{O_2} difference. Whether or not the latter contributes to maintaining the oxygen flux during hypoxia is unknown. Finally, recent studies (49) indicate that arterial hypoxia increases capillary permeability in the intestine. Thus, in the previous reports, increased PS and K_f could be due to increased capillary permeability rather than capillary recruitment.

Although the effects of arterial hypoxia on the intestinal vasculature appear to be mediated directly by low oxygen levels, indirect effects on blood flow could result from hypoxia-induced changes in intestinal tonus and motility (56). The effects of arterial hypoxia can also be mimicked by intraarterial infusions of cyanide (10).

REACTIVE HYPEREMIA

Three different mechanisms could contribute to the characteristic overshoot in blood flow that follows arterial occlusion: metabolic vasodilation, myogenic reactions, and a refilling and passive distension of the vasculature (Fig. 2). However, a preponderance of the evidence supports the metabolic mechanism. The metabolic model predicts that the vasodilation and capillary recruitment in response to arterial occlusion should cause an overshoot in both tissue P_{O_2} and oxygen extraction upon the release of an occlusion. These predictions have, in general, been confirmed in skeletal muscle but not thoroughly studied in the intestine. In skeletal muscle (16), the postocclusive capillary recruitment has been detected by measurements of PS and K_f. Furthermore, the overshoot in tissue P_{O_2} predicted by mathematical modeling has been confirmed by microelectrode studies (26). Further support for a metabolic mechanism is the observation that both the magnitude and the duration of the reactive hyperemic response are related to the duration of occlusion (33). The magnitude of the reactive hyperemia with arterial occlusion alone is greater than that observed with simultaneous arterial and venous occlusions (33). This observation could be explained by erythrocytes exiting from the tissues during arterial occlusion, thus reducing the oxygen stores during the ischemic period, or by the maintained vascular transmural pressures during simultaneous arterial and venous occlusion. This effect would minimize myogenic contributions to the vasodilation upon release of the occlusion.

The bulk of the evidence indicates that intestinal vascular responses during venous occlusion or elevated venous pressure result primarily from a myogenic mechanism. For further discussion of venous pressure and the myogenic mechanism, see Chapter 4.

The metabolic scheme predicts vasodilation secondary to a tissue P_{O_2} reduction or to the

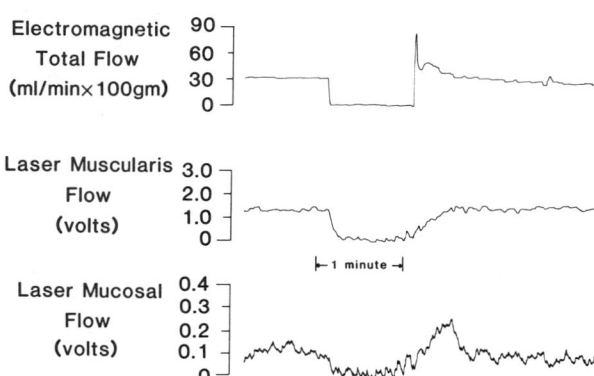

FIG. 2. Reactive hyperemia. In an isolated loop of canine intestine, occluding the mesenteric artery for 60 sec evoked a reactive hyperemia shown as total flow measured with an electromagnetic flow probe on the mesenteric artery. Tracings from two laser-Doppler blood flowmeters show that reactive hyperemia occurred in the mucosa but not in the muscularis. (Shepherd and Riedel, *unpublished observations*).

accumulation of vasodilator metabolites. Tissue P_{O_2} reductions (18) and purine metabolite accumulations (34) have both been observed during arterial occlusion in the small intestine. These are discussed below in greater detail under "Vasodilator Metabolites."

FUNCTIONAL OR METABOLIC HYPEREMIA

To test the metabolic theory of local control, it would be desirable to increase the intestine's requirement for oxygen and measure the attendant vasodilation, capillary recruitment, and oxygen consumption rate. Many such experiments have been carried out in skeletal muscle (12). However, the appropriate means through which intestinal oxygen demands can be increased without producing other complex effects has turned into a difficult question. The increased blood flow that follows the ingestion of a mixed meal can be called a functional or postprandial hyperemia, but this is a complex response involving not only local mechanisms but also possibly nervous and humoral factors. A detailed discussion of postprandial hyperemia can be found in Chapter 8.

At present there are two means available to produce relatively uncomplicated increases in intestinal oxygen demands: increased temperature (29) and intraluminal glucose (43,60,62). Evidence from bioassay and cross-perfusion studies (5) indicates that a functional hyperemia due entirely to local mechanisms occurs in isolated gut loops when their lumens are perfused with simple, nonlipid solutes such as glucose.

In response to glucose-stimulated oxygen demands, the metabolic theory predicts vasodilation and capillary recruitment. The vasodilation, although mild, is well documented (5,43,59), and the increased oxygen extraction that invariably occurs is attended by increases in K_f (43). Furthermore, if glucose is instilled into gut loops perfused at constant blood flow (43), the increases in oxygen extraction are associated with increased PS (^{86}Rb) as shown in Fig. 3. The vascular responses to glucose appear to be solely the result of increased oxygen demand, because other explanations have been easily disproven. For example, mannitol and 2-deoxyglucose, hexoses that are not actively transported, fail to increase blood flow. The simple presence of glucose, the hypertonicity of some of the glucose solutions that have been studied, and glucose catabolism are inadequate explanations. In support of the latter conclusion is the observation that 3-O-methylglucose (a form of glucose that is actively transported but not metabolized) increased oxygen uptake and blood flow (10). Finally, the rate of intestinal oxygen uptake and the fluid absorption accompanying solute transport are significantly correlated. In fact, the oxygen cost of a given volume of absorbed fluid depends on the specific solute transported (59).

As stated earlier, test meals containing protein or fat apparently elicit complex responses that involve the release of vasoactive agents and changes in capillary permeability (3,61). However, the vascular responses elicited by luminal glucose seem to be due entirely to local mechanisms, since the venous blood from such gut loops, when recirculated, does not vasodilate adjacent gut segments (5). Although the data from microsphere studies are contradictory (10), the glucose-induced hyperemia may even be confined to the mucosa. In summary, the active transport of glucose and other nonlipid solutes appears to increase oxidative requirements and elicit the predicted vasodilation and capillary recruitment.

PRESSURE-FLOW AUTOREGULATION

If autoregulation is defined as "the intrinsic ability of an organ to regulate blood flow in accordance with its metabolic demands," each of the phenomena we previously discussed, namely, reactive hyperemia, functional hyperemia, and hypoxic vasodilation, could be considered examples of autoregulation. However, a more restrictive definition of autoregulation is "the intrinsic ability of an organ to maintain a relatively constant blood flow despite imposed changes in perfusion pressure" (21). If we accept the more restrictive definition for the present discussion, it can be fairly stated that

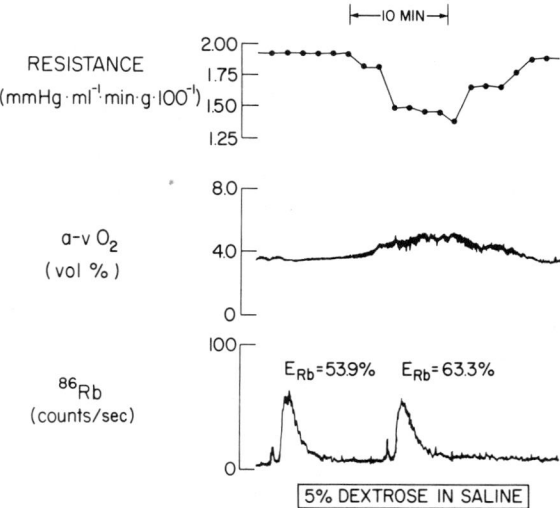

FIG. 3. Metabolic vasodilation. In an isolated gut loop perfused at constant blood flow, intraluminal glucose increased oxygen uptake as shown in the arteriovenous oxygen difference record (a-v O_2). At constant flow, the metabolic "hyperemia" is seen as a fall in perfusion pressure and vascular resistance. Washout curves *(lower tracing)* show Rb^{86} extraction increased with metabolic rate. (From Shepherd, ref. 43, with permission).

autoregulation in the intestine is not the intense phenomenon seen in some other organs such as the kidneys, since a reduction in perfusion pressure is usually accompanied by a reduction in blood flow, whereas resistance falls by modest amount. Figure 4 shows a pressure-flow relationship indicative of exceptional intestinal autoregulation. Autoregulation in the intestine is also a labile phenomenon and is infrequently present in preparations in which pumps and external perfusion circuits are extensively employed. Early studies (19–24) have tentatively established the essentially intrinsic or local nature of the autoregulatory phenomenon. The site of the resistance changes evoked by a reduction in arterial pressure occur in the precapillary resistance vessels while venous resistance actually rises. The local nature of the response has been further established by experiments with nerve blocking agents, chronically denervated intestine, sympatholytic agents, intraarterial cyanide, and nonblood perfusates.

The major observation made in the last 10 years is that the metabolic rate of the intestine has a profound effect on the efficacy of pressure-flow autoregulation. Early studies in skeletal and cardiac muscle suggested a relationship between pressure-flow autoregulation and the metabolic rate of these tissues (16,25), indicating that the effectiveness of the flow control system in response to reduced perfusion pressure depended on the prevailing venous oxygen content. Granger and Shepherd (15) hypothesized that the physiological basis for such a

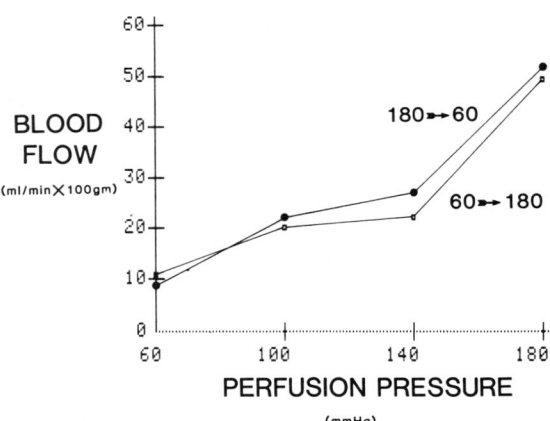

FIG. 4. Pressure-flow curve. In an isolated loop of canine small bowel, raising and lowering arterial pressure while measuring the steady state flow after each pressure step resulted in a pressure-flow relationship indicative of excellent autoregulation. (Shepherd and Riedel, *unpublished observations.*)

relationship between autoregulation and venous oxygen content could be that precapillary sphincters are more sensitive than resistance vessels to tissue hypoxia. When such an assumption was included in the computer model of metabolic control, it predicted a more powerful autoregulatory response to reduced arterial pressure if (a) the resting blood flow level was low, (b) arterial oxygen saturation was below normal, or (c) the metabolic rate was high. The reason for this prediction is that in response to a small reduction in the oxygen availability-to-demand ratio, the more sensitive precapillary sphincters and a passive widening of the capillary-to-cell P_{O_2} difference maintain tissue oxygenation by increasing oxygen extraction, whereas the contribution by the feedback loop controlling blood flow is relatively minor (see Fig. 1). If, however, the venous oxygen reserve is reduced, the contribution of the flow-controlling mechanism becomes more significant and the contribution of oxygen extraction declines. These predictions of the metabolic model have been systematically studied in both skeletal muscle (12) and intestine (13,44,53). In isolated gut loops, pressure-flow autoregulation was enhanced by high metabolic rates induced by intraluminal solutes. As Fig. 5 shows, pressure-flow autoregulation was totally absent in control loops; when arterial pressure was reduced, augmented oxygen extraction was the only means utilized to maintain tissue oxygenation. In fact, passive vascular recoil was the primary flow response, that is, flow fell proportionately more than perfusion pressure. By contrast, during the hypermetabolic state induced by intraluminal solutes, oxygen extraction was already relatively high, and each of the previously passive gut loops began to actively autoregulate its blood flow in response to the same pressure perturbation (44).

Enhanced pressure-flow autoregulation has also been demonstrated in the superior mesenteric artery of intact dogs (13,36). The ability of the intact intestine to autoregulate was compared to animals fed before the experiment and in fasted preparations. In fed preparations, intestinal blood flow remained relatively constant as perfusion pressure was lowered from 125 to 40 mm Hg. Although oxygen delivered to the tissues of the small bowel was well regulated in both fasted and fed preparations down to perfusion pressure as low as 30 mm Hg, the relative contribution of blood flow to the maintenance of adequate oxygenation was dependent on the control level of oxygen extraction. In fasted preparations, intestinal venous oxygen content was high, and increased oxygen extraction was the major mechanism for maintaining oxygen uptake, whereas in fed preparations, the venous oxygen content was lowered by the increased metabolic demands of absorption. Thus, the contribution of local flow regulation became more important in maintaining intestinal oxygenation. These findings and those in isolated gut segments show that a metabolic control system is indeed involved in intestinal autoregulation. They also probably explain, in part, the contradictory early reports about the presence or absence of autoregulation in the intestine. Although the myogenic theory also predicts vasodilation in response to reduced arterial pressure, it is difficult to envision how a purely myogenic mechanism could account for the relationship between intestinal metabolic rate and the efficacy of pressure-flow autoregulation.

OXYGEN UPTAKE: THE CONTROLLED VARIABLE

Although circulatory physiologists have focused attention primarily on the flow-controlling ability of the intestine, more investigations have recently examined the ability of the gut to maintain its oxygen uptake (28,29). Particularly in the last 5 years, intestinal oxygen consumption has been measured as blood flow was altered by pump-perfusion or by infusing vasodilators. Because of the complexity of the vascular beds in the gut, neither of these two approaches necessarily yields straightforward results. In fact, some vasodilators depress intestinal O_2 uptake in gut loops perfused at constant flow, and a number of contradictory findings have been reported regarding the effects of various vasodilators on intestinal oxygen consump-

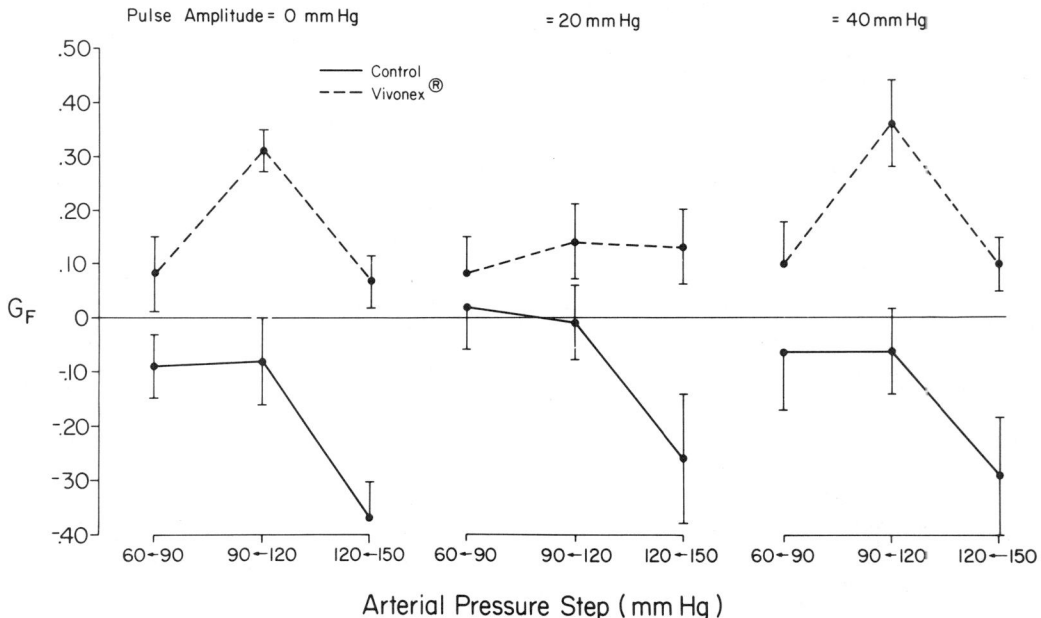

FIG. 5. Effect of increased metabolic rate and pulse pressure on autoregulation. Closed-loop gain (G_F, defined below) is plotted for each arterial pressure step. G_F was calculated as follows: $G_F = 1 - [(\Delta F/F) \div (\Delta P/P)]$. Here P and F are the pressure and flow before the step change in pressure (ΔP) and the resulting change in flow (ΔF). Defined this way, $G_F = 0$ in a rigid system in which flow changes exactly in proportion to pressure. Negative G_F indicate passive vascular distension predominants, whereas positive values denote that active autoregulation minimized the flow change for a given ΔP. Note that in isolated canine gut loops, autoregulation was weak or absent in control group, whereas active autoregulation occurred in the hypermetabolic state labeled Vivonex. Changing the amplitude of the arterial pressure pulse to sensitize myogenic reactivity did not systematically alter autoregulation expressed as G_F. (From Shepherd and Riedel, ref. 53.)

tion during constant pressure perfusion (see Chapter 32). Vasodilators such as isoproterenol and adenosine (54) cause a maldistribution of blood flow, apparently depress total and regional oxygen uptake, and defeat the local mechanism's ability to optimize tissue oxygenation and the distribution of capillary perfusion. Therefore, we will consider the oxygen uptake versus blood flow relationship obtained by altering perfusion pressure (pump-perfusion).

Figure 6 depicts the relationship between canine intestinal oxygen uptake and blood flow (29). As Fig. 6 shows, oxygen consumption remains essentially constant until blood flow falls to a critical level at approximately 35 ml/min/100 g. Three factors could contribute to the maintenance of oxygen uptake under these conditions. First, mitochondrial oxygen uptake and P_{O_2} obey a Michaelis-Menton relationship. Therefore, if the cell P_{O_2} is normally above the critical P_{O_2} below which oxygen uptake is P_{O_2}-dependent, a fall in cell P_{O_2} during the reduction in blood flow would not alter O_2 uptake until the critical P_{O_2} is reached. Second, the cell P_{O_2} could fall thus maintaining both the capillary-to-cell P_{O_2} difference and, therefore, the oxygen flux to the cells. Third, the recruitment of previously unperfused capillaries would maintain the O_2 flux by increasing capillary surface area and by shortening the diffusion distance. Of these possibilities, only the latter has readily lent itself to investigation.

Figure 7 shows the predicted relationship between capillary density and intestinal blood flow *(left panel)*. As the lower curve in Fig. 7 shows, if the oxygen demands of the tissue are constant

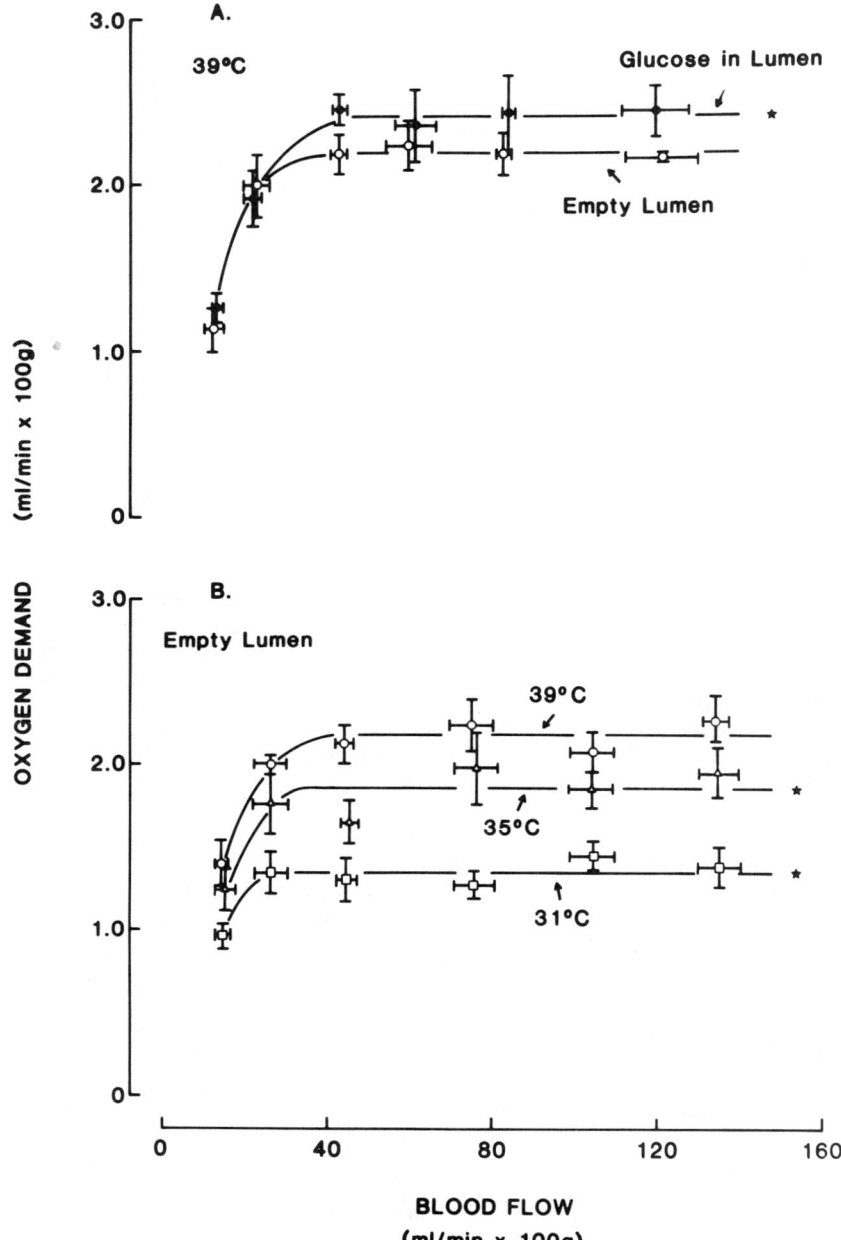

FIG. 6. Relationship between oxygen consumption and blood flow. Note that intestinal oxygen uptake is essentially independent of blood flow above a critical blood flow of approximately 35 ml/min/100 g. **A:** Glucose in lumen of canine ileum shifted the curve upward, increasing oxygen demands. **B:** Increased temperature raises the plateau in this relationship obtained in pump-perfused canine ileum. (From Kvietys et al., ref. 29, with permission.)

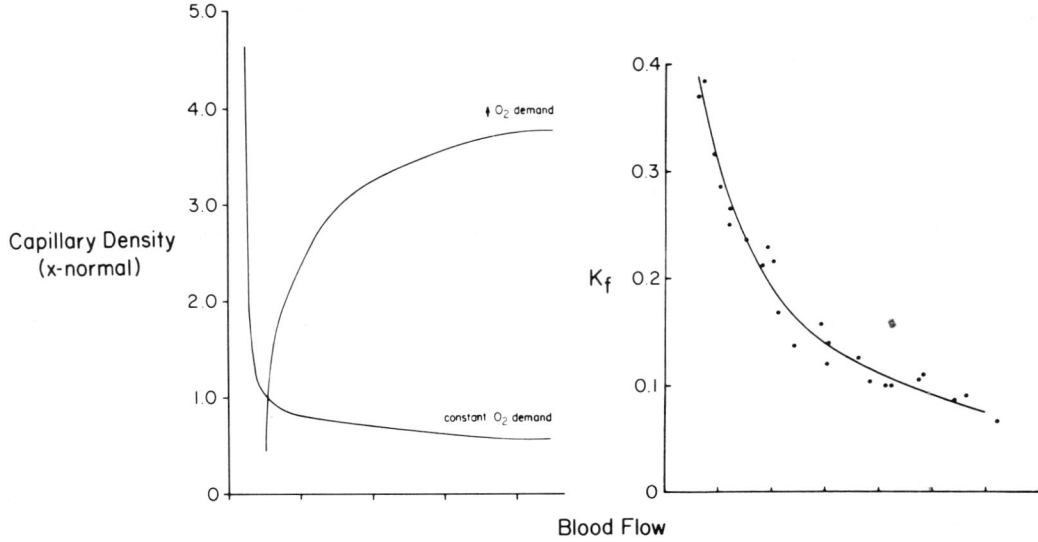

FIG. 7. Theoretical relationship between blood flow and capillary density **(left)** is compared with animal data **(right)**. Note that, if a metabolic feedback mechanism is assumed to regulate capillary density, the relationship between capillary density and blood flow depends on the means used to change blood flow. If oxygen demands of tissue increase, metabolic feedback causes both flow and capillary density to increase concomitantly. However, if tissue demands are constant, lowering blood flow then causes capillary recruitment. The latter relationship is confirmed by measured capillary filtration coefficients (K_f) **(right)**. (Simulation from model in Shepherd and Granger, ref. 48; animal data from Granger et al., ref. 9, with permission.)

and blood flow is reduced mechanically, capillary density and blood flow are inversely related with recruitment occurring as perfusion falls. Note that this prediction was confirmed experimentally *(right panel)* by measuring K_f, which increased during mechanically reduced blood flow (9). Further support for the view that capillary recruitment contributes to the constancy of oxygen uptake is the finding that PS and K_f are significantly correlated with the arteriovenous oxygen difference (as an index of oxygen extraction) under a variety of experimental conditions (9).

The chief value of these studies is that they have provided evidence that capillary recruitment contributes to the maintenance of a practically constant oxygen uptake and that they have identified the critical blood flow below which oxygen uptake becomes flow-limited. In fact, results from some early studies may have to be reinterpreted because control blood flow values were apparently already at the critical point. We feel that systematic studies of the oxygen uptake versus blood flow relationship under other experimental circumstances could possibly provide further insight into the adequacy of tissue oxygenation under physiological and pathophysiological conditions. For example, hemodilution (hematocrit = 20%) apparently reduces oxygen availability so drastically that intestinal oxygen consumption becomes flow-dependent throughout the physiological range (50). Such studies have also led to the tentative conclusion that there is an optimum hematocrit above and below which intestinal oxygenation is less than maximal (52).

CANDIDATE VASODILATOR METABOLITES

In general, the overall behavior of the resistance and exchange vessels in isolated gut loops agrees with the metabolic model's simulations of autoregulation, hypoxic vasodilation, functional hyperemia, and reactive hyperemia. Nevertheless, the signal that serves to couple the intestine's metabolic demands to its vascular regulators is still unknown. Numerous substances with known vasodilatory properties have been nominated as candidate vasodilators in the intestinal circulation. Substances that exhibit demonstrable vasodilator effects on the mesenteric circulation include potassium, hydrogen ion, carbon dioxide, adenosine, and the adenine nucleotides. Other possibilities include hyperosmolality, the prostaglandins (which are abundant in the intestine), and serotonin. Finally, the gastrointestinal hormones could act as local, or even as recirculating, vasodilators. For discussion of evidence implicating the gastrointestinal hormones and constituents of chyme in postprandial hyperemia, see Chapters 8 and 10.

Before any metabolite can be accepted as a mediator of local vascular control, its temporal and quantitative release into the intestinal interstitium must be correlated with the particular hyperemic response. Furthermore, when exogenous agents are injected intraarterially, their vasodilatory properties should be sufficiently potent to mimic their proposed *in vivo* role. However, it seems quite possible that several substances could function in concert as vasodilator metabolites.

It is instructive to examine several of the more thoroughly studied candidate vasodilator metabolites. *Hypercapnia*, for example, is a mild vasodilator in the intestine (56). Moreover, CO_2 levels change in a direction consistent with the metabolic model. However, P_{CO_2} must be changed beyond the physiological range to cause vasodilation sufficient to account for the commonly observed hyperemias. Furthermore, hypercapnia apparently has a paradoxical effect on capillary density, that is, K_f falls during hypercapnia (57). Whether or not this apparent capillary derecruitment has any effect on the ability of the small bowel to maintain its oxygenation has not been studied. Another curious property of hypercapnia is that it apparently does not diminish the myogenic reactivity of resistance vessels in response to venous pressure elevation. Thus, these data suggest that hypercapnia is unlikely to be an important contributor to the metabolic feedback signal.

By contrast, stronger evidence implicates *adenosine* as a metabolic vasodilator. Adenosine administered intraarterially is a potent vasodilator (32), but the adenosine-blocker, theophylline, does not alter the control blood flow, nor does it affect autoregulation in control gut loops (14). These data indicate that adenosine plays little role if any in determining basal vascular resistance in the intestine. Theophylline also does not block the hyperemia induced by placing predigested dog food in the intestinal lumen. Furthermore, dipyridamole (an inhibitor of adenosine re-uptake) does not vasodilate the empty intestine. Thus, these data and others indicate that adenosine does not participate in the response to moderate increases in oxygen demands or to moderate hypoxia. However, with more severe hypoxia adenosine may indeed be involved as a causative agent. Adenosine levels in venous blood increase fourfold following a 60-sec arterial occlusion (34). The reactive hyperemia thus produced lasts only half as long with theophylline. Furthermore, the enchanced autoregulation during high metabolic rates is attenuated by theophylline, and dipyridamole causes a 25% enhancement in the hyperemia induced by predigested dog food (14). Thus, adenosine may be involved in the vasodilation produced by more severe challenges to intestinal oxygen homeostasis but not during moderate adjustments. Additional findings somewhat inconsistent with adenosine's potential role as a feedback signal are that it depresses PS and K_f (11), acts selectively to vasodilate the muscularis, and, when administered intraarterially, reduces mucosal blood flow (54).

Hypoxia is a potent vasodilator both *in vivo* and *in vitro* and could possibly serve as the feedback signal. However, it is not clear that perivascular P_{O_2} values have as great an effect as blood P_{O_2} on the tone of the microvessels. Nevertheless, microelectrode measurements of P_{O_2} in the intestinal mucosa show that tissue P_{O_2} falls during the absorption of glucose (2). The time course of glucose absorption and the fall in P_{O_2} in intestinal villi are consistent with a causal relationship. In addition, the decrease in Po_2 from 15 to 7 mm Hg is in the range in which hypoxia relaxes vascular smooth muscle *in vitro*. These findings, therefore, are all consistent with tissue Po_2 serving as the metabolic feedback signal. Other findings are more problematic. The perivascular Po_2 rises rather than falls near the upstream submucosal arterioles in which a considerable portion of the glucose-induced vasodilation occurs. See Chapter 12 for further discussion of tissue Po_2.

REGIONAL DIFFERENCES IN LOCAL CONTROL

The tissues that comprise the bowel wall, the mucosa, the submucosa, and muscularis differ not only in their functions but also in the properties of their vascular beds. The mucosa with its greater oxygen demands and its absorptive specialization receives the greater portion of intramural blood flow, and it has the more numerous and the more permeable capillaries (see Chapter 2). Because of the difficulties that have plagued the methods for fractionating blood flow within the gut wall and because of uncertainties about the spatial resolution of these techniques, relatively little is known of how the three regional vascular beds differ in their abilities to control their perfusion; however, the few studies available have yielded interesting and sometimes contradictory results.

In *reactive hyperemia* microsphere measurements suggest that relatively uniform increases in blood flow occur throughout the feline gut wall only for an occlusion period of 60 sec, but lengthening the duration of occlusion results in a hyperemia predominantly in the muscularis (37). Presumably, the longer durations of arterial occlusion stimulate intestinal motility because it is well known that ischemia stimulates motility. Thus, the greater hyperemia in the muscularis with longer (>60 sec) occlusions could result from the increased oxygen demands required by muscular contractions. More recent studies (51,55), in which regional perfusion was measured by laser-Doppler velocimetry, contradict the microsphere data for short (<60 sec) occlusions. As Fig. 2 shows, the laser technique registers a pronounced reactive hyperemia in the mucosa following a 60-sec occlusion, but practically no reactive hyperemia is seen at the muscularis-serosal surface. The explanation for the contradictory results with these two techniques is not apparent. The microsphere method is difficult to apply during the nonsteady flow of reactive hyperemia, and it measures microsphere accumulation in the tissue physically dissected from the gut and in which radioactivity is counted. By contrast, the laser technique provides a continuous flow signal and is easier to use in such nonsteady conditions, but the precise volume of tissue from which the flow signal arises is unknown. The laser method probably measures "villus" flow, but hard data are not available to support this tentative conclusion.

Autoregulation is also apparently more pronounced in the mucosa. Measurements of "villus blood flow" with washout techniques (30) indicate marked reductions in arterial pressure hardly affect "villus blood flow." Thus, the autoregulatory ability of vessels in the villi may exceed the autoregulatory capacity of the gut wall as a whole. If this conclusion sustains further investigation, a redistribution of flow to the more metabolically active mucosa during solute absorption could explain, in part, the enhanced autoregulation seen during high metabolic rates.

In *functional hyperemia* inconsistent results with microsphere measurements of the intramural distribution of intestinal blood flow have been reported. Investigators using 7 to 10 μm spheres find that following feeding blood flow increases throughout the bowel wall, whereas others using 13 to 15 μm spheres reported that the hyperemia is restricted to the mucosal layer (5,10). Preliminary studies with laser-Doppler velocimetry confirmed the increased mucosal flow with glucose (Vivonex), and that blood flow in the muscularis is unchanged during solute-induced hyperemia. (Shepherd and Riedel, *unpublished observations*). The regional differences in vascular responses to hypercapnia and hypoxia have not been studied. Finally, during increased motility, a functional hyperemia analogous to the exercise hyperemia of skeletal muscle has been reported to occur in the muscularis (4). However, the relationship between intestinal blood flow and motility is complex and is discussed elsewhere (4,39; Chapter 9).

FUTURE DIRECTIONS

Although our crystal ball is probably no better than the reader's, we would like to speculate about directions that studies of local control might profitably take in the future. A relatively unexplored area is the interaction between myogenic and metabolic mechanisms. Neither the metabolic nor the myogenic theory adequately explains all the findings indicative of local control, yet neither theory can be ruled out. On the contrary, strong evidence supports both the myogenic reactivity of intestinal microvessels and a link between the intestine's metabolic demands and its vasculature. This stalemate between the two theories has led to the proposal of the dual or unified theory (7,23), according to which both types of mechanisms participate in local control, and the relative contributions of the two mechanisms depend on experimental conditions.

Even though only a few studies have examined the interaction between myogenic and metabolic mechanisms, they have already led to contradictory data. For example, arterial hypoxia may either attenuate (57) or have no effect (42) on the myogenic vasoconstriction evoked by raising venous pressure. Similarly, the effect of increased metabolic rate on myogenic responses is unclear. In one study (13), increasing metabolic rate attenuated the vasoconstriction evoked by venous pressure; however, in another report (44), myogenic responses were absent in controls but appeared when the metabolic rate increased. Pulsatile arterial pressure apparently sensitizes the myogenic mechanism because vasoconstrictor responses to elevated venous pressure are observed more frequently, and they have a greater magnitude if arterial pressure is pulsatile rather than steady (42). One study (53) attempted to determine the relative contributions of myogenic and metabolic mechanisms to autoregulation in response to reduced arterial pressure. As Fig. 5 shows, the amplitude of the arterial pressure pulse has no systematic effect on the ability of the gut to regulate flow in response to step-changes in mean arterial pressure. By contrast, increasing the metabolic rate significantly increased the ability of isolated gut loops to regulate flow in response to the same step-reduction in mean arterial pressure. These data therefore support the conclusion that under the conditions of the experiment, metabolic feedback makes greater contributions than the myogenic mechanism to autoregulation. In view of the paucity and inconsistency of the data, future studies should more systematically examine the interaction between myogenic and metabolic mechanisms.

Several other relatively unexplored aspects of the intestine could possibly lead to progress in our understanding of our local control. First, *in vitro* studies precisely define the metabolic characteristics and the oxygen demands of each of the tissues within the gut wall. As mentioned earlier, these tissues may differ in the efficacy of their local control mechanisms. Therefore, better methods to fractionate the intramural distribution of blood flow and perhaps techniques that would apply the Fick principle to determine the oxygen consumption rates of the separate circulations *in vivo*, if technologically feasible, could lead to significant advances. At this writing, all the evidence for capillary recruitment in the intestine is indirect, that is, from PS and K_f measurements in isolated preparations. However, in skeletal muscle, direct quantitative observations of capillary recruitment have been made with intravital microscopy. Such observations in the intestine would greatly strengthen the oxygen delivery version of the metabolic theory because of the quantitatively significant contribution that capillary recruitment makes to the control of tissue oxygenation. A second important factor in the oxygen delivery version is that intracellular P_{O_2} can fall, thus widening the capillary-to-cell P_{O_2} gradient. If techniques less cumbersome than the microelectrode could be developed to determine an intracellular P_{O_2}

representative of the intestinal tissues, the role of the capillary-to-cell PO_2 gradient could be explored. Finally, as mentioned earlier, the directional changes in tissue PO_2 measured with microelectrodes are consistent with the metabolic hypothesis in the villi but not in the submucosal vessels that participate in functional hyperemia. The possibility of "ascending vasodilation" has not been examined in the intestinal circulation.

In summary, we predict that progress will depend on both investigative innovation and technological advances. If the basic metabolism of mucosal and muscularis cells and their mechanisms for producing ATP can be delineated and if better methods can be devised for measuring blood flow and metabolic rate within each of the tissues that comprise the gut wall, our understanding of the metabolic mechanisms regulating the intestinal circulation will continue to increase.

REFERENCES

1. Baez, S., Laidlaw, Z., and Orkin, L. R. (1974): Localization and measurement of microvascular and microcirculatory responses to venous pressure elevation in the rat. *Blood Vessels*, 11:260–276.
2. Bohlen, H. G. (1980): Intestinal tissue PO_2 and microvascular responses during glucose exposure. *Am. J. Physiol.*, 238:H164–171.
3. Borgstrom, B., and Laurell, C. B. (1953): Studies on lymph and lymph-protein during absorption of fat and saline by rats. *Acta Physiol. Scand.*, 29:264–280.
4. Chou, C. C., and Grassmick, B. (1978): Motility and blood flow distribution within the wall of the gastrointestinal tract. *Am. J. Physiol.*, 235:H34–H39.
5. Chou, C. C., Hsieh, C. P., Yu, Y. M., Kvietys, P., and Yu, L. C. (1976): Localization of mesenteric hyperemia during digestion in dogs. *Am. J. Physiol.*, 230:583–589.
6. Folkow, B. (1949): Intravascular pressure as a factor regulating the tone of the small vessels. *Acta Physiol. Scand.*, 17:289–310.
7. Folkow, B. (1964): Description of the myogenic hypothesis. *Circ. Res. (Suppl.)*, 14:279–285.
8. Gaskell, W. H. (1877): On the changes of blood stream in muscle through stimulation of their nerves. *J. Anat.*, 11:360.
9. Granger, D. N., Kvietys, P. R., and Perry, M. A. (1982): Role of exchange vessels in the regulation of intestinal oxygenation. *Am. J. Physiol.*, 242:G570–G574.
10. Granger, D. N., Richardson, P. D. I., Kvietys, P. R., and Mortillaro, N. A. (1980): Intestinal blood flow. *Gastroenterology*, 78:837–863.
11. Granger, D. N., Valleau, J. D., Parker, R. E., Lane, R. S., and Taylor, A. E. (1978): Effects of adenosine on intestinal hemodynamics, oxygen delivery, and capillary fluid exchange. *Am. J. Physiol.*, 235:H707–719.
12. Granger, H. J., Goodman, A. H., and Granger, D. N. (1976): Role of resistance and exchange vessels in local microvascular control of skeletal muscle oxygenation in the dog. *Circ. Res.*, 38:379–385.
13. Granger, H. J., and Norris, C. P. (1980): Intrinsic regulation of intestinal oxygenation in the anesthetized dog. *Am. J. Physiol.*, 238:H836–843.
14. Granger, H. J., and Norris, C. P. (1980): Role of adenosine in local control of intestinal circulation in the dog. *Circ. Res.*, 46:764–770.
15. Granger, H. J., and Shepherd, A. P., Jr. (1973): Intrinsic microvascular control of tissue oxygen delivery. *Microvasc. Res.*, 5:49–72.
16. Granger, H. J., and Shepherd, A. P. (1979): Dynamics and control of the microcirculation. In *Advances in Biomedical Engineering*, Vol. 7, edited by J. H. U. Brown, pp. 1–63. Academic Press, Inc., New York.
17. Hinshaw, L. B. (1962): Arterial and venous pressure-resistance relationships in perfused leg and intestine. *Am. J. Physiol.*, 203:271–274.
18. Inberg, M. V., Havia, T., Arola, M. K., and Niinikoski, J. (1974): Effect of oxygen breathing on jejunal tissue gas tensions during superior mesenteric arterial occlusion. *Scand. J. Gastroenterol.*, 9:337–342.
19. Johnson, P. C. (1960): Autoregulation of intestinal blood flow. *Am. J. Physiol.*, 199:311–318.
20. Johnson, P. C. (1964): Origin, localization, and homeostatic significance of autoregulation in the intestine. *Circ. Res. (Suppl.)*, 14(I):225–232.
21. Johnson, P. C. (1964): Review of previous studies and current theories of autoregulation. *Circ. Res. (Suppl.)*, 15(I):2–9.
22. Johnson, P. C. (1965): Effect of venous pressure on mean capillary pressure and vascular resistance in the intestine. *Circ. Res.*, 16:294–300.
23. Johnson, P. C. (1967): Autoregulation of blood flow in the intestine. *Gastroenterology*, 52:435–441.
24. Johnson, P. C., and Hanson, K. M. (1966): Capillary filtration in the small intestine of the dog. *Circ. Res.*, 19:766–773.
25. Jones, R. D., and Berne, R. M. (1964): Intrinsic regulation of skeletal muscle blood flow. *Circ. Res.*, 14:126–128.
26. Klabunde, R. E., and Johnson, P. C. (1977): Capillary velocity and tissue PO_2 changes during reactive hyperemia. *Am. J. Physiol.*, 233:H379–383.
27. Krogh, A. (1918): The number and distribution of capillaries in muscles with calculations of the oxygen pressure head necessary for supplying the tissue. *J. Physiol.*, 52:409–515.
28. Kvietys, P. R., and Granger, D. N. (1982): Relation between intestinal blood flow and oxygen uptake. *Am. J. Physiol.*, 242:G202–G208.
29. Kvietys, P. R., Perry, M. A., and Granger, D. N. (1983): Intestinal capillary exchange capacity and oxygen delivery-to-demand ratio. *Am. J. Physiol.* 245:G635–G640.
30. Lundgren, O., and Svanvik, J. (1973): Mucosal hemodynamics in the small intestine of the cat during

reduced perfusion pressure. *Acta Physiol. Scand.*, 88:551–563.
31. Lutz, J., Henrich, H., and Bauereisen, E. (1975): Oxygen supply and uptake in the liver and the intestine. *Pflügers Arch.*, 360:7–15.
32. Mailman, D., Pawlik, W., Shepherd, A. P., Tague, L. L., and Jacobson, E. D. (1977): Cyclic nucleotide metabolism and vasodilation in canine mesenteric artery. *Am. J. Physiol.*, 232:H191–196.
33. Mortillaro, N. A., and Granger, H. J. (1977): Reactive hyperemia and oxygen extraction in the feline small intestine. *Circ. Res.*, 41:859–865.
34. Mortillaro, N. A., and Mustafa, S. J. (1978): Possible role of adenosine in the development of intestinal post-occlusion reactive hyperemia. *Fed. Proc. (Abstr.)*, 37:874.
35. Mortillaro, N. A., and Taylor, A. E. (1976): Interaction of capillary and tissue forces in the cat small intestine. *Circ. Res.*, 39:348–358.
36. Norris, C. P., Barnes, G. E., Smith, E. E., and Granger, H. J. (1979): Autoregulation of superior mesenteric flow in fasted and fed dogs. *Am. J. Physiol.*, 237:H174–177.
37. Parker, R. E., and Granger, D. N. (1979): Effect of graded arterial occlusion on ileal blood flow distribution. *Proc. Soc. Exp. Biol. Med.*, 146–149.
38. Richardson, P. D. I., and Granger, D. N. (1981): Capillary filtration coefficient as a measure of perfused capillary density. In: *Measurement of Blood Flow: Applications to the Splanchnic Circulation*, edited by D. N. Granger and G. B. Bulkley, pp. 319–336. Williams & Wilkins, Baltimore.
39. Scott, J. B., and Dabney, J. M. (1964): Relation of gut motility to blood flow in the ileum of the dog. *Circ. Res. (Suppl.)*, 14(I):234–239.
40. Shepherd, A. P. (1977): Myogenic responses of intestinal resistance and exchange vessels. *Am. J. Physiol.*, 233:H547–554.
41. Shepherd, A. P. (1978): Intestinal oxygen consumption and ^{86}Rb extraction during arterial hypoxia. *Am. J. Physiol.*, 234:E248–251.
42. Shepherd, A. P. (1978): Effect of arterial pulse pressure and hypoxia on myogenic responses in the gut. *Am. J. Physiol.*, 235:H157–H161.
43. Shepherd, A. P. (1979): Intestinal capillary blood flow during metabolic hyperemia. *Am. J. Physiol.*, 237:E548–E554.
44. Shepherd, A. P. (1980): Intestinal blood flow autoregulation during foodstuff absorption. *Am. J. Physiol.*, 239:H156–H162.
45. Shepherd, A. P. (1981): Intestinal capillary exchange capacity and oxygen uptake rate: Applications of indicator dilution principles. In: *Measurement of Blood Flow: Applications to the Splanchnic Circulation*, edited by D. N. Granger and G. B. Bulkley, pp. 289–317. Williams & Wilkins, Baltimore.
46. Shepherd, A. P. (1982): Role of capillary recruitment in the regulation of intestinal oxygenation. *Am. J. Physiol.*, 242:G435–G441.
47. Shepherd, A. P. (1982): Local control of intestinal oxygenation and blood flow. *Annu. Rev. Physiol.*, 44:13–27.
48. Shepherd, A. P., and Granger, H. J. (1973): Autoregulatory escape in the gut: A systems analysis. *Gastroenterology*, 65:77–91.
49. Shepherd, A. P., Perry, M. A., Kvietys, P. R., and Granger, D. N. (1984): Effect of hypoxia and histamine on feline intestinal capillary permeability. *Fed. Proc. (Abstr.)*, 43:311.
50. Shepherd, A. P., and Riedel, G. L. (1981): The intestinal O_2 uptake vs. blood flow relationship and the optimal hematocrit for O_2 transport. *Fed. Proc. (Abstr.)*, 40:491.
51. Shepherd, A. P., and Riedel, G. L. (1982): Continuous measurement of intestinal mucosal blood flow by laser-Doppler velocimetry. *Am. J. Physiol.*, 242:G668–G672.
52. Shepherd, A. P., and Riedel, G. L. (1982): Optimal hematocrit for oxygenation of canine intestine. *Circ. Res.*, 51:233–240.
53. Shepherd, A. P., and Riedel, G. L. (1982): Effects of pulsatile pressure and metabolic rate on intestinal autoregulation. *Am. J. Physiol.*, 242:H769–775.
54. Shepherd, A. P., and Riedel, G. L. (1983): Laser Doppler velocimetric (LDV) studies of intestinal blood flow during selective vasodilation. *Microvasc. Res. (Abstr.)*, 23:256.
55. Shepherd, A. P., and Riedel, G. L. (1983): Regional differences in intestinal reactive hyperemia studied by laser Doppler velocimetry. *Physiologist (Abstr.)*, 26:A18.
56. Sidky, M. M., and Bean, J. W. (1951): Local and general alterations of blood CO_2 and influence of intestinal motility on intestinal blood flow. *Am. J. Physiol.*, 167:413.
57. Svanvik, J., Tyllstrom, J., and Wallentin, I. (1968): The effects of hypercapnia and hypoxia on the distribution of capillary blood flow in the denervated intestinal vascular bed. *Acta Physiol. Scand.*, 74:543–551.
58. Texter, E. C., Jr., Merrill, S., Schwartz, M., Van Derstrappen, G., and Haddy, F. S. (1962): Relationship of blood flow to pressure in the intestinal bed of the dog. *Am. J. Physiol.*, 202:253–256.
59. Valleau, J. D., Granger, D. N., and Taylor, A. E. (1979): Effect of solute-coupled volume absorption on oxygen consumption in the cat ileum. *Am. J. Physiol.*, 236:E198–E203.
60. Van Heerden, P. D., Wagner, H. N., Jr., and Kaihara, S. (1968): Intestinal blood flow during perfusion of the jejunum with hypertonic glucose in dogs. *Am. J. Physiol.*, 215:30–33.
61. Wollin, A., and Jaques, L. B. (1973): Plasma protein escape from the intestinal circulation to the lymphatics during fat absorption. *Proc. Soc. Exp. Biol. Med.*, 142:1114–1117.
62. Yu, Y. M., Yu, L. C., and Chou, C. C. (1975): Distribution of blood flow in the intestine with hypertonic glucose in the lumen. *Surgery*, 78:520–525.

Myogenic and Venous-Arteriolar Responses in Intestinal Circulation

Paul C. Johnson

Department of Physiology, University of Arizona College of Medicine, Tucson, Arizona 85724

The myogenic response, a property possessed by certain blood vessels, causes them to constrict following an elevation of transmural pressure. The response may be transient; a brief constriction may follow a sudden elevation of transmural pressure. The response may also be sustained; a prolonged elevation of pressure may produce an equally prolonged constriction of the vessel. There is substantial evidence for both types of response in the intestinal circulation.

TRANSIENT MYOGENIC RESPONSE

This response may be seen with a single step change in arterial pressure, as following release of arterial occlusion or with the periodic pressure changes of the normal arterial pressure pulse. In respect to the former, the myogenic response may be the cause of the secondary rise in vascular resistance and fall in blood flow in an isolated intestinal loop following a steep rise in arterial pressure as shown in Fig. 1 (14). In this case, a damped oscillation of the resistance vessels is evident following the pressure change. The secondary constriction of the resistance vessels is presumably due to the pressure rise, although it might also be ascribed to the sudden rise in flow, which would wash out vasoactive metabolites or increase tissue oxygen tension. The rapidity of the response argues against such a flow-dependent mechanism, but a contribution from this source cannot be entirely ruled out.

Studies at the microcirculatory level by Pollock (21) provide further insight into the un-

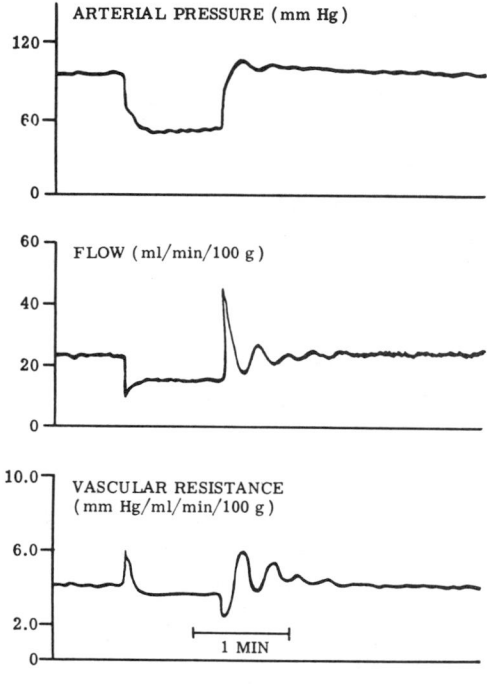

FIG. 1. Blood flow and vascular resistance in an isolated loop of dog intestine during step changes in arterial pressure. Vascular resistance was computed continuously from the instantaneous arterial-venous pressure difference divided by the instantaneous blood flow. (From Johnson, ref. 13, with permission.)

derlying mechanism. Shown in Fig. 2 is the red cell velocity recording from a mesenteric capillary during a sudden change of arterial pressure. In this study, arterial pressure to an isolated, perfused cat mesentery preparation (17) was initially reduced, and blood flow autoregulation caused capillary flow, as measured by red cell

49

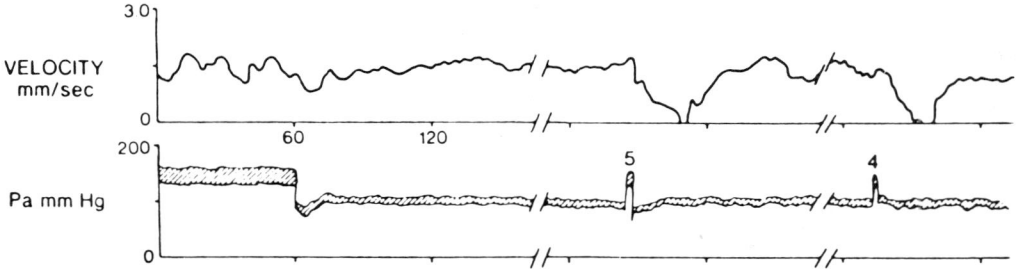

FIG. 2. Red cell velocity in cat mesenteric capillary recorded by the dual slit method during step changes in arterial pressure. Initially mean arterial pressure was reduced from 145 to 100 mm Hg. Subsequently arterial pressure was elevated by 40 to 50 mm Hg for 5 sec or 4 sec as indicated in the figure. Time intervals on horizontal axis *(vertical marks)* are 1 min. (From Pollack, ref. 21, with permission.)

velocity, to return to the initial level. Note that there is almost no rise in capillary flow during a brief (4 or 5 sec) 40 to 50 mm Hg arterial pressure elevation, but there is a very pronounced fall in flow a few seconds later. The fall in flow is presumably due to constriction at some level of the precapillary circulation. The lack of an initial hyperemia seems to mitigate against a washout of vasodilator metabolites or an overshoot of tissue oxygen tension as being responsible for the vascular response and prolonged flow stoppage. In this study, we also noted that when arterial pressure is increased slowly, red cell velocity in the capillaries remains constant because of an autoregulatory response, but there is no sudden flow stoppage.

In certain vascular beds, rhythmic arterial pulsation also causes arteriolar constriction. Mellander and Arvidsson (20) and Rovick and Robertson (22) have shown in skeletal muscle that arterial pulsation causes a substantial increase in vascular resistance compared with nonpulsatile perfusion at the same mean pressure. The matter has not been studied extensively in the intestine, but available evidence indicates pulsatile perfusion pressure does not increase vascular resistance. In the course of a study on the influence of pulse pressure on the vascular response to venous pressure elevation in the gut, Shepherd (25) found no difference in vascular resistance under control conditions whether steady or pulsatile perfusion was employed (Table 3 in ref. 25). The reason for this difference between gut and skeletal muscle circulation is not readily apparent.

SUSTAINED MYOGENIC RESPONSE

Several lines of evidence suggest that intestinal resistance vessels respond to a sustained rise in transmural pressure with a maintained constriction. Like many other vascular beds, the intestinal circulation exhibits autoregulation of blood flow. When arterial pressure to the isolated, perfused intestinal loop of the dog was reduced from 120 to 80 mm Hg, vascular resistance fell by 10% to 20% (12). Blood flow fell modestly, and, as a consequence of the maintained O_2 consumption, venous O_2 was decreased. To determine if the fall in the venous oxygen level was implicated in autoregulation, the animal was ventilated with an oxygen-rich gas mixture that elevated arterial O_2 content. The venous O_2 content returned to control levels, but vascular resistance did not. This study indicates that reduction of tissue O_2 content is probably not the cause of the vasodilation with arterial pressure reduction. Other studies showed that the vasodilation was not associated with a change in tonus of the intestinal wall or motility as determined from a balloon placed in the intestinal lumen (12). In addition, intraarterial infusion of procaine in quantities sufficient to abolish the vasoconstrictor effect of sympathetic nerve stimulation did not affect autoregulation of blood flow. These studies provide evidence, largely by elimination of other mechanisms, that the resistance vessels of the intestine are sensitive to intravascular pressure.

A variety of other studies provide additional evidence in support of a myogenic response of intestinal resistance vessels to intravascular pressure elevation. As noted above, the principal focus of experimentation on the mechanism of autoregulation of blood flow in the intestine has been to distinguish between metabolic or flow-dependent and myogenic or pressure-dependent mechanisms. When arterial pressure is altered, flow and intravascular pressure change in the same direction and thus tend to produce similar effects on vascular resistance. However, these two mechanisms can be dissociated by elevating venous pressure, which reduces blood flow by decreasing the arteriovenous pressure difference. If vascular tone is flow-dependent, this procedure should cause dilation of the arterioles. At the same time, venous pressure elevation should increase intravascular pressure in the resistance vessels, especially those nearest the capillary network. If a myogenic response is dominant, vascular resistance should rise. Conversely, if a metabolic mechanism is dominant, vascular resistance should fall. Experimental studies have shown a preponderant constriction of the intestinal resistance vessels in this circumstance, suggesting that the myogenic response is dominant (11,23).

A key question in these studies is whether the venous pressure elevation is indeed causing a myogenic constriction of the arterial vessels or whether some other mechanism is involved. A prominent alternative possibility is an arteriovenous reflex. Andrews et al. (1) showed increased frequency of afferent action potentials in nerves from the small intestine when portal venous pressure was elevated. They also showed increased efferent discharge to the intestine, which was abolished by section of the intestinal nerves. It was not determined if this spinal reflex was concerned with blood flow regulation, but it must be considered a possibility.

The role of the above-mentioned spinal reflex in the response to venous pressure elevation would obviously depend on the conditions of the study. Typically, hemodynamic studies in the intestine involve surgical isolation of an intestinal loop, in the course of which the nerves are severed. Also, intraarterial infusion of procaine or phenoxybenzamine in sufficient quantities to abolish the constrictor response to sympathetic nerve stimulation does not diminish the vascular response to venous pressure elevation in isolated preparations (11). The latter studies appear to eliminate a spinal cord mediated venous-arteriolar reflex as well as a local reflex mediated by the intramural sympathetic nerves. Under conditions in which the nerve supply is intact, a spinal reflex must still be considered a possible explanation for the observed vasoconstriction.

The relative importance of metabolic and myogenic factors appears to depend on initial conditions. Lutz and Henrich (19) found that the constrictor response to venous pressure elevation in the isolated intestine was highly dependent on initial arterial pressure and rate of flow. Below an arterial pressure of 50 mm Hg and above a pressure of 170 mm Hg, there was no constriction with venous pressure elevation. The lack of response at the low arterial pressure may be due to reduced flow and tissue O_2 levels, whereas at the higher pressure it may represent the inability of the arteriolar smooth muscle to maintain active tension against a strong stretching force.

Shepherd (24) has shown that the resistance increase in isolated segments of dog small intestine during venous pressure elevation is dependent on volume flow rate. When an isolated intestinal segment was perfused at a constant flow of 35 ml/min × 100 g tissue, intestinal vascular resistance rose 28% when venous pressure was elevated from 0 to 20 mm Hg. However, when the initial flow rate was 23 ml/min × 100 g tissue, vascular resistance fell 14% with the same 20 mm Hg rise in venous pressure. Tissue oxygen consumption was about 30% lower at the low perfusion rate. The lower O_2 uptake suggests that the altered tissue metabolism, presumably extant in these circumstances, caused release of vasodilator metabolites, which overpowered local myogenic mechanisms. However, initial vascular resistance was not reduced in the group with lower initial flow.

The influence of arterial blood oxygen levels on the venous-arteriolar response in the intestine was also studied by Shepherd (25). Reduction of arterial Po_2 from 106 to 46 mm Hg did not alter the constrictor response to venous pressure elevation even though the arterial hypoxia reduced initial vascular resistance by about 33%. This result is surprising, considering the abolition of response at low arterial pressures and flows cited above. In a separate study, Shepherd (26) found that O_2 consumption was reduced 26% under these conditions of hypoxia. This is about the same reduction as seen in the low flow state. Under hypoxic conditions, the initial blood flow was higher than that found in the normoxic state. One possible explanation for the lack of an effect of arterial hypoxia on the venous-arteriolar response is that this procedure caused sufficient arteriolar dilation to better distribute blood flow to the capillaries and maintain a more uniform tissue Po_2 in the various layers of the intestine than was the case in the reduced flow state. In the reduced flow state, however, O_2 consumption rose with venous pressure elevation from 70% to about 90% of that seen at normal flows. The complete abolition of the response to venous pressure elevation at reduced flow seems hardly ascribable to such a small deprivation of O_2 supply.

Alternatively, the washout of vasodilator metabolites may be a more critical factor than tissue Po_2 as such, and the higher flow in the hypoxic state may provide better washout. Since O_2 consumption was reduced to virtually the same extent by low flow and arterial hypoxia, the difference in flow is the only obvious explanation for the difference in behavior. Arterial pressure in the two preparations was about the same (63.2 ± 4.3 mm Hg in the hypoxic state as compared to 67.5 ± 9.4 mm Hg in normoxia at reduced flow). In addition, we note that in Shepherd's experiments with arterial hypoxia (25), the response to venous pressure elevation was not reduced even when blood flow was not allowed to rise as the arterial O_2 content was lowered. Under these conditions arterial pressure fell from 87 to 63 mm Hg owing to hypoxic vasodilation. Resistance still increased 26% under hypoxic conditions when venous pressure was elevated and flow held constant as compared to a 23% increase under normoxic circumstances. From these observations, it appears that arterial pressure per se is not a critical factor in the venous-arteriolar response. It seems possible that attenuation and abolition of the venous-arteriolar response as arterial pressure is reduced (19) is due to the reduction of flow rather than the decrease in pressure. In this regard, it may be noted that pulsatile arterial pressure increases the frequency of occurrence and the magnitude of the constrictor response to venous pressure elevation (25,27). Since pulsatile arterial pressure per se does not increase vascular resistance, the effect of the pulsatile pressure may be to provide a more uniform flow distribution in the capillary networks.

These studies indicate that the arteriolar response to venous pressure elevation is highly sensitive to blood flow but rather insensitive to tissue Po_2 levels. Presumably, with further reduction of arterial Po_2 a point would be reached at which oxygen levels are too low to sustain an active response of the arterioles.

The level at which flow begins to influence the response to venous pressure elevation may vary with the preparations used. Our intestinal preparations (11,23) showed resistance changes similar to Shepherd's with venous pressure elevation, although the initial blood flow at normal arterial pressure was only about 20 ml/min × 100 g tissue, which is actually less than the flow rate that Shepherd found abolished the response to venous pressure elevation. The initial vascular tone in our preparations was approximately 75% greater, since the flow in Shepherd's preparation at a normal perfusion pressure was about 35 ml/min × 100 g tissue. The experimental conditions of the two studies were also substantially different. In our studies, the venous outflow was cannulated, but the artery was left intact. In Shepherd's study, the isolated loop was either perfused with blood by a peristaltic pump or the animal was rendered areflexic, and arterial flow was monitored with an electromagnetic flow meter. Possibly under the conditions of pump perfusion, the flow distribution to the various tissue layers was different than under the conditions of our study. As Gore (9) has pointed out, the intestinal circulation is in fact three circulations, supplying submucosa, mucosa, and muscularis layers, respectively, with presumably somewhat different control mechanisms in each type of tissue. The initial capillary pressure is different in each layer (9), and the profile of the pressure change would vary in each vascular bed with venous pressure elevation. It should also be noted that under conditions of pump perfusion autoregulation of blood flow in the intestine appears to be less pronounced than when the arterial vessels to the intestine are intact or when they are replaced with a minimum of external circuitry, that is, polyethylene tubing (12).

Microcirculatory studies (principally on mesentery) also provide evidence that the arterioles constrict in a sustained fashion to a maintained rise in intravascular pressure and that the response may be modulated somewhat by flow. When arterial pressure to the isolated cat mesentery preparation is reduced, the arterioles dilate, even when the flow in these vessels remains at control levels or increases because of the arteriolar dilation (17).

Overall, there does not appear to be a close relation between flow and arterial pressure in the individual arterioles, although mean flow may fall modestly when arterial pressure is reduced from 100 to 60 mm Hg. When flow in an arteriole is stopped by occlusion downstream with a micropipette, the arteriole dilates, indicating a sensitivity of the vessel to flow (17). However, subsequent reduction of arterial pressure to the preparation causes further dilation. Comparison of the dilation seen with arterial pressure reduction from 100 to 60 mm Hg with that seen when flow is reduced by the same amount by partial occlusion downstream (which should not alter pressure, while reducing flow) reveals that about one-fourth of the arteriolar dilation in the mesentery could be ascribed to flow reduction. The remainder was presumably due to reduction of the intravascular pressure stimulus for the myogenic response. Further analysis of the flow sensitivity of the mesenteric arteriole obtained from partial microocclusion indicates that flow changes alone would produce a modest degree of autoregulation (17). However, the effect would logically be somewhat more pronounced if flow were reduced in the surrounding vessels as well.

Several microcirculatory studies have been done under no-flow conditions to assess more directly the response of arterioles to pressure per se. One of these involved flow stoppage by microocclusion of an arteriole in the isolated cat mesentery, followed by reduction of arterial pressure to the preparation (Fig. 3). Under these conditions, the arteriole dilated almost to the same extent as when arterial pressure was reduced during free flow. It is noteworthy that although the microocclusion itself caused substantial dilation of the arteriole, it did not reduce the magnitude of arteriolar dilation with subsequent pressure reduction. These data may be taken as evidence that a portion of the initial vascular tone is sensitive only to arteriolar blood flow and a fraction is sensitive only to arteriolar transmural pressure. One assumption that must be noted in the foregoing interpretation is that the response of the occluded arteriole is determined wholly by pressure and flow within the arteriole under study. However, if flow in the surrounding vessels influences the tissue metabolic activity adjacent to the vessel under study, or if constrictor or dilator responses in adjacent vessels are transmitted to the vessel under study, the findings are subject to other interpretations. We will return to this point later.

A related type of study has been to stop flow completely in the vascular bed and raise static intravascular pressure. This study was first performed in the rat mesoappendix by Baez (2), who found that the arteriole became smaller as static intravascular pressure was elevated. Similar results were obtained in cat mesentery (17). These studies provide perhaps the most definitive evidence that the arterioles respond to a pressure stimulus per se, although the stimulus cannot be localized specifically to the vessel under study.

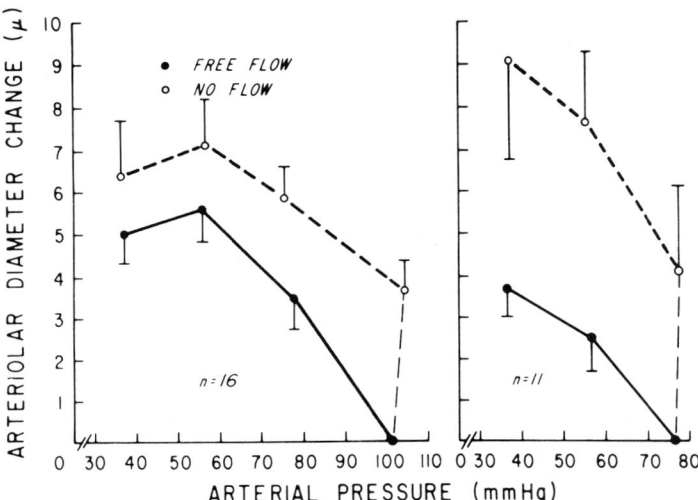

FIG. 3. Diameter changes in mesenteric arterioles during stepwise changes in arterial pressure under conditions of free flow and no flow. (From Johnson and Intaglietta, ref. 17, with permission.)

Microcirculatory studies also provide evidence for arteriolar constriction with venous pressure elevation. In studies of capillary flow (as determined by red cell velocity) in the mesentery, a periodic flow pattern was found at normal arterial and venous pressure (3). When arterial pressure was lowered, red cell velocity fell and then returned to control levels. The flow periodicity (presumably due to arteriolar or precapillary sphincter vasomotion) ceased when arterial pressure was reduced and then resumed when venous pressure was elevated. Accompanying the resumption of vasomotion was a sustained fall in red cell velocity. These data suggest that vasomotion is highly dependent on intravascular pressure but not flow. Further evidence was obtained by Baez et al. (3), who found a graded constrictor response to venous pressure elevation in the arteriolar network, with the small, distal arterioles showing the greatest constriction and the larger vessels upstream displaying lesser constriction. This finding is consistent with the myogenic mechanism, for one would expect a stronger response in the distal arterioles where the pressure rise would be greater.

As noted above, it seems reasonable to expect that the magnitude of arteriolar myogenic response would depend on the magnitude of the pressure change in the arteriole under study. In a recent series of experiments on the isolated perfused cat mesentery (5), we simultaneously measured pressure, diameter, and red cell velocity in the arcade arterioles while raising either arterial or venous pressure. One of the striking features of our findings was the considerable variation among individual vessels in the magnitude of the rise in arteriolar pressure with a fixed step increase in arterial or venous pressure, as shown in Fig. 4. In several instances, arteriolar pressure was essentially unchanged. Despite this variability in the local stimulus for the myogenic response, the magnitude of constriction was about the same in all vessels as is also apparent in Fig. 4. This dissociation of local pressure change and response argues against a local pressure stimulus as the sole determinant of the constriction evoked by elevation of arterial or venous pressure.

This type of study also enables us to compare the effectiveness of arterial and venous pressure elevation in inducing vasoconstriction In earlier pressure-flow studies on the intestinal loop (13), it was noted that the resistance increase with venous pressure elevation was about nine times greater than with the same increment of arterial pressure. This finding is unexpected, because the blood flow fall with venous pressure eleva-

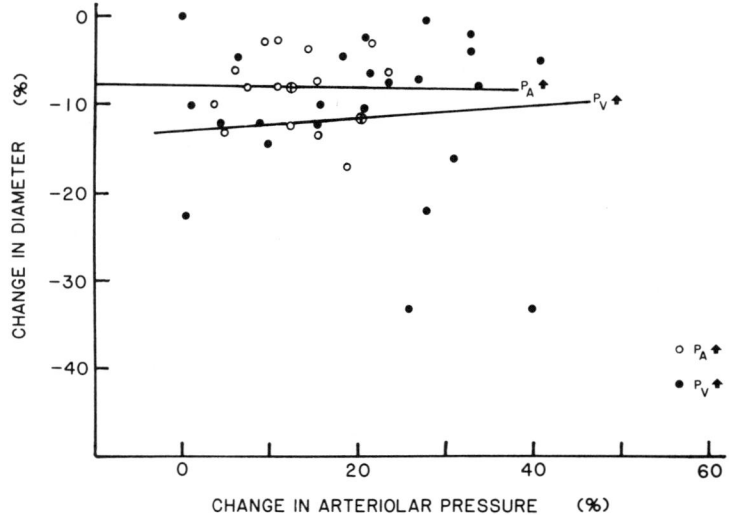

FIG. 4. Diameter and pressure changes in mesenteric arterioles during a single step change in arterial or venous pressure. (Data replotted from Burrows and Johnson, ref. 5.)

tion should attenuate the constrictor response. It was postulated that venous pressure elevation increased pressure in the distal arterioles disproportionately and induced a strong myogenic response in those vessels. In the microcirculatory studies cited above (5) and shown in Fig. 4, it was possible to compare the response to venous and arteriolar pressure elevation for the same increase in arteriolar pressure. The arteriolar constriction during the two procedures was not significantly different when expressed in terms of the rise in arteriolar pressure (1.8 μm/ 10 mm Hg for venous pressure elevation as compared with 1.2 μm/10 mm Hg for arterial pressure elevation). This comparison suggests that the greater pressure rise in the distal arterioles may be a principal reason for the greater resistance increase to a given increment of venous pressure. However, as noted above, because flow falls with venous pressure elevation and increases slightly with arterial pressure elevation, one would expect less constriction when venous pressure is elevated with the same increase in arteriolar pressure. The lack of a significant difference may indicate either that (a) the mesenteric arteriole is not sensitive to local blood flow or (b) venous pressure elevation involves additional mechanisms that elicit arteriolar constriction in addition to a local myogenic response. One additional mechanism may be a local venous-arteriolar reflex, although, for reasons cited previously, this seems unlikely in the isolated intestinal loop. A second possibility is that the arterioles more distal to the ones under study (which were in the arcade network and are not immediately adjacent to the capillary network) experienced a greater stimulus and transmitted a constrictor response to the vessels upstream.

The influence of blood flow on the response to changes in intravascular pressure is complex. As noted above, Shepherd (24) found that a modest decrease in total flow to the intestine abolished the constrictor response to venous pressure elevation, but this could not be ascribed to accompanying tissue hypoxia, since arterial hypoxia failed to weaken the response. When venous pressure is elevated, the overall blood flow falls, but the changes are quite variable among arterioles. The relations among arteriolar volume flow, diameter, and internal pressure for individual arterioles of cat mesentery were studied during a step-elevation of venous pressure (5). Shown in Fig. 5 are the changes in volume flow and diameter on the horizontal

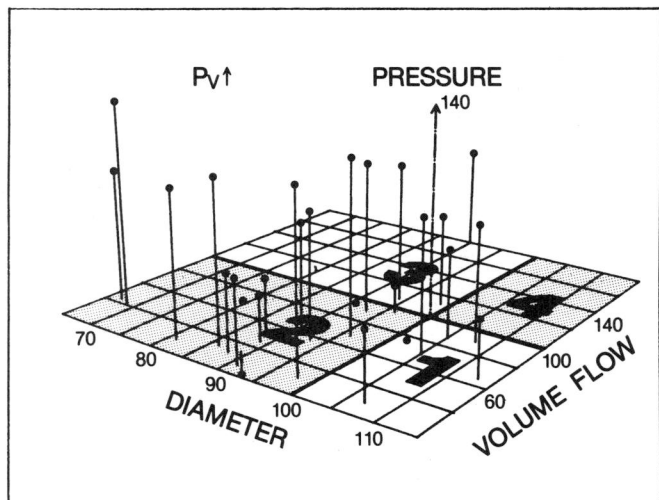

FIG. 5. Diameter, calculated volume flow, and intravascular pressure in the mesenteric arterioles following a step increase in venous pressure. All values are expressed as percentage of control. All responses but one were above the horizontal plane, which represents the initial pressure. The responses may be classified according to the octant in which they fell as discussed in the text. (From Burrows and Johnson, ref. 5, with permission.)

axes as a function of the increase in arteriolar pressure plotted on the vertical axis.

As shown in Fig. 5, 24% of the vessel responses were found within octant #1. These responses are consistent with flow dependence but not pressure dependence because the vessels dilated when pressure rose and volume flow fell. Most of the remaining vessel responses (61%) were found in octant #2, where the vessels constricted when pressure rose and volume flow fell. This is consistent with a pressure-dependent but not with a flow-dependent response. Most of the remaining responses (11%) fell in octant #3, where both flow and pressure rose with constriction. This response is consistent with either mechanism. Overall, flow rose in 11% of the vessels and fell in 89% when venous pressure was increased by about 20 mm Hg. Presumably, differences among vessels in the magnitude of constriction to venous pressure elevation and differences among local networks in the magnitude of flow redistribution allow flow in some vessels to rise while total flow is falling.

Associated with arteriolar constriction to venous pressure elevation is generally a reduction in capillary filtration coefficient (K_f) as determined by whole organ techniques. K_f may fall by 75% as venous pressure is elevated from 0 to 15 mm Hg (16). Since K_f is measured by increasing venous pressure by a fixed increment, the measurement technique itself probably has some influence on the value obtained. For this reason, it would appear advisable to utilize as small an increment of pressure as feasible, consistent with obtaining reliable K_f measurements. The fall in K_f with venous pressure elevation could be due to flow stoppage in the capillary network or reduction in flow to the point where filtration is somewhat flow-limited. If the fall in K_f with venous pressure elevation were due solely to flow stoppage, three-fourths of the capillaries must experience such flow stoppage when venous pressure was elevated from 0 to 15 mm Hg. This would cause a dramatic change in the flow patterns in the capillary networks. Examples of complete flow stoppage were seen in individual capillaries of the mesentery (18) with venous pressure elevation, but the effect overall was not quantitatively equivalent to the aforementioned change in K_f. Such a change would require about a twofold increase in flow in the remaining capillaries, since flow does not fall to the same degree as K_f. Such an increase seems unlikely. On the other hand, there is evidence that flow distribution through the intestine is altered. Granger et al. (10) found that flow to the mucosal-submucosal layer fell from 82% of total flow to 51% when venous pressure was elevated from 0 to 20 mm Hg. The filtration coefficient of muscularis capillaries is higher than that of the mesenteric capillaries (8), and the filtration coefficient of mucosal capillaries is probably higher than that of the other two tissues. The observed shift of flow away from the mucosal layer (assuming it is accompanied by a decrease in the number of capillaries with blood flow) with venous pressure elevation would reduce K_f in the absence of any change in overall flow. Although the exact effect on K_f would depend on the relative filtration coefficients of the various layers, such a shift could possibly account for much of the observed reduction in K_f. It must be noted, however, that the percentage decrease in number of capillaries with flow must be greater in the layer with the highest filtration coefficient than the observed percentage change in K_f, assuming that the other layers also have significant filtration capabilities.

The nature of the myogenic response is still largely unknown. Several theories that have been advanced may explain most facets of the observed behavior. The basic observation is that the arteriole constricts with transient or sustained elevation of internal pressure. The vascular smooth muscle cell appears to act as a sensor as well as an effector when responding to pressure changes. The transient myogenic response can be ascribed to stretch of the smooth muscle cell, a stimulus that leads typically to contraction in several types of smooth muscle (6). The stretch presumably causes deformation of the cell membrane and possibly depolarization or change in membrane permeability. This response appears to be quite important in arterioles of skeletal muscle, where evidence indicates that this normal arterial pulse provides a repetitive stimulus that leads to a sustained contraction (20,22). As noted above, Shepherd (25) found little evidence that the arterial pulse increased vascular resistance in the intestine, although pulsatile arterial pressure appeared to enhance the constrictor response to venous pressure elevation.

The mechanism for the sustained myogenic response is more difficult to conceptualize. The initial stretch with pressure elevation could lead to stretch of the smooth muscle cell, which in turn would cause a contraction for reasons stated above. However, when the smooth muscle cell shortens to its initial length or to less than its initial length as seen in the arterioles, the initial deformation would no longer be present. Thus, the sustained contraction when elevated pressure is maintained cannot be explained on the basis of elongation of the smooth muscle cell. Several authors have suggested that the arteriolar smooth muscle responds to changes in wall tension or wall stress as defined by the Laplace relationship (for review, see 15). This hypothesis is difficult to test directly, but simultaneous measurements of pressure and diameter in arterioles of the bat wing and cat mesentery provide some support for this concept. However, when the responses of individual arterioles in cat mesentery are examined during venous pressure elevation, there is no evidence that the wall tension is closely regulated (5). Rather, the constriction appears to be more closely related to the average rise in arteriolar pressure and wall tension than to the specific change in the vessel under study. These data suggest that changes in other regions of the vascular network may be equally important. Thus, the myogenic response may be a network phenomenon as well as a local phenomenon. In this respect, we note that spontaneous vasomotion spreads from vessel to vessel in cat mesentery *(unpublished observations)*. This spread would provide a mechanism for a myogenic response in one vessel to be communicated to adjacent vessels. This would also explain our observation that the response to pressure elevation was not related to local pressure changes (Fig. 4). However, if such a response were transmitted without decrement throughout the arteriolar network, it is possible that a few vessels that were strongly stimulated by pressure elevation could cause strong contraction throughout the bed. Baez's observation (3) that venous pressure elevation led to a graded degree of response from small to large arterioles is not consistent with this suggestion. It seems more likely that the spread of vasomotion is localized and is perhaps decremental in nature. Observations in support of the latter suggestion have been made by A. Colantuoni, S. Bertuglia, and M. Intaglietta in the skin microcirculation of the unanesthetized Syrian Golden Hamster *(personal communication)*. They found that the frequency of spontaneous vasomotion was different in arterioles of different size, but some transmission was evident between branching levels, being greatest between adjacent branches. Reduction of arterial pressure in cat mesentery usually causes reduction in vasomotor frequency, a finding that could be interpreted as due to loss of the pressure stimulus (4).

The morphological basis for a tension- or wall stress-related myogenic response is not known. It can be speculated that when the smooth muscle cell shortens to less than its original length, the elevated tension or stress causes a sustained deformation of some portion of the cell. The arrangement of the myofilaments in the smooth muscle cell is different from the skeletal muscle fiber in several important respects. For example, the site of attachment to the cell membrane is at the dense bodies on the internal surface of the membrane as shown in Fig. 6 (7). These anchoring points would presumably be areas of increased stress or tension in the membrane itself, where the degree of deformation locally might well depend on the circumferential forces and not on the overall length of the cell. Areas of membrane indentation in the vicinity of the dense bodies, as are apparent in Fig. 6, could conceivably be deformed in relation to the tension transmitted through the dense body from the myofibril to the surrounding tissue.

On the basis of the concepts presented above, a rather speculative model of the myogenic response of an arteriolar network (based on cat mesentery) may be presented. Elevation of arterial or venous pressure would lead to elevation of pressure in the arteriolar network and, in turn, to stretch of the arteriolar smooth muscle cell. This would lead to a transient contraction

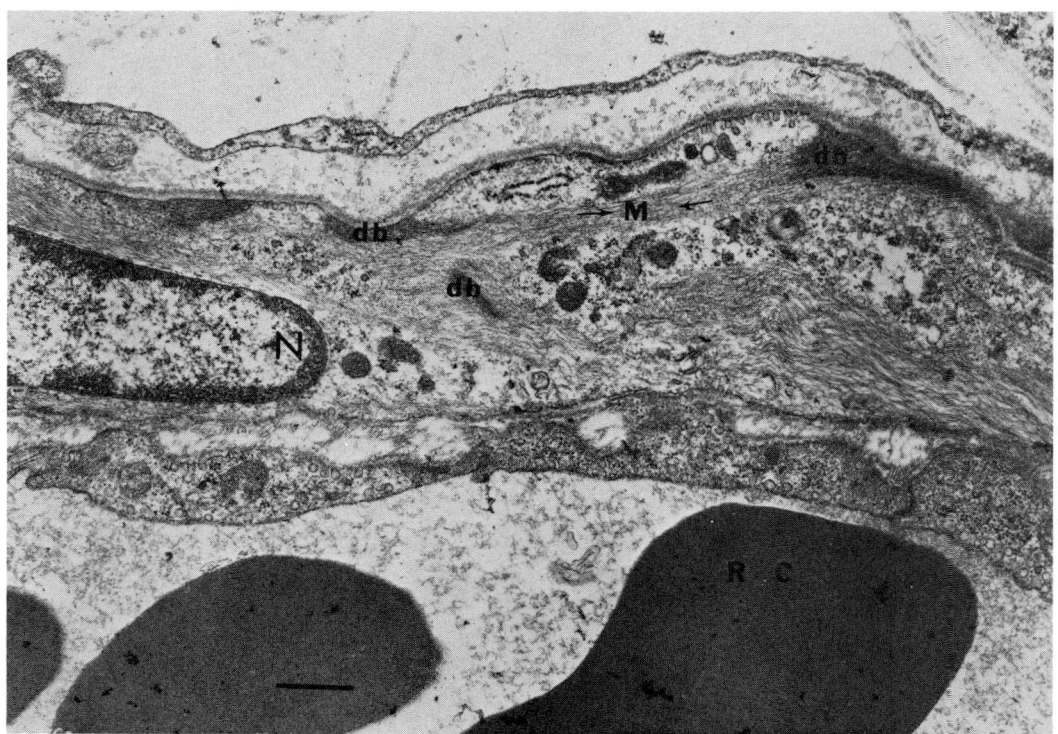

FIG. 6. Myofibril (M) in vascular smooth muscle cell with dense body (db) sites of attachment to the plasma membrane. Also shown are the smooth muscle cell nucleus (N) and a red cell (RC), the latter in the vessel lumen. Scale bar: 0.5 μm (From Carlson et al., ref. 7, with permission.)

owing to the general stretch of the cell membrane, causing membrane depolarization or change in membrane permeability that would lead to activation of the contractile machinery. When the smooth muscle cell returns to its original length, deformation of the membrane in the vicinity of the dense bodies persists because of the increased tension borne by the myofibrils. As the cell contracts further, wall tension decreases because of the Laplace relationship ($T = P \times r$) and reaches a steady state when the increased circumferential tension or wall stress provides just sufficient error signal to maintain a sustained shortening of the smooth muscle cell. This response is transmitted to adjacent cells and to adjacent arteriolar branches, providing a somewhat uniform response at any arteriolar level. Because of the transmission of the response, the pressure change in the local network is more important than in the vessel itself. This transmitted response is decremental in nature and provides for different degrees of response at the several levels of the arteriolar network, depending on the pressure change in that level of the network. Flow changes in each vessel exert some influence on the above response with flow reduction causing some attenuation of the myogenic response and flow elevation augmenting it.

ACKNOWLEDGMENTS

Supported by NIH grants HL 15390, HL 07249, and HL 17421. The technical assistance of Evelyn Gradillas and secretarial support of Lura Hanekamp and Peggy Hawbaker are gratefully acknowledged.

REFERENCES

1. Andrews, C. J. H., Andrews, W. H. H., and Orbach, J. (1972): A sympathetic reflex elicited by distension of the mesenteric venous bed. *J. Physiol.*, 266:119–131.
2. Baez, S. (1968): Bayliss response in the microcirculation. *Fed. Proc.*, 27:1410–1415.
3. Baez, S., Laidlaw, Z., and Orkin, L. R. (1974): Localization and measurement of microvascular and microcirculatory responses to venous pressure elevation in the rat. *Blood Vessels*, 11:260–276.
4. Burrows, M. E., and Johnson, P. C. (1981): Diameter, wall tension, and flow in mesenteric arterioles during autoregulation. *Am. J. Physiol.*, 241 *(Heart Circ. Physiol.*, 10):H829–H837.
5. Burrows, M. E., and Johnson, P. C. (1983): Arteriolar responses to elevation of venous and arterial pressures in cat mesentery. *Am. J. Physiol.*, 245:H796–H807.
6. Burnstock, G., and Prosser, C. L. (1960): Response of smooth muscles to quick stretch; relation of stretch to conduction. *Am. J. Physiol.*, 198:921–925.
7. Carlson, E. C., Burrows, M. E., and Johnson, P. C. (1982): Electron microscopic studies of cat mesenteric arterioles: A structure-function analysis. *Microvasc. Res.*, 24:123–141.
8. Gore, R. W. (1982): Fluid exchange across single capillaries in rat intestinal muscle. *Am. J. Physiol.*, 242 *(Heart Circ. Physiol.*, 11):H268–H287.
9. Gore, R. W., and Bohlen, H. G. (1977): Microvascular pressures in rat intestinal muscle and mucosal villi. *Am. J. Physiol.*, 233(6):H685–H693.
10. Granger, D. N., Richardson, P. D. I., and Taylor, A. E. (1979): Volumetric assessment of the capillary filtration coefficient in the cat small intestine. *Pfluegers Arch.*, 381:25–33.
11. Johnson, P. C. (1959): Myogenic nature of increase in intestinal vascular resistance with venous pressure elevation. *Circ. Res.*, 6:992.
12. Johnson, P. C. (1960): Autoregulation of intestinal blood flow. *Am. J. Physiol.*, 199(2):311–318.
13. Johnson, P. C. (1964): Origin, localization, and homeostatic significance of autoregulation in the intestine. *Circ. Res. (Suppl.)*, 15(1):225–232.
14. Johnson, P. C. (1976): Autoregulation of blood flow in the intestine. *Gastroenterology*, 52:435–441.
15. Johnson, P. C. (1980): The myogenic response. In: *Physiology Handbook*, edited by D. F. Bohr, A. P. Somlyo, and H. V. Sparks, executive editor Stephen R. Geiger, Chapt. 15, pp. 409–442. American Physiological Society, Bethesda.
16. Johnson, P. C., and Hanson, K. M. (1966): Capillary filtration in the small intestine of the dog. *Circ. Res.*, 19:766–773.
17. Johnson, P. C., and Intaglietta, M. (1976): Contributions of pressure and flow sensitivity to autoregulation in mesenteric arterioles. *Am. J. Physiol.*, 231:1686–1698.
18. Johnson, P. C., and Wayland, H. (1967): Regulation of blood flow in single capillaries. *Am. J. Physiol.*, 212:1405–1415.
19. Lutz, J., and Henrich, H. (1970): Gefaesskontraktionen in situ bei druck und stromkonstanter Perfusion der intestinalen Strombahn und ihre Abhaengigkeit vom Ausgangsdruck. *Pfluegers Arch.*, 319:68–81.
20. Mellander, S., and Arvidsson, S. (1974): Possible 'dynamic' component in the myogenic vascular response related to pulse pressure distension. *Acta Physiol. Scand.*, 90:283–285.
21. Pollock, G. P. (1975): *Reactive Hyperemia in Cat Mesentery Capillaries.* Doctoral Dissertation. University of Arizona.
22. Rovick, A. A., and Robertson, P. A. (1964): Interaction of mean and pulse pressures in the circulation of the isolated dog tongue. *Circ. Res.*, 15:208–215.
23. Selkurt, E. E., and Johnson, P. C. (1958): Effect of acute elevation of portal venous pressure on mesen-

23. teric blood volume, interstitial fluid volume and hemodynamics. *Circ. Res.*, 6:592–599.
24. Shepherd, A. P. (1977): Myogenic responses of intestinal resistance and exchange vessels. *Am. J. Physiol.*, 233(5):H547–H554.
25. Shepherd, A. P. (1978): Effect of arterial pulse pressure and hypoxia on myogenic responses in the gut. *Am. J. Physiol.*, 235(2):H157–H161.
26. Shepherd, A. P. (1978): Intestinal O_2 consumption and ^{86}Rb extraction during arterial hypoxia. *Am. J. Physiol.*, 234:E248–E251, or *Am. J. Physiol.: Endocrinol. Metab. Gastrointest. Physiol.*, 3:E248–E251.
27. Shepherd, A. P., and Riedel, G. L. (1982): Effect of pulsatile pressure and metabolic rate on intestinal autoregulation. *Am. J. Physiol.*, 242(11):H769–H775.

Neural Control and Autoregulatory Escape

Clive V. Greenway

Department of Pharmacology and Therapeutics, University of Manitoba, Winnipeg R3E OW3, Canada

Although local nervous mechanisms influencing blood flow occur within the gut wall, extrinsic innervation of intestinal arterioles involves sympathetic vasoconstrictor pathways with preganglionic fibers mainly in the splanchnic nerves and postganglionic fibers accompanying the superior mesenteric artery. Stimulation of these sympathetic fibres causes an initial vasoconstriction followed by return of the flow towards the control level in spite of maintained nerve stimulation. This phenomenon, called "autoregulatory escape," is characterized by a fading of the initial vasoconstriction in the arterioles but not in precapillary sphincters or venules in spite of continued sympathetic nerve stimulation. Evidence is presented that it involves relaxation of the same vessels that were initially constricted. It is unaltered by beta-receptor blocking agents. Although tachyphylactic responses to norepinephrine infusions *in vivo* and *in vitro* have been described, it has not been clearly established that these responses have the same characteristics and mechanism as autoregulatory escape. The mechanism of autoregulatory escape remains unknown but could involve either release of an unknown vasodilator substance secondary to sympathetic nerve stimulation or a cellular mechanism that results in inability of the arteriolar smooth muscle to maintain its contraction in response to the neurotransmitter. Intestinal vasoconstriction mediated by the sympathetic nerves involves the action of the neurotransmitter norepinephrine on alpha-1 and alpha-2 postsynaptic receptors, but the transmitter does not reach beat-receptors unless its release is increased by nonselective alpha-blockers such as phenoxybenzamine. Although the role of the splanchnic nerves in control of splanchnic blood volume is well established, the role of these nerves in controlling intestinal blood flow is not clear, since in experimental situations their effects are often overshadowed by the effects of circulating vasopressin and angiotensin.

INNERVATION OF INTESTINAL ARTERIOLES

Most studies on neural control of intestinal blood flow have examined the vasoconstrictor responses to direct electrical stimulation of either the preganglionic sympathetic nerves (splanchnic nerves) or the postganglionic fibers accompanying the superior mesenteric artery. The postganglionic fibers innervating the blood vessels are predominantly sympathetic noradrenergic nerves (1,23,75). The sympathetic vasoconstrictor supply to the vascular bed of the celiac artery is almost entirely through the splanchnic nerves. However, the vascular bed of the superior mesenteric artery receives a small but significant number of sympathetic fibers from the lumbar region of the spinal cord. These fibres do not run in the splanchnic nerves (9). Thus, section of the splanchnic nerves does not completely denervate the intestinal blood vessels in the dog.

Extrinsic cholinergic nerves of vagal origin supply the intestine, but they do not cause vascular responses. Gastric vasodilatation accompanies the acid secretion caused by vagal stimulation; however, it is not known whether this vasodilatation is caused directly by vasodilator nerves or whether it is secondary to secretion and increased metabolism (50). Vagotomy has no effect on superior mesenteric arterial flow (80). Moreover, Kewenter (45) found that stimulation of the vagi below the level of the heart did not alter intestinal vascular resistance despite the use of a wide variety of stimulus parameters. In addition, no responses to vagal stimulation were unmasked after guanethidine. Therefore, vagal nerves do not appear to convey any specific vasodilator fibers to the intestinal blood vessels.

The possible modulation of sympathetic noradrenergic responses by presynaptic cholinergic receptors (81) has not been studied in the intestinal vascular bed. In the hepatic arterial bed, infusions of acetylcholine inhibited, but vagal stimulation had no effects, on responses to sympathetic nerve stimulation. This suggests that presynaptic cholinergic receptors exist but are not innervated (C. V. Greenway, *unpublished observations*).

Electrical field stimulation or mechanical mucosal stimulation increased intestinal blood flow. These responses were not affected by extrinsic autonomic denervation but were blocked by tetrodotoxin and lidocaine, suggesting a local intramural nervous pathway (2–5). Since these responses were blocked by 2-bromo-LSD and mimicked by injections of 5-hydroxytryptamine (5-HT), the involvement of tryptaminergic nerves was considered. However, since intestinal 5-HT was localized in the enterochromaffin cells (1) and since 5-HT itself acts via a nervous mechanism to produce vasodilatation (4), the transmitter acting on the smooth muscle cells remains unknown. Vasoactive intestinal polypeptide (VIP) is a likely candidate (12,16). VIP was released into the portal blood when the intestinal mucosa was stimulated and when close intraarterial injections of 5-hydroxytryptamine were given to anesthetized cats. Tetrodotoxin blocked both this VIP release and the vasodilator response (16).

These data, although far from conclusive, suggest that the central nervous system controls intestinal blood flow solely via sympathetic noradrenergic fibers acting directly on the smooth muscle cells of the arterioles. However, it remains possible that sympathetic noradrenergic effects on neurones of the intramural nervous plexuses may modulate the direct effects through nervous pathways mediated by polypeptides. Most of the studies to be described were carried out in anesthetized, surgically operated animals, and they show wide variations in baseline blood flows and responses to nerve stimulation. Anesthesia, surgery, and alterations in gut motility may influence the vascular responses to neural activity (10,54).

EFFECTS OF SYMPATHETIC NERVE STIMULATION ON INTESTINAL BLOOD FLOW

The classic work by Mellander (57) in skeletal muscle established the pattern for the later studies on the intestinal bed. The hind-quarters of cats anesthetized with chloralose-urethane were isolated to allow measurement of arterial and venous pressures, blood flow, and total organ volume. Stimulation of the lumbar sympathetic trunks at frequencies within the physiological range (0.5–16 Hz) produced a frequency-dependent vasoconstriction that was well maintained for the duration of stimulation. The capillary filtration coefficient initially decreased but subsequently returned to control values in spite of maintained nerve stimulation, and capillary pressure decreased. These studies demonstrated that in skeletal muscle at constant perfusion pressure, blood flow can be directly controlled by the sympathetic innervation, that responses are proportional to frequency of stimulation, and that they are well maintained for many minutes.

Folkow and his co-workers (20) conducted similar studies on the intestinal vascular bed. In anesthetized cats a portion of ileum was isolated, and the remainder of the intestine was removed. The mesenteric vein was cannulated to allow measurement of blood flow and control of venous pressure. The organ blood volume was determined with a plethysmograph. The mesenteric artery and its surrounding nerves were intact, and the splanchnic nerves were prepared for stimulation after removal or denervation of the adrenal glands. Electrical stimulation of the splanchnic nerves produced an initial frequency-dependent vasoconstriction, but this was followed within 2 min by a recovery of the flow towards the control level in spite of maintained nerve stimulation (Fig. 1). This was the original and now classical description of autoregulatory escape. The capillary filtration coefficient decreased at the onset of nerve stimulation and remained decreased, suggesting that the precapillary sphincters remained constricted throughout nerve stimulation. Mean capillary pressure was unchanged from the prestimulatory control level during the steady state phase after escape. In the early experiments, organ blood volume decreased but then tended to recover as blood flow recovered during autoregulatory escape. In these experiments, venous pressure was low and volume effects secondary to flow changes were large. When the experiments were repeated with mesenteric vein pressures closer to the normal values of portal pressure, the decrease in organ blood volume was well maintained for the duration of stimulation (20,61). Thus, the phenomenon of autoregulatory escape was seen in the arterioles controlling blood flow but not in the precapillary sphincters or capacitance vessels. Subsequent work demonstrated that autoregulatory escape occurred with postganglionic mesenteric nerve stimulation (18,31) and could not therefore involve mechanisms in autonomic ganglia.

DESCRIPTION OF AUTOREGULATORY ESCAPE

Because fading responses or tachyphylaxis can be induced in many different situations, it is necessary to precisely describe autoregulatory escape before we attempt to delineate the sites where it occurs and its possible mechanisms. True autoregulatory escape has the following characteristics. It occurs only in arteriolar smooth muscle and not in venous smooth muscle. At the time when arteriolar resistance is recovering towards the control level, the venous or capacitance response is well maintained (Fig. 1). It occurs during reflex activation (35,59) as well as during direct electrical stimulation of the sympathetic nerves. It occurs at all frequencies of stimulation. Thus, it is not due to stimulating the nerves at unphysiological rates. During the steady state response, flow is usually 58% to 75% of control (71). However, in some animals flow may recover to above the control level, indicating inhibition of the basal arteriolar tone (20,31). Cessation of stimulation is followed by a pronounced poststimulatory hyperemia even after prolonged (30 min) periods of nerve stimulation during which flow is close to the control level (13,20,31). In preparations where autoregulatory escape is small, the poststimulatory hyperemia is also small (13,82). These char-

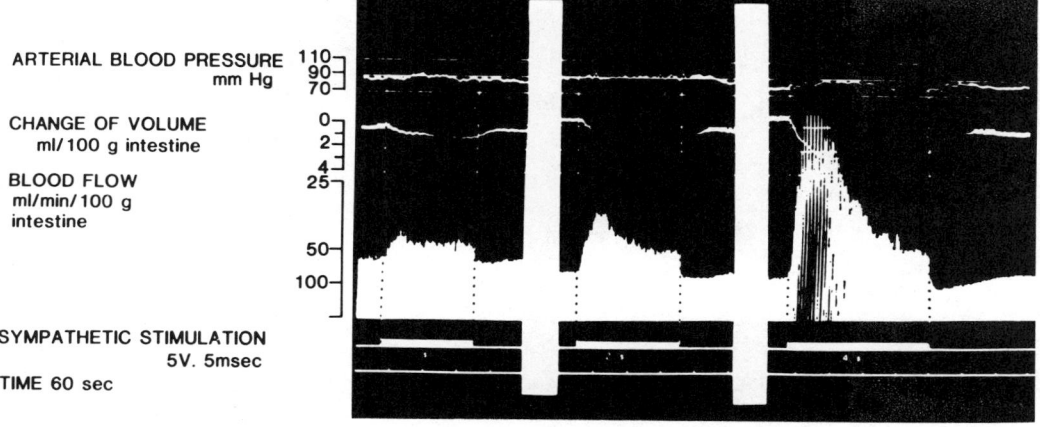

FIG. 1. The classical picture of autoregulatory escape in the intestinal bed perfused at constant inflow pressure in anesthetized cats. Note also the well-maintained venous response (change in volume) and the poststimulatory hyperemia. (From Folkow et al., ref. 20, with permission.)

acteristics indicate that some effect of nerve stimulation is maintained throughout the stimulation period, and that the poststimulatory hyperemia is not reactive (secondary to a reduction in total flow). It occurs during constant pressure or constant flow perfusion of the vascular bed (13,49). If the bed is perfused at constant pressure, the response is elicited as an initial fall followed by a recovery in the flow, whereas if the bed is perfused at constant flow, the response is elicited as an initial increase followed by a decrease towards control in the perfusion pressure. It is unaltered after administration of beta-receptor blocking agents (Fig. 2). This excludes the involvement of interactions between alpha- and beta-receptors (64). It is also unaltered after atropine (31).

SITES OF AUTOREGULATORY ESCAPE

Although this chapter is primarily concerned with intestinal resistance vessel responses to nerve stimulation, discussion of autoregulatory escape requires consideration of other vascular sites where it is seen. Proposed explanations should be tenable in all the organs in which autoregulatory escape is seen.

Sympathetic Nerve Stimulation

Autoregulatory escape as described above was demonstrated in the small intestine of cats (18, 20,21,31,37,47,49,77,82), dogs (74, G. Oshiro and C. V. Greenway, *unpublished observations*) and humans (42). It was demonstrated in the hepatic arterial bed in cats (18,27,30,46) but not in dogs (30). Escape occurred in the renal vascular bed in cats but a poststimulatory hyperemia was not seen (11,43,49). Escape does not occur in skeletal muscle (35,57) or adipose tissue (60). In the spleen a weak, slowly developing escape was seen (28). Escape occurred in a preparation of intestinal mesentery and lymph nodes after removal of the intestine (48), in the gastric microcirculation of rats (34), and in the colonic microcirculation of cats (41). In isolated perfused intestinal loops, responses to sympathetic stimulation were of the same size as those seen in intact animals after escape had occurred, but the classic picture of an initial vasoconstriction followed by recovery was not seen (71,73).

Norepinephrine Infusions *In Vivo* and *In Vitro*

The occurrence of autoregulatory escape during norepinephrine infusions is controversial and

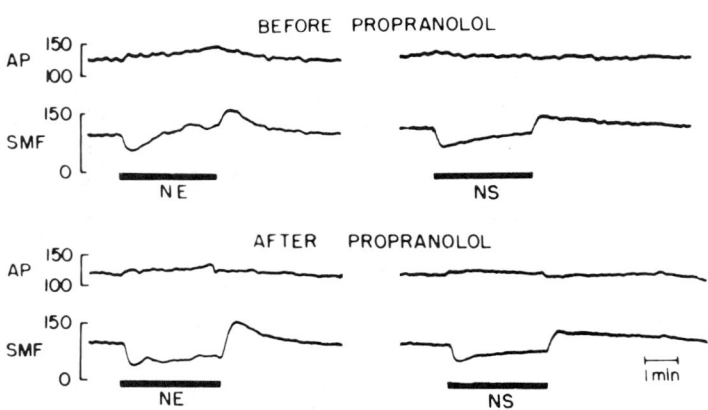

FIG. 2. Comparison of effects of intramesenteric arterial infusion of norepinephrine (NE, 1 μg/min) and stimulation of mesenteric periarterial nerves (NS) before and after intravenous propranolol (0.5 mg/kg) in anesthetized cats. AP, mean systemic arterial pressure (mm Hg); SMF, mean flow in superior mesenteric artery (ml/min). Note that before propranolol the degree of escape during norepinephrine infusion is greater than that during nerve stimulation. After propranolol, escape during norepinephrine infusion is impaired but that during nerve stimulation is unaffected. (From Ross, ref. 64, with permission.)

nonspecific causes of fading have not been excluded. In the intestine of cats and dogs, escape during norepinephrine infusions has been demonstrated (33,62–65,70,78). It may be greater (64) or less (13,37,49,82) than during nerve stimulation, and it may be reduced or abolished by propranolol (63–65,78). In the experiment illustrated in Fig. 2, escape was greater during norepinephrine infusion than during nerve stimulation, but after propranolol escape during norepinephrine became similar to that during nerve stimulation (64). Escape during norepinephrine infusions was not significant in the baboon (44) but was present and unaffected by propranolol in rats (40). In the kidney of cats, escape during norepinephrine infusion was small or absent (43,49). In the hepatic arterial bed in cats, escape that was not blocked by propranolol was seen during intraarterial infusions of norepinephrine (27,68) but not during intravenous infusions (27). This unexpected dependence on route of administration of norepinephrine has been confirmed recently (C. V. Greenway, *unpublished observations*).

In vitro, mesenteric arterial rings or perfused artery segments showed escape to norepinephrine (17,38,39,66,67). However, other drugs also showed escape, notably vasopressin (17,39), which does not show escape *in vivo* (13). Further confusion is added by the recent observation that isolated mesenteric resistance vessels of rats do not show escape in response to electrical stimulation (58).

These various fading responses to norepinephrine and other drugs have not been proved to be related to autoregulatory escape as seen in response to nerve stimulation in anesthetized animals. Therefore, it is not yet possible to decide with certainty whether autoregulatory escape occurs only when norepinephrine is released in the vicinity of nerve varicosities or whether it also occurs when all the smooth muscle is bathed in norepinephrine. This would clearly be useful information to delineate the mechanism.

MECHANISM OF AUTOREGULATORY ESCAPE

The criteria for autoregulatory escape set out earlier allow exclusion of some possible mechanisms. Since autoregulatory escape occurs at low frequencies of stimulation, does not occur in simultaneously recorded venous responses, and is seen after reflex activation of the sympathetic nerves, it is unlikely that failure of the nerve stimulation or transmitter depletion are responsible. Thus, it appears to be a genuine physiological phenomenon and not an experimental artifact. The flow can recover to above the control level during escape and a poststimulatory hyperemia is seen even after a 30-min stimulation during which flow recovered and remained close to the control level. Increasing the frequency of nerve stimulation after escape has developed causes a further vasoconstriction, which then itself shows escape (27). These data suggest autoregulatory escape is not simply a disappearance of the vasoconstriction, and any type of desensitization of alpha-receptors (36) is unlikely (72).

In early studies, Folkow and his co-workers (14,19,21,82) suggested autoregulatory escape involved a redistribution of flow within the intestine, possibly by opening submucosal shunt vessels. This explanation was organ-specific but at that time, autoregulatory escape in other organs had not been described. This hypothesis has not been supported by subsequent work. Neither microspheres (29) nor microscopy (33) demonstrated shunt vessels in the intestinal submucosa. Submucosal vessels appeared to continue into the mucosa. Microspheres trapped in the submucosa were subsequently redistributed into the mucosa when the vascular bed was dilated (29,51,52). The distribution of blood flow in the intestine (31,42,65), gastric wall (34), and liver (30) is unchanged throughout the responses to nerve stimulation and norepinephrine infusion, and the oxygen consumption of the liver and intestine return towards the control level during autoregulatory escape (46,47). However, one recent study suggests significantly greater escape in the mucosa than in the muscularis in dogs (74). In man, the vasoconstriction was somewhat more pronounced in the muscularis than in the mucosa-submucosa, but the redistribution was small (42). Measurement of vessel diameter by microscopy confirmed that autoregulatory escape occurred in the vessels that showed initial constriction (33). Microvascular pressure studies were also unable to demonstrate a major redistribution of flow within the intestine during sympathetic nerve stimulation. Indeed, these data suggested that the primary site of sympathetic vasoconstriction was upstream from the division of the vessels into the parallel mucosa-submucosa and muscle circuits (6,7,24). However, since blood flow was not recorded, it is not certain that autoregulatory escape occurred in these studies in rats.

It should be noted that although these observations strongly suggest that a flow redistribution is not the cause of autoregulatory escape, they do not invalidate the hypothesis proposed by Svanvik (42,77) that a flow redistribution occurs within the intestinal mucosa from the crypts to the villi and that this may alter mucosal function in important ways. This is a separate phenomenon, which occurs only within the intestinal mucosa and which appears to be unrelated to autoregulatory escape.

There now seems little doubt that, as originally suggested by Richardson and Johnson (62), autoregulatory escape involves relaxation of the same vessels that originally constricted (69). This relaxation could be due to a specific substance released directly or indirectly by sympathetic nerve stimulation or a failure of arteriolar smooth muscle to maintain its contraction. These hypotheses will now be considered.

If autoregulatory escape is due to direct or indirect release of a specific substance by sympathetic nerve stimulation, this substance must be produced in the vicinity of the arterioles only in organs that show escape. It must not be produced, or the smooth muscle must be insensitive, in the precapillary sphincters and venules. The substance must be a highly effective antagonist to norepinephrine. Autoregulatory escape is unaffected by propranolol (see above), by atropine, antihistamines, and indomethacin (31). We have recently shown it is unaltered in the presence of naloxone, an opiate receptor blocker (Seaman and C. V. Greenway, *unpublished observations*). However, it remains possible that an unknown substance exists. Shepherd and Granger (72) have modeled a possible interaction between neural vasoconstriction and a vasodilator metabolite produced by the parenchymal cells. Their results suggest such a mechanism is feasible. Neural release of a vasodilator substance within the vessel wall is also feasible. Electrical field stimulation of strips of pulmonary artery constricted by norepinephrine produced a relaxation mediated by an unknown diffusible substance produced in the endothelium (22). Production of such a substance and its slow diffusion into the media could explain autoregulatory escape. It would be interesting to know if autoregulatory escape occurs in the pulmonary vascular bed.

Other possible mechanisms involve failure of the arteriolar smooth muscle to maintain its contraction. *In vitro*, substitution of sodium by lithium or substitution of chloride by iodide, perchlorate, or isoethionate abolished escape to norepinephrine in cat mesenteric arterial rings. These observations led Ross (66) to suggest fading of propagated activity. However, if failure of propagated activity is responsible for autoregulatory escape, it is not at present clear why it occurs only in certain arterioles. Failure of the arteriolar smooth muscle to maintain its contraction could be due to intracellular Na accumulation as demonstrated in taenia coli (8) or to fading of calcium-spike activity (67). However, such failure does not appear to occur during nerve stimulation in isolated mesenteric resistance vessels from rats (58).

In summary, until autoregulatory escape can be demonstrated unequivocally in isolated preparations and in response to norepinephrine infusions, the most likely hypothesis is the production of a vasodilator antagonist to norepinephrine either within the vessel wall or by parenchymal cells of the organ.

ADRENERGIC RECEPTOR SUBTYPES

Adrenergic receptor mechanisms have been reviewed recently (36) and are currently undergoing intensive study. It is well established that the mesenteric arterioles have both alpha- and beta-receptors, and the effects of epinephrine, norepinephrine, and isoproterenol on mesenteric vascular resistance have been reviewed in the context of their overall actions on the circulation (25). Isoproterenol produces an intestinal vasodilatation mediated by beta-2 receptors (79) whereas norepinephrine produces a vasoconstriction mediated through both alpha-1 and alpha-2 receptors (see below). Epinephrine may produce a brief constriction followed by vasodilation when given as a bolus injection, but when infused it produces a sustained vasodilatation in man, cat, and baboon but perhaps not in dog (see ref. 25). The question of which receptors are involved in neural responses has been reexamined recently (61). Since phenoxybenzamine reverses the effects of sympathetic nerve stimulation from intestinal vasoconstriction to vasodilatation, it appeared initially that the transmitter acted on both alpha and beta receptors and that the net response was a balance of these actions. However, it is now known that alpha-blockers such as phenoxybenzamine increase the release and overflow of transmitter, presumably by inhibiting presyn-

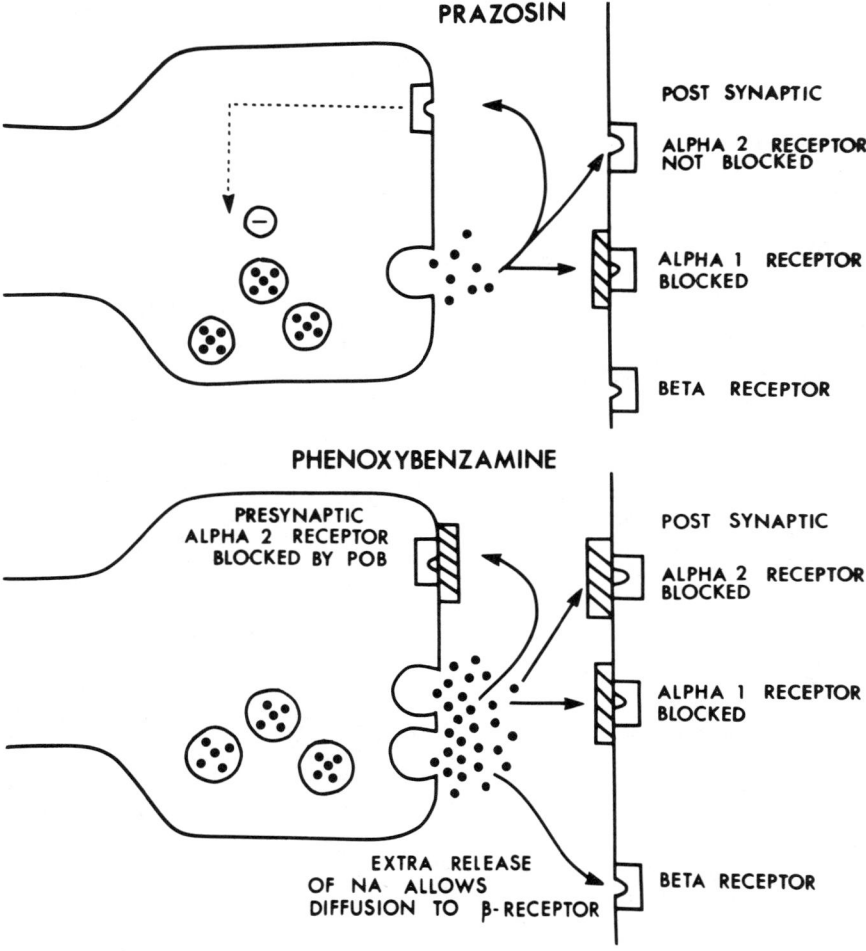

FIG. 3. Diagrammatic illustration of the hypothesis that after prazosin, the postsynaptic alpha-1 receptor is blocked but norepinephrine (NA) release is unchanged, whereas after phenoxybenzamine (POB), both pre- and postsynaptic alpha receptors are blocked and norepinephrine release is increased, allowing diffusion to the beta-receptors in the mesenteric vascular bed. (From Patel et al., ref. 61, with permission.)

aptic alpha-2 receptors. Since beta-blockers have no significant effects on the responses to nerve stimulation in the absence of alpha-blockers (see Fig. 2), it now appears that the transmitter does not reach the beta-receptors unless the release and overflow are enhanced by a non-selective alpha-blocker as illustrated in Fig. 3 (61). This hypothesis has been confirmed by work on isolated mesenteric arterial strips (32).

Alpha-receptors have been divided into alpha-1 and alpha-2 subtypes. Initially, it was suggested that postsynaptic receptors were of the alpha-1 type and presynaptic receptors were alpha-2. More recently, it has become apparent that postsynaptic receptors may be of both types (76). In anesthetized cats, the intestinal vasoconstrictor and local blood volume responses to sympathetic nerve stimulation were reduced but not abolished in the presence of prazosin (61). Pressor responses to splanchnic nerve stimulation in anesthetized cats were reduced more by yohimbine than by prazosin (15). These results indicate that both alpha-1 and alpha-2 postsynaptic receptors mediate the responses to sympathetic nerve stimulation in this vascular bed. The role of the presynaptic receptors in neural control of intestinal blood flow has not yet been studied.

ROLE OF EXTRINSIC INNERVATION IN INTESTINAL VASCULAR RESPONSES

It is beyond the scope of this chapter to review the role of the splanchnic innervation in complex vascular responses such as hemorrhage, exercise, and shock (see Chapters 13, 14). However, it seems worth pointing out that although the role of the splanchnic nerves in mediating blood volume redistribution is well established (26), the importance of these nerves in blood flow responses remains to be elucidated (73). The occurrence of autoregulatory escape and the marked responses of the intestinal bed to other endogenous vasoconstrictors such as angiotensin and vasopressin make it difficult to detect any portion of the total flow response that might be attributed to the sympathetic innervation. In an extensive series of experiments in cats, McNeill and his co-workers showed that intestinal vasoconstriction following hemorrhage or diuretic-induced volume-depletion was mediated by endogenous release of vasopressin and angiotensin. A role for the sympathetic innervation could not be detected (53,55). Similarly, they showed that the mesenteric vasoconstriction caused by surgery was mediated by these endogenous hormones rather than by the innervation (54,56).

At present it does not appear possible to attribute any intestinal vasocontrictor response *in vivo* solely to activity of the sympathetic innervation. The splanchnic nerves appear to be much more important in controlling other aspects of the splanchnic vascular bed than they are in controlling intestinal blood flow.

ACKNOWLEDGMENTS

Work from my laboratory was supported by grants from the Medical Research Council of Canada and the Manitoba Heart Foundation.

REFERENCES

1. Ahlman, H., Enerback, L., Kewenter, J., and Storm, B. (1973): Effects of extrinsic denervation on the fluorescence of monoamines in the small intestine of the cat. *Acta Physiol. Scand.*, 89:429–435.
2. Biber, B., Fara, J., and Lundgren, O. (1973): Intestinal vasodilatation in response to transmural electrical field stimulation. *Acta Physiol. Scand.*, 87:277–282.
3. Biber, B., Fara, J., and Lundgren, O. (1973): Intestinal vascular responses to 5-hydroxytryptamine. *Acta Physiol. Scand.*, 87:526–534.
4. Biber, B., Fara, J., and Lundgren, O. (1974): A pharmacological study of intestinal vasodilator mechanisms in the cat. *Acta Physiol. Scand.*, 90:673–683.
5. Biber, B., Lundgren, O., and Svanvik, J. (1971): Studies on the intestinal vasodilatation observed after mechanical stimulation of the mucosa of the gut. *Acta Physiol. Scand.*, 82:177–190.
6. Bohlen, H. G., and Gore, R. W. (1979): Microvascular pressures in rat intestinal muscle during direct nerve stimulation. *Microvasc. Res.*, 17 27–37.
7. Bohlen, H. G., Henrich, H., Gore, R. W., and Johnson, P. C. (1978): Intestinal muscle and mucosal blood flow during direct sympathetic stimulation. *Am. J. Physiol.*, 235:H40–H45.
8. Bose, D. (1975): Mechanism of mechanical inhibition of smooth muscle by ouabain. *Br. J. Pharmacol.*, 55:111–116.
9. Brooksby, G. A., and Donald, D. E. (1970): Sympa-

thetic outflow from spinal cord to splanchnic circulation of the dog. *Am. J. Physiol.*, 219:1429–1433.
10. Chou, C. C. (1982): Relationship between intestinal blood flow and motility. *Annu. Rev. Physiol.*, 44:29–42.
11. Coote, J. H., Johns, E. J., MacLeod, V. H., and Singer, B. (1972): Effect of renal nerve stimulation, renal blood flow and adrenergic blockade on plasma renin activity in the cat. *J. Physiol. (Lond.)*, 226:15–36.
12. Costa, M., and Furness, J. B. (1982): Neuronal peptides in the intestine. *Br. Med. Bull.*, 38:247–252.
13. Dresel, P., and Wallentin, I. (1966): Effects of sympathetic vasoconstrictor fibres, noradrenaline and vasopressin on the intestinal vascular resistance during constant blood flow or blood pressure. *Acta Physiol. Scand.*, 66:427–436.
14. Dresel, P., Folkow, B., and Wallentin, I. (1966): Rubidium86 clearance during neurogenic redistribution of intestinal blood flow. *Acta Physiol. Scand.*, 67:173–184.
15. Drew, G. M., and Whiting, S. B. (1979): Evidence for two distinct types of postsynaptic alpha adrenoceptors in vascular smooth muscle in vivo. *Br. J. Pharmacol.*, 67:207–215.
16. Eklund, S., Fahrenkrug, J., Jodal, M., Lundgren, O., Schaffalitzky De Muckadell, O. B., and Sjoqvist, A. (1980): Vasoactive intestinal polypeptide, 5-hydroxytryptamine and reflex hyperaemia in the small intestine of the cat. *J. Physiol. (Lond.)*, 302:549–557.
17. Fara, J. W., and Ross, G. (1972): Escape from drug-induced constriction of isolated arterial segments from various vascular beds. *Angiologica*, 9:27–33.
18. Fasth, S., Hulten, L., and Nordgren, S. (1980): Adjustments of hepatic and small intestine blood flow on selective vasoconstrictor fibre stimulation. *Acta Physiol. Scand.*, 110:343–350.
19. Folkow, B. (1967): Regional adjustments of intestinal blood flow. *Gastroenterology*, 52:423–432.
20. Folkow, B., Lewis, D. H., Lundgren, O., Mellander, S., and Wallentin, I. (1964): The effect of graded vasoconstrictor fibre stimulation on the intestinal resistance and capacitance vessels. *Acta Physiol. Scand.*, 61:445–457.
21. Folkow, B., Lewis, D. H., Lundgren, O., Mellander, S., and Wallentin, I. (1964): The effect of the sympathetic vasoconstrictor fibres on the distribution of capillary blood flow in the intestine. *Acta Physiol. Scand.*, 61:458–466.
22. Frank, G. W., and Bevan, J. A. (1983): Electrical stimulation causes endothelium-dependent relaxation in lung vessels. *Am. J. Physiol.*, 244:H793–H798.
23. Furness, J. B., and Costa, M. (1980): Types of nerves in the enteric nervous system. *Neuroscience*, 5:1–20.
24. Furness, J. B., and Marshall, J. M. (1973): Constrictor responses and flow changes in the rat mesenteric microvasculature resulting from the stimulation of paravascular nerves. *Bibl. Anat.*, 12:404–409.
25. Greenway, C. V. (1981): Mechanisms and quantitative assessment of drug effects on cardiac output with a new model of the circulation. *Pharmacol. Rev.*, 33:213–251.
26. Greenway, C. V. (1983): Role of splanchnic venous system in overall cardiovascular homeostasis. *Fed. Proc.*, 42:1678–1684.
27. Greenway, C. V., Lawson, A. E., and Mellander, S. (1967): The effects of stimulation of the hepatic nerves, infusions of noradrenaline and occlusion of the carotid arteries on liver blood flow in the anesthetized cat. *J. Physiol. (Lond.)*, 192:21–41.
28. Greenway, C. V., Lawson, A. E., and Stark, R. D. (1968): Vascular responses of the spleen to nerve stimulation during normal and reduced blood flow. *J. Physiol. (Lond.)*, 194:421–433.
29. Greenway, C. V., and Murthy, V. S. (1972): Effects of vasopressin and isoprenaline infusions on the distribution of blood flow in the intestine; criteria for the validity of microsphere studies. *Br. J. Pharmacol.*, 46:177–188.
30. Greenway, C. V., and Oshiro, G. (1972): Comparison of the effects of hepatic nerve stimulation on arterial flow, distribution of arterial and portal flows and blood content in the livers of anaesthetized cats and dogs. *J. Physiol. (Lond.)*, 227:487–501.
31. Greenway, C. V., Scott, G. D., and Zink, J. (1976): Sites of autoregulatory escape of blood flow in the mesenteric vascular bed. *J. Physiol. (Lond.)*, 259:1–12.
32. Guimaraes, S., Paiva, M. Q., and Moura, D. (1982): Evidence for existence of distinct biophases for alpha and beta adrenoceptors in the vascular tissue. *J. Cardiovasc. Pharmacol.*, 4:S58–S62.
33. Guth, P. H., Ross, G., and Smith, E. (1976): Changes in intestinal vascular diameter during norepinephrine vasoconstrictor escape. *Am. J. Physiol.*, 230:1466–1468.
34. Guth, P. H., and Smith, E. (1975): Escape from vasoconstriction in the gastric microcirculation. *Am. J. Physiol.*, 228:1893–1895.
35. Hadjiminas, J., and Oberg, B. (1968): Effects of carotid baroreceptor reflexes on venous tone in skeletal muscle and intestine of the cat. *Acta Physiol. Scand.*, 72:518–532.
36. Heinsimer, J. A., and Lefkowitz, R. J. (1982): Adrenergic receptors: Biochemistry, regulation, molecular mechanism and clinical implications. *J. Lab. Clin. Med.*, 100:641–658.
37. Henrich, H. (1973): Adjustment behavior of adrenergic-induced vasoconstrictions in the intestinal circulation of the cat. *Angiologica*, 10:233–247.
38. Henrich, H., and Biester, J. (1973): Localization of vascular adjustments in the intestinal vascular bed. *Bibl. Anat.*, 11:428–433.
39. Henrich, H., and Lutz, J. (1971): Vascular escape-phenomenon in the intestinal circulation and its induction by different vasoconstrictor agents. *Pfluegers Arch.*, 329:82–94.
40. Henrich, H., Singbartl, G., and Biester, J. (1974): Adrenergic-induced vascular adjustments - initial and escape reactions. I. Influence of beta-adrenergic blocking agents on the intestinal circulation of the rat (in vivo). *Pfluegers Arch.*, 346:1–12.
41. Hulten, L. (1969): Extrinsic nervous control of colonic motility and blood flow. An experimental study in the cat. *Acta Physiol. Scand. (Suppl.)*, 335:1–116.
42. Hulten, L., Lindhagen, J., and Lundgren, O. (1977): Sympathetic nervous control of intramural blood flow in the feline and human intestines. *Gastroenterology*, 72:41–48.

43. Johansson, B., Sparks, H., and Biber, B. (1970): The escape of the renal blood flow response during sympathetic nerve stimulation. *Angiologica*, 7:333–343.
44. Kerr, J. C., Reynolds, D. G., and Swan, K. G. (1978): Adrenergic stimulation and blockade in mesenteric circulation of the baboon. *Am. J. Physiol.*, 234:E457–E462.
45. Kewenter, J. (1965): The vagal control of the jejunal and ileal motility and blood flow. *Acta Physiol. Scand.*, (Suppl.),65:251:1–68.
46. Lautt, W. W. (1977): Effect of stimulation of hepatic nerves on hepatic O_2 uptake and blood flow. *Am. J. Physiol.*, 232:H652–H656.
47. Lautt, W. W., and Graham, S. A. (1977): Effect of nerve stimulation on pre-capillary sphincters, oxygen extraction, and hemodynamics in the intestines of cats. *Circ. Res.*, 41:32–36.
48. Lundgren, O., and Wallentin, I. (1964): Local chemical and nervous control of consecutive vascular sections in the mesenteric lymph nodes of the cat. *Angiologica*, 1:284–296.
49. Lutz, J., and Henrich, H. (1973): Comparison of the vascular escape phenomenon in the intestinal and renal circulation under nerval and humoral induction. *Pflüegers Arch.*, 339:37–48.
50. Martinson, J. (1965): The effect of graded vagal stimulation on gastric motility, secretion and blood flow in the cat. *Acta Physiol. Scand.*, 65:300–309.
51. Maxwell, L. C., Shepherd, A. P., and Riedel, G. L. (1982): Vasodilation or altered perfusion pressure moves 15-micron spheres trapped in the gut wall. *Am. J. Physiol.*, 243:H123–H127.
52. Maxwell, L. C., Shepherd, A. P., Riedel, G. L., and Morris, M. D. (1981): Effect of microsphere size on apparent intramural distribution of intestinal blood flow. *Am. J. Physiol.*, 241:H408–H414.
53. McNeill, J. R. (1974): Intestinal vasoconstriction following diuretic-induced volume depletion: role of angiotensin and vasopressin. *Can. J. Physiol. Pharmacol.*, 52:829–839.
54. McNeill, J. R., and Pang, C. C. Y. (1982): Effect of pentobarbital anesthesia and surgery on the control of arterial pressure and mesenteric resistance in cats: role of vasopressin and angiotensin. *Can. J. Physiol. Pharmacol.*, 60:363–368.
55. McNeill, J. R., Stark, R. D., and Greenway, C. V. (1970): Intestinal vasoconstriction after hemorrhage: roles of vasopressin and angiotensin. *Am. J. Physiol.*, 219:1342–1347.
56. McNeill, J. R., Wilcox, W. C., and Pang, C. C. Y. (1977): Vasopressin and angiotensin: reciprocal mechanisms controlling mesenteric conductance. *Am. J. Physiol.*, 232:H260–H266.
57. Mellander, S. (1960): Comparative studies on the adrenergic neuro-hormonal control of resistance and capacitance blood vessels in the cat. *Acta Physiol. Scand. (Suppl.)*, 50(176):1–86.
58. Nilsson, H., and Folkow, B. (1982): Vasoconstrictor nerve influence on isolated mesenteric resistance vessels from normotensive and spontaneously hypertensive rats. *Acta Physiol. Scand.*, 116:205–208.
59. Oberg, B. (1964): Effects of cardiovascular reflexes on net capillary fluid transfer. *Acta Physiol. Scand. (Suppl.)*, 62(229):1–98.
60. Oberg, B., and Rosell, S. (1967): Sympathetic control of consecutive vascular sections in canine subcutaneous adipose tissue. *Acta Physiol. Scand.*, 71:47–56.
61. Patel, P., Bose, D., and Greenway, C. V. (1981): Effects of prazosin and phenoxybenzamine on alpha and beta receptor mediated responses in intestinal resistance and capacitance vessels. *J. Cardiovasc. Pharmacol.*, 3:1050–1059.
62. Richardson, D. R., and Johnson, P. C. (1969): Comparison of autoregulatory escape and autoregulation in the intestinal vascular bed. *Am. J. Physiol.*, 217:586–590.
63. Ross, G. (1967): Effects of epinephrine and norepinephrine on the mesenteric circulation of the cat. *Am. J. Physiol.*, 212:1037–1042.
64. Ross, G. (1971): Escape of mesenteric vessels from adrenergic and non-adrenergic vasoconstriction. *Am. J. Physiol.*, 221:1217–1222.
65. Ross, G. (1971): Effects of norepinephrine infusions on mesenteric arterial blood flow and its tissue distribution. *Proc. Soc. Exp. Biol. Med.*, 137:921–924.
66. Ross, G. (1975): Norepinephrine vasoconstrictor escape in isolated mesenteric arteries. *Am. J. Physiol.*, 228:1652–1655.
67. Ross, G., and Belsky, J. (1978): Effects of tetraethylammonium and manganese on mesenteric vasoconstrictor escape. *Proc. Soc. Exp. Biol. Med.*, 159:390–393.
68. Ross, G., and Kurrasch, M. (1969): Adrenergic responses of the hepatic circulation. *Am. J. Physiol.*, 216:1380–1385.
69. Shanbour, L. L., and Jacobson, E. D. (1971): Autoregulatory escape in the gut. *Gastroenterology*, 60:145–148.
70. Shehadeh, Z., Price, W. E., and Jacobson, E. D. (1969): Effects of vasoactive agents on intestinal blood flow and motility in the dog. *Am. J. Physiol.*, 216:386–392.
71. Shepherd, A. P. (1979): Intestinal O_2 uptake during sympathetic stimulation and partial arterial occlusion. *Am. J. Physiol.*, 236:H731–H735.
72. Shepherd, A. P., and Granger, H. J. (1973): Autoregulatory escape in the gut: A systems analysis. *Gastroenterology*, 65:77–91.
73. Shepherd, A. P., Johnson, J. M., and Proppe, D. W. (1981): Interaction of nervous and local control of the intestinal circulation. *Adv. Physiol. Sci*, 9:201–210.
74. Shepherd, A. P., and Riedel, G. L. (1983): Effect of sympathetic stimulation on intestinal mucosal blood flow studied by laser Doppler velocimetry. *Int. Congr. Physiol., Sydney, Australia*.
75. Silva, D. G., Ross, G., and Osborne, L. W. (1971): Adrenergic innervation of the ileum of the cat. *Am. J. Physiol.*, 220:347–352.
76. Starke, K., and Docherty, J. R. (1982): Types and functions of peripheral alpha-adrenoceptors. *J. Cardiovasc. Pharmacol.*, 4:S3–S7.
77. Svanvik, J. (1973): Mucosal hemodynamics in the small intestine of the cat during regional sympathetic vasoconstrictor activation. *Acta Physiol. Scand.*, 89:19–29.
78. Swan, K. G., and Reynolds, D. G. (1971): Effects of

intraarterial catecholamine infusions on blood flow in the canine gut. *Gastroenterology*, 61:863–871.
79. Taira, N., and Yabuuchi, Y. (1977): Profile of beta-adrenoceptors in femoral, superior mesenteric and renal vascular beds of dogs. *Br. J. Pharmacol.*, 59:577–583.
80. Tibblin, S., Burns, G. P., Hahnloser, P. B., and Schenk, W. G. (1969): The influence of vagotomy on superior mesenteric artery blood flow. *Surg. Gynecol. Obstet.*, 129:1231–1234.
81. VanHoutte, P. M., and Levy, M. N. (1980): Prejunctional cholinergic modulation of adrenergic neurotransmission in the cardiovascular system. *Am. J. Physiol.*, 238:H275–H281.
82. Wallentin, I. (1966): Studies on intestinal circulation. *Acta Physiol. Scand. (Suppl.)*, 69(279):1–38.

Control of Capacitance Vessels

Carl F. Rothe

Department of Physiology, Indiana University Medical Center, Indianapolis, Indiana 46223

CHARACTERISTICS OF SPLANCHNIC VASCULAR CAPACITANCE

Splanchnic vascular capacitance contributes to cardiovascular homeostasis by providing, under conditions of stress, a rapid transfer of blood to or from these peripheral vessels to the heart. The influence, similar to a change in total blood volume, changes the end-diastolic volume of the right ventricle and thus may modify cardiac function (see Chapter 13). The nature and importance of active and passive changes in capacitance vessel volume are but cursorily mentioned in current physiology textbooks, but several recent reviews describe and evaluate the role of the venous system (24,26,34,55,57,68). The vasculature of the splanchnic bed contains 20% to 40% of the total blood volume (7,26,27,31,52,70) and so provides a potentially large blood reservoir to contribute importantly in the control of arterial blood pressure and in the compensation for blood pooling or loss (12).

Folkow and Mellander (21) considered the venous system an integrated unit serving the cardiovascular system as a whole, but this simplifying concept may not be true. The large conduit veins and the capacitance vessels of skeletal muscle are less responsive than those of the viscera. Smooth muscles in the walls of cutaneous veins are controlled primarily by thermoregulatory mechanisms (55,57,62,63). Embryological differences in the genesis of the veins of body wall and extremities and the veins of the splanchnic bed may account for differences in responsiveness (37).

Although "splanchnic" refers to all organs within the abdomen, the kidney and reproductive organs are not considered here because relatively little is known about their vascular capacitance properties. Only a small fraction of the total blood volume is present in these organs. The gravid uterus and placenta, however, are potentially of great importance. Because the venous outflow of the intestinal tract, stomach, and spleen go to the liver via the portal vein, the vascular resistances of the liver and pressures in the liver markedly influence the blood volume in these organs. Rowell (Chapter 13), Donald (15,16), and Greenway (26) have recently reviewed the circulation of the splanchnic bed.

Vascular capacitance is not easily quantified (34,55,56). Blood vessels contain blood at zero transmural pressure. This is the unstressed volume. In practice, it is estimated by extrapolation of the pressure-volume relationship under the operating conditions to zero transmural pressure (Fig. 1). This is feasible because the intestinal vascular pressure-volume relationship is reasonably linear over a venous pressure range of 3 to 35 mm Hg (58). Increasing the transmural pressure distends the vessels. The slope of the volume-pressure relationship is the compliance (C) at a specific transmural pressure:

$$C = \Delta V / \Delta P$$

For comparison to other studies, the unit of compliance should be normalized to a kilogram of tissue or body weight. The vascular capacity (in ml/kg tissue) is the unstressed volume plus the product of the distending pressure and compliance, if the compliance may reasonably be considered constant over the physiological range.

Blood volume compensation by the veins occurs by two major mechanisms: (a) *passive* elastic recoil or distension related to changes in transmural pressure from changes in upstream or downstream pressure or from changes in flow

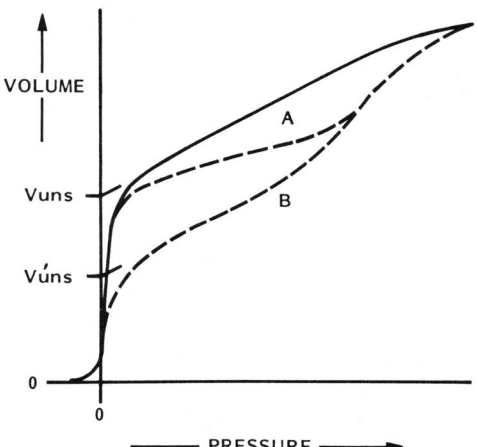

FIG. 1. Vascular pressure-volume relationship. Vuns is the unstressed volume, calculated by linear extrapolation of the pressure-volume curve to the volume at zero transmural pressure. *(A)* Relationship from venoconstriction that causes a reduced compliance without a change in unstressed volume. *(B)* Relationship from venoconstriction that causes a reduced unstressed volume (V'uns) without a change in compliance (slope of curve) over the physiologic pressure range. (From Rothe, ref. 56, with permission.)

and (b) *active* venoconstriction or venodilation from changes in vascular smooth muscle tension.

Active venoconstriction, induced by sympathetic nerve activity or circulating catecholamines or other vasoactive drugs, increases vessel wall tension that increases transmural pressure or decreases contained volume, or produces some combination of both. As shown in Fig. 1, active venoconstriction may cause a decrease in compliance with no change in unstressed volume, as shown by curve A or it may cause a decrease in unstressed volume (to V' uns) with no change in compliance over the normal venous pressure range, as shown by curve B. Typically, some combination of both reduced compliance and reduced unstressed volume occurs. Experimental evidence clearly indicates that active venoconstriction can reduce unstressed volume with little change in vascular compliance (e.g., 69). Thus, a measure of the volume response to a test change in venous pressure, that is, the compliance, does not adequately measure the magnitude of active vascular changes. Possible changes in unstressed volume must also be measured (34,55–57). Measuring dynamic changes in *total* blood volume or the volume of any organ is difficult.

Because there is a finite resistance to blood flow along the vasculature between the right atrium and the major capacitance vessels buried within the tissue of various organs, a change in flow changes the pressure gradient along the vessels and thus alters the internal pressure in the upstream small veins and venules. The magnitude depends on concomitant changes in downstream pressure. As a consequence, there is a passive elastic distension or recoil. The passive flow effect on vascular volume is large and important. A rapid (less than 30 sec) hemorrhage of about 25 ml/kg will reduce the normal canine cardiac output of about 125 ml/kg-min to zero by reducing the effective filling pressure to zero (18,59). Assuming a linear relationship, this amounts to about 0.2 ml/1 ml/min change in flow. The 25 ml/kg of hemorrhaged blood comes primarily from passive elastic recoil of the vasculature and heart. Some reflex venoconstriction occurs during the approximately 30 sec required for a massive hemorrhage. With reflexes blocked by hexamethonium and cardiac output controlled with a pump, Numao and Iriuchijima (49) reported a sensitivity to the flow of about 0.25 ml/ml/min. With reflexes intact, compensation occurs, and so the vascular volume changed nearly 0.5 ml/1 ml/min of forced change in cardiac output (49). The passive flow effect for the splanchnic bed is about 0.2 ml/ml/min (9,15). Increasing the resistance to inflow to the splanchnic bed, to reduce the blood inflow, allows up to 40% of the contained volume to be expelled by passive elastic recoil (15). For the liver, the flow effect averages 0.066 ml/ml/min (3). For segments of the small intestine, it averages 0.061 ml/ ml/min (60).

Increased sympathetic outflow does not necessarily reduce flow as vascular volume is actively changed. Liver lobe thickness of unanesthetized dogs does not change with exercise (29). Changing carotid sinus pressure of vagotomized dogs between 240 and 40 mm Hg induced a 36% reduction in liver volume, a 167 mm Hg increase in arterial blood pressure, a 26% increase in hepatic arterial flow, and only a 3% increase in portal venous flow. The flow changes were opposite to the direction of volume change, because vascular resistance changed relatively less than the arterial pressure (11). Thus, volume can be decreased even though the flow increases. With a more physiologic stress, such as hemorrhage, the arterial pressure decrease would cause the withdrawal of carotid sinus activity and an increased sympathetic outflow. Thus, the passive effect of a flow reduction would add to the active reduction in hepatic vascular volume.

In summary, blood volume compensation can occur by passive or active mechanisms acting on the splanchnic blood vessels. Both appear to be important. Active changes in venous tone result from changes in compliance or unstressed volume. Changes in vascular compliance seem to be minor.

Because the densities of blood, tissue, and tissue fluids are similar and because the walls of the abdomen hold the contents in a similar position as posture is changed, the effect of gravity is minimized relative to the large effect on capacitance vessels of the limbs. On the other hand, diaphragmatic and abdominal wall muscle contraction will increase the pressure on the abdominal contents to impede the entering flow of blood and aid outflow to the heart. In the intact active animal, changes in peritoneal pressure can have marked influence on the volume of blood in the splanchnic bed. How much is not known.

Electrical stimulation of the splanchnic nerves of cats causes nearly 30% of the splanchnic volume to be mobilized (26). This volume accounts for about 10% of the total blood volume. Stimulating the left thoracic splanchnic nerve of dogs at 15 Hz expels about 15 ml/kg BW of blood from the abdomen (8). The response is rapid, with more than half being expelled within 30 sec. Because stimulation at 2 Hz causes the mobilization of about 75% of this volume, it would appear that the normal sympathetic nerve activity is low (8). However, the vascular smooth muscle response to synchronous electrical stimulation may differ markedly from that of naturally occurring sympathetic activity. Even at 6 Hz, an active plus passive expulsion of about 110 ml blood/kg liver (about half the total) was found in dogs and cats (28). The spleen of the dog contributes a large (ca. 30%) fraction of the active response to sympathetic stimulation (10,17,69). However, the spleen of humans and cats is less important than in dogs as a blood reservoir.

Following *hemorrhage* in humans, about 50% of the lost volume comes from the splanchnic bed (52). In dogs, nearly 70% of the blood volume lost is from the splanchnic bed (8,26,27). In cats, the liver and intestines contribute about 50% of the blood volume change during hemorrhage or transfusion (26,27). However, in response to hemorrhage of dogs, only about 14% of the shed volume comes from the liver (10). Much of this is from passive elastic recoil related to reduced flow and pressure. In people subjected to stress such as standing, exercise, hemorrhage or hyperthermia, reflex change in splanchnic blood flow and thus passive capacitance vessel compensation appear to be more important than in dogs (61–63,70, Chapter 13).

Changing the *carotid sinus pressures* between about 50 and 250 mm Hg elicits a 5 to 6 ml/kg body weight increase in abdominal volume (8,31,43). In vagotomized dogs with autoperfused livers, decreasing the carotid sinus pressure in steps from 240 to 40 mm Hg induced a 4.9 ml/kg body weight hepatic blood volume decrease (11). Most of this volume reduction was considered by Carneiro and Donald (11) to be from active decreases in vascular volume that could be independent of decreases in blood flow. Under other conditions, the passive flow effect accounts for two-thirds of the total (9,15). Because the splanchnic blood volume change was only half of that induced by maximal splanchnic nerve stimulation (11,15), there may be other types of stress that could elicit a larger capacitance vessel response. Although the majority of the overall capacitance vessel response to canine carotid sinus pressure changes appears to be in the splanchnic bed (31), a maximal total circulatory response of about 12 ml/kg body weight suggests that other beds, such as the cardiopulmonary, are also important.

In dogs, stimulating the carotid or aortic chemoreceptors with venous blood elicits a small venoconstriction (ca. 1 ml/kg) of the abdominal vasculature as well as vasoconstriction (e.g., 32,33).

In humans, changes in splanchnic vascular conductance during stress are large, accounting for about a third of the change in total peripheral conductance (39,64,65). The flow change presumably induces a large volume redistribution. With progressively greater lower body negative pressure, the splanchnic blood flow starts to decrease with a decrease in right atrial pressure but before a significant change in mean or pulsatile aortic blood pressure, suggesting a sensitive cardiopulmonary volume receptor system (39).

The *cardiopulmonary receptors* contribute about 37% of the total hepatic volume decrease induced by withdrawal of both carotid and cardiopulmonary receptor inhibition of sympathetic outflow (11). Stimulation of high-threshold afferent fibers in the vagi of cats at 2 to 4 Hz caused hepatic vascular dilation that was abolished by cutting the splanchnic nerves. Balloon inflation in the left atrium or ventricle had no effect (26). Quantitative data relating changes in atrial pressure to splanchnic capacitance responses are not yet available. As Greenway (26) has noted, advances in our understanding of the reflex control of splanchnic blood volume reservoir await techniques for measuring this volume with minimal surgical intervention and anesthetic attenuation.

INTESTINAL VASCULAR CAPACITANCE

Because the intestinal tract changes in function and character between the stomach and anus and because the muscularis function is so different from that of the mucosal layer, intestinal vascular capacitive functions may also vary along the length of the intestinal bed.

Intestinal Volume

The intestinal bed comprises about 5% to 6% of the body weight (27). In dogs, the duodenum to descending colon weight averaged 2.8% of the body weight (17). The intestinal blood content of monkeys, dogs, cats, and rats is, at zero arterial and venous pressures, about 40 ml/kg of tissue (1,19). Indicator dilution techniques, used at normal arterial and venous pressures, suggest that the small intestinal blood volume is about 100 ml/kg body weight (10,33,51,58,60). In the dog ileum perfused at about 1,000 ml/min-kg tissue weight, the blood volume averaged 174 ml/kg of tissue (17). Using an erythrocyte washout method, the volume was estimated as 149 ml/kg (17). Estimates as high as 290 ml/kg (36) and 390 ml/kg (14) tissue have been reported. Greenway et al. (27) assumed 10% of the total blood volume to be in the intestinal bed; Horvath et al. (36) estimated that 40% of splanchnic blood volume and 8.7% of the total blood volume was in the mesenteric bed. The intestinal bed is a blood reservoir of potential but uncertain magnitude.

Intestinal Compliance: Passive Effects

The vascular compliance of segments of canine small intestine is about 2.5 ml/mm Hg-kg tissue weight (38,41,47,58,60,67), a value similar to that of the systemic vasculature as a whole (55). The pressure-volume relationship over the physiologic range of pressures (5–25 mm Hg) is remarkably linear (41,47,58). Our studies, which used the mean transit time of indocyanine-green-labeled blood proteins, suggest a zero-flow intestinal volume of about 60 ml/kg tissue. This was obtained by a quadratic extrapolation of blood volume to zero flow at a venous pressure of 10 mm Hg (60). Because the vascular volume is about 100 ml/kg tissue at normal flows, the difference (100 − 60 = 40 ml/kg) is the amount of blood available by passive recoil when blood flow is stopped (17,60). Yet more blood may be expelled from the intestinal bed (10 mm Hg times 2.5 ml/mm Hg-kg = 25 ml/kg) when the portal venous pressure is reduced to zero. The blood remaining

$(100 - 40 - 25 = 35$ ml/kg) is the unstressed volume. Thus, about two-thirds of the blood volume of the intestine may be expelled by passive elastic recoil if flow and pressure are reduced to zero. Under control conditions, the effect of flow changes on intestinal blood volume may be predicted with a linear equation (60):

Volume (ml/kg tissue) = 74.3 (ml/kg) + 0.061 Flow (ml/min-kg)

Studies of vascular compliance are complicated by the difficulty of partitioning an estimated volume change between the blood volume distending the vasculature and the volume of fluid crossing capillaries into the interstitial space (25,58). The vascular volume change is virtually complete in 30 sec or less, whereas transcapillary filtration is slower. Stress relaxation or contraction of the vessel walls is also slow, but this delayed compliance (stress-relaxation) accounts for only 15% to 20% of the volume change at 10 min following a change in canine intestinal venous pressure (38). In these studies, an indicator dilution technique was used to measure the vascular volume.

Estimating the pressure drop from the outlet vein to the capacitance vessels is uncertain (58). The investigator cannot assume that 100% of a venous pressure change is transmitted to the capacitance vessels. In fact, Johnson (40), using autoperfused dog small intestine, found that only 62% of a small venous pressure change is transmitted to the capillaries. The major capacitance vessels are downstream from the capillaries. Thus, an appreciably higher fraction of a pressure change must be transmitted to them. At high pressures, effective venous conductance increases because the diameters of the vessels are increased. Thus, a greater fraction of a pressure change is transmitted upstream. However, Johnson's equation ($P_{cap} = 9.7 + 0.62\ P_V$) suggests that, at a venous pressure (P_V) of 25.5 mm Hg, the canine intestinal capillary pressure (P_{cap}) will also be 25.5 mm Hg, and so the venous resistance would have to be zero. Mortillaro and Taylor (48) reported for cat intestine an equation with an intercept of 9.3 mm Hg and a slope of 0.69. This equation predicts that the capillary pressure equals the venous pressure at 30 mm Hg. With no pressure drop from capillaries to veins and continuing blood flow, the venous resistance must be zero. Other mechanisms must be involved at venous pressures greater than about 25 mm Hg, because this conclusion is not reasonable. The pressure drop from mucosal or muscularis capillaries to small veins of rat intestine is only 3 to 5 mm Hg (4,23). Schmid-Schönbein (66) suggests that the majority of the postcapillary resistance is in the immediate postcapillary venules, whereas the pressure drop across the larger venules and small veins, continuing over 40% of the total blood volume, is much less. Thus, at least 80% and possibly over 90% of a change in conduit vein pressure is transmitted to the capacitance vessels within an organ (58).

Gore and Bohlen (22) found that the cat mesentery capillary pressure was relatively insensitive to changes in systemic arterial pressure. This would suggest that the mechanism acting to maintain a constant capillary pressure, as arterial pressure is changed, would tend to maintain the venular pressure in these vessels also.

Stimulation of Sympathetic Nerves

Maximal sympathetic stimulation may mobilize 4% of the *total body* blood volume from the intestinal bed, as Greenway and Lister have reported (27), but others suggested only 2% as the maximum (16). Intestinal vasoconstriction, by reducing portal vein blood flow and portal venous pressure, may be equally important in the passive mobilization of blood from the compliant vasculature of the liver.

Stimulation of the sympathetic nerves of cat intestine can expel up to 40% of the contained volume (20). With dog ileum stimulated maximally at 15 Hz, 56% (105 ml blood/kg tissue) was expelled (17). At a stimulation rate of 2 Hz, only 27% of the maximal amount was expelled. Constriction of the intestinal veins is by a combination of active venoconstriction and passive elastic recoil related to the reduced blood flow. In contrast to the autoregulatory escape of the resistance vessels, venoconstriction is maintained throughout a 5- to 10-min stimulation period (8,16,17,50) but not indefinitely (46). Using constant flow perfusion and supramaximal sympathetic stimulation, the amount of blood that can be expelled increases, if the inflow is increased (17).

Stimulation of sympathetic nerve to rat small intestine at 4 to 16 Hz caused a 5% to 15% reduction in venular diameter (5). There was little change in venular pressure with low-frequency stimulation (4 and 8 Hz) that caused 10% reductions in venular diameter (and a 20% reduction in volume). At 16 Hz, the diameter reduction was about 15% (28% volume reduction), but some of the reduced diameter would have been related to the reduced pressure from arteriolar constriction and reduced flow.

Reflex Control of Intestinal Capacitance

In 1918, Hooker (35) studied the canine large intestine and found that stimulation of sensory nerves, nerves to intestine, or asphyxia caused an elevation of venous pressure during periods when both arteries and veins were clamped. Öberg (50), in 1964, reported that a reduction in carotid sinus pressure in cats induced a larger change in intestinal blood volume per kilogram of tissue than in hindquarter blood volume, but further studies led to the conclusion that the intestinal veins are only moderately involved in the baroreceptor reflexes (30). Bilateral carotid occlusion induced only an 0.7 ml/kg tissue (5.5%) decrease in intestinal blood volume, but the mesenteric venous pressure increased 2 mm Hg (10). This would tend to increase the blood volume passively. Chemoreceptor stimulation causes a reflex constriction of the portal vein (2). Stimulation of the hypothalamic "defence" area of cats caused expulsion of 30% to 40% of the intestinal blood volume (13). Carotid occlusion of the rat seems to have no effect on intestinal venular diameters (6).

From his review of the literature, Lautt (45) has tentatively concluded that the arterial baroreceptors do not activate the venous smooth muscles of the intestines of dogs and cats. To date, however, no quantitative data are available in any species relating active venoconstriction of the intestinal bed to various carotid sinus or aortic arch pressures, or to changes in blood pH or gas composition.

Myogenic and *venoarteriolar* responses of the intestinal vasculature are covered in Chapter 4.

Hemorrhage

The intestinal capacitance vessels are not critically involved in irreversible hemorrhagic shock. A lack of consistent weight change of a vascularly isolated segment of canine small intestine led Johnson and Selkurt (42) to conclude that intravascular pooling of blood is not a necessary feature of hemorrhagic shock. However, they and others found sloughing of mucosal cells, frank hemorrhage, and fluid losses (42,53,54).

In response to hemorrhage, about 5% to 7% of the shed blood volume comes from the canine intestinal bed compared to about 15% of the shed volume coming from the liver and about 30% from the spleen. The change in intestinal blood volume in response to severe hemorrhage is about 10 times that from carotid occlusion (10). In the cat, the intestinal tract contributes about 30% of the hemorrhaged volume (27). In both species, the splanchnic bed contributes about half of the shed blood. Both resistance and capacitance responses appear to wane in the intestine of cats subjected to prolonged severe hemorrhagic hypotension (46). During hemorrhage, venules of rat intestine constrict (6), but this may be a passive response to reduced flow.

In summary, the intestinal bed provides a small, but significant, reservoir function to compensate for blood volume changes.

Drugs and Hormones

Norepinephrine infusions (50 μg/min-kg tissue) cause a 13 to 15 ml/kg decrease in contained intestinal blood volume at a constant flow and only a small reduction in vascular compliance (38,60). Norepinephrine may cause the capacitance vessels of cats to dilate as well as to constrict, depending on the initial venous pressure (44). Blocking beta-receptors with propranolol has no effect, but alpha blockade with dihydroergotoxin elicits dilatory responses only, especially in the range of 10 to 15 mm Hg.

Isoproterenol (100 µg/liter blood) causes a 242% increase in canine vascular conductance, but only a small (12%) increase in volume and no change in compliance at constant flow (60).

Papaverine (2 mg/min-kg tissue) increases the unstressed volume of canine jejunal segments by 38 ml/kg tissue, but induces little change in compliance (38).

Areas of Future Research

Although the intestinal capacitance vessels apparently contribute to arterial pressoreceptor, cardiopulmonary volume receptor, and chemoreceptor reflexes, quantitative details are sparse. Because of the large reservoir capacity of the liver, compared to the intestinal bed, the entire splanchnic bed should be studied as a whole to quantify the importance of these tissues in cardiovascular homeotasis. Furthermore, because the spleen of the dog is so large, relative to that of most species (16,55,57), it should be excluded or its contribution evaluated separately if dogs are used.

The role of spinal reflexes or myogenic responses of the capacitance vessels of the intestinal bed is unknown. The quantitative effect of changes in peritoneal pressure on blood volume distribution is unclear.

Very little is known about reflex control of the splanchnic vascular capacitance without anesthesia. In humans, splanchnic compensation seems to be important during hemorrhage, exercise, or heat loads, but few measures of changes in splanchnic vascular volume have been made (52,70). An accurate, atraumatic technique for the measure of splanchnic vascular volume is needed.

ACKNOWLEDGMENTS

The suggestions and advice of my colleagues are gratefully acknowledged, as is the help of Helen Glancy. The project was supported in part by US PHS grant HL07723.

REFERENCES

1. Altman, P. L., and Dittmer, D. S. (1971): *Respiration and Circulation*, pp. 383–385. Fed. Am. Soc. Exp. Biol., Bethesda.
2. Auden, R. M., and Donald, D. E. (1975): Reflex responses of the isolated in situ portal vein of the dog. *J. Surg. Res.*, 18:35–42.
3. Bennett, T. D., and Rothe, C. F. (1981): Hepatic capacitance responses to changes in flow and hepatic venous pressure in dogs. *Am. J. Physiol.*, 240:H18–H28.
4. Bohlen, H. G., and Gore, R. W. (1977): Comparison of microvascular pressures and diameters in the innervated and denervated rat intestine. *Microvasc. Res.*, 14:251–264.
5. Bohlen, H. G., and Gore, R. W. (1979): Microvascular pressures in rat intestinal muscle during direct nerve stimulation. *Microvasc. Res.*, 17:27–37.
6. Bohlen, H. G., Hutchins, P. M., Rapela, C. E., and Green, H. D. (1975): Microvascular control in intestinal mucosa of normal and hemorrhaged rats. *Am. J. Physiol.*, 229:1159–1164.
7. Bradley, S. E., Marks, P. A., Reynell, P. C., and Meltzer, J. (1953): Circulating splanchnic blood volume in dog and man. *Trans. Assoc. Am. Physicians*, 66:294–302.
8. Brooksby, G. A., and Donald, D. E. (1971): Dynamic changes in splanchnic blood flow and blood volume in dogs during activation of sympathetic nerves. *Circ. Res.*, 29:227–238.
9. Brooksby, G. A., and Donald, D. E. (1972): Release of blood from the splanchnic circulation in dogs. *Circ. Res.*, 31:105–118.
10. Carneiro, J. J., and Donald, D. E. (1977): Blood reservoir function of dog spleen, liver, and intestine. *Am. J. Physiol.*, 232:H67–H72.
11. Carneiro, J. J., and Donald, D. E. (1977): Change in liver blood flow and blood content in dogs during direct and reflex alteration of hepatic sympathetic nerve activity. *Circ. Res.*, 40:150–158.
12. Chien, S. (1967): Role of the sympathetic nervous system in hemorrhage. *Physiol. Rev.*, 47:214–288.
13. Cobbold, A., Folkow, B., Lundgren, O., and Wallentin, I. (1964): Blood flow, capillary filtration coefficients and regional blood volume responses in the intestine of the cat during stimulation of the hypothalamic 'defence' area. *Acta Physiol. Scand.*, 61:467–475.
14. Delorme, E. J., Macpherson, A. I. S., Mukherjee, S. R., and Rowlands, S. (1951): Measurement of the visceral blood volume in dogs. *Q. J. Exp. Physiol.*, 36:219–231.
15. Donald, D. E. (1981): Mobilization of blood from the splanchnic circulation. In: *Hepatic Circulation in Health and Disease*, edited by W. W. Lautt, pp. 193–202. Raven Press, New York.
16. Donald, D. E. (1983): Splanchnic circulation. In: *Handbook of Physiology, The Cardiovascular System*, edited by J. T. Shepherd and F. M. Abboud, sect. 2, vol. III, chapt. 7, pp. 219–240. American Physiological Society, Bethesda.
17. Donald, D. E., and Aarhus, L. L. (1974): Active and passive release of blood from canine spleen and small intestine. *Am. J. Physiol.*, 227:1166–1172.

18. Drees, J. A., and Rothe, C. F. (1974): Reflex venoconstriction and capacity vessel pressure-volume relationships in dogs. *Circ. Res.*, 34:360–373.
19. Everett, N. B., Simmons, B., and Lasher, E. P. (1956): Distribution of blood (Fe^{59}) and plasma (I^{131}) volumes of rats determined by liquid nitrogen freezing. *Circ. Res.*, 4:419–424.
20. Folkow, B., Lewis, D. H., Lundgren, O., Mellander, S., and Wallentin, I. (1964): The effect of graded vasoconstrictor fibre stimulation on the intestinal resistance and capacitance vessels. *Acta Physiol. Scand.*, 61:445–457.
21. Folkow, B., and Mellander, S. (1964): Veins and venous tone. *Am. Heart J.*, 68:397–408.
22. Gore, R. W., and Bohlen, H. G. (1975): Pressure regulation in the microcirculation. *Fed. Proc.*, 34:2031–2037.
23. Gore, R. W., and Bohlen, H. G. (1977): Microvascular pressures in rat intestinal muscle and mucosal villi. *Am. J. Physiol.*, 233:H685–H693.
24. Gow, B. S. (1980): Circulatory correlates: Vascular impedance, resistance, and capacity. In: *Handbook of Physiology. The Cardiovascular System*, edited by D. F. Bohr, A. P. Somlyo, and H. V. Sparks, Jr., sect. 2, vol. II, chapt. 14, pp. 353–408. American Physiological Society, Bethesda.
25. Granger, D. N., Richardson, P. D. I., and Taylor, A. E. (1979): Volumetric assessment of the capillary filtration coefficient in the cat small intestine. *Pflüegers Arch.*, 381:25–33.
26. Greenway, C. V. (1983): Role of splanchnic venous system in overall cardiovascular homeostasis. *Fed. Proc.*, 42:1678–1684.
27. Greenway, C. V., and Lister, G. E. (1974): Capacitance effects and blood reservoir function in the splanchnic vascular bed during non-hypotensive haemorrhage and blood volume expansion in anaesthetized cats. *J. Physiol.*, 237:279–294.
28. Greenway, C. V., and Oshiro, G. (1972): Comparison of the effects of hepatic nerve stimulation on arterial flow, distribution of arterial and portal flows and blood content in the livers of anaesthetized cats and dogs. *J. Physiol.*, 227:487–501.
29. Guntheroth, W. G., and Mullins, G. L. (1963): Liver and spleen as venous reservoirs. *Am. J. Physiol.*, 204:35–41.
30. Hadjiminas, J., and Öberg, B. (1968): Effects of carotid baroreceptor reflexes on venous tone in skeletal muscle and intestine of the cat. *Acta Physiol. Scand.*, 72:518–532.
31. Hainsworth, R., and Karim, F. (1976): Responses of abdominal vascular capacitance in the anaesthetized dog to changes in carotid sinus pressure. *J. Physiol.*, 262:659–677.
32. Hainsworth, R., Karim, F., McGregor, K. H., and Rankin, A. J. (1983): Effects of stimulation of aortic chemoreceptors on abdominal vascular resistance and capacitance in anaesthetized dogs. *J. Physiol.*, 334:421–431.
33. Hainsworth, R., Karim, F., McGregor, K. H., and Wood, L. M. (1983): Response of abdominal vascular resistance and capacitance to stimulation of carotid chemoreceptors in anaesthetized dogs. *J. Physiol.*, 334:409–419.
34. Hainsworth, R., and Linden, R. J. (1979): Reflex control of vascular capacitance. In: *Cardiovascular Physiology III*, edited by A. C. Guyton and D. B. Young, chapt. 3, pp. 67–124. University Park Press, Baltimore.
35. Hooker, D. R. (1918): The veno-pressor mechanism. *Am. J. Physiol.*, 46:591–598.
36. Horvath, S. M., Kelly, T., Folk, G. E., Jr., and Hutt, B. K. (1957): Measurement of blood volumes in splanchnic bed of the dog. *Am. J. Physiol.*, 189:573–575.
37. Ishikawa, N., Ichikawa, T., and Shigei, T. (1980): Possible embryogenetical differences of the dog venous system in sensitivity to vasoactive substances. *Jpn. J. Pharmacol.*, 30:807–818.
38. Johns, B. L., and Rothe, C. F. (1978): Delayed vascular compliance and fluid exchange in the canine intestine. *Am. J. Physiol.*, 234:H660–H669.
39. Johnson, J. M., Rowell, L. B., Niederberger, M., and Eisman, M. M. (1974): Human splanchnic and forearm vasoconstrictor responses to reductions of right atrial and aortic pressures. *Circ. Res.*, 34:515–524.
40. Johnson, P. C. (1965): Effect of venous pressure on mean capillary pressure and vascular resistance in the intestine. *Circ. Res.*, 16:294–300.
41. Johnson, P. C., and Hanson, K. M. (1963): Relation between venous pressure and blood volume in the intestine. *Am. J. Physiol.*, 204:31–34.
42. Johnson, P. C., and Selkurt, E. E. (1958): Intestinal weight changes in hemorrhagic shock. *Am. J. Physiol.*, 193:135–143.
43. Karim, F., Hainsworth, R., and Pandey, R. P. (1978): Reflex responses of abdominal vascular capacitance from aortic baroreceptors in dogs. *Am. J. Physiol.*, 235:H488–H493.
44. Kudriashov, Y. A. (1977): Peripheral mechanisms of the small intestine capacitance vessel responses to noradrenalin. *Sechenov Physiol. J. USSR*, 63:557–564.
45. Lautt, W. W. (1980): Hepatic nerves: A review of their functions and effects. *Can. J. Physiol. Pharmacol.*, 58:105–123.
46. Lundgren, O. (1983): Role of splanchnic resistance vessels in overall cardiovascular homeostasis. *Fed. Proc.*, 42:1673–1677.
47. Lutz, J. (1969): Hämodynamische Eigenschaften und Gefässreaktionen der intestinalen Strombahn. *Arch. Kreislauff.*, 59:99–152.
48. Mortillaro, N. A., and Taylor, A. E. (1976): Interaction of capillary and tissue forces in the cat small intestine. *Circ. Res.*, 39:348–358.
49. Numao, Y., and Iriuchijima, J. (1977): Effect of cardiac output on circulatory blood volume. *Jpn. J. Physiol.*, 27:145–156.
50. Öberg, B. (1964): Effects of cardiovascular reflexes on net capillary fluid transfer. *Acta Physiol. Scand.*, 62:S229:1–98.
51. Polosa, C., and Hamilton, W. F. (1963): Blood volume and intravascular hematocrit in different vascular beds. *Am. J. Physiol.*, 204:903–909.
52. Price, H. L., Deutsch, S., Marshall, B. E., Stephen, G. W., Behar, M. G., and Neufeld, G. R. (1966): Hemodynamic and metabolic effects of hemorrhage

in man, with particular reference to the splanchnic circulation. *Circ. Res.*, 18:469–474.
53. Rothe, C. F. (1966): Cardiac and peripheral failure in hemorrhagic shock treated with massive transfusions. *Am. J. Physiol.*, 210:1347–1361.
54. Rothe, C. F. (1970): Heart failure and fluid loss in hemorrhagic shock. *Fed. Proc.*, 29:1854–1860.
55. Rothe, C. F. (1983): The venous system; physiology of the capacitance vessels. In: *Handbook of Physiology. The Cardiovascular System*, edited by J. T. Shepherd and F. M. Abboud, sect. 2, vol. III, chapt. 13, pp. 397–452. American Physiological Society, Bethesda.
56. Rothe, C. F. (1983): Measurement of circulatory capacitance and resistance. In: *Techniques in the Life Sciences*, Cardiovascular Physiology (Vol. P3), edited by P. J. Linden. Elsevier, Amsterdam. *(In press).*
57. Rothe, C. F. (1984): Reflex control of the veins and vascular capacitance. *Physiol. Rev. (In press).*
58. Rothe, C. F., Bennett, T. D., and Johns, B. L. (1980): Linearity of the vascular pressure-volume relationship of the canine intestine. *Circ. Res.*, 47:551–558.
59. Rothe, C. F., and Drees, J. A. (1976): Vascular capacitance and fluid shifts in dogs during prolonged hemorrhagic hypotension. *Circ. Res.*, 38:347–356.
60. Rothe, C. F., Johns, B. L., and Bennett, T. D. (1978): Vascular capacitance of dog intestine using mean transit time of indicator. *Am. J. Physiol.*, 234:H7–H13.
61. Rowell, L. B. (1973): Regulation of splanchnic blood flow in man. *Physiologist*, 16:127–142.
62. Rowell, L. B. (1974): Human cardiovascular adjustments to exercise and thermal stress. *Physiol. Rev.*, 54:75–159.
63. Rowell, L. B. (1975): The splanchnic circulation. In: *The Peripheral Circulations*, edited by R. Zelis, pp. 163–192. Grune & Stratton, New York.
64. Rowell, L. B. (1983): Cardiovascular aspects of human thermoregulation. *Circ. Res.*, 52:367–379.
65. Rowell, L. B., Detry, J.-M. R., Blackmon, J. R., and Wyss, C. (1972): Importance of the splanchnic vascular bed in human blood pressure regulation. *J. Appl. Physiol.*, 32:213–220.
66. Schmid-Schönbein, H. (1972): Blood rheology in the microcirculation. *Pflüegers Arch.*, 336:S84–S87.
67. Selkurt, E. E., and Johnson, P. C. (1958): Effect of acute elevation of portal venous pressure on mesenteric blood volume, interstitial fluid volume and hemodynamics. *Circ. Res.*, 6:592–599.
68. Shepherd, J. T., and Vanhoutte, P. M. (1975): *Veins and Their Control*. Saunders, Philadelphia.
69. Shoukas, A. A., MacAnespie, C. L., Brunner, M. J. and Watermeier, L. (1981): The importance of the spleen in blood volume shifts of the systemic vascular bed caused by the carotid sinus baroreceptor reflex in the dog. *Circ. Res.*, 49:759–766.
70. Wade, O. L., Combes, B., Childs, A. W., Wheeler, H. O., Cournand, A., and Bradley, S. E. (1956): The effect of exercise on the splanchnic blood flow and splanchnic blood volume in normal man. *Clin. Sci.*, 15:457–463.

Countercurrent Exchange Mechanisms in the Small Intestine

*Mats Jodal, **Ulf Haglund, and *Ove Lundgren

*Department of Physiology, University of Göteborg, S-400 33 Göteborg, Sweden; and **Department of Surgery, University of Lund, Malmö General Hospital, S-214 01 Malmö, Sweden

The existence of a countercurrent exchanger in the small intestine is based on the vascular arrangement in the villi. Therefore, in the first part of this chapter the vascular anatomy in different mammals is surveyed. The functional implications of the exchanger are reviewed in the remainder of the chapter.

ANATOMICAL CONSIDERATIONS

The shape of the intestinal villus varies in different species from a slender finger-like structure to a broad-based leaf-like appearance. However, the basic vascular arrangement, described as "fountain-like" by Spanner (52), is similar in all types of animals studied, including man (see Fig. 1). This vascular arrangement was described in the classical works by Heller (24), Mall (43), and Spanner (52) [for a review, see Patzelt (45)]. Their findings have been confirmed in later reports (27,56,58). The arterial supply to the villus is composed of one or two vessels originating from the submucosal vascular network. These vessels run unbranched centrally in the lamina propria (43), and they lack a smooth muscle coat in the upper two-thirds of the villus (Fig. 2). At the villus tip, the arterial vessels branch into a dense subepithelial capillary network that collects into venules at different levels in the villus (Fig. 1).

Some reports concerning monkey (46), dog (22), mouse (8), and cat (9) give a picture of the vascular anatomy that is opposite to the one described above. According to these reports, several arteries arborize at the villus base into a subepithelial capillary network that, close to the villus tip, converges into a central draining vein. However, with the possible exception of monkey (46), the evidence favors the concept of a central arterial supply. It should be stressed, however, that the functional implications described below are identical regardless of whether the central vessel is an arterial or a venous one. Thus, the discussions below are carried out assuming the central vessel to be arterial.

From this description, it seems clear that the villus vascular anatomy principally is a hairpin arrangement in which the main directions of the blood flow in the two limbs of the loop are opposite to each other (Fig. 1). This also holds true when the basal parts of the villus may receive their arterial supply from the crypt capillary network as proposed by Ganon et al. (14,15). However, such a blood flow pattern is consistent neither with the capillary P_{O_2} values measured along the villus by Bohlen (4) nor with the model for villus blood flow proposed by Levitt et al. (37). Therefore, the anatomical prerequisites for a villus countercurrent exchanger may exist in all species studied.

The efficiency of a villus countercurrent exchanger depends on several morphological factors, such as the diffusion distances between the two limbs in the exchanger and the surface area and the permeability characteristics of the vessels constituting the countercurrent exchanger (see below). Information is sparse concerning the diffusion distances. Lundgren (40) calculated from histological data reported by Schriever (48) that the intervascular distance in the slender, finger-like feline villi was about 20 μm. In

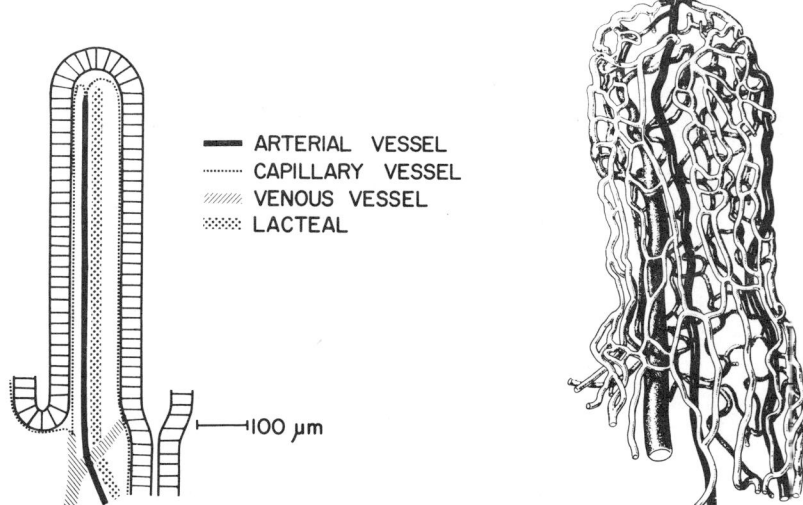

FIG. 1. Schematic vascular anatomy of a cat villus *(left)* and of a human villus *(right)*. In the human villus, *black* denotes arterial vessels and *gray* venous ones. (From Lundgren, ref. 40, and Spanner, ref. 52, with permission.)

other species, such as rabbit and rat, in which the villus cross-section has an ellipsoid form, the mean intervascular distance may be somewhat longer, but precise information is presently not available.

The general permeability characteristics of the villus capillaries resemble those of other organs; the capillaries are highly permeable to lipid-soluble compounds. Thus, the rate of transcapillary diffusion depends mainly on capillary surface area. In the cat, surface area has been calculated to be 2.45 $m^2 \times 100$ g^{-1} villi. The surface area of the central arterial vessel can be estimated to be about 10% of this value (3). The transcapillary movement of water-soluble solutes depends on the presence of water filled "pores" in the capillary wall. Villus capillaries are of the fenestrated type that have been estimated to have a hydraulic conductivity about 20 times greater than the continuous capillaries in the muscularis layer. However, their permeability to large hydrophilic solutes seems to be remarkably similar to continuous capillaries (41). This implies that the size of each pore may be the same in the two types of capillaries, but the number of pores may vary. With regard to intestinal countercurrent exchange, it is also important to point out that the fenestrations of the capillaries always face the epithelial cells (see below). The central arterial vessel of the villus has an intact endothelium with no fenestrae and an intact basal membrane (Fig. 2). Whether or not this vessel possesses an interendothelial "small pore" system is not known.

GENERAL THEORETICAL CONSIDERATIONS

The anatomical description above implies the possible presence of an intestinal countercurrent exchanger in the villi of the species studied. However, if the anatomical structure is to function as a countercurrent exchanger, the time for diffusion must not be too long in relation to mean transit time through the hairpin loops of the villi. The diffusion time is influenced by such factors as exchange area, diffusion distance, and the vascular permeability to the solute in question. In cats, the plasma mean transit times in the villi have been determined with an indicator dilution method (2). Figure 3 shows mean transit times in the central vessel, in the capillary network, and in the whole hairpin loop of cat villi (3,42). The ratio between the blood volumes in the central arterial vessel and the subepithelial capillaries was assumed to be 1:4 at "rest" and 1:9 during vasodilatation induced pharmacologically and during reduced blood flow caused by partial occlusion of the superior mesenteric artery (55). The mean transit times should be compared to the diffusion times in Fig. 4. In this figure, the theoretically calculated times required for reaching diffusion equilibrium between the outer surface of a cylinder and its center are shown for various radii of the cylinder. Diffusion was assumed to occur freely in water, and the diffusion constant was set to 10^{-5} cm^2/sec. The shaded area indicates the mean transit times of plasma in the subepithelial capillary network recorded at varying intestinal blood flows in the cat (Fig. 3).

Comparing Figs. 3 and 4 makes it clear that even at maximal vasodilatation there may be a considerable diffusion exchange from the capillary network to the central vessel. The diffusion equilibrium is facilitated by the fact that the diffusion occurs from the outer surface towards the center of the cylinder. However, the exchange diffusion from the central vessels towards the outer surface of the cylinder is hampered by the short transit time of blood in the central vessel (a small fraction of the overall transit time shown in Fig. 3).

EXPERIMENTAL OBSERVATIONS AND FUNCTIONAL IMPLICATIONS

The extravascular cross-diffusion of a solute in a countercurrent exchanger cannot be demonstrated directly with techniques presently available. Therefore, the possible presence of a countercurrent exchange mechanism in the small intestine (or in any other organ) must be shown indirectly by demonstrating the expected effects of the exchanger. Thus, experimental demonstrations of the functional implications (reviewed below) represent evidence for the countercurrent hypothesis. For each experimental "proof" an alternative explanation may be suggested; however, the countercurrent hypothesis is the only mechanism that adequately explains *all* the experimental findings.

As previously mentioned, countercurrent exchange may take place from the capillary network to the central vessel or vice versa (see Fig. 5). These two types of exchange are discussed separately below.

Diffusion from Capillaries to the Central Arterial Vessel

An easily diffusible solute may be delayed in its net absorption from the lumen if it diffuses from the extensive subepithelial capillary network to the central arterial vessel (*left panel*, Fig. 5). This brings the compound back towards the villus tip and delays its entrance into the venous drainage. Theoretical treatments of intestinal countercurrent exchange with regard to absorption have been performed by Winne (57) and by Levitt et al. (37). In these reports, a simplified arrangement of the intestinal countercurrent exchanger is used to evaluate its importance for absorption of various solutes. Absorption is assumed to take place in the apical part of the villus, and the exchange area is presumed to occur in the lower part of the villus. Winne (57) derived the following equation, which we have modified from his Eq. 33:

$$J_{net} = \frac{C_l - C_p}{\dfrac{1}{k_i A_i} + \dfrac{1}{a\alpha FE} + \dfrac{R}{a\alpha F}}, \quad (1)$$

where

$$E = 1 - e^{-\dfrac{k_c A_c}{a\alpha F}} \quad (2)$$

and

$$R = \frac{P_e A_e}{a\alpha F}. \quad (3)$$

J_{net} = net flux of solute across intestinal epithelium; C = concentration of solute in intestinal lumen (l) and in plasma (p); k = permeability coefficient for solute across intestinal epithelium (i) and capillary wall (c); A = area of intestinal epithelium (i), of capillaries (c), and of exchange area (e); α = fraction of total intestinal blood flow (F) diverted to the "absorptive" mucosa; a = the relationship between the solute

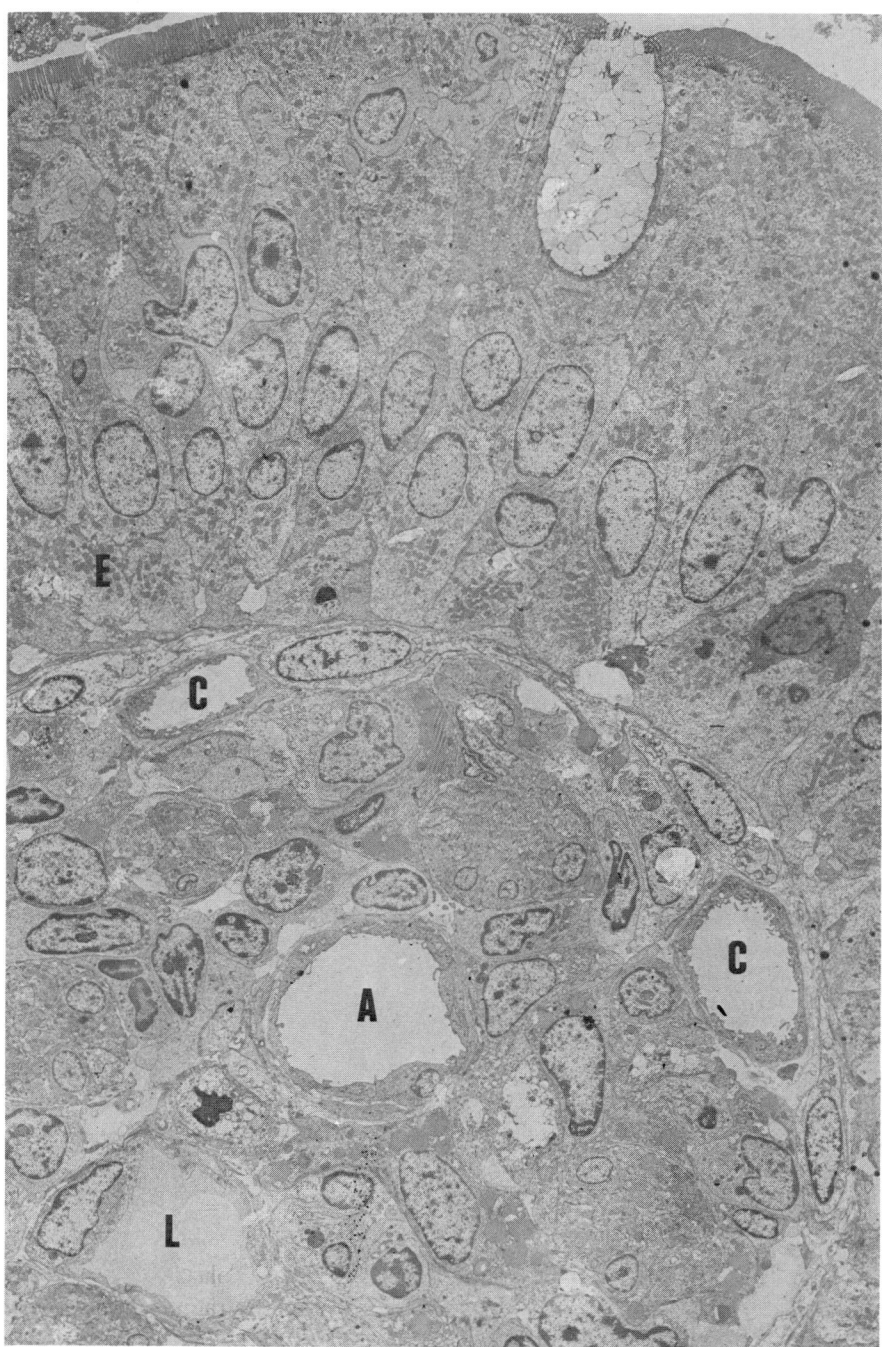

FIG. 2. Left: Low-power electron micrograph of transversely sectioned cat intestinal villus. The figure demonstrates the topographical relationships among the lacteal (L), the central arteriole (A), and the subepithelial capillaries (C). (E) Epithelium. ×1,400. **Right:** Electron micrograph of the central arteriole in a cat intestinal villus sectioned about halfway between tip and base. The vessel lumen is lined by several endothelial cells joined by overlapping junctions *(arrowheads)*. Outside the periendothelial basal lamina *(arrow)*, an incomplete layer of cells (M) appears to be a transition form between smooth muscle cells and pericytes. A felt-like meshwork of filaments *(asterisk)* separates the vessel from the stromal cells of the villus. ×6,200. (The micrographs were produced by Dr. Bengt R. Johansson, Department of Anatomy, University of Göteborg, Sweden.)

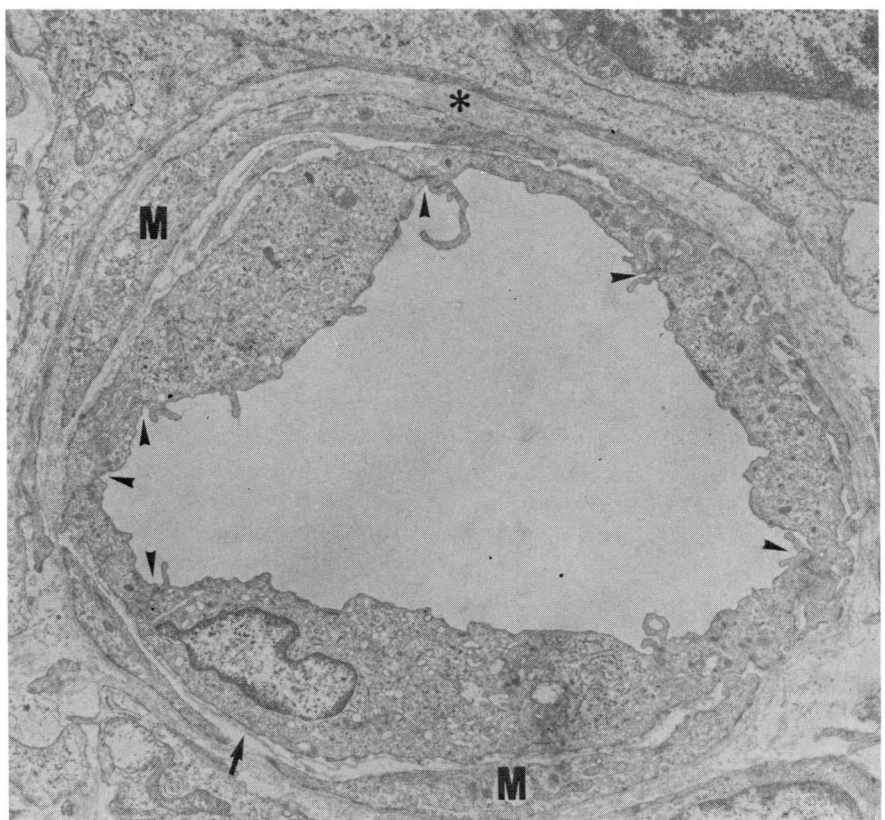

FIG. 2. *(continued)*

concentration in blood to that in plasma; and P_e = permeability coefficient of the exchange region.

Equations 1 to 3 were developed from several assumptions. Transport from the villus was assumed to occur exclusively via the blood stream and the solute was presumed to be metabolically inert. No recirculation of the absorbed solute was considered to take place, that is, C_p was constant. Furthermore, the permeability coefficient for lumen to plasma transport was assumed to be identical to that for transport in the opposite direction. Fluid transfer across the intestinal epithelium was also considered to be negligible when compared to the volume flow of blood in the villi.

Although Eq. 1 may be an oversimplified description of the physiological interaction between the rate of passive solute absorption and blood flow, it does identify some important factors. First, the absorption rate obviously must be proportional to the solute concentration difference between intestinal lumen and capillary. Second, one may look upon the denominator of Eq. 1 as a "resistance" to absorption. Three resistances in series sum to yield the "resistance to absorption." The first factor $(1/k_iA_i)$ represents the epithelial "resistance" to diffusion. The second term $(1/a\alpha FE)$ quantitates the resistance offered by the blood flow and the capillary wall.

Countercurrent exchange represents a third resistance to absorption of passively transported solutes. The more pronounced the exchange (large R) the lower the rate of net absorption is. The extent of exchange, in turn, depends on the area (A_e) and the "permeability" (P_e) of the exchange region. The latter factor is determined by sev-

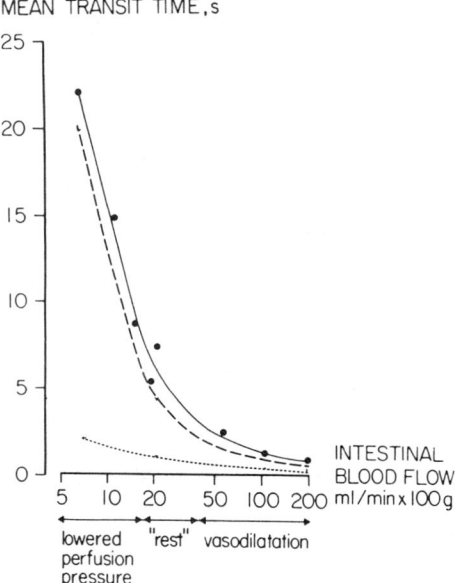

FIG. 3. Plasma mean transit time in cat villi at varying total intestinal blood flows. *(Solid line)* Transit time through the whole villus; it was constructed from actual measurements *(closed circles)* (3,42). *(Dashed line)* Calculated transit time for plasma in the subepithelial capillary network. *(Dotted line)* Corresponding values for transit times in the central arterial vessel. Note that the scale of the abscissa is logarithmic.

eral parameters, such as the intervascular distance and capillary permeability to the solute. Substituting

$$F = \frac{V}{\bar{t}} \quad (4)$$

(V = blood volume; $\bar{t}$ = mean transit time) into the third term in the denominator of Eq. 1 yields

$$\frac{R}{a\alpha F} = \frac{P_e A_e}{a^2 \alpha^2 F^2} = \frac{P_e A_e (\bar{t})^2}{a^2 \alpha^2 V^2}. \quad (5)$$

Equation 5 reveals the importance of the mean transit time for the efficiency of the exchanger. The shorter the mean transit time, the smaller the value of Eq. 5, the less the resistance offered by the exchanger, and the higher the rate of absorption. An increased regional blood volume, according to Eqs. 1 and 5, makes countercurrent exchange of a quickly diffusible solute less efficient in hindering net blood transport. However, a larger blood volume may, in many situations, imply the opening up of more perfused capillaries, which, in turn, may increase the area of the exchange region (A_e) and also reduce the mean diffusion distance (P_e). The interdependence of blood flow and mean transit time makes it difficult to decide which factor is rate-limiting for the absorption of highly diffusible solutes.

The first experimental evidence for a countercurrent "delay" of intestinal absorption of lipophilic solutes was reported by Kampp and Lundgren (33), who showed that the elimination

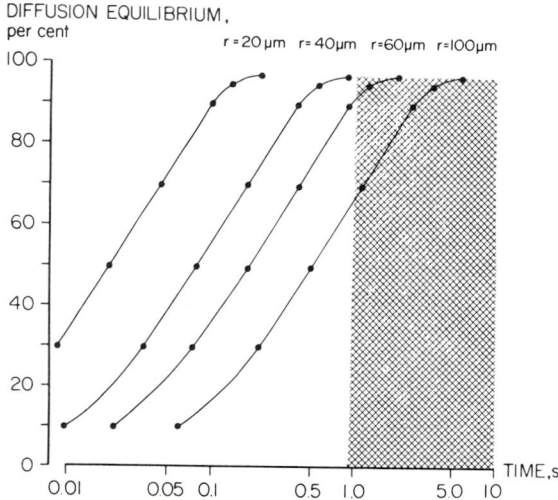

FIG. 4. The theoretically calculated times for reaching diffusion equilibrium between the outer surface of a cylinder and its center at varying radii of the cylinder *(r)*. Diffusion was assumed to occur freely in water, the diffusion constant being 10^{-5} cm$^2 \times$ s^{-1}. The calculations are based on Fig. 217 in Davson (13). The shaded area indicates the range of the calculated plasma mean transit times in the subepithelial capillary network recorded at varying total intestinal blood flow (see Fig. 3).

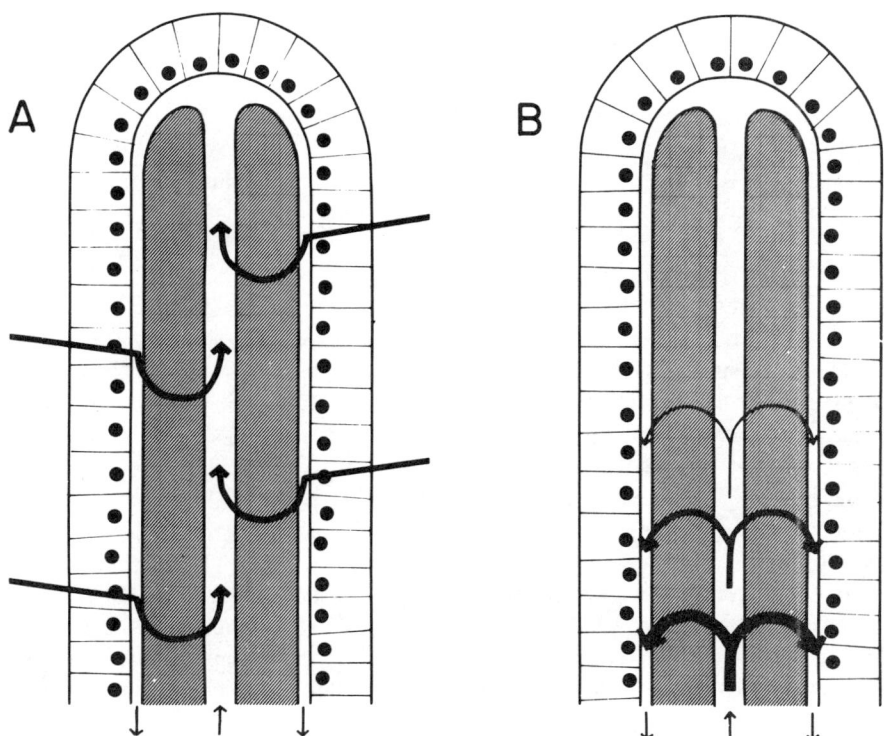

FIG. 5. Functional implications of the intestinal countercurrent exchanger (40). Intervascular distance is exaggerated for sake of clarity. For details, see text.

of ^{85}Kr from the small intestinal mucosa was surprisingly slow. In fact, it was slower than the washout rate from the muscle layer despite the fact that the vascular density is higher in the mucosa than in the muscle. From this and other observations, Lundgren (40) concluded that the slow elimination of krypton from the villi was due to a countercurrent exchanger.

Further evidence for a countercurrent mechanism was provided by Hamilton et al. (22), Bond et al. (7) (who studied the dog), and our subsequent studies in the cat (32,35,40). Bond et al. (7) studied the absorption rates of four different gases from the canine intestine. Villus blood flow was estimated with the microsphere technique. Knowing villus flow and the blood solubility of the different gases, they calculated a theoretical absorption rate for each gas. However, the observed rates were only about 20% of the calculated values. The discrepancy between calculated and observed rates of gas absorption was ascribed to the action of a villus countercurrent exchanger. By using carbon monoxide at low concentrations, the authors ruled out a luminal diffusion limitation.

Using a completely different technique, Jodal et al. (32) arrived at the same conclusion for krypton absorption in the feline gut. They also provided evidence that the degree of distension of the intestine influenced the rate of krypton absorption. When the gut is not distended, only the tips of the villi are in "functional contact" with the intestinal contents, but in the distended state the intervillus spaces are more accessible to the tracer. Hence, when the intestine is not distended, the villus exchanger is long and highly efficient, slowing rate of gas absorption.

Quantitatively, Bond et al. (7) estimated the percentage of the initially absorbed gas shunted in the canine countercurrent exchanger at "resting" blood flow. Their values were 84% for H_2, 87% for He, 84% for CH_4, and 56% for ^{133}Xe.

Similarly, Jodal et al. (32) estimated the exchanger to be 100% effective for ^{85}Kr at "rest," that is, in an unexpanded cat small bowel krypton escaped only by diffusion past the exchanger into the deeper parts of the mucosa where no exchanger exists.

Levitt and co-workers (6,38) have also investigated the possible existence of an intestinal countercurrent exchanger in the rat and rabbit. These authors could not obtain any support for a countercurrent exchange of gases in the small intestine in these two species. This observation may be explained by the gases reaching the bases of the villi, thereby circumventing the exchanger, since the villi are less densely packed, at least in the rabbit (7). This proposal is supported by our observation of a villus tip osmolality of 600 to 900 mOsm/kg H_2O in the rat and the rabbit, suggesting the presence of a countercurrent multiplier (D.-A. Hallbäck et al., *unpublished observations*).

With regard to hydrophilic compounds, Kampp et al. (36) made some observations that suggest that such substances of low molecular weight (e.g., urea) may be trapped in the exchanger, although to a smaller extent than lipophilic compounds. The difference between lipophilic and hydrophilic compounds is explained by the lower capillary permeability to water-soluble compounds.

Carbon dioxide is a physiological metabolite that is lipid soluble and of small molecular mass. From the foregoing discussion of other gases, it seems reasonable to assume that CO_2 is also trapped in the exchanger and delayed in its elimination from the gut lumen. A high CO_2 tension in the intestinal contents has also been reported by several research groups (23,25,47), but it is difficult, if not impossible, to differentiate *in vivo* between a delayed elimination of CO_2, produced by the epithelial cells, and an active transport of bicarbonate ions.

Fatty acids represent a group of substances with varying lipid solubility, the intestinal absorption of which is rather complex. It is generally accepted that the short-chain fatty acids (those with fewer than 10 to 12 carbon atoms) are absorbed from the mammalian small intestine mainly via the blood, whereas the long-chain fatty acids are predominantly transported via the lymph as triglycerides in chylomicrons. This partition between blood and lymph is usually explained in terms of the rapid esterification of the long-chain fatty acids in the apical parts of the epithelial cells, whereas this would not be the case with the short-chain fatty acids (12).

The different routes of lipid absorption may also be explained, in part, by the intestinal countercurrent mechanism. The exchanger may hinder net transport of the lipid-soluble, long-chain fatty acids more efficiently than the predominantly water-soluble, pore-restricted short-chain fatty acids. Such a mechanism would work together with the intracellular enzymes to provide them with a high substrate concentration. Experimental support for this hypothesis was presented by Jodal et al. (16,30,31). The proposed hypothesis implies that the transcapillary movement of long-chain fatty acids from the intravascular albumin molecules to the extracellular space or vice versa should be rapid. Model experiments on tumor cells and observations on myocardial tissue seem to support this assumption (53,54).

Diffusion from the Central Arterial Vessel to Capillaries

As depicted in Fig. 5 *(right panel)*, a solute may diffuse from the central arterial vessel to the subepithelial capillary network, provided that a concentration gradient exists between these vessels and that the solute can easily diffuse from one vessel to another. This mechanism tends to increasingly impair net blood transport of the solute towards the tips of the villi. Since the vascular wall represents a diffusion barrier to water-soluble but not to lipid-soluble compounds, it seems reasonable that lipophilic solutes will be most efficiently excluded from the villi when approaching them via the blood. However, the efficiency of the countercurrent exchanger in hindering net blood transport is much lower when approaching the exchanger from the "tissue" side rather than the "luminal" side (see discussion above).

Experimental support for such an extravascular shunting in the villi has been reported in the cat for the lipid-soluble solutes oxygen (34), krypton (32,35,55), and antipyrine (36) and, to some extent, for the water-soluble compounds urea and rubidium (36). The experimental approaches in these studies varied and the reader is referred to the survey by Lundgren (41) for a summary.

In autoradiographic experiments, Kampp et al. (36) investigated the distribution of ^{14}C-methyl-antipyrine in the intestinal tissue 5 to 10 sec after a close intraarterial injection of the tracer. At resting blood flow, the radioactivity was found almost exclusively in the crypt region and at the villus base, but during vasodilation there was a more or less homogeneous distribution of labeled antipyrine throughout the mucosa. This finding indicates that antipyrine reached the villus tips more easily when blood flow was high and transit time short.

Oxygen is a functionally more significant solute than antipyrine. Two observations suggest that oxygen is also shortcircuited in the exchanger. Kampp et al. (34) demonstrated that oxygen appears 1 to 2 sec earlier on the venous side than labeled red cells after i.a. injection during resting conditions. Because of their axial position in vessels, red cells pass through a vascular bed faster than plasma. Thus, the even earlier appearance of oxygen was taken as evidence for its extravascular shortcircuiting in the villus exchanger. Such shunting of oxygen in the intestinal countercurrent exchanger implies that villus tissue Po_2 decreases from the base towards the tip of the villi.

The postulated oxygen gradient along the villus has been demonstrated in the rat by Bohlen (4) with oxygen microelectrodes. During absorption of a glucose-free luminal solution, Bohlen measured a Po_2 around 26 mm Hg at the villus base and about 13 mm Hg at the tips. Adding glucose to the luminal solution reduced oxygen tension nearly to zero at the tip. Hence, the villus tips are relatively hypoxic, a fact that is important to transport mechanisms dependent on cellular metabolism.

Figure 4 shows that increasing blood flow makes the countercurrent exchanger less efficient. In fact, we have shown that shunting of oxygen does not occur in the cat when total intestinal blood flow reaches high values (above 150 $ml \times min^{-1} \times 100\ g^{-1}$). Oxygen shunting is probably small even at a flow rate of 60 $ml \times min^{-1} \times 100\ g^{-1}$, because it was not possible to demonstrate any early appearance of oxygen on the venous side above that flow level (34).

Lowering arterial blood pressure profoundly alters intestinal hemodynamics and increases the efficiency of the exchanger. Oxygen is then efficiently hindered in its net transport into the villi. The hemodynamics at low perfusion pressure and the functional consequences of the exchange of oxygen are discussed in detail in Chapter 25.

The Intestinal Countercurrent Multiplier

The intestinal countercurrent exchanger may also function as a so-called multiplier. This hypothesis is based on the countercurrent arrangement of the villus vasculature and on the presence of active solute pumps along the basolateral membrane of the epithelial cells (Fig. 6). These pumps may increase osmolality in the subepithelial capillary network as depicted in the left panels of Fig. 7. For example, it is now believed that the sodium-potassium exchange taking place in the plasma membrane of most cells involves the concomitant pumping of 3 Na ions out of the cell and 2 K ions into the cell (49). Furthermore, the fenestrated parts of the capillary wall, in all probability containing the pores, always face the epithelial cells (8,10,26).

An exchange may occur between the limbs of the vascular loops in the villi as shown in the middle panels of Fig. 7. This may be accomplished in two ways: the solute may diffuse along its concentration difference to the central vessel or water, driven by osmotic forces, may move in the opposite direction. The latter mechanism seems more likely to dominate, since most actively transported solutes are polar compounds of lower plasma membrane permeability than water (Fig. 6). In Fig. 7, such an exchange

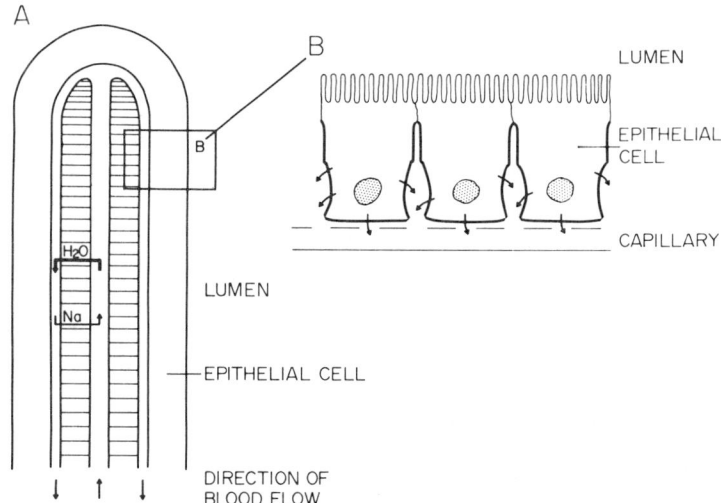

FIG. 6. Proposed mechanism of countercurrent multiplication. The active transport of sodium along the basolateral plasma membranes of the enterocytes *(arrows on panel B)* produces, at each point along the villus, a plasma sodium concentration difference between the central arterial vessel and the subepithelial capillary network. The hairpin loop arrangement in the intestinal villi allows this comparatively small concentration difference to be multiplied along the length of the villus, creating the rising tissue osmolality indicated by the increased number of horizontal lines in panel A. Countercurrent multiplication is probably accomplished mainly via the transfer of water from the central vessel to the capillaries *(thick arrow in panel A)* secondary to the osmotic forces created by the augmented capillary sodium concentration. The movement of sodium along its concentration gradient may, however, also occur to some extent *(thin arrow in panel A)*. Note that the pore-containing (fenestrated) part of the villus capillaries always faces the enterocytes. The relative magnitude of the pore area is exaggerated in panel B for clarity. The proposed mechanisms are accompanied by osmolality changes in the blood and probably in the epithelium, but these are not indicated in the figure.

has been illustrated, assuming that the capillary volume amounts to about 10% of the villus core volume.

The third aspect of countercurrent multiplication requires flowing blood (right panels of Fig. 7). Of course, *in vivo* all the three requirements are met: active solute transport, exchange and blood flow occur simultaneously. Figure 7 only illustrates principles; the osmolality values given are arbitrary and not measured values.

Figure 7 also illustrates the factors determining the efficiency of the countercurrent multiplier, that is, the osmolality profile along the villus length. The new variable compared to the passive countercurrent exchanger (see Eqs. 1, 3) is the so-called single effect, that is, the capacity of the enterocytes to increase villus capillary plasma osmolality. The magnitude of this single effect depends on the solute transport capacity of the enterocytes and on the hydraulic conductivity of the epithelium. It is important to realize that these factors are complex variables and, furthermore, probably vary significantly along the villus length. For example, villus epithelial hydraulic conductivity is lower than that of the crypts (44). Besides changes in the single effect, the efficiency of the countercurrent multiplier is also affected by the permeability characteristics of the exchanger, including intervascular diffusion distances. Finally, blood flow is important, since vasodilation may "wash out" the osmolality gradient (17,28).

The countercurrent multiplication hypothesis has been substantiated by studies of the osmolality and ionic composition of the villus. In one study, efforts were made to determine the concentration of electrolytes along the villus length. Haljamäe et al. (17) estimated the amount of

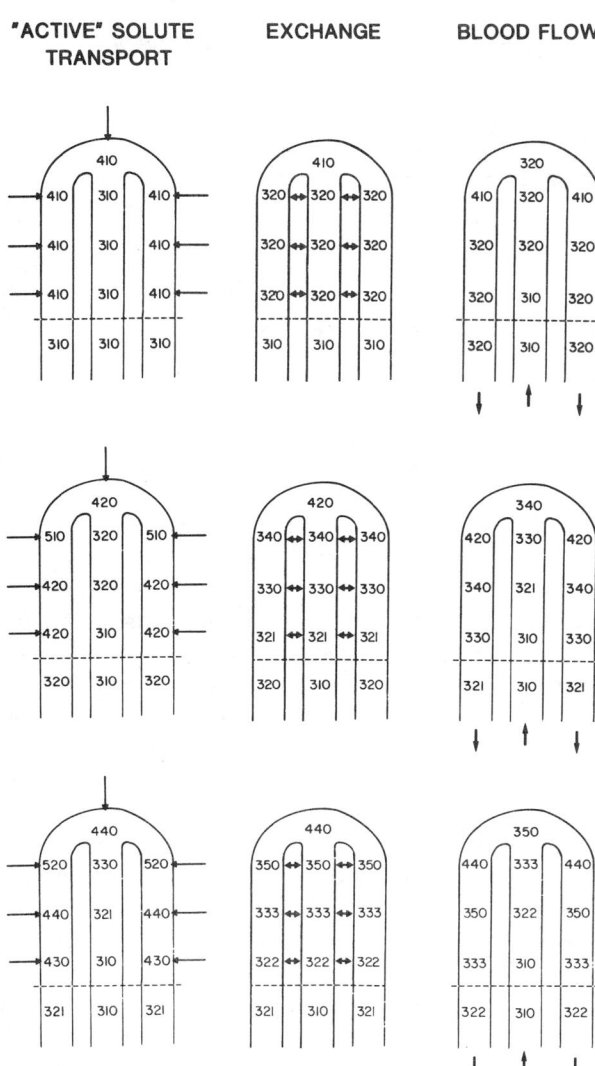

FIG. 7. Three components of countercurrent multiplication in intestinal villi. Countercurrent exchange is assumed to occur only above the *dashed line*. Figures indicate arbitrary, not measured, osmolality values (mOsm × kg^{-1} H$_2$O). Active transport of a hypertonic solution increases osmolality in the subepithelial capillaries *(left)*, leading to an exchange of solute and water *(middle*; see Fig. 6). Vascular osmolality after the exchange was calculated assuming that the capillary volume constituted 1/10th of the total villus core volume. Blood flow, the third component of the multiplication, is also shown *(right)*.

sodium per unit weight tissue protein. They found that the amount of sodium (per unit weight tissue protein) exhibited a steep gradient along the length of the villus, the tip to base ratio being about 3:1. This suggests the existence of a high extracellular sodium concentration at the tip. This conclusion was substantiated in a direct way by Bohlen (5). Using a sodium-sensitive microelectrode, he demonstrated that the sodium concentration at the villus tip of a rat was approximately double that found in the submucosa when the luminal perfusate contained glucose. The presence of high chloride concentration in the villus core of rabbit villi (59) is also in agreement with the findings of Haljamäe et al. (17).

In experiments with a cryoscopic technique, the presence of a multiplier was further corroborated by the demonstration of a hyperosmolar tissue compartment in the cat villus (18–21,28). During absorption of an isotonic glucose electrolyte solution at a "resting" blood flow, osmolality increased from base to tip, the tip osmolality being about three times greater than that of the base. An osmolality gradient of the same type as in the cat, although less pronounced, was demonstrated in the human gut (18). Table 1 summarizes results obtained in the

TABLE 1. *Tip and mean osmolality (mOsm × kg^{-1} H$_2$O) in various portions of intestinal villi in man and cat*

	Tip	From 5–30% of villus length	From 5–50% of villus length	Whole villus
Man				
Jejunum, "rest" ($n = 7$)	677 ± 43	562 ± 36	510 ± 35	467 ± 31
Ileum, "rest" ($n = 16$)	716 ± 31	585 ± 23	526 ± 20	491 ± 16
Cat				
Jejunum, "rest" ($n = 6$)	838 ± 83	590 ± 34	514 ± 20	429 ± 9
Jejunum, cholera ($n = 6$)	717 ± 55	579 ± 35	522 ± 28	439 ± 17

Mean ± SE. n = number of observations.

cat and man at "rest" with the cryoscopic method. Included in Table 1 are data obtained in cat intestinal segments extirpated 3 hr after exposing them to cholera toxin (20). These segments showed only a small decrease in tissue osmolality. Changes in tissue osmolality consistent with the countercurrent multiplication hypothesis were also observed, that is, vasodilatation and ischemia decreased the villus hyperosmolality (28).

The values given in Table 1 include only observations made in a "randomized" manner. In the early part of our studies, we chose those villi that, in a frozen cross-section, showed the highest tip osmolality. Therefore, osmolality values in our first report (28) are higher than those reported later. From these observations, one may conclude that villi differ in their efficiency as countercurrent multipliers. A similar observation was reported by Bohlen (4) with regard to the countercurrent exchange of oxygen.

It has been demonstrated repeatedly that water can be absorbed in the absence of or even against a lumen-to-plasma osmolality difference (50). To explain such experimental findings, Curran inferred the presence of a hyperosmolar tissue compartment. Curran's model was based on a thermodynamic analysis, and it was proved to work in model experiments (11). According to Curran, this hyperosmolar compartment should be located in the close vicinity of the epithelial cell (50). On the basis of the observations reported above, Jodal et al. (28) proposed that the demonstrated villus hyperosmolar region represents the tissue compartment necessary for explaining intestinal water absorption *in vivo*. This conclusion was corroborated in the cat by demonstrating a direct correlation between intestinal fluid transport and villus osmolality (21).

The upper parts of the villi represent that part of the intestinal epithelium that is in most "efficient" contact with the luminal contents. When the intestinal lumen is perfused with an isotonic Krebs-glucose solution, a gradient of tissue- (upper third of villus) to-lumen osmolality of about 400 mOsm/kg H$_2$O is present. This is clearly a large pressure difference. If a solute can exert its full osmotic force, 400 mOsm × kg^{-1} H$_2$O would equal about 10 atm, or around 7,500 mm Hg. Most of the hyperosmolality in the villi is probably made up of sodium chloride. Using a value of 0.6 as a rough estimate of the intestinal reflection coefficient for sodium chloride, we calculated that an osmotic pressure head of about 4,500 mm Hg would be present across the epithelial lining at the villus tip. With such large forces involved in the transport of water across the villus epithelium, one may propose that the villi are the chief site of fluid absorption *in vivo*. The flux of water into the lumen would occur predominantly in the crypts during physiological conditions. It seems also reasonable to propose that the brisk flow of water influences the epithelial transport of other solutes partly via a "solvent drag" effect and partly by influencing the thickness of the unstirred layer adjacent to the epithelial cells. A considerable villus tissue hyperosmolality was also demonstrated in cholera (see Table 1). Since it theoretically is unlikely that the villi are secreting structures with such a high osmolality, net fluid secretion in this secretory state probably emanates from the crypts of Lieberkühn. These studies and other investigations in our laboratory strongly suggest that villi are absorbing structures during most physiological and pathophysiological situations and that net fluid transport in the small intestine is regulated by varying the secretory volume from the crypts.

According to Curran's model, hydrostatic pressure is increased in the hyperosmolar tissue compartment. The change in osmolality along the length of the villus is therefore probably accompanied by a corresponding hydrostatic gradient, which creates the pressure head for the flow of lymph in the central lacteal. It may be assumed that the villus hyperosmolality is increased during digestive work and, consequently, the hydrostatic gradient along the villus. Such a mechanism may, in part, explain the increase of lymph flow seen with food intake. In fact, several reports seem to indicate that up to 50% of the volume of fluid absorbed is transported away from the villi via the lymphatics (1,29,51).

Bohlen (5) recently reported an interesting further functional implication of the countercurrent multiplier. Using an ion-selective microelectrode, he demonstrated that adding glucose to the luminal perfusate (presumably augmenting rate of sodium uptake) increased sodium concentration in villi and, after a certain time lag, also increased the sodium concentration in the submucosa from about 140 to approximately 180 mM. Concomitantly, the submucosal arterial vessels dilated, thus allowing increased blood flow in the villi. Hence, the countercurrent multiplier may indirectly be responsible for at least part of the functional hyperemia of the gut by producing a vasodilatory hyperosmolality in the submucosa.

The presence of a countercurrent multiplier may also influence the Starling forces across the subepithelial villus capillaries. This may occur in several ways. If countercurrent multiplication occurs as depicted in Fig. 6, that is, by water leaving the central arterial vessel, the plasma protein concentration must increase correspondingly along the villus length. This implies that the plasma oncotic pressure at the villus tip must be high. Furthermore, the interstitial hydrostatic pressure is probably also increased as discussed above. However, none of these variables have been measured so far in the villus vessels.

CONCLUSIONS

The vascular arrangement in the villi of most species including man, is consistent with presence of a countercurrent exchanger. This mechanism has several interesting functional consequences. It delays the absorption of highly diffusible solutes such as gases. The exchanger influences the oxygen delivery to the villi, making their tips being relatively hypoxic compared to the villus base. The exchanger may also function as a multiplier producing a high tissue osmolality, which probably is partly responsible for the fluid uptake from the intestine *in vivo*. Although the major functional implications of the intestinal countercurrent exchanger have been studied, we still lack important information concerning details of the countercurrent mechanisms in the small intestine.

REFERENCES

1. Barrowman, J., and Roberts, K. B. (1967): The role of the lymphatic system in the absorption of water from the intestine of the rat. *Q. J. Exp. Physiol.*, 52:19–30.
2. Biber, B., Lundgren, O., Stage, L., and Svanvik, J. (1973): An indicator-dilution method for studying intestinal hemodynamics in the cat. *Acta Physiol. Scand.*, 87:433–447.
3. Biber, B., Lundgren, O., and Svanvik, J. (1973): Intramural blood flow and blood volume in the small intestine of the cat as analyzed by an indicator-dilution technique. *Acta Physiol. Scand.*, 87:391–403.
4. Bohlen, H. G. (1980): Intestinal tissue P_{O_2} and microvascular responses during glucose exposure. *Am. J. Physiol.*, 7:H164–H171.
5. Bohlen, H. G. (1982): Na^+-induced intestinal interstitial hyperosmolality and vascular responses during absorptive hyperemia. *Am. J. Physiol.*, 242:H785–H789.
6. Bond, J. H., Levitt, D. G., and Levitt, M. D. (1974): Use of inert gases and carbon monoxide to study the possible influence of countercurrent exchange on passive absorption from the small bowel. *J. Clin. Invest.*, 54:1259–1265.
7. Bond, J. H., Levitt, D. G., and Levitt, M. D. (1977): Quantitation of countercurrent exchange during passive absorption from the dog small intestine. *J. Clin. Invest.*, 59:308–318.

8. Casley-Smith, J. R. (1971): Endothelial fenestrae in intestinal villi: Differences between the arterial and venous ends of the capillaries. *Microvasc. Res.*, 3:49–68.
9. Casley-Smith, J. R., Donoghue, P. J., and Crocker, K. W. J. (1975): The quantitative relationships between fenestrae in jejunal capillaries and connective tissue channels: Proof of "tunnel-capillaries." *Microvasc. Res.*, 9:78–100.
10. Clementi, F., and Palade, G. E. (1969): Intestinal capillaries. I. Permeability to peroxidase and ferritin. *J. Cell. Biol.*, 41:33–58.
11. Curran, P. F., and Macintosh, J. R. (1962): A model system for biological water transport. *Nature*, 193:347–348.
12. Davenport, H. W. (1977): *Physiology of the Digestive Tract*. Year Book Medical Publishers, Chicago.
13. Davson, H. (1970): *A Textbook of General Physiology*, 4th ed., vol. I. J. & A. Churchill, London.
14. Gannon, B. J., Gore, R. W., and Rogers, P. A. W. (1980): Dual blood supplies to intestinal villi of rabbit and rat. *Microvasc. Res.*, 19:247.
15. Gannon, B. J., Gore, R. W., and Rogers, P. A. W. (1981): Is there an anatomical basis for a vascular countercurrent mechanism in rabbit and human intestinal villi? *Biomed. Res.*, 2:235–241.
16. Haglund, U., Jodal, M., and Lundgren, O. (1973): An autoradiographic study of the intestinal absorption of palmitic and oleic acid. *Acta Physiol. Scand.*, 89:306–317.
17. Haljamäe, H., Jodal, M., and Lundgren, O. (1973): Countercurrent multiplication of sodium in intestinal villi during absorption of sodium chloride. *Acta Physiol. Scand.*, 89:580–593.
18. Hallbäck, D.-A., Hultén, L., Jodal, M., Lindhagen, J., and Lundgren, O. (1978): Evidence for the existence of a countercurrent exchanger in the small intestine in man. *Gastroenterology*, 74:683–690.
19. Hallbäck, D.-A., Jodal, M., and Lundgren, O. (1979): Importance of sodium and glucose for the establishment of a villous tissue hyperosmolality by the intestinal countercurrent multiplier. *Acta Physiol. Scand.*, 107:89–96.
20. Hallbäck, D.-A., Jodal, M., and Lundgren, O. (1979): Effects of cholera toxin on villous tissue osmolality and fluid and electrolyte transport in the small intestine of the cat. *Acta Physiol. Scand.*, 107:239–249.
21. Hallbäck, D.-A., Jodal, M., and Lundgren, O. (1980): Villous tissue osmolality, water and electrolyte transport in the cat small intestine at varying luminal osmolalities. *Acta Physiol. Scand.*, 110:95–100.
22. Hamilton, J. D., Dawson, A. M., and Webb, J. (1967): Limitation of the use of inert gases in the measurement of small gut mucosal blood flow. *Gut*, 8:509–521.
23. Hamilton, J. D., Dawson, A. M., and Webb, J. P. W. (1968): Observations upon small gut "mucosal" pO_2 and pCO_2 in anesthetized dogs. *Gastroenterology*, 55:52–60.
24. Heller, A. (1872): Über die Blutgefässe des Dünndarmes. *Ber. sächs. Ges. Wiss.*, 24:165–171.
25. Herrin, R. C. (1937): Ammonia content, pH and carbon dioxide tension in the intestine of dogs. *J. Biol. Chem.*, 118:459–470.
26. Horstmann, E. (1966): Über das Endothel der Zottenkappilaren im Dünndarm des Meerschweinchen und des Menschen. *Z. Zellforsch.*, 72:364–369.
27. Jacobson, L. F., and Noer, R. F. (1952): The vascular pattern of the intestinal villi in various laboratory animals and man. *Anat. Rec.*, 114:85–101.
28. Jodal, M., Hallbäck, D.-A., and Lundgren, O. (1978): Tissue osmolality in intestinal villi during luminal perfusion with isotonic electrolyte solutions. *Acta Physiol. Scand.*, 102:94–107.
29. Jodal, M., Hallbäck, D.-A., Svanvik, J., and Lundgren, O. (1975): A method for the continuous study of net water transport in the feline small bowel. *Acta Physiol. Scand.*, 95:441–447.
30. Jodal, M., and Lundgren, O. (1973): Studies on the in vivo absorption of butyric acid in the small intestine of the cat. *Acta Physiol. Scand.*, 89:327–333.
31. Jodal, M., and Lundgren, O. (1973): The distribution of absorbed ^3H-palmitic acid in the intestinal villi of the cat during various circulatory conditions. *Acta Physiol. Scand.*, 89:318–326.
32. Jodal, M., Svanvik, J., and Lundgren, O. (1977): The importance of the intestinal countercurrent exchanger for ^{85}Kr absorption from the feline gut. *Acta Physiol. Scand.*, 100:412–423.
33. Kampp, M., and Lundgren, O. (1966): Evidence for countercurrent exchange in intestinal villi. *Acta Physiol. Scand. (Suppl.)*, 68(277):103.
34. Kampp, M., Lundgren, O., and Nilsson, N. J. (1968): Extravascular shunting of oxygen in the small intestine of the cat. *Acta Physiol. Scand.*, 72: 396–403.
35. Kampp, M., Lundgren, O., and Sjöstrand, J. (1968): On the components of the Kr^{85} wash-out curves from the small intestine of the cat. *Acta Physiol. Scand.*, 72:257–281.
36. Kampp, M., Lundgren, O., and Sjöstrand, J. (1968): The distribution of intravascularly administered lipid soluble and lipid insoluble substances in the mucosa and the submucosa of the small intestine of the cat. *Acta Physiol. Scand.*, 72:469–480.
37. Levitt, D. G., Bond, J. H., and Levitt, M. D. (1980): Use of a model of small bowel mucosa to predict passive absorption. *Am. J. Physiol.*, 2:G23–G29.
38. Levitt, M. D., and Levitt, D. G. (1973): Use of inert gases to study the interaction of blood flow and diffusion during passive absorption from gastrointestinal tract of the rat. *J. Clin. Invest.*, 52:1852–1862.
39. Levitt, D. G., Sircar, B., Lifson, N., and Lender, E. J. (1979): Model for mucosal circulation of rabbit small intestine. *Am. J. Physiol.*, 6:E373–E382.
40. Lundgren, O. (1967): Studies on blood flow distribution and countercurrent exchange in the small intestine. *Acta Physiol. Scand. (Suppl.)*, 303:1–42.
41. Lundgren, O. (1984): Blood flow in the gastrointestinal tract. In: *Handbook of Physiology*, edited by E. M. Renkin and C. Michel *(in press)*.
42. Lundgren, O., and Svanvik, J. (1973): Mucosal hemodynamics in the small intestine of the cat during reduced perfusion pressure. *Acta Physiol. Scand.*, 88:551–563.
43. Mall, J. P. (1888): Die Blut- und lymphwege im Dünndarm des Hundes. *Abh. sächs. Ges. Wiss.*, 14:153–189.
44. Madara, J. L., Trier, J. S., and Neutra, M. R. (1980):

Structural changes in the plasma membrane accompanying differentiation of epithelial cells in human and monkey small intestine. *Gastroenterology*, 78:963–975.
45. Patzelt, V. (1936): Der Darm. *Handbuch der mikroskopischen Anatomie des Menschen.*, 5:(3) 1–448.
46. Reynolds, D. G., Brim, J., and Sheehy, T. W. (1967): The vascular architecture of the small intestinal mucosa of the monkey. *Anat. Rec.*, 159:211–218.
47. Rune, S. J. (1972): Acid-base parameters of duodenal contents in man. *Gastroenterology*, 62:533–539.
48. Schriever, O. (1899): *Die Darmzotten der Haussäugetiere*. Thesis, Giessen.
49. Schultz, S. G. (1981): Homocellular regulatory mechanisms in sodium-transporting epithelia: Avoidance of extinction by "flush-through." *Am. J. Physiol.*, 241:F579–F590.
50. Schultz, S. G., and Curran, P. F. (1968): Intestinal absorption of sodium chloride and water. In: *Handbook of Physiology. Alimentary Canal*, edited by C. F. Code, sect. 6, vol. III, chapt. 66, pp. 1245–1275. American Physiological Society, Washington, D.C.
51. Simmonds, W. J. (1954): The effect of fluid, electrolyte and food intake on thoracic duct lymph flow in unanaesthetized rats. *Aust. J. Exp. Biol. Med. Sci.*, 32:285–300.
52. Spanner, R. (1932): Neue Befunde über die Blutwege der Darmward und ihre funktionelle Bedeutung. *Morph. Jb.*, 69:394–454.
53. Spector, A. (1971): Metabolism of free fatty acids. *Prog. Biochem. Pharmacol.*, 6:130–176.
54. Spitzer, J. J. (1974): Effect of lactate infusion on canine myocardial free fatty acid metabolism in vivo. *Am. J. Physiol.*, 226:213–217.
55. Svanvik, J. (1973): Mucosal blood circulation and its influence on passive absorption in the small intestine. An experimental study in the cat. *Acta Physiol. Scand. (Suppl.)*, 385:1–44.
56. Swan, K. G., Spees, E. K., Reynolds, D. G., Kerr, J. C., and Zinner, M. J. (1978): Microvascular architecture of anthropoid primate intestine. *Circ. Shock*, 5:375–382.
57. Winne, D. (1975): The influence of villous counter current exchange on intestinal absorption. *J. Theor. Biol.*, 53:145–176.
58. Winne, D. (1977): The vasculature of the jejunal villus. In: *Intestinal Permeation*, edited by M. Kramer and F. Lauterbach, pp. 56–57. Excerpta Medica, Amsterdam.
59. Zeuthen, T., and Monge, C. (1975): Intra- and extracellular gradients of electrical potential and ion activities of the epithelial cells of the rabbit ileum *in vivo* recorded by microelectrodes. *Phil. Trans. B.*, 71:277–281.

Postprandial Mesenteric Hyperemia

John W. Fara

ALZA Corporation, Palo Alto, California 94304

Shortly after the ingestion of a meal, blood flow to the gastrointestinal tract increases, and over the next 3 to 6 hr it remains elevated at levels approaching 100% to 150% of normal (10, 14,24,25,31,32,34,38,47,51,59–61). The occurrence and mechanism of this postprandial hyperemia have received much investigative attention in recent years, and one can now point to a number of factors that are thought to mediate this hemodynamic response to food. This chapter focuses on the cardiovascular changes accompanying the ingestion and digestion of food and on the mechanisms thought to be responsible.

Although suggestions were made in the early 1900s that the drowsiness one feels after a meal may be due to a redistribution of blood away from the brain to the intestine, it was not until the 1930s that measurements were first made to quantify cardiovascular events during digestion. During this time, Herrick and co-workers (21,38) reported some of the first *in vivo* measurements of an increase in superior mesenteric blood flow in awake dogs following a meal. Utilizing the thermostromuhr, they observed that blood flow in the carotid, coronary, femoral, and superior mesenteric arteries increased for up to 5 hr after a meal. These studies were thus interpreted to indicate that increased blood flow to the intestine during the meal was not due to a redistribution away from other organs. Indeed, Gladstone (35) postulated that this increase may be accounted for by the 25% increase in cardiac output he measured in man after a heavy meal. At the same time Herrick et al. (38) also suggested that a mechanism for postprandial mesenteric vasodilatation may be the release and action of a secretogogue elaborated by the gastrointestinal tract.

Studies on mesenteric blood flow were not pursued for some time after that except for a few scattered reports in the literature during the 1950s. However, in the late 1960s comprehensive studies were undertaken to investigate the entire hemodynamic response pattern during food intake and digestion. During this time, studies by Reininger and Sapirstein in the rat (51), by Fronek and Stahlgren in the dog (32), and by Vatner et al. also in the dog (59) showed that there was a selective increase in superior mesenteric blood flow after a meal.

The basic finding that digestive organ blood flow increases after food intake has now been confirmed in numerous species, and it has stimulated interest in both basic and clinical research settings to elucidate the mechanism. Postprandial mesenteric hyperemia has been reported in humans (9,47), other primates (58,61), dogs (8,10,30–32,34,38,59,60), cats (24,25), sheep (18,20), and rats (51). These studies, performed largely over the past 10 to 15 years, have focused on two basic areas: (a) the overall cardiovascular changes associated with a meal, including blood flow to organs within and outside of the gastrointestinal tract, for instance, colon, stomach, brain, muscle, and (b) the mechanism(s) of postprandial mesenteric vasodilatation.

GENERAL CARDIOVASCULAR CHANGES DURING DIGESTION

It is now fairly well documented that even before food reaches the stomach, cardiovascular changes occur in preparation for the arrival of the meal. However, during this anticipatory period only a small increase in superior mesenteric blood flow occurs. An increase of considerably greater magnitude occurs later and appears to require the presence of food in the stomach and intestine.

Studies in both dogs and primates have shown that cardiac output, heart rate, and aortic pressure increase during the anticipatory and digestive period (32,59–61), but there is little change in mesenteric vascular resistance (31,32). At the same time, resistance in the renal vascular bed increases (60,61) and that in the limbs reportedly either increases (32) or decreases (32,60,61). As one might predict, there are probably also local blood flow changes to the salivary glands during ingestion; however, this has only been documented in sheep (18). The majority of these cardiovascular changes during the anticipatory period reportedly occur for only a few minutes, after which the cardiovascular system returns toward control. Once food enters the stomach and intestine, however, the entire mesenteric hemodynamic response pattern emerges.

Within 3 to 5 min after the arrival of food in the gastrointestinal tract, blood flow to the stomach and intestine begins to increase. Additionally, cardiovascular responses in other organs are evoked to support this increase. The latency and duration of these responses depend to a considerable extent on the type and quantity of the meal, with high-fat and protein-containing foods producing the most profound and sustained intestinal hyperemia (25,54,61). Carbohydrates are less effective (9,61), but their effects may depend on the quantity ingested or instilled. In general, the mesenteric vasodilation reaches its maximum some 30 to 90 min after food enters the intestine and lasts 4 to 6 hr depending on the nature and quantity of the meal. These characteristics have been carefully studied in anesthetized cats (25) and conscious dogs (8,10,31,32,34,59–61).

During this time, blood flow to other vascular beds is either increased, decreased, or in some cases unchanged. In sheep, for example, blood flow to the spleen, heart, kidneys, and brain is reportedly unchanged during a meal, whereas flow to adipose tissue decreases (18,20). This postprandial reduction in adipose tissue blood flow also occurs in the dog, in which again brain, heart and adrenal gland blood flow are unaltered (34). Blood flow to various regions within the brain, namely, cerebellum, cortex, hypothalamus, medulla, pituitary, and thalamus, also does not change during this time (34). Thus, blood flow is apparently not redistributed within the brain during digestion.

Renal blood flow decreased during digestion in two studies (60,61); however, Reihardt et al. (50) reported an increase of around 40% in kidney blood flow after a meal. This occurred with both high- and low-sodium diets but may be due to the high fluid volume ingested by the animals in this study. In cats, renal blood flow is unaltered during food-elicited mesenteric hyperemia (25).

In the limbs and skeletal muscle, blood flow is either unchanged (25,34) or decreased (32,60,61), but this may depend on the amount of exercise during digestion (31,58).

The large mesenteric vascular response to a meal may be accomplished either by an increase in cardiac output or a redistribution of blood away from other vascular beds to the gut. As the reader has probably gathered, there is some confusion whether or not blood flow is redirected selectively to the mesentery. This conflict may reflect differences between species and the varied methods used over the years to record blood flow. Early studies indicated that postprandial mesenteric hyperemia was accompanied by increased cardiac output (51). More recently, however, increased cardiac output has only been associated with the anticipatory period prior to arrival of food in the gut (32,59,61). Current evidence thus indicates that postprandial mesenteric hyperemia is confined to organs in which digestion is occurring. It is suggested that small changes in the vascular resistance of several organs together with small, hard-to-measure increases in cardiac output may contribute to this rather selective response.

CARDIOVASCULAR CHANGES IN MESENTERIC ORGANS

The postprandial increase in superior mesenteric blood flow is not shared equally by all the mesenteric organs; it is selective to those participating in digestion (14,25,34). Even within the intestine itself, various regions are perfused to different degrees (34). Similarly, the introduction of food into the stomach of the conscious dog increases blood flow only in the celiac artery (14). Likewise, fatty acids placed in the colon of dogs elicit an organ-specific colonic hyperemia (41). Furthermore, of the rise in superior mesenteric blood flow elicited by food in the intestine, little or none is distributed to the stomach and colon (8,25). However, this increased flow is shared more or less equally by the small intestine and pancreas, as Fig. 1 shows. Additionally, as a result of the increase in portal blood flow draining the mesenteric circulation, total hepatic blood flow increases postprandially. However, hepatic artery flow does not change (1,18,20,34).

Within sequential segments of the small intestine, all regions are not perfused equally at any one time (14,25,63). For example, Chou et al. (14) demonstrated that intraduodenal placement of food increases blood flow in the superior mesenteric artery but does not alter celiac flow or blood flow to an isolated jejunal segment (see Table 1).

At the local intestinal level, the nature of the food material in the lumen is the determinant of the vascular response. For example, Kvietys et al. (43) demonstrated that luminal osmolarity over the range 180 to 1,000 osmoles/kg is not a significant factor in contributing to local hyperemia, but the concentration of the nutrient is. When chyme was analyzed for its local hyperemia-stimulating activity, the partially digested fats and carbohydrates were especially effective; undigested food elicited no response (16). Additionally, bile apparently plays an important role in the intestinal response to food (16,40). Whereas bile in the jejunum has no effect by itself, bile enhances the hyperemic effect of digested food (16). By contrast, bile salts alone elicit hyperemia in the ileum (42).

The selectivity of postprandial hyperemia extends to the various layers of the gut wall; differences in blood flow distribution exist among the mucosa, submucosa, and muscularis. Using radioactively labeled microspheres, Chou et al. (14,15) showed the local distribution of microspheres within jejunum favored the mucosa

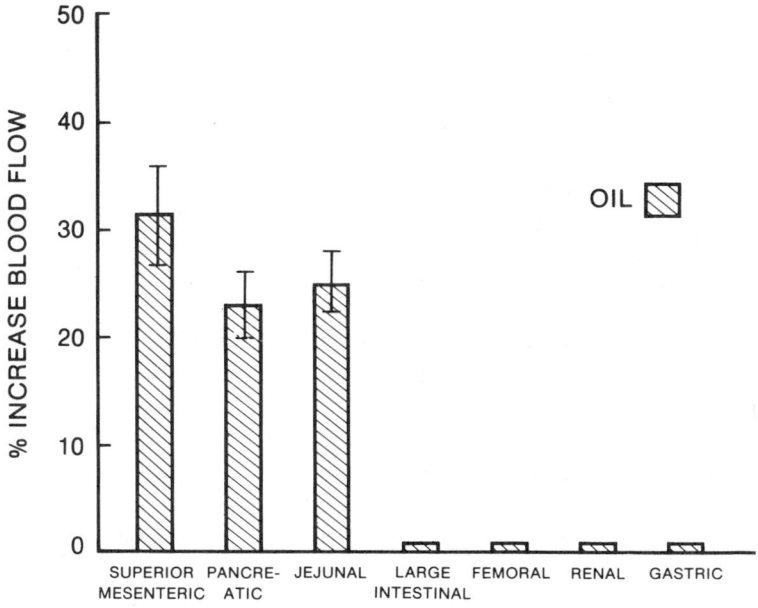

FIG. 1. The percent increase in blood flow in various vascular beds of the anesthetized cat when small amounts of corn oil are instilled into the duodenum. (From Fara et al., ref. 25, with permission.)

TABLE 1. *Selective increase in blood flow to jejunal segments containing nonabsorbable polyethylene glycol (PEG) or food*

	PEG	Food	Empty
	^{141}Ce cpm/g tissue		
Whole wall	4,015 ± 355	6,004 ± 816[a]	4,734 ± 546
Mucosa	4,303 ± 414	6,770 ± 759[a]	5,240 ± 628
Submucosa	1,647 ± 230	2,101 ± 370	1,966 ± 345
Muscle-serosa	4,412 ± 547	5,930 ± 1,574	4,774 ± 1,137
	^{85}Sr cpm/g tissue		
Whole wall	1,204 ± 126	1,627 ± 209[a]	1,359 ± 158
Mucosa	1,294 ± 152	1,857 ± 224[a]	1,497 ± 206
Submucosa	597 ± 106	696 ± 129	631 ± 116
Muscle-serosa	1,267 ± 157	1,485 ± 317	1,357 ± 254

Values are mean ± SE. Blood flow was determined by distribution of radioactively labeled microspheres.
[a]Value statistically different from the corresponding value for PEG at $p < 0.05$.
From Chou et al. (14), with permission.

(Table 1). This preferential distribution to mucosa was also reported by Gallavan et al. (34). On the other hand, blood flow to the muscularis layer does not change over the first 90 min after a meal (34), during which time superior mesenteric blood flow increases over 100%. Postprandial gastric and colonic hyperemia are also attributed to increased mucosal flow (8,34). Thus, it appears that mesenteric postprandial hyperemia is quite selective in its distribution to regions that are closely tied to digestive and absorptive processes, and that the mucosal region receives the largest share of the increase.

MECHANISM OF THE MESENTERIC VASCULAR RESPONSE TO FOOD

Much investigative attention has been paid to the mechanism of postprandial mesenteric hyperemia. Various mediators of this response have been proposed: These include hormonal and humoral factors (2,3,12,14,16,22–29, 33,40,55), general and local vasodilator reflexes (12,24,59), and metabolic changes associated with absorption (12,14,24,25,43,49,55).

The possible role of hormonal component in postprandial mesenteric hyperemia was suggested in 1967 by Burns and Schenk (10), who found that intravenous infusions of secretin and gastrin increased superior mesenteric blood flow. Moreover, systemically administered secretin and cholecystokinin (CCK) increase both small intestinal and superior mesenteric blood flow (13,24,25,27,52,53) and pancreatic blood flow (19,25,29). Also, the intravenous infusion of gastric inhibitory peptide mimics the mesenteric vascular response observed following the ingestion of hypertonic glucose (26), and systemic gastrin infusions also increase blood flow or decrease vascular resistance in stomach (45), gastric mucosa (39,56), and duodenum (13). Furthermore, secretin and CCK reportedly redistribute blood flow within the intestinal wall with CCK eliciting a preferential increase in blood flow to the mucosa (23). Neurotensin, which also increases intestinal blood flow, is postulated to regulate flow specifically within the muscle layer of the ileum (2).

Thus, many of the well-characterized gastrointestinal peptides have mesenteric vascular effects. However, the extent to which they are responsible for postprandial mesenteric hyperemia is not well understood because the concentrations released after a meal have not been correlated with the regional vascular responses. Of all the peptides closely studied, CCK emerges as a viable mediator of mesenteric hyperemia, for in addition to the mesenteric blood flow changes observed following the introduction of food and various substances into the gut, other recognized CCK-mediated responses also occur in the gastrointestinal tract (Table 2). This has led to the hypothesis that this peptide in particular probably contributes to postprandial intestinal hyperemia (13,23,25). Vascular effects of the gastrointestinal hormones are discussed in detail in Chapter 10.

During digestion, motility of the gastrointestinal tract increases to mix and propel the chyme. Although various relationships have been described between motility and blood flow, little is actually known about the relative contribution of motility to postprandial mesenteric hyperemia. The effect of motility on blood flow is discussed in Chapter 9 and has also been reviewed recently (11). However, the increased motility observed after a meal and also elicited by intravenous administration of CCK (25) may contribute to postprandial hyperemia. Additionally, a portion of the increased oxygen consumption reported to occur in the intestine after food (25) may be accounted for by increased motility, but active transport processes during digestion and absorption are also postulated to account for this (49,55,57). Increased metabolism may also contribute to the increased pancreatic blood flow observed after intraluminal instillation of food and food components (25).

These mesenteric vascular responses to food are not modified by pharmacological sympathetic blockade or acute splanchnicectomy (25,59). These findings diminish the possibility that the response is secondary to a selective inhibition of sympathetic vasoconstrictor activity or to an adrenergic effect mediated through β-receptors in the mesenteric vessels. Additionally, the reported absence of food-induced mesenteric vasodilatation after atropine (25,59) is compatible with the partial involvement of a hormonal mechanism, for cholinergic blockade reportedly prevents the release of CCK (62). Furthermore, at the local level, jejunal hyperemia induced by intraluminal bile-oleic acid is unaffected by cholinergic blockade (44). Therefore, if a nervous component is involved, one would have to postulate a nonadrenergic, noncholinergic mechanism.

Because postprandial mesenteric hyperemia is localized to regions in which food is present or in which digestive processes are occurring, for example, pancreas, one can postulate that in addition to changes in metabolism, other local events may contribute to the hyperemia. Indeed, gentle mechanical stimulation of the gut elicits mesenteric vasodilatation (4), an effect thought to be mediated by the release and action of 5-dihydroxytryptamine (5-HT) either locally or through a myenteric reflex (3). Investigators have attributed the blood flow response seen after ingestion or intestinal instillation of hyper-

TABLE 2. *Range of vascular, pancreatic, and biliary responses after intraduodenal instillation of different agents*

Intraduodenal agent	Latency Δ SMF, min	SMF, % Δ	Gall bladder pressure, Δ mm Hg	Pancreatic enzyme output, % Δ	Pancreatic vol, % Δ	Bile vol, % Δ
Control		(27 ± 1.4 mg/min)	(1–2 mm Hg)	(0)	(0.02–0.09 ml/min)	(0.04 ml/min)
Milk (3–5 ml) 5 Corn oil (fat) (0.5–2 ml) 18	7–20	15–59[a]	0.5–3[a]	50–100[a]	0–15	0–15
L-Phenylalanine 7	1–5	10–30[a]	1–3[a]	25–60[a]	2–14	2–14
	1–2	12–20[a]	0	0	10–30	0–10
HCl 6	3–5	27–49[a]	3–5[a]	20–40[a]	50–200[a]	30–50[a]

Numbers in brackets = number of trials. Δ = change in the measured variable; in all cases an increase (+). (Values in parentheses): absolute control values; means ± SE or range. SMF = superior mesenteric blood flow.
[a]Significant change ($p < 0.01$).
From Fara et al. (25), with permission.

tonic glucose to direct vascular effects of hypertonicity on vascular smooth muscle (12), and although there is little evidence that intraluminal osmolarity per se contributes significantly to mesenteric hyperemia as discussed earlier, there is good support for an osmotic contribution from the absorbed nutrients. Presumably, this is by a direct action on the local vasculature. In rat, for example, Bohlen (7) postulates that hyperosmolarity in intestinal villus and submucosa during glucose and sodium absorption initiates microvessel dilatation. This mechanism has been invoked for this response in other species as well (12,14,34,43,63). Furthermore, the availability of oxygen during active absorption is thought to also play a role (5,6).

In addition to these osmotic and metabolic mechanisms, the release and action of a variety of endogenous chemical substances have been implicated in mesenteric hyperemia. These include 5-HT and bradykinin (3), prostacyclin and prostaglandins (28,33), and adenosine (37).

In the stomach, histamine release and action have long been implicated in the control of blood flow (46), and recently a possible role of H_2 receptors in intestinal vasodilatation has been reported during continuous histamine infusion (48). However, with specific regard to postprandial mesenteric hyperemia, Chou and Siregar (17) showed that the effect of histamine is mediated primarily by the H_1-receptors. In their study, a 30% food-induced increase in mesenteric blood flow was reduced to 15% after H_1-receptor blockade. This reduction was unaffected by concomitant H_2-receptor blockade. Thus, histamine does play a role in the regulation of the mesenteric circulation in general (36), and as a contributor in postprandial hyperemia. However, the study of Chou and Siregar (17) certainly points to the involvement of other mechanisms as well.

Finally, there is evidence that these locally released substances have direct relaxing effects on intestinal vascular smooth muscle (3,22). Thus, when released, such agents as CCK, 5-HT, and histamine may produce their vascular action before being degraded or absorbed into the circulation.

In conclusion, a number of mechanisms have been proposed to explain postprandial mesenteric hyperemia. Of these, humoral and metabolic factors appear particularly important; each of them has its own characteristics and appeal as a regulatory mechanism. In the overview, however, it is apparent that no one factor alone accounts for this well-integrated response. Rather, it probably involves a combination of events.

ACKNOWLEDGMENT

The author gratefully thanks Ms. Kera Alexander for her skillful assistance in the preparation of this manuscript.

REFERENCES

1. Anderson, M. F., Drake-Bailey, C., and Knutti, J. W. (1982): Measurement of hepatic blood flow in conscious dogs at rest after feeding by a new, totally implanted, pulsed Doppler ultrasonic flowmeter. *Gastroenterology*, 82:1008.
2. Baca, I., Mittmann, U., Feurle, G. E., Haas, M., and Muller, Th. (1981): Effect of neurotensin on regional intestinal blood flow in the dog. *Res. Exp. Med. (Berl.)*, 179:53–58.
3. Biber, B., Fara, J., and Lundgren, O. (1974): A pharmacological study of intestinal vasodilator mechanism in the cat. *Acta Physiol. Scand.*, 90:673–683.
4. Biber, B., Lundgren, O., and Svanvick, J. (1971): Studies on the intestinal vasodilatation observed after mechanical stimulation of the mucosa of the gut. *Acta Physiol. Scand.*, 82:177–190.
5. Bohlen, H. G. (1980): Intestinal tissue PO_2 and microvascular responses during glucose exposure. *Am. J. Physiol.*, 238:H164–H171.
6. Bohlen, H. G. (1980): Intestinal mucosal oxygenation influences absorption hyperemia. *Am. J. Physiol.*, 239:H489–H493.
7. Bohlen, H. G. (1982): Na^+-induced intestinal interstitial hyperosmolarity and vascular responses during absorptive hyperemia. *Am. J. Physiol.*, 242:H785–H789.
8. Bond, J. H., Prentiss, R. A., and Levitt, M. D. (1979): The effects of feeding on blood flow to the stomach, small bowel, and colon of the conscious dog. *J. Lab. Clin. Med.*, 93:594–599.
9. Brandt, J. L., Castleman, L., Ruskin, H. D., Greenwald, J. J., and Kelley, J. (1955): The effect of oral protein and glucose feeding on splanchnic blood flow and oxygen utilization in normal and cirrhotic subjects. *J. Clin. Invest.*, 34:1017–1025.
10. Burns, G. P., and Schenk, W. G. (1969): Effect of digestion and exercise on intestinal blood flow and cardiac output. *Arch. Surg.*, 98:790–794.
11. Chou, C. C. (1982): Relationship between intestinal blood flow and motility. *Annu. Rev. Physiol.*, 44:29–42.

12. Chou, C. C., Burns, T. D., Hsieh, C. P., and Dabney, J. M. (1972): Mechanism of local vasodilation with hypertonic glucose in the jejunum. *Surgery*, 71:380–387.
13. Chou, C. C., Hsieh, C. P., and Dabney, J. M. (1977): Comparison of vascular effects of gastrointestinal hormones on various organs. *Am. J. Physiol.*, 232:H103–H109.
14. Chou, C. C., Hsieh, C. P., Yu, Y. M., Kvietys, P., Yu, L. C., Pittman, R., and Dabney, J. M. (1976): Localization of mesenteric hyperemia during digestion in dogs. *Am. J. Physiol.*, 230:583–589.
15. Chou, C. C., and Kvietys, P. R. (1981): Physiological and pharmacological alterations in gastrointestinal blood flow. In: *The Measurement of Splanchnic Blood Flow*, edited by G. B. Bulkley and D. N. Granger, pp. 475–509. Williams and Wilkins, Baltimore.
16. Chou, C. C., Kvietys, P., Post, J., and Sit, S. P. (1978): Constituents of chyme responsible for postprandial intestinal hyperemia. *Am. J. Physiol.*, 235:H677–H682.
17. Chou, C. C., and Siregar, H. (1982): Role of histamine H_1- and H_2-receptors in postprandial intestinal hyperemia. *Am. J. Physiol.*, 243:G248–G252.
18. Dobson, A., Barnes, R. J., and Comline, R. S. (1981): Changes in the sources of hepatic portal blood flow with feeding in the sheep. *Physiologist*, 24:15.
19. Dorigotti, L., and Glasser, A. H. (1968): Comparative effects of caerulein, pancreozymia, and secretin on pancreatic blood flow. *Experientia*, 24:806–807.
20. Edelstone, D. I., and Holzman, I. R. (1981): Gastrointestinal tract O_2 uptake and regional blood flows during digestion in conscious newborn lambs. *Am. J. Physiol.*, 241:G289–G293.
21. Essex, H. E., Herrick, J. R., Baldes, E. J., and Mann, F. C. (1936): Blood flow in the circumflex branch of the left coronary artery of the intact dog. *Am. J. Physiol.*, 117:271–279.
22. Fara, J. W. (1975): Effects of gastrointestinal hormones on vascular smooth muscle. *Am. J. Dig. Dis.*, 20:346–353.
23. Fara, J. W., and Madden, K. S. (1975): Effect of secretin and cholecystokinin on small intestinal blood flow distribution. *Am. J. Physiol.*, 229:1365–1370.
24. Fara, J. W., Rubinstein, E. H., and Sonnenschein, R. R. (1969): Visceral and behavioral responses to intraduodenal fat. *Science*, 166:110–111.
25. Fara, J. W., Rubinstein, E. H., and Sonnenschein, R. R. (1972): Intestinal hormones in mesenteric vasodilation after intraduodenal agents. *Am. J. Physiol.*, 223:1058–1067.
26. Fara, J. W., and Salazar, A. M. (1978): Gastric inhibitory polypeptide increases mesenteric blood flow. *Proc. Soc. Exp. Biol. Med.*, 158:446–448.
27. Fasth, S., Filipsson, S., Hulten, L., and Martinson, J. (1972): The effect of the gastrointestinal hormones on intestinal motility and blood flow. *Experientia*, 29:982–984.
28. Fondacaro, J. D., and Jacobson, E. D. (1981): The role of prostacyclin (PGI_2) in metabolic hyperemia. *Prostaglandins*, S21:25–32.
29. Frogge, J. D., Heimrech, A. S., and Thal, A. P. (1970): Metabolic and hemodynamic effects of secretin and pancreozymin on the pancreas. *Surgery*, 68:498–502.
30. Fronek, A. (1970): Combined effect of carotid sinus hypotension and digestion on splanchnic circulation. *Am. J. Physiol.*, 219:1759–1762.
31. Fronek, K., and Fronek, A. (1970): Combined effect of exercise and digestion on hemodynamics in conscious dogs. *Am. J. Physiol.*, 218:555–559.
32. Fronek, K., and Stahlgren, L. H. (1968): Systemic and regional hemodynamic changes during food intake and digestion in nonanesthetized dogs. *Circ. Res.*, 23:687–692.
33. Gallavan, R. H., and Chou, C. C. (1982): Prostaglandin synthesis inhibition and postprandial intestinal hyperemia. *Am. J. Physiol.*, 242:G140–G146.
34. Gallavan, R. H., Chou, C. C., Kvietys, P. R., and Sit, S. P. (1980): Regional blood flow during digestion in the conscious dog. *Am. J. Physiol.*, 238:H220–H225.
35. Gladstone, S. A. (1935): Cardiac output and related functions under basal and post prandial conditions—a clinical study. *Arch. Surg.*, 55:533–546.
36. Granger, D. N., Richardson, P. D. I., Kvietys, P. R., and Mortillaro, N. A. (1980): Intestinal blood flow. *Gastroenterology*, 78:837–863.
37. Granger, H. J., and Norris, C. P. (1980): Role of adenosine in local control of intestinal circulation in the dog. *Circ. Res.*, 46:764–770.
38. Herrick, J. F., Essex, H. E., Mann, F. C., and Baldes, E. J. (1934): The effect of digestion on blood flow in certain blood vessels of the dog. *Am. J. Physiol.*, 108:621–628.
39. Jacobson, E. D., Linford, R. H., and Grossman, M. I. (1966): Gastric secretion in relation to mucosal blood flow studied by a clearance technic. *J. Clin. Invest.*, 45:1–13.
40. Kvietys, P. R., Gallavan, R. H., and Chou, C. C. (1980): Contribution of bile to postprandial intestinal hyperemia. *Am. J. Physiol.*, 238:G284–G288.
41. Kvietys, P. R., and Granger, D. N. (1981): Effect of volatile fatty acids on blood flow and oxygen uptake by the dog colon. *Gastroenterology*, 80:926–969.
42. Kvietys, P. R., McLendon, J. M., and Granger, D. N. (1981): Postprandial intestinal hyperemia: Role of bile salts in the ileum. *Am. J. Physiol.*, 241:G469–G477.
43. Kvietys, P. R., Pittman, R. P., and Chou, C. C. (1976): Contribution of luminal concentration of nutrients and osmolality to postprandial intestinal hyperemia in dogs. *Proc. Soc. Exp. Biol. Med.*, 152:659–663.
44. Kvietys, P. R., Wilborn, W. H., and Granger, D. N. (1981): Effect of atropine on bile-oleic acid-induced alterations in dog jejunal hemodynamics, oxygenation, and net transmucosal water movement. *Gastroenterology*, 80:31–38.
45. Laureta, H. C., Chou, C. C., and Texter, E. C., Jr. (1965): Effects of gastrointestinal hormones on total resistance of gastric circulation. *Clin. Res.*, 13:256.
46. Naitove, A., and Colby, E. D. (1967): Gastric hemodynamic responses to histamine. *Gastroenterology*, 52:1139.
47. Norryd, C., Denker, H., Lunderquist, A., Olin, T., and Tylen, U. (1975): Superior mesenteric blood flow during digestion in man. *Acta Chir. Scand.*, 141:197–202.
48. Pawlik, W., Tague, L. L., and Tepperman, B. L. (1977): Histamine H1 and H2 receptor vasodilation of canine intestinal vasculature. *Am. J. Physiol.*, 233:E219–E224.
49. Pawlik, W. W., Fondacaro, J. D., and Jacobson, E. D.

(1980): Metabolic hyperemia in canine gut. *Am. J. Physiol.*, 239:G12–G17.
50. Reihardt, H. W., Kaczmarczyk, G., Fahrenhorst, K., Blendinger, I., Gatzka, M., Kuhl, U., and Riedel, J. (1975): Postprandial changes in renal blood flow. Studies on conscious dogs on a high and low sodium intake. *Pfluegers Arch.*, 354:287–297.
51. Reininger, E. J., and Sapirstein, L. A. (1957): Effect of digestion on distribution of blood flow in the rat. *Science*, 126:1176.
52. Richardson, P. D. I. (1976): The actions of natural secretin on the small intestinal vasculature of the anaesthetized cat. *Br. J. Pharmacol.*, 58:127–135.
53. Ross, G. (1970): Cardiovascular effects of secretin. *Am. J. Physiol.*, 218:1166–1170.
54. Siregar, H., and Chou, C. C. (1982): Relative contribution of fat, protein, carbohydrate and ethanol to intestinal hyperemia. *Am. J. Physiol.*, 242:G27–G31.
55. Sit, S. P., Nyhof, R., Gallavan, R., and Chou, C. C. (1980): Mechanisms of glucose-induced hyperemia in the jejunum. *Proc. Soc. Exp. Biol. Med.*, 163:273–277.
56. Swan, K. G., and Jacobson, E. D. (1967): Gastric blood flow and secretion in conscious dogs. *Am. J. Physiol.*, 212:891–896.
57. Valleau, J. D., Granger, D. N., and Tayler, A. E. (1979): Effect of solute-coupled volume absorption on oxygen consumption in cat ileum. *Am. J. Physiol.*, 236:E198–E203.
58. Vatner, S. F. (1978): Effects of exercise and excitement on mesenteric and renal dynamics in conscious unrestrained baboons. *Am. J. Physiol.*, 234:H210–H214.
59. Vatner, S. F., Franklin, D., and Van Citters, R. L. (1970): Mesenteric vasoactivity associated with eating and digestion in the conscious dog. *Am. J. Physiol.*, 219:170–174.
60. Vatner, S. F., Franklin, D., and Van Citters, R. L. (1970): Coronary and visceral vasoactivity associated with eating and digestion in the conscious dog. *Am. J. Physiol.*, 219:1380–1385.
61. Vatner, S. F., Patrick, T. A., Higgins, C. B., and Franklin, D. (1974): Regional circulatory adjustments to eating and digestion in conscious unrestrained primates. *J. Appl. Physiol.*, 36:524–529.
62. Wang, C. C., and Grossman, M. I. (1951): Physiological determination of the release of secretin and pancreozymin from intestine of dogs with transplanted pancreas. *Am. J. Physiol.*, 164:527–545.
63. Yu, Y. M., Yu, L. C. C., and Chou, C. C. (1975): Distribution of blood flow in the intestine with hypertonic glucose in the lumen. *Surgery*, 78:520–525.

Intestinal Blood Flow and Motility

Joseph D. Fondacaro

*Smith Kline and French Laboratories
Philadelphia, Pennsylvania 19101*

The physiology of the gastrointestinal system is classically divided into three major functions: motility, secretion, and absorption. An adequate blood supply is necessary for the optimal performance of these essential functions. The mechanical activities of the intestinal musculature that provide for the mixing and propulsion of food are integral components of the total digestive process. Contractions of the visceral smooth muscle of the intestine produce varying alterations in mesenteric blood flow depending on the intensity of contraction. These mechanical events can also change the distribution of blood flow within the wall of the gut. Conversely, alterations in blood flow to the bowel can influence visceral smooth muscle activity.

Several intrinsic and extrinsic factors affect the relationship between intestinal motility and blood flow. Such factors include extravascular compression, smooth muscle cell metabolism, vagal tone, neurohumoral substances including the gastrointestinal hormones, venous pressure, pharmacological agents and the P_{O_2} of mesenteric arterial blood. The elucidation of the influence of these factors has been slow in developing, for little attention has been given to the subject in recent years. The lack of progress can be attributed to limitations in the methods for simultaneously studying intestinal blood flow and motility (75). Nevertheless, some understanding has been gained and reviews on this subject have been published recently (11,13,75).

The purpose of this chapter is to review the effects of intestinal motility on gut blood flow and vice versa. The influence of different types of motor patterns on blood flow will be explored along with the effects of various intrinsic and extrinsic factors on blood flow and motility. The reader may wish to review the unique anatomical relationship between the intestinal musculature and circulation (31).

EFFECTS OF MOTILITY ON BLOOD FLOW

Rhythmic and tonic contractions of the intestinal smooth musculature produce various patterns of intestinal motility. These well-defined but differing patterns of motility in turn evoke various responses from the intestinal circulation. Also, the means by which these motility patterns are induced, that is, luminal distention or nerve stimulation, can modify the response of the mesenteric vasculature.

Rhythmic Versus Tonic Contractions

Rhythmic contractions of the intestinal musculature appear to have a paradoxical effect on intestinal blood flow. When rhythmic contractions are mild, there is usually no change observed in mean blood flow to the intestine. However, instantaneous blood flow undergoes cyclic changes that parallel the rhythmicity of the contractions (13,38,57). Venous outflow and vascular resistance increase, but arterial inflow decreases during contraction. The relaxation phase produces the opposite effects on these parameters (13,38,39,51,57,64). The mechanism by which these mild rhythmic contractions influence the hemodynamics of the mesenteric vasculature is unknown. However, Chou and Gallavan (13) and Pytkowsk and Michalowski (57) have reported that with rhythmic contractions of greater amplitude (so that basal luminal pressure increases), mean blood flow to the intestine decreases. This is what one would expect, since increased luminal pressure would produce an increase in gut wall tension and mechanical compression of blood vessels. However, these same investigators report an increase in blood flow to the gut accompanying high-amplitude rhythmic contractions. The mechanism responsible for this increase is unclear but Chou (11) has suggested that since oxygen consumption increases during this perturbation, active hyperemia and the release of dilator metabolites may be responsible for the observed increase in blood flow during high-amplitude contractions.

Unlike the response to rhythmic contractions, mesenteric blood flow demonstrates a more predictable pattern in response to tonic contractions of the intestinal musculature. In general, blood flow decreases and vascular resistance increases during tonic contractions. This relationship has been observed whether the visceral muscle activity is spontaneous or drug-induced (8,12,39,57,64,65). Furthermore, Kachelhoffer et al. (39) have shown that a positive linear correlation exists between increases in luminal pressure associated with tonic contractions and increases in vascular resistance. Pytkowsk and Michalowski (57) also demonstrated an inverse relationship between tonic contractions and mean blood flow. These responses and the resultant effects on hemodynamic parameters are most likely due to mechanical compression. There is some evidence, however, that a paradoxical effect may also be present. Chou and Gallavan (13) have reported that tonic contractions that are accompanied by strong rhythmic contractions and an increase in oxygen consumption can produce a vasodilator response with a decrease in vascular resistance.

Recent studies have attempted to determine the distribution of blood flow within the intestinal wall during various motility patterns. Investigators have frequently used the distribution of radioactively labeled microspheres to determine the distribution and redistribution of blood flow within the gut wall. The method is simple, consistent, and reproducible, but the validity of the technique has been questioned (34,68). Using this method, Chou and Grassmick (14) reported that rhythmic contractions accompanied by hyperemia result in an increase in muscularis flow with no change in mucosal-submucosal blood flow. This occurred whether the mild rhythmic contractions were induced by luminal distension or by handling the intestine. Schwaiger et al. (62) found that over 90% of the total mesenteric blood flow is distributed to the mucosa-submucosa in both conscious and anesthetized dogs. This was reduced to 78% during surgical manipulation of the gut that produced rhythmic contractions of the musculature.

In contrast, tonic contractions of the intestine reduce total mesenteric blood flow and mucosal-submucosal fractional flow. Blood flow to the muscularis remains unaltered (11). Therefore, during tonic contractions, the fractional blood flow to the muscularis increases. This suggests that the blood flow to the mucosa-submucosa is susceptible to mechanical compression, whereas flow to the muscularis appears to escape this influence. Another explanation for this centers on the interplay of various factors influencing blood flow to the visceral smooth muscle.

Walus and Jacobson (75) and Chou and Gallavan (13) have presented diagrams explaining the influence of various factors on the relationship between motility and blood flow. Rhythmic contractions of the intestinal musculature can be induced by nerve stimulation, chemical agents, or luminal distension. As discussed above, if rhythmic contractions are mild with only a small increase in luminal pressure, a hyperemia results that may be a consequence of increased metabolic activity of the muscle tissue. However, when the force of rhythmic contractions increases, compression of blood vessels occurs, thus reducing blood flow. This would also simultaneously reduce O_2 supply to the tissue and suppress the active hyperemia (13). If this reduced blood flow accompanies luminal distension, receptive relaxation brings about a reduction of the vascular compression effect and a return of the active hyperemic response. These factors, along with autoregulatory mechanisms, would tend to return blood flow to normal levels. Also playing a role in this scheme are local venoarteriolar responses that tend to enhance the increase in vascular resistance that accompanies extravascular compression. Likewise, local nervous reflexes tend to augment the vasodilation produced by active hyperemia and the autoregulatory response.

Tonic contractions of the intestinal musculature usually compromise blood flow because of a pronounced increase in transmural pressure. This would tend to offset any vasodilatory influence of increased smooth muscle metabolism. However, autoregulatory escape has been observed under these conditions with flow gradually increasing towards control (73).

Not to be overlooked in this scheme are the direct effects of nerve stimulation and the action of blood-borne vasoactive agents on the vascular and visceral smooth muscle. Similarly, chemical agents may influence mucosal cell metabolism and alter total intestinal blood flow (13) while also changing intestinal motor activity.

It is difficult to predict which factor or factors have the dominant influence on intestinal blood flow and motility at any moment. It is likely that the net effect represents the algebraic sum of several of these factors.

Luminal Distension

The distension of the intestinal wall induces various response patterns from the visceral musculature. These motor responses, in turn, may alter the distribution of blood flow within the gut wall as well as total blood flow to the intestine. Studies of the relationship between luminal distension and blood flow may be useful in assessing the pathophysiology of mesenteric ischemia that accompanies intestinal obstruction. However, the experimental method by which luminal distension is produced must be carefully chosen, as it will influence the vascular response. The hemodynamic effects of luminal distension are also discussed in Chapter 27.

Hanson (36) studied the hemodynamic effects of distension in the canine intestine. Using stepwise increases in luminal pressure produced by 50-ml injections of mineral oil, he showed that the initial response to the first few inflation steps was a brief increase in blood flow with a return to control within 1 min. As distension increased so that luminal pressure approached and exceeded 100 mm Hg, blood flow to the gut segment was reduced by 50%. Although flow returned to control level, the time to recovery was prolonged several minutes compared with the response to the first few inflations. Using saline as the inflation medium, Chou and Grassmick (14) also showed that mild distension of the gut to a maximum of 25 mm Hg increased total blood flow. This increase in flow to the distended segment was due to an increase in blood flow to the muscularis; flow to the mucosa-submucosa was unaltered. Again, augmented flow during mild distension was transient and the return of flow to control levels coincided with a return to control of intraluminal pressure, suggesting that receptive relaxation is most likely involved. Although Chou and Dabney (12) have reported that vascular resistance decreases as compliance of the gut wall increases, active hyperemia associated with the rhythmic contractions noted during these experiments may also play an important role (13).

Earlier, Brobmann et al. (8,9), using isolated canine small bowel segments, showed that increasing intraluminal pressure to 40 mm Hg reduced both arterial and venous flows. They suggested that increasing intraluminal pressure raised vascular resistance and depressed arterial inflow. Venous outflow initially increased but rapidly fell below control level because of compression of veins by contracting visceral muscle. Arterial flow gradually returned to normal. Since recovery in this case was probably due to receptive relaxation, hemodynamic readjustments could likely have been prevented if elevated luminal pressure had been maintained. However, it is also possible that active hyperemia contributes to the return of flow to control level.

Stepwise increases in intraluminal pressure from 50 to 100 mm Hg produce stepwise decreases in blood flow (13,51). Further increases in pressure do not proportionally reduce flow. Chou and Gallavan (13) and Ohman (51) report an increase in venous PO_2 during high intraluminal pressures and suggest that residual blood flow still traversing this vascular bed is perfusing low or nonnutritive vessels. Pytkowsk et al. (57) and Semba et al. (64) both observed that once the tonic contractions that accompany large increases in intraluminal pressure subside, a hyperemia occurs. They suggest that myogenic and metabolic factors account for this hemodynamic response.

As noted earlier, distension of the gut has notable effects on the distribution of blood flow within the intestinal wall. Ruf and colleagues (59), studying segments of small and large bowel in piglets, demonstrated that ischemia produced by inflation of the gut with air to 15 to 45 mm Hg was confined to the mucosa-submucosa. Fractional blood flow to the muscularis (measured with microspheres) actually increased during this perturbation. Further increases in luminal pressure to 60 mm Hg reduced total blood flow by 75% and depressed mucosal-submucosal flow by 80%, but muscularis flow was only reduced 20% to 25% in both the large and the small bowel. No attempt was made to correlate the blood flow response to intestinal motor activity because closed abdominal preparations were used. However, one must assume that motor activity was increased to some degree with inflation of the gut lumen. These studies support the idea stated earlier that the vascular compartment of the mucosa is more susceptible to the mechanical influence of contraction than is that of the muscularis.

Effects of Nerve Stimulation

The influence of the nervous system on gastrointestinal motility involves three major types of nerves, namely, the extrinsic autonomic nervous system, the intrinsic neurons of the myenteric plexus, and visceral afferent nerves that synapse with both the extrinsic and the intrinsic networks. Signals that traverse these nerves can either increase or decrease gastrointestinal motility and blood flow.

Within the extrinsic network, parasympathetic stimulation, that is, the vagus nerve, generally increases motor activity of the visceral smooth muscle. However, some evidence exists for vagal inhibitory pathways to the gut (76). Sympathetic stimulation mediated through the mesenteric plexus reduces intestinal blood flow and inhibits intestinal motility. The myenteric plexus, an intricate network of neurons and nerve fibers, not only relays and modifies signals from the central nervous system but also influences muscular and vascular activity within the gut via local reflex activity. All these nervous components and their transmitter substances could profoundly affect the relationship between gastrointestinal motility and blood flow.

Early reports suggested that stimulation of the vagus nerve causes both mesenteric vasoconstriction and vasodilation (75). However, since vagal stimulation increases the motor function of the intestine, the concomitant hyperemia may have resulted from increased visceral smooth muscle metabolism and the release of vasodilator metabolites (27). Therefore, one cannot presume dilator nerves exist in the vagus simply because mesenteric vasodilation occurs with vagal stimulation.

Although vagal fibers appear to be uniformly distributed in the proximal and distal small bowel, Kewenter (41) has shown that direct cervical vagal stimulation increases motility in the feline jejunum but does not significantly increase ileal motility. Intestinal blood flow was not appreciably altered in these experiments until high stimulating frequencies were used and a mild vasodilation was observed. No evidence of vagal inhibitory fibers could be obtained with cervical stimulation. Kewenter also demonstrated that intrathoracic and subdiaphragmatic vagal stimulation induced either excitatory or inhibitory motor responses in the jejunum and ileum. The inhibitory responses were caused by activation of high threshold fibers and were accompanied by a decrease in intestinal blood flow. This decrease in blood flow may be due to vagally mediated systemic hypotension, which may in itself depress intestinal motor activity.

However, according to Kock (42), intestinal blood flow has to be reduced 25% to 30% of resting flow before motility of the gut is inhibited. Therefore, the most likely explanation for this reduced blood flow is mechanical compression of the mucosal vascular compartment.

Kewenter (41) also showed that direct stimulation of the splanchnic sympathetic nerves produced a prompt decrease in ileal motility and a vasoconstriction of the intestinal vasculature. This perturbation, however, had little effect on jejunal motility. Intravenous infusion of norepinephrine significantly inhibited jejunal and ileal motility and produced mesenteric vasoconstriction. There was no evidence of direct vagal innervation of intestinal blood vessels. Vagotomy in humans and dogs reduces intestinal peristalsis but does not alter segmental activity (58). Intestinal blood flow has been reported to decrease (3) or not change (28) after vagotomy. Grayson (33) has suggested the reduced blood flow following vagotomy may be due, in part, to elimination of the pumping action of intestinal contractions on capacitance vessels, and Ballinger (3) proposes that direct sympathetic innervation is responsible for this reduction in flow.

The parasympathetic postganglionic neurotransmitter acetylcholine (ACh) is a potent vasodilator and a stimulant of intestinal motility. However, the dilator response may be indirect, resulting from vasodilator metabolites released from contracting visceral smooth muscle (75). Also, the route of administration of ACh produces different effects depending on the experimental setting. Systemic infusion reduces blood flow (30) through a combination of increased mechanical impedance by contracting viscera and through hypotension created by reduced cardiac function. Walus et al. (73) demonstrated that infusion of ACh directly into the canine mesenteric artery augments ileal motility and blood flow. Similar results had been reported previously (4,6,8,41,56).

The response of blood flow to ACh infusion is not always consistent (Fig. 1). In some cases, flow initially increases with motility, but returns to control by the end of a 10-min infusion (73). This return may reflect classic autoregulatory escape or a response to compression produced by sustained tonic visceral contraction. In other cases, the blood flow response is delayed and shows a reciprocal relationship with motility (Fig. 1 and ref. 73). High doses of ACh produce strong, tonic contractions that diminish blood flow. In all cases, intestinal oxygen consumption is unaltered. Atropine blocks the motor but not the vascular response (4). This argues against a direct effect of ACh on mesenteric vascular smooth muscle in favor of an indirect action through release of dilator metabolites from contracting visceral smooth muscle. When ACh is infused intraarterially into segments of small intestine perfused at constant flow, the initial increase in perfusion pressure coincident with increased motor activity (56,63) is followed by a dilator response (6).

In summary, sympathetic stimulation causes predictable effects on intestinal motility and blood flow. Direct vagal stimulation has fairly reproducible effects on intestinal motor function. However, the response of the intestinal vasculature to increased vagal activity is paradoxical. Other factors, including mechanical influences, systemic hemodynamics, and visceral muscle metabolism, modify this vascular response. Blood flow distribution within the gut is also modified by nerve stimulation and vasoactive transmitters.

EFFECTS OF CHEMICAL AGENTS

The activity of vascular and visceral smooth muscle can be influenced by chemicals released locally or borne in the blood from other organ systems. The net effect of these substances *in vivo* depends on the sensitivity of the muscle tissue they influence and the magnitude of the response that is elicited. Thus, a vasodilator substance that would ordinarily increase mesenteric blood flow may also stimulate tonic contractions of the gut that could markedly increase vascular resistance. Likewise, large increases in flow could be seen with a less-potent vasodi-

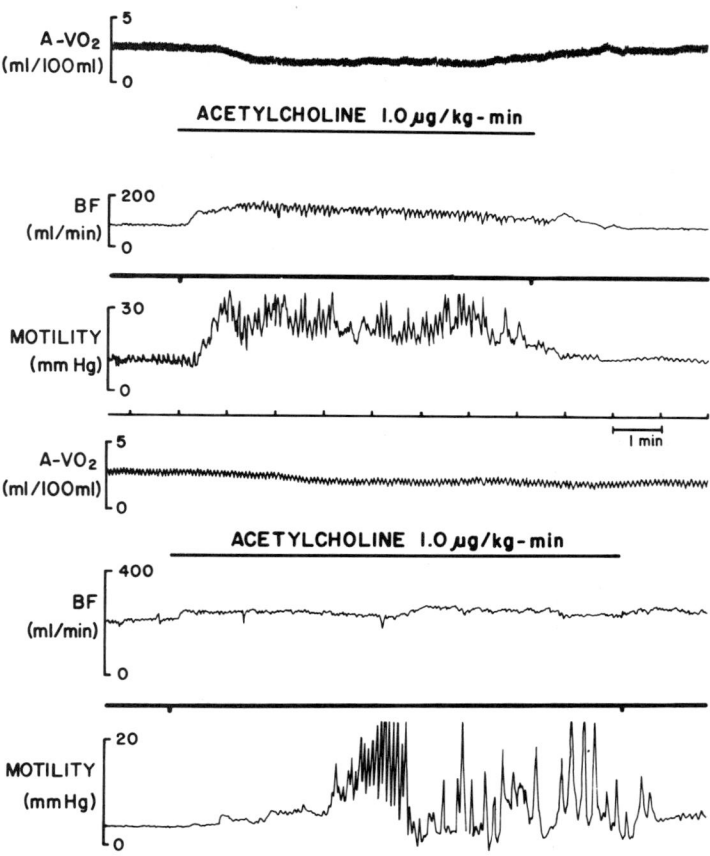

FIG. 1. Effects of intraarterial acetylcholine on intestinal blood flow (BF), arteriovenous oxygen content difference (A-V_{O_2}) and motility under constant pressure perfusion. Note that acetylcholine increases both blood flow and motility. (From Walus et al., ref. 73, with permission.)

lator if the substance administered also initiates mild rhythmic contraction with accompanying release of dilator metabolites. The effects of various endogenous and exogenous chemical agents on intestinal motility and blood flow are presented in Table 1.

In a recent study, Walus et al. (73) investigated the effects of intraarterial administration of several of these agents on total mesenteric blood flow, fractional muscularis flow, motility, oxygen extraction, and oxygen consumption (V_{O_2}). Infusion of ACh at 0.1 µg/kg-min did not significantly alter any of these parameters. Higher doses produced significant dose-dependent increases in total flow, muscularis flow, and motility, whereas oxygen extraction decreased and V_{O_2} was unchanged. The effects of ACh have already been discussed in the previous section on nerve stimulation.

Prostaglandin D_2 (PGD_2) and methionine-enkephalin (met-enkephalin) both increase total mesenteric blood flow, muscularis flow, and motility when infused intraarterially into the mesenteric vascular bed (Fig. 2). However, PGD_2 reduces oxygen extraction and V_{O_2} whereas met-enkephalin increases V_{O_2} without altering oxygen extraction. Also, the hyperemic response produced by PGD_2 was delayed and appeared to commence when the motor activity began to decline. This suggests that the direct vasodilator response to PGD_2 was offset by the initial strong mechanical effect of motility and was not revealed until the compression effect began to wane.

TABLE 1. *Effect of various chemical agents on intestinal motility and blood flow*

Agent	Effect on motility	Effect on blood flow	Ref.
Acetylcholine	Increase	Increase	13,26,38,73
Adrenergics	Decrease	Decrease	13
Angiotensin II	Increase	Decrease	38,73
Bradykinin	Increase	Variable	12–14,22–25,38,67
Ca^{2+}			
(low doses)	Decrease	Decrease	13,17
(high doses)	Increase	Decrease	72
Ca^{2+} antagonists	Decrease	Increase	72
Carbon dioxide	Decrease	Increase	4
Endotoxin	Increase	Variable	49
Gastrin and CCK	Increase	Increase	7,20,21,53,61,69
Glucagon	Decrease	Increase	69,75
Histamine	Increase	Increase	38,62,74
K^+			
(low doses)	Decrease	Increase	13,17,21
(high doses)	Increase	Decrease	13,17,21
Methacholine	Increase	Decrease	75,77
Methionine-enkephalin	Increase	Increase	54,55,73
Mg^{2+}	Decrease	Increase	13,15,17
Morphine	Increase	No change	18,37,45,54,55,73
Physostigmine	Increase	Decrease	14
Prostaglandin D_2	Increase	Increase	73
Prostaglandin $F_{2\alpha}$	Increase	Decrease	67,73
Secretin	Decrease	Variable	13,53,69
Serotonin	Variable	Variable	1,5,12,13,37
Somatostatin	Decrease	Decrease	43,75
Substance P			
(low doses)	No change	Increase	60
(high doses)	Increase	Increase	46,60
Vasoactive intestinal polypeptide			
(stomach)	Decrease	Increase	19
(colon)	Increase	Increase	19
Vasopressin	Variable	Decrease	61,66

Conversely, intraarterial infusions of angiotensin II and prostaglandin $F_{2\alpha}$ ($PGF_{2\alpha}$) increase intestinal motor activity and decrease total blood flow (Fig. 3). In both cases, the vasoconstrictor response preceded the motor response, and evidence of autoregulatory escape of blood flow was noted. This suggests a possible mechanism by which these agents increase motor activity. Since partial ischemia and hypoxia are known to transiently increase motor activity (13), the initial reduction in blood flow and oxygen delivery may have brought about the increase in motility. With gradual escape from the vasoconstrictor response and an increase in oxygen extraction (which is also delayed) (Fig. 3), increased motor activity could be sustained through direct stimulation of visceral smooth muscle by these agents. However, Vo_2 only increased with $PGF_{2\alpha}$ infusion and muscularis flow only increased with angiotensin II, so the exact mechanism remains unknown.

Morphine produced a dose-dependent increase in motor activity without altering total ileal blood flow, oxygen extraction or Vo_2 (73). However, there appeared to be a redistribution of flow away from the muscularis at the highest dose used (0.1 μg/kg-min). This parameter was not examined at other doses of morphine. Figure 4 illustrates the delay in onset of motor activity and the lack of change in total blood flow and arterial pressure (and thus mesenteric vascular resistance) during morphine infusion.

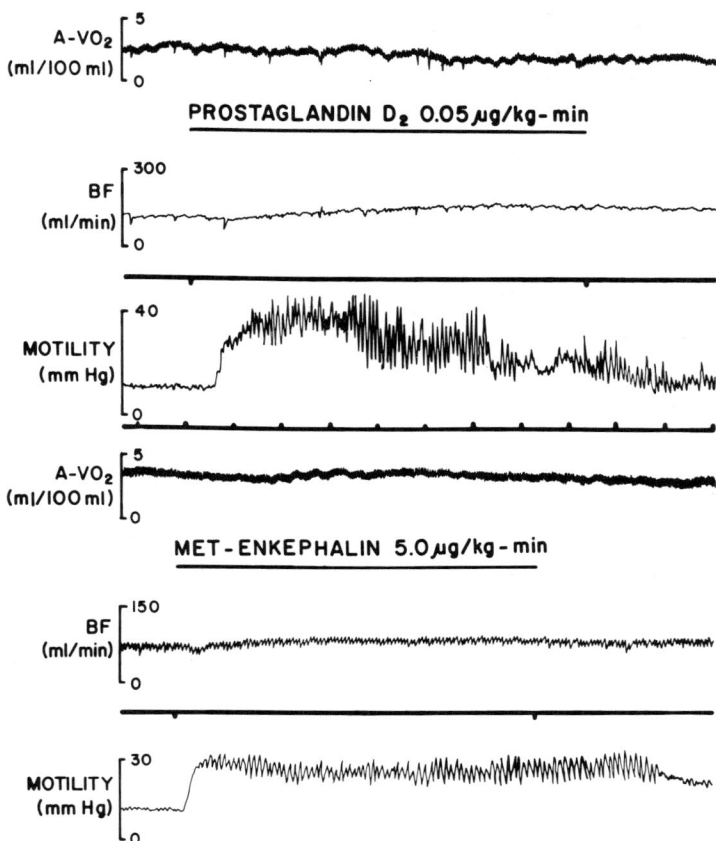

FIG. 2. Effects of prostaglandin D_2 *(upper tracings)* and methionine-enkephalin *(lower tracings)* on A-V_{O_2}, BF, and intestinal motility. Note the motor response preceding the flow response. Note also that these agents, like acetylcholine, increase both blood flow and motility. For definition of abbreviations, see legend to Fig. 1. (From Walus et al., ref. 73, with permission.)

These studies suggest that, unless a direct vascular response is masked by the visceral activity, the mesenteric vasculature is devoid of opiate receptors. This conclusion is supported by the lack of a direct vascular effect on intraarterial infusion of met-enkephalin (Fig. 2 and ref. 73) and the demonstration that the response of mesenteric arterial strips to KCl *in vitro* was unaltered in the presence of met-enkephalin (29).

There appears to be no distinct relationship between intestinal blood flow and motility that can be elucidated with experimental administration of vasoactive agents. As seen in Table 1, responses are varied even between agents that are chemically similar. With varying responses of motility, total blood flow, fractional flow, and V_{O_2}, it is perhaps best that these agents and others be evaluated for their separate effects on flow and motility. Conclusions drawn regarding a relationship between the flow and motor responses to a given agent should be left to speculation.

EFFECTS OF BLOOD FLOW ON MOTILITY

Thus far we have seen that blood flow through the intestinal vascular bed can be altered by various motor patterns of the gut. However, if a change in mesenteric blood flow is the initial event, the intestinal musculature may not always respond but may remain unaffected by altered blood flow. These responses are important

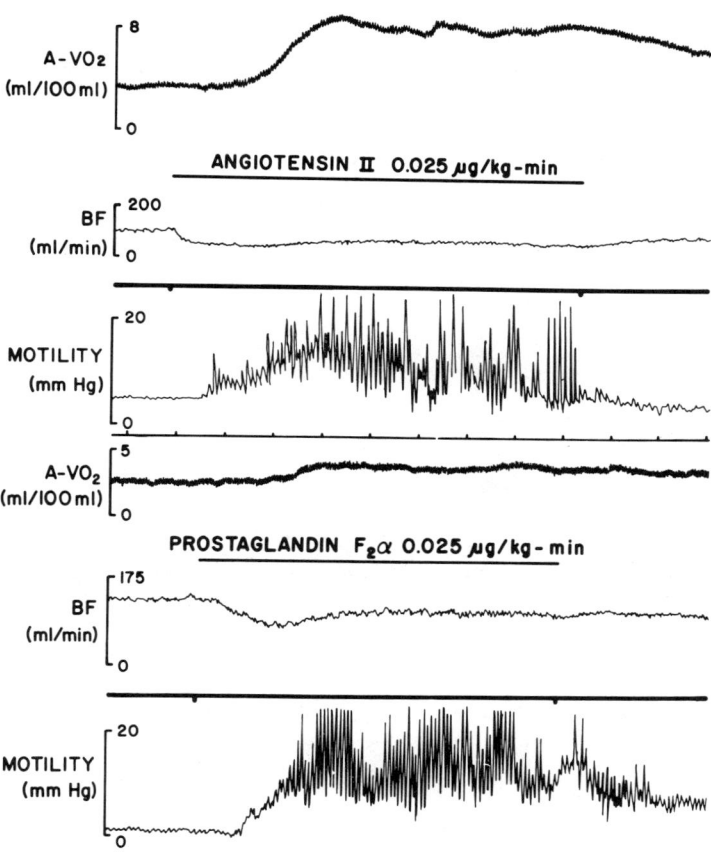

FIG. 3. Effects of intraarterial angiotensin II *(upper tracings)* and prostaglandin $F_{2\alpha}$ *(lower tracings)*. Note that these agents depress blood flow but increase motility. For definition of abbreviations, see legend to Fig. 1. (From Walus et al., ref. 73, with permission.)

in our understanding of the pathophysiology of intestinal ischemia and its therapy.

Intestinal motor activity is not altered by an increase in intestinal blood flow. Chou and Dabney (12) have shown that, in pump-perfused segments of bowel, doubling blood flow does not significantly change intestinal motility. However, reductions in flow or oxygen content of blood can have profound effects on both the electrical and contractile activities of the gut. A biphasic change in motility follows ischemia and hypoxia. Arterial occulsion of an intestinal gut segment produces a prompt but transient increase in spike potentials and contractions lasting up to 5 min (10,13,35). A similar response occurs with a 75% reduction in inhaled oxygen (48). Following the hypermotile response, motility subsides and the musculature becomes quiescent. Partial ischemia or a 50% reduction in inhaled O_2 produce only the hypermotile phase, with muscular activity of the gut returning to control within 5 min. Because tetrodotoxin prevents the initial stimulatory phase, Chou and Gallavan (13) have proposed that local intrinsic nerves mediate the response.

Reduced blood flow to one portion of the gut may alter motility of the entire small bowel through intrinsic reflex activity. Nylander and Wikstrom (50) found that moderate ileal ischemia augmented gastric emptying and decreased intestinal transit in the rat. After 24 hr, the inflammatory response was noted at the ischemic site and motility of the entire bowel was markedly reduced. By contrast, severe is-

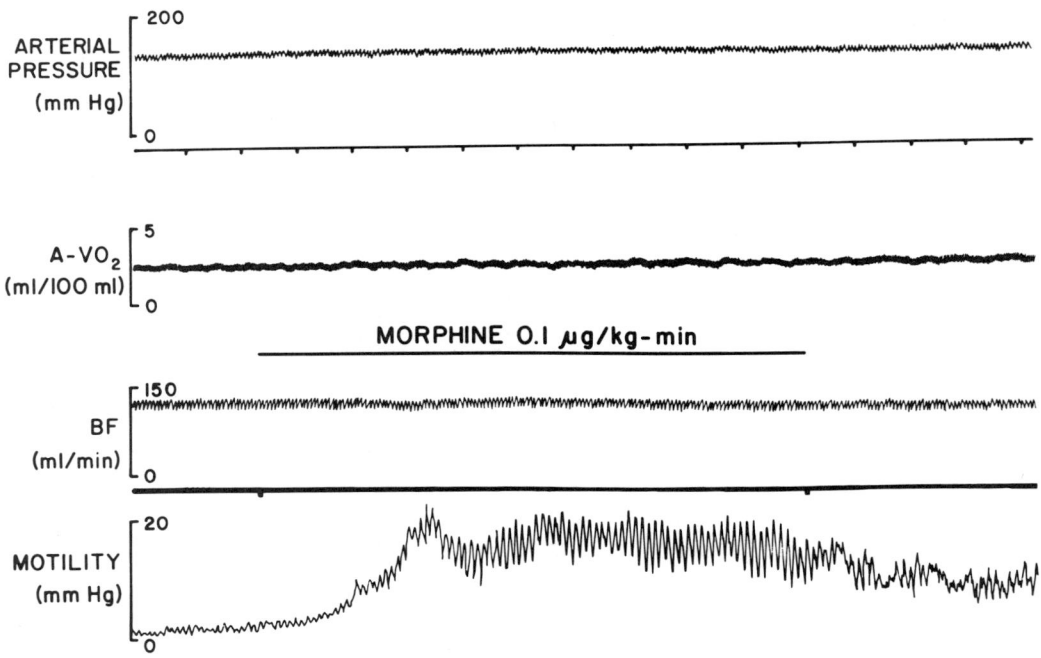

FIG. 4. Effect of intraarterial morphine on motility. Note the lack of change in blood flow, A-VO_2 and arterial pressure. (From Walus et al., ref. 73, with permission.)

chemia produced an immediate cessation of gastric emptying and a slowing of wave propagation within the visceral muscle.

The duration of the ischemic insult appears to be a critical factor in the restoration of normal motor activity of the intestine upon reperfusion. In the study by Cabot and Kohastu (10), ischemia of an intestinal segment for up to 3 hr in the dog did not prevent the return of normal electrical and spontaneous mechanical activity of the segment upon recirculation. Kessler and Linden (40) made the same observation. However, total ischemia for 4 hr prevented the return of motility following reperfusion (10,35). This lack of motility was characterized by Szurszewski and Steggerda (70,71) as an uncoupling of intestinal slow waves and a decrease in their frequency.

Intestinal necrosis induced by mesenteric vascular insufficiency begins in the mucosa (62). Two hours of total ischemia in the dog small bowel causes exfoliated epithelial cells at the villus tips (2). Transmission electron microscopy reveals severe architectural alterations of the microvilli (2). However, as noted above, ischemia of up to 3 hr has minimal effect on nerve and muscle activity in the gut. Chou (11) has suggested that the intestinal musculature is more resistant to ischemic damage than the mucosa because of its lower metabolic rate. Furthermore, it appears as though an intact myenteric plexus is critical to normal motility. Ischemia longer than 3 hr alters the frequency of myogenic pacemaker activity and causes asynchrony of muscular contractions in both the ischemic segment and adjacent areas (75).

Kyi and Daniel (44) have reported that muscle strips obtained from ischemic bowel showed no rhythmic activity and a reduced contractile response to methacholine. Normal responses were observed when the nerves to these segments were stimulated. The initial changes may be due to alterations in electrolyte balance within these excitable tissues. Ischemia and anoxia increase visceral smooth muscle cell Na^+, Ca^{2+}, and Cl^-, but depress K^+ and Mg^{2+} (11). Severe or prolonged intestinal ischemia may produce profound changes in permeability of the sarcolemma, thus causing an abnormal redistribution of electrolytes, so that the enzyme-mediated membrane pumps fail to maintain the membrane potential. Consequently, the reported changes in synchrony and pacemaker activity resulting from ischemia of the bowel can be accounted for by altered smooth muscle excitability, impulse conduction, and excitation-contraction coupling processes that are dependent on a normal electrolyte distribution across plasma membranes.

In summary, the small intestinal musculature responds to reductions in both blow flow and the oxygen content of arterial blood. Initial changes in motility are biphasic in nature with a cessation of activity during continued ischemia. Although the visceral musculature appears to be less sensitive to ischemia and hypoxia than the mucosa, if the duration of the ischemic insult is substantial, profound effects on motility are noted. These effects appear to depend primarily on the degree of damage of the myenteric plexus within the smooth muscle layer. However, changes in electrolyte distribution across visceral sarcolemmal membranes can account for many of the disturbances seen with reduced blood flow to the intestine. Thus, it appears as though changes in motility with initial alterations in intestinal blood flow are less predictable than the changes in blood flow brought on by altered intestinal motor activity.

SUMMARY

It is apparent that intestinal motility can influence mesenteric blood flow. Furthermore, we now have some understanding of how various motor patterns alter blood flow distribution and oxygen consumption within the intestinal tissue. Mild rhythmic contractions may increase total mesenteric blood flow, primarily owing to release of dilator metabolites. Also, vascular compression during contraction may offset any dilator response. An increase in blood flow under these conditions is generally seen as an increase in fractional flow to the muscularis, whereas flow to the mucosa is either reduced by mechanical compression or not altered. Certainly the mucosal blood vessels are more susceptible to extravascular compression than vessels in the muscularis. With more forceful rhythmic activity and with tonic contractions, total intestinal blood flow decreases largely because of substantial increases in extravascular compression. Many other factors influence the vascular response to forceful contractions, making assessment of the relationship between flow and motility difficult in the experimental setting.

Distension of the intestinal wall will elicit rhythmic or tonic contractions of the intestinal musculature depending on the degree of distension. Blood flow responses are generally the same as those described above. However, the added factor of receptive relaxation may alter the temporal pattern of the vascular response.

An intricate network of nerves and synapses is involved in the moment-to-moment modification of intestinal motor activity. This adds to the difficulty in characterizing the relationship between intestinal motility and blood flow when nerve stimulation is used. Likewise, the use of chemical agents to assess this relationship is controversial because of the varied direct and indirect vascular and visceral effects that are possible with administration of such agents.

Finally, changes in intestinal motor activity are less tightly coupled to initial alterations in mesenteric blood flow. Ischemia of the bowel has profound effects on motility, but these effects are varied, depending on the degree of ischemia and the portion of bowel to which the ischemic insult is directed.

Further studies of the blood flow–motility relationship are warranted. Modern methodology and technology permit the use of conscious animal models for the more meaningful study of this relationship. An accurate description of these events and their regulatory influences could prove vital for the future therapeutic approach to gastrointestinal disorders involving the circulatory and visceral smooth muscle systems.

REFERENCES

1. Adar, R., and Salzman, E. W. (1974): Serotonin and the mesenteric circulation. *Pr. Med. J.*, 2:444.
2. Ashraf, M., Lepera, R., and Fondacaro, J. D. (1982): Surface ultrastructure changes in dog small intestinal mucosa following ischemia. *Scand. Electron Microsc.*, 11:797–803.
3. Ballinger, W. F., Dadulla, R. T., and Camishion, R. C. (1965): Mesenteric blood flow following total and selective vagotomy. *Surgery*, 57:409–413.
4. Bean, J. W., and Sidky, M. M. (1958): Intestinal blood flow as influenced by vascular and motor reactions to acetylcholine and carbon dioxide. *Am. J. Physiol.*, 194:512–518.
5. Biber, B., Fara, J., and Lundgren, O. (1973): Intestinal vascular responses to 5-hydroxytryptamine. *Acta Physiol. Scand.*, 87:526–534.
6. Boatman, D. L., and Brody, M. J. (1983): Effects of acetylcholine on the intestinal vasculature of the dog. *J. Pharmacol. Exp. Ther.*, 142:185–191.
7. Bowen, J. C., Pawlik, W., Fang, W. F., and Jacobson, E. D. (1975): Pharmacologic effects of gastrointestinal hormones on intestinal oxygen consumption and blood flow. *Surgery*, 78:515–519.
8. Brobmann, G. F., Jacobson, E. D., and Brecher, G. A. (1970): Intestinal vascular response to gut pressure and acetylcholine in vitro. *Angiologica*, 7:129–139.
9. Brobmann, G. F., Jacobson, E. D., and Brecher, G. A. (1970): Effects of distension and acetylcholine on intestinal blood flow in vivo. *Angiologica*, 7:140–146.
10. Cabot, R. M., and Kohastu, S. (1978): The effects of ischemia on the electrical and contractile activities of the canine small intestine. *Am. J. Surg.*, 136:242–246.
11. Chou, C. C. (1982): Relationship between intestinal blood flow and motility. *Annu. Rev. Physiol.*, 44:29–42.
12. Chou, C. C., and Dabney, J. M. (1967): Interrelation of ileal wall compliance and vascular resistance. *Am. J. Dig. Dis.*, 12:1198–1208.
13. Chou, C. C., and Gallavan, R. H. (1982): Blood flow and intestinal motility. *Fed. Proc.*, 41:2090–2095.
14. Chou, C. C., and Grassmick, B. (1978): Motility and blood flow distribution within the wall of the gastrointestinal tract. *Am. J. Physiol.*, 235:H34–H39.
15. Dabney, J. M., Scott, J. B., and Chou, C. C. (1966): Intestinal vascular resistance as affected by the biphasic response of smooth muscle to the potassium ion. *Physiologist*, 9:163.
16. Dabney, J. M., Scott, J. B., and Chou, C. C. (1967): Action of adenosine and ATP on ileal wall tension and blood flow. *Physiologist*, 10:150.
17. Dabney, J. M., Scott, J. B., and Chou, C. C. (1967): Effects of cations on ileal compliance and blood flow. *Am. J. Physiol.*, 212:835–839.
18. Daniel, E. E. (1968): Pharmacology of the gastrointestinal tract. In: *Handbook of Physiology: Alimentary Canal*, edited by C. F. Code, pp. 2267–2324. American Physiological Society, Washington, D.C.
19. Eklund, S., Jodal, M., Lundgren, O., and Sjoqvist, A. (1979): Effects of vasoactive intestinal polypeptide on blood flow, motility and fluid transport in the gastrointestinal tract of the cat. *Acta Physiol. Scand.*, 105:461–468.
20. Fara, J. W., Rubenstein, E. H., and Sonnenschen, R. R. (1972): Intestinal hormones in mesenteric vasodilation after intradrodenal agents. *Am. J. Physiol.*, 233:1058–1067.
21. Fasth, S., Fiupsson, S., Hulten, L., and Martinson, J. (1973): The effect of the gastrointestinal hormones on small intestinal motility and blood flow. *Experientia*, 29:982–984.
22. Fasth, S., and Hulten, L. (1972): Neurohumal regulation of motility and blood flow in the colon. *Experientia*, 28:1447–1448.
23. Fasth, S., and Hulten, L. (1973): The effect of bradykinin on intestinal motility and blood flow. *Acta Chir. Scand.*, 139:699–705.
24. Fasth, S., and Hulten, L. (1973): The effect of bradykinin on the consecutive vascular sections of the small and large intestine. *Acta Chir. Scand.*, 139:707–715.
25. Fasth, S., Hulten, L., Johnson, B. J., Nordgren, S., and Zeithin, L. J. (1978): Mobilization of colonic kallikrein following pelvic nerve stimulation in the atropinized cat. *J. Physiol.*, 285:471–478.
26. Fasth, S., Hulten, L., and Nordgren, S. (1980): Evidence for a dual pelvic nerve influence on large bowel motility in the cat. *J. Physiol.*, 298:159–169.
27. Folkow, B. (1955): Nervous control of the blood vessels. *Physiol. Rev.*, 35:629–663.
28. Folkow, B., Lewis, D. H., Lundgren, O., Mellander, S., and Wallentin, L. (1964): The effect of graded vasoconstrictor fibre stimulation on intestinal resistance and capacitance vessels. *Acta Physiol. Scand.*, 61:445–457.
29. Fondacaro, J. D., DiSalvo, J., and Jacobson, E. D. (1981): Effects of diltiazem, nifedipine and metenkephalin on mesenteric vascular smooth muscle. *Clin. Res. (Abstr.)*, 29:823A.
30. Gotse, T. (1940): Die Bedeutung der Blutgefässe und des Herzen für die Regulierung des Blutdruckes. *Arch. Exp. Pathol. Pharmacol.*, 195:26–42.
31. Granger, D. N., and Buckley, G. B., editors (1981): *Measurements of Blood Flow; Application to the Splanchnic Circulation*. Williams and Wilkins, Baltimore.
32. Granger, D. N., Kvietys, P. R., Mortillaro, N. A., and Taylor, A. E. (1980): Effect of luminal distension on intestinal transcapillary fluid exchange. *Am. J. Physiol.*, 239:G516–G523.
33. Grayson, J. (1974): The gastrointestinal circulation. In: *Gastrointestinal Physiology*, edited by E. D. Jacobson and L. L. Shanbour, pp. 105–138. University Park Press, Baltimore.
34. Greenway, C. V., and Murthy, V. S. (1972): Effects of vasopressin and isoprenaline infusions on the distribution of blood flow in the intestine; criteria for the validity of microsphere studies. *Br. J. Pharmacol.*, 46:177–188.
35. Guisan, Y. J., Hreno, A., and Gurd, F. N. (1975): Effect of acute ischemia on the motility of the small bowel in the awake dog. *Eur. Surg. Res.*, 7:23–33.
36. Hanson, K. (1973): Hemodynamic effects of distension of the dog small intestine. *Am. J. Physiol.*, 225:456–460.

37. Hashimoto, K., and Kumakura, S. (1965): The pharmacological features of the coronary, renal, mesenteric and femoral arteries. *Jpn. J. Physiol.*, 15:540–551.
38. Jacobson, E. D., Brobmann, G. F., and Brecher, G. A. (1970): Intestinal motor activity and blood flow. *Gastroenterology*, 58:575–579.
39. Kachelhoffer, J., Pousse, A., Marescaux, J., Iturizaga, M., and Grenier, J. F. (1978): Effects of motility and luminal distension on dog small intestine hemodynamics. *Eur. Surg. Res.*, 10:184–193.
40. Kessler, E., and Linden, G. (1964): Die Postischämische Kontracktur des Darmes. *Frankf. Z. Pathol.*, 73:363–379.
41. Kewenter, J. (1965): The vagal control of the jejunal and ileal motility and blood flow. *Acta Physiol. Scand. (Suppl.)*, 251:1–68.
42. Kock, N. G. (1959): An experimental analysis of mechanisms engaged in reflex inhibition of intestinal motility. *Acta Physiol. Scand. (Suppl.)*, 164:1–54.
43. Konturek, S. J., Krol, R., Pawlik, W., Tasler, J., Thor, P., Walus, K. M., and Schally, A. V. (1978): Pharmacology of somatostatin. In: *Gut Hormones*, edited by S. R. Gloom, pp. 457–467. Churchill Livingstone, Edinburgh.
44. Kyi, J. K. J., and Daniel, E. E. (1970): The effects of ischemia on intestinal nerves and electrical slow waves. *Am. J. Dig. Dis.*, 15:959–981.
45. Leaman, D. M., Levenson, L., Zelis, R., and Shiroff, R. (1978): Effects of morphine on splanchnic blood flow. *Br. Heart J.*, 40:569–571.
46. Lembeck, F., and Hettich, R. (1969): Comparative study of the effects of substance P on blood pressure, salivatory functions and intestinal motility. *Naunyn Schmiedebergs Arch. Pharmacol.*, 265:216–224.
47. Lifson, N. (1979): Fluid secretion and hydrostatic relationships in the small intestine. In: *Mechanisms of Intestinal Secretion*, edited by H. J. Binder, pp. 249–261. Liss, New York.
48. Meissner, A., Bowes, K. L., and Sarna, S. K. (1976): Effects of ambient and stagnant hypoxia on the mechanical and electrical activity of the canine upper jejunum. *Can. J. Surg.*, 19:316–321.
49. Meyer, M. W., and Visscher, M. B. (1962): Partial analysis of segmental resistance in intestinal vessels after endotoxin. *Am. J. Physiol.*, 202:913–918.
50. Nylander, G., and Wikstrom, S. (1968): Propulsive gastrointestinal motility in regional and graded ischemia of the small bowel. An experimental study in rats. I. Immediate results. *Acta Chir. Scand. (Suppl.)*, 385:1–67.
51. Ohman, U. (1975): Studies on small intestinal obstruction. Blood circulation in obstructed and artificially distended small intestine in the cat. *Acta Chir. Scand. (Suppl.)*, 452.
52. Ohman, U. (1976): Blood flow and oxygen consumption in the feline small intestine: Responses to artificial distension and intestinal obstruction. *Acta Chir. Scand.*, 142:329–333.
53. Pawlik, W., Bowen, J. C., and Jacobson, E. D. (1977): Vasoactive and metabolic effects of gastrointestinal hormones in the intestine. *Mat. Med. Pol.*, 31:151–154.
54. Pawlik, W. W., Walus, K. M., and Fondacaro, J. D. (1980): Effects of methionine-enkephalin on intestinal circulation and oxygen consumption. *Proc. Soc. Exp. Biol. Med.*, 165:26–31.
55. Pawlik, W. W., Walus, K. M., Konturek, S. J., Coy, D. H., and Schally, A. V. (1977): Effect of enkephalin on intestinal circulation. *Proc. 23rd Int. Congr. Physiol. Sci. Paris*, 13:584.
56. Price, W. E., Shehadeh, Z., Thompson, G. H., Underwood, L. D., and Jacobson, E. D. (1969): Effects of acetylcholine on intestinal blood flow and motility. *Am. J. Physiol.*, 216:343–347.
57. Pytkowsk, B., and Michalowski, J. (1977): Motility and blood flow-dependent absorption of amino acids in canine small intestine. *Eur. J. Clin. Invest.*, 7:79–86.
58. Roth, H. P., and Beams, A. J. (1959): The effects of vagotomy on the motility of the small intestine. *Gastroenterology*, 36:452–458.
59. Ruf, W., Suehiro, G. T., Suehiro, A., Pressler, V., and McNamara, J. J. (1980): Intestinal blood flow at various intraluminal pressures in the piglet with closed abdomen. *Ann. Surg.*, 191:157–163.
60. Schrauwen, E., and Houvenaghel, A. (1979): Influence of substance P on mesenteric hemodynamics in the pig. *Arch. Int. Pharmacodyn. Ther.*, 242:315–317.
61. Schuurkes, J. A. J., and Charbon, G. A. (1978): Motility and hemodynamics of the canine gastrointestinal tract. Stimulation by pentagastrin, cholecystokinin and vasopressin. *Arch. Int. Pharmacodyn. Ther.*, 236:214–227.
62. Schwaiger, M. M., Fondacaro, J. D., and Jacobson, E. D. (1979): Effects of glucagon, histamine and perhexiline on the ischemic canine mesenteric circulation. *Gastroenterology*, 77:730–735.
63. Scott, J. B., and Dabney, J. M. (1964): Relation of gut motility and blood flow in the ileum of the dog. *Circ. Res. (Suppl.)*, 15(1):234–239.
64. Semba, T., Kazumoto, F., and Fujii, Y. (1971): The influence of rhythmic and tonic contractions of the small intestine on blood flow through the intestinal segment. *Jpn. J. Physiol.*, 21:1–145.
65. Sidky, M., and Bean, J. W. (1958): Influence of rhythmic and tonic contraction of intestinal muscle on blood flow and blood reservoir capacity in dog intestine. *Am. J. Physiol.*, 193:386–392.
66. Shapiro, H., and Britt, L. G. (1972): The action of vasopressin on the gastrointestinal tract. A review of the literature. *Am. J. Dig. Dis.*, 17:649–667.
67. Shehadeh, Z., Price, W. E., and Jacobson, E. D. (1969): Effects of vasoactive agents on intestinal blood flow and motility in the dog. *Am. J. Physiol.*, 216:386–392.
68. Shepherd, A. P., Jr., Maxwell, L. C., and Jacobson, E. D. (1981): Limitations of the microsphere technique to fractionate intestinal blood flow. In: *Measurement of Splanchnic Blood Flow; Application to the Splanchnic Circulation*, edited by D. N. Granger, and G. B. Buckley, pp. 195–200. Williams and Wilkins, Baltimore.
69. Svanik, J., and Lundgren, O. (1977): Gastrointestinal circulation. In: *International Review of Physiology, vol. 12, Gastrointestinal Physiology II*, edited by R. Crane, pp. 1–34. University Park Press, Baltimore.

70. Szurszewski, J., and Steggerda, F. R. (1968): The effect of hypoxia on the electrical slow wave of the canine small intestine. *Am. J. Dig. Dis.*, 13:168–177.
71. Szurszewski, J., and Steggerda, F. R. (1968): The effect of hypoxia on the mechanical activity of the canine small intestine. *Am. J. Dig. Dis.*, 13:178–185.
72. Walus, K. M., Fondacaro, J. D., and Jacobson, E. D. (1981): Effects of calcium and its antagonists on the canine mesenteric circulation. *Circ. Res.*, 48:692–700.
73. Walus, K. M., Fondacaro, J. D., and Jacobson, E. D. (1981): Hemodynamic and metabolic changes during stimulation of ileal motility. *Dig. Dis. Sci.*, 26:1069–1077.
74. Walus, K. M., Fondacaro, J. D., and Jacobson, E. D. (1981): A further characterization of histamine H_1 and H_2 effects and blockade in canine intestinal circulation. *Dig. Dis. Sci.*, 26:1542–1549.
75. Walus, K. M., and Jacobson, E. D. (1981): Relation between small intestine motility and circulation. *Am. J. Physiol.*, 241:G1–G15.
76. Wood, J. D. (1981): Physiology of the enteric nervous system. In: *Physiology of the Gastrointestinal Tract*, edited by L. R. Johnson, pp. 1–37. Raven Press, New York.
77. Zeigler, M. G., Barton, R. W., and Swan, K. G. (1973): Mesenteric blood flow and small intestinal motility in the dog. *Surgery*, 73:649–656.

Gastrointestinal Hormones and Intestinal Blood Flow

C. C. Chou, M. J. Mangino, and D. R. Sawmiller

Departments of Physiology and Medicine, Michigan State University, East Lansing, Michigan 48824

Cardiovascular effects of the gastrointestinal hormones were first observed by Bayliss and Starling in 1902 when they discovered secretin (5). Intravenous injection of an acid extract of the small intestine caused not only a copious pancreatic secretion but also a considerable fall in the blood pressure. Although they attributed the vasodepressor effect of the extract to its impurities, many recent studies have shown that some hormones secreted from the small intestine are potent vasodilators.

All of the 10 gastrointestinal hormones reviewed in this chapter, except somatostatin, are vasodilators in the small intestine. To determine whether or not a particular hormone plays a role in the regulation of intestinal blood flow under physiological conditions, we have constructed Table 1. The calculated or measured blood concentration of a hormone at the minimal infusion that induced vasodilation (Table 1, see "Minimal effect") can be compared with the serum concentrations the hormone achieved after a meal. In addition, if a study examined dose-response relationships, the maximum dose reported and its effect are shown in Table 1 as "Maximum effects." Some studies employed only one infusion rate. The responses are expressed as percentage changes from control values either quoted from the original paper or calculated from actual flow values. Papers that did not indicate infusion rates or quantitative responses were excluded from this chapter and are not shown in Table 1. Effects of the hormones on other variables such as capillary filtration coefficient (K_f), oxgyen uptake ($\dot{V}O_2$), motility, blood flow to the mucosa, submucosa, muscularis (muscle), and absorptive site (Abs. site F), as well as tissue volume are shown in the Miscellaneous column. Because various species respond differently to a given hormone, the species used are also indicated in Table 1. Most studies were performed under anesthesia. Many studies with cholecystokinin (CCK) and secretin utilized tissue extracts; the source of these hormones is also shown, since extracts differ in their effects. Many older studies are not included in this chapter because of limitation in space. Some original articles are quoted indirectly from papers that cited the original articles.

CCK

CCK decreases intestinal vascular resistance (R) and increases intestinal blood flow (F) in the anesthetized cat, dog, and pig (6,7,10,14,16,18). The minimal infusion rates that produced vasodilation were about 1.0 U/kg/hr i.v. of 17% pure CCK (Karolinska Institute) (14), 0.05 U/min i.a. (equivalent to 0.1 µg/min based on 0.5 U/µg) of 17% pure CCK (Karolinska Institute) (10), 0.1 µg/min i.a. of 95% pure CCK (18), and 0.01 µg/min i.a. of a synthetic CCK-octapeptide (18). The minimal infusion rates required to produce vasodilation in these studies are therefore similar. At these infusion rates, CCK produced a 10% to 17% increase in intestinal blood flow or a 9% decrease in vascular resistance (Table 1). The increase in the blood concentration of CCK during the infusion can easily be calculated in the constant flow preparation. A local intraarterial infusion of CCK at 0.05 U/min increased local arterial blood CCK concentration by about 2.5 mU/ml (equivalent to about 5 ng/ml) (10). Postprandial serum CCK concentrations have been reported

TABLE 1. *Vascular effects of gastrointestinal hormones in the small intestine*

Horm. infusion rtes	Minimal effects		Maximum effects			Ref., species
	Dose	% changes	Dose	% changes	Misc.	
CCK						
Extract (K.I.)						
i.v.	1.1 U/k/hr	+10% F	4.3 U/k/hr	+60% F	+Motility	15, cat
i.v.	1.0 U/k/hr	+15% F	6.5 U/k/hr	+85% F	+$\dot{V}_{O_2}$ +Mucosal F −Submucosal F	14, cat
Extract (K.I.)						
i.a.	0.05–0.2 U/k/min	+60% F	3 to 4 U/k/min	+150% F	+K_f +Tissue vol.	6,14, cat
i.a.	0.05 U/min	−9% R	0.2 U/min	−40% R	+Motility	10, dog
Extract (K.I.), 95% pure						
i.a.	0.1 μg/min	+17% F	5 μg/min	+85% F		18, pig
Synthetic Squibb, CCK-OP						
i.a.	0.01 μg/min	+10% F	0.5 μg/min	+100% F		18, pig
i.a.			0.1 μg/k/min[a]	+45% F[a]	+$\dot{V}_{O_2}$ 23%	7, dog
Secretin						
Extract (K.I.)						
i.v.	4 U/k/hr	−10–25% R	1–10 U	−28–48% R	Motility NC	36, cat
i.v.	1.34 U/k/hr	+11% F	4.7 U/k/hr	+54% F	+$\dot{V}_{O_2}$	15, cat
i.v.	2 U/k/hr	+20% F	11 U/k/hr	+70% F	−Mucosal F +Submucosal F	14, cat
Extract (Boots)						
i.v.	6 U/k/hr	NC	30 U/k/hr	+65% F	+K_f	34, cat
Extract (K.I.)						
i.a.	0.2 U/min	−6% R	2 U/min	−47% R	Motility NC	10, dog
i.a.			3–12 U/k/hr[a]	+60% F[a]	+K_f +Tissue vol.	6, cat
i.a.			1.8 enh/k/min[a]	+150% F[a]	+Motility NC	16, cat
i.a. (95% pure)	3 μg/min	+5% F	10 μg/min	+33% F		18, pig
Synthetic						
i.a.	0.03 μg/k	NC	0.3 μg/k	NC	+$\dot{V}_{O_2}$ NC	7, dog
Gastrin						
Pentagastrin						
i.v.	1 μg/min	NC	0.1 μg/k/min[a]	NC[a]	−K_f 46%	33, cat
i.v.			10 μg/m	NC	−Abs. site F	28, dog
i.a.			3 μg/k/min[a]	+50% F[a]	+Motility	16, cat
i.a.			0.5 μg/k/min[a]	+55% F[a]	+$\dot{V}_{O_2}$ 35%	7, dog

	i.a.	1 μg/min	−8% R	−23% R	+Motility	10, dog
	i.a.	1 μg/min	+13% F	+35% F		18, pig
Glucagon						
	i.v.	0.01 μg/k	+11% F	NC[a]		33, cat
	i.v.			+180% F	−K$_f$ 55%	43, dog
	i.v.			+230% F[a]		43, C-dog
	i.a.			+80% F[a]	+V̇O$_2$ 40%	7, dog
	i.a.			+250% F[a]	−Motility	17, cat
	i.a.	4 μg/min	+8% F	+28% F		18, pig
	i.a.	0.05 μg/k/min	+12% F	+26% F	+V̇O$_2$	31, dog
	i.a.	1 μg/min	−R	−55% R		37, dog
	i.a.			+98% F[a]	See text	20, cat
VIP						
	i.v.	1.75 ng/min	−F	+100% F[a]	+Hepatic F	29, dog
	i.v.			−5% F[a]	−Abs. site F	44, dog
	i.v.			−F		26, dog
	i.a.			+34% F[a]	−Absorption	38, dog
	i.a.	0.017 nM/min	+30% F	+50% F	+Secretion	12, cat
Enkephalins						
	i.a.	0.03 μg/k/min	+4% F	+23% F	+Muscle F	32, dog
					+Motility	
					+V̇O$_2$	
	i.a.			+8%[a]	+V̇O$_2$	48, dog
					+Muscle F	
Morphine						
	i.v.	0.01 mg/k	+17%	+38%	Total F NC	27, dog fasted
			Abs. site F.	Abs. site F		
	i.v.	0.01 mg/k	+24%	+100%		27, dog fed
			Abs. site F.	Abs. site F		
Somatostatin						
	i.v.	0.2 μg/k/min	−20% F	−30% F	−Portal V F	39, dog
Neurotensin						
	i.v.	2.5 pM/k/min	+100% Muscle F	+300% Muscle F	Mucosa F NC	5, dog
	i.a.	12.5 pM/k/min	+9.5% F	+22% F	+V̇O$_2$	25, dog
Substance P						
	i.v.	0.3 ng/k/min	+102% F	+171% F		21, dog
GIP						
	i.v.	10/ng/k/min	NC	+45% F		3, dog

K.I., Karolinska Institute; U, unit; K, Kg; F, if no adjective preceding F, it indicates total intestinal blood flow; +, increase; −, decrease; NC, no changes; ABS, absorptive; K_f, capillary filtration coefficient; OP, octapeptide; C-dog, conscious dog; Portal V, portal vein; +V̇O$_2$, oxygen uptake.
[a]Only one infusion rate in these studies.

to increase from a basal value of 26 to 700 pg/ml to 0.5 to 8 ng/ml (47) or an increment of 1.2 to 2.5 mU/ml above basal values in men (10). In dogs, serum CCK increased by 16.4 ng/ml during duodenal instillation of amino acids (10). Therefore, it seems reasonable to conclude that CCK may play a role in the regulation of intestinal blood flow under physiological conditions. Other indirect evidence also supports this conclusion. The cardiovascular changes during digestion are confined to vasodilation in the small intestine (11). As shown in Fig. 1, CCK markedly reduces duodenal and jejunal vascular resistance but does not significantly alter the vascular resistance of the muscle, skin, kidney, forelimb, heart, and spleen when blood CCK concentration is increased between 2 and 10 mU/ml. Although gastrin has dose-response curves similar to those of CCK, the blood gastrin concentration necessary to vasodilate the small intestine significantly is considerably above the physiological range (see section on gastrin). Secretin, on the other hand, produced similar vasodilation in the eight above mentioned vascular beds (Fig. 1, also see section on secretin).

At infusion rates 5 to 10 times the minimum vasodilatory dose, CCK increases flow 50% to 85% above control and reduces resistance by 40% (Table 1). At infusion rates 20 to 50 times the minimal rate, CCK increases flow 100% to 150% above control values. CCK also increases intestinal K_f, oxygen uptake, and motility, and it redistributes intestinal blood flow in favor of the mucosa (Table 1).

SECRETIN

Intravenous infusions of secretin (Karolinska Institute) at 1 to 2 U/kg/hr increased blood flow 10% to 20% (14,15); 4 U/kg/hr decreased resistance by 10% to 25% (36) in anesthetized cats. However, secretin made by Boots (Boots Pharmaceutical, Inc., Shreveport, Louisiana), infused at 6 U/kg/hr, had no effect on intestinal blood flow in anesthetized cats (34). This discrepancy is probably due to the different sources of secretin used. At higher doses, that is, 4.7 and 11 U/kg/hr, secretin (Karolinska Institute) increased flow by 54% and 70%, respectively, in anesthetized cats (14,15).

The minimum doses of secretin producing vasodilation upon intraarterial administration were 0.2 U/min of pure natural secretin, which produced a 6% decrease in intestinal vascular resistance in a constant flow preparation in the anesthetized dog (10), and 3 µg/min of 95% pure secretin (Karolinska Institute), which produced a 5% increase in flow in the anesthetized pig (18). The calculated minimal increase in blood concentration required to produce vasodilation in the small intestine was about 10 mU/ml. The increments in serum secretin during duodenal instillation of acid, the strongest stimulator of secretin release, are only about 0.3 to 0.6 mU/liter (10) and 12 pM/ml (equivalent to about 36 ng/ml). Therefore, it appears unlikely that secretin is involved in the regulation of intestinal blood flow under physiological conditions. This conclusion is supported by the finding that synthetic secretin infused at 0.03 to 0.3 µg/kg/min i.a. has no vascular or metabolic effects (7). Furthermore, although secretin is a potent vasodilator, it vasodilates nondigestive organs as well as the small intestine (Fig. 1).

At high intraarterial infusion rates, the changes in vascular resistance or flow ranged from 33% to 60% (Table 1), and the highest reported increase in flow was produced by intraarterial infusion of secretin at 1.8 enh/kg/min (16). Unlike CCK, secretin does not appear to alter intestinal motility (10,15,16) or oxygen uptake (7). However, it does increase K_f and tissue volume, and it redistributes flow away from the mucosa to the submucosa (6,14,34).

GASTRIN

The studies included in this review all used pentagastrin. In the anesthetized cat, intrave-

FIG. 1. Comparison of vasodilator effects of cholecystokinin (CCK) **(top)**, gastrin **(middle)**, and secretin **(bottom)** in 8 vascular beds. (From Chou et al., ref. 10, with permission.)

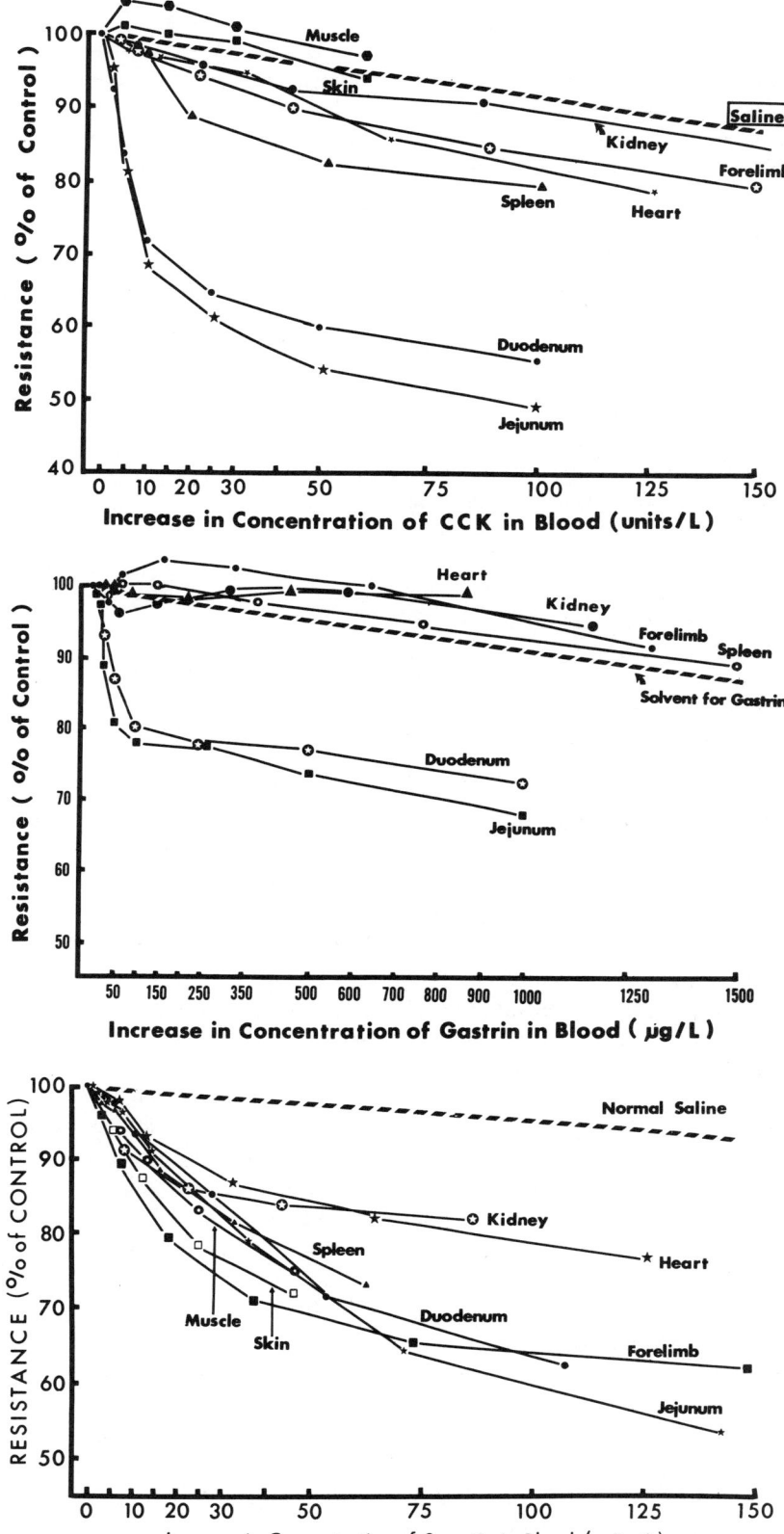

nous infusion of pentagastrin (Peptavlon, Ayerst, N.Y.) at 0.1 μg/kg/min had no effect on jejunal blood flow or jejunal vascular resistance but decreased K_f (33). In the anesthetized dog, pentagastrin 1 and 10 μg/min i.v. did not significantly alter total intestinal blood flow but depressed "absorptive-site blood flow" in fasted dogs (28). The decrease in absorptive-site flow was associated with an increase in the secretory flux of Na, a decrease in the absorptive flux of water, and thus a net decrease in the absorption of Na and water. Absorptive-site flow was unchanged by pentagastrin in fed dogs. These effects, however, are most likely pharmacological. The minimal local intraarterial infusion rate required to produce vasodilation in the small intestine is 1 μg/min pentagastrin made by Ayerst Laboratories (10) and ICI (Imperial Chemical Industries, Cheshire, England) (18). At this dose, it produced an 8% decrease in resistance and a 13% increase in flow (Table 1). The calculated increase in the blood gastrin (10) concentration was 25 to 50 ng/ml (equivalent to 32–65 pmoles/ml). This concentration range is 125 to 250 times greater than the postprandial serum gastrin concentration, 160 to 200 pg/ml (10). It is possible that the vasoactivity of G-34 and G-17, the two major forms of gastrin found in blood, may be greater than the vasoactivity of pentagastrin, but the 125- to 250-fold differences between the minimum vasodilatory concentration and the postprandial serum concentrations seem to indicate that gastrin does not play a role in the postprandial blood flow response in the small intestine. Gastrin, however, may play a physiological role in the regulation of gastric mucosal blood flow (47).

At higher infusion rates, gastrin produced a 35% to 50% increase in intestinal blood flow and a 23% decrease in vascular resistance; the vasodilator effect is therefore smaller than those of CCK and secretin (Table 1). Gastrin also increases intestinal motility and oxygen uptake at high infusion rates and depresses K_f at a dose that did not alter blood flow (33).

GLUCAGON

Pancreatic glucagon is a potent vasodilator; it increases intestinal blood flow to as much as 250% of the control value (Table 1). The minimal intraarterial infusion rate required to produce vasodilator effects was about 0.5 μg/min or 0.05 μg/kg/min (31,37). At this infusion rate, the calculated increments in blood glucagon concentration were about 20 μg/ml or 8 μg/ml. The increments in plasma glucagon concentration after protein or fat meals are about 75 to 100 pg/ml (45). The potent vasodilator effect of pancreatic glucagon in the small intestine therefore seems to be pharmacological. Glucagon also increases oxygen uptake but decreases both intestinal motility and K_f (Table 1). At a dosage that had no effect on blood flow, glucagon reduced jejunal K_f by 55% (31).

Glucagon exerts significant effects on intestinal secretion. At a dose that did not alter net volume secretion (0.05 μg/kg/min), glucagon not only increased flow by 98% but also produced a 560% increase in lymph flow. In addition, glucagon increased K_f, capillary pressure, intestinal tissue volume, and interstitial fluid pressure (20). These microcirculatory effects may be the mechanism of glucagon-induced intestinal secretion. Whether glucagon plays a significant role in regulating the intestinal microcirculation under physiological conditions is doubtful, since the minimum effective doses appear to be pharmacological.

VASOACTIVE INTESTINAL POLYPEPTIDE

Vasoactive intestinal polypeptide (VIP) is a vasodilator in the small intestine when large doses are given intravenously (29,38). VIP in lesser amounts, however, decreases intestinal blood flow (both total and absorptive site flows) and increases hepatic blood flow (26,44). The largest vasodilator response observed was at a dose of 3 μg/kg i.v., which increased total intestinal blood flow twofold (29). This effect was abolished by splanchnic nerve denervation but not by vagotomy. A decrease in intestinal blood flow of 5% was observed at 0.36 μg/kg/min i.v., but this appeared to result from a concomitant drop in mesenteric perfusion pressure (44). A decrease in absorptive site blood flow was also observed at low infusion rates, 1.75 to 175 ng/min i.v. (26). When guanethidine or atropine was administered with the later dose of VIP, the vascular effects were altered. With guanethidine, VIP had no significant effect on total blood flow but still depressed absorptive site flow (175 ng/min). With atropine, VIP (17.5 ng/min) had no significant effect on absorptive site blood flow, but total flow fell below control (26). Therefore, vascular effects of intravenous infusion of VIP may be mediated by other factors. VIP at 1.0 μg/kg/min i.a. increased blood flow 17.3%, oxygen uptake 15.2%, and intestinal secretion in the cat ileum (19). In contrast to cholera-toxin, theophylline, and prostaglandin E_1, which produced a significant positive correlation between increases in oxygen uptake and net volume secretion, the increases in intestinal secretion produced by VIP were not significantly correlated with increases in oxygen uptake (19).

The minimal infusion rate required to produce vasodilation was 0.017 nM/min (0.05 μg/min) i.a. This dose increased the arterial plasma VIP concentration to 4.9 nM/liter and also depressed net fluid absorption (12). At an arterial plasma VIP concentration of 2.0 nM/liter, VIP did not alter flow but still decreased net fluid absorption. At plasma concentrations above 0.5 μM/liter, a net intestinal secretion was observed. A 40% to 50% increase in flow was observed when arterial plasma VIP concentration ranged between 0.15 and 0.45 μM/liter. Mechanical stimulation of the mucosal surface increased blood flow 40% to 50% but increased arterial and venous plasma VIP concentrations only by 10 and 100 pM/liter, respectively (13). This effect is presumably due to stimulation of intramural nerves. The nervous release of VIP into the bloodstream, therefore, was only 1/10,000 of the arterial VIP concentration needed to induce quantitatively similar vasodilation with intraarterial VIP infusions. Therefore, VIP may play a physiological role in the gastrointestinal tract as a neurotransmitter but not as a circulating hormone. Significant increases in plasma VIP levels were not observed in human subjects after normal feeding (30), but intraduodenal placement of HCl, fat, and ethanol did cause increases in plasma VIP (40).

OPIATE AGONISTS

Opiate receptor agonists such as morphine, endorphins, met-enkephalin, and leu-enkephalin increase gastrointestinal blood flow (27,32,48,49). The minimal infusion rate of met-enkephalin to increase blood flow in the canine intestine was 0.03 μg/kg/min i.a. and the dose that produced maximum vasodilation was 0.5 μg/kg/min (32). The latter induced increases in intestinal blood flow, arteriovenous oxygen difference, oxygen uptake, and intestinal motility of 23%, 33%, 58%, and 10%, respectively (32,48). In dogs, a redistribution of blood flow also seems to be a salient vascular effect of exogenous opiate agonists. In the gastric vascular bed, met-enkephalin (1–64 nM/kg/hr i.a.) caused a dose-dependent increase in total blood flow with a larger increase to the mucosal layer (49). In the intestinal vascular bed, met-enkephalin (0.5 μg/kg/min i.a.) increased total blood flow only 23%, but flow to the muscularis increased 50% (32). Morphine, on the other hand, at doses of 0.01 to 1.0 mg/kg i.v., produced 17% to 100% increases in absorptive site flow without altering total flow (27). The vascular responses to exogenous opiates may result, in part, from their effects on oxidative metabolism, intestinal motor activity, and glandular function (27,32,48,49).

SOMATOSTATIN

Intravenous bolus injections of somatostatin at 0.5 to 100 μg produced a decrease in portal venous blood flow, no change in hepatic arterial flow, and no change or a modest fall (14–20%) in the flow through the superior mesenteric artery in the anesthetized dog (23). The maximum decrease in portal venous flow was 40% to 50% of control. In normal human subjects, intravenous infusion of somatostatin at 10 μg/min for 1 hr reduced total hepatic blood flow by 30% (46).

A significant decrease in flows through the superior mesenteric and pancreaticoduodenal arteries by 15% to 25% of control was also observed during intravenous infusions of somatostatin at 0.2 μg/kg/min in the dog. The infusion did not affect blood flow in the left gastric artery, portal vein, or hepatic artery (39). At 2 μg/kg/min i.v., somatostatin increased hepatic artery flow by 5% but depressed flows through the superior mesenteric artery, left gastric artery, and portal vein by 25% to 35% of control. The responses occurred within 1 to 2 min after the onset of the infusions, and had a duration of approximately 6 min (39). In two dogs, 1-min infusions of somatostatin at 15 μg/kg/min produced effects similar to those observed with 2 μg/kg/min, with two exceptions: hepatic artery flow seemed to be unaffected or slightly decreased, and the responses were of longer duration. These doses are markedly higher than the physiological range. The portal and femoral venous plasma somatostatin concentrations increase from basal levels of 49 and 25 pg/ml to 113 and 54 pg/ml, respectively, after ingestion of 500 ml canned food in the conscious dog (9). Therefore, the vascular effects of exogenous somatostatin seem to be pharmacological.

NEUROTENSIN

Intravenous infusion of neurotensin (36 ng/kg/min) raised superior mesenteric artery blood flow to a maximum 2 to 4 min after infusion. The initial vasodilation was followed by a slight and variable vasoconstriction (35). The vascular effects of intravenous infusions of synthetic neurotensin on muscularis and mucosal blood flows of the duodenum, jejunum, and ileum have also been studied (4). The percentage changes shown in Table 1 are those in the ileum. In the study cited, intravenous infusion of 20 to 40 pM/kg/min increased blood flow to the muscularis of the duodenum, jejunum, ileum, and colon without effect on mucosal flow. The maximum dilation was found to be a 300% increase in flow to the muscularis (i.v. infusion of neurotensin at 20 pM/kg/min). At 40 pM/kg/min, the increased flow was only 200% above control. The ileal muscularis is most responsive to neurotensin. At 2.5 pM/kg/min, blood flow to only the muscularis of the ileum rose significantly above control. At this infusion rate, the increase in the plasma neurotensin concentration is comparable to that observed after feeding (4). Neurotensin, therefore, may play a role in the regulation of ileal blood flow after feeding. Neurotensin also increases oxygen uptake and motility of the ileum. Local intraarterial infusion at 12.5 and 50 pM/kg/min increased blood flow, motility, and oxygen uptake (+ 25% and + 28%) of the canine ileum (25) (Table 1). It is interesting to note that the concentrations of immunoreactive neurotensin are higher in the ileum than the other sections of the gastrointestinal tract (47).

SUBSTANCE P

Substance P has been classified as the most powerful vasodilator on a molar basis in the mesenteric vascular bed (41). In the dog, intravenous infusion of substance P at 0.3 and 14.4 ng/kg/min increased superior mesenteric artery blood flow as much as 102% and 171%, respectively (21). The vascular response was significantly smaller if the same dose of substance P was given into the portal vein. Rapid hepatic clearance of substance P could account for the difference. In the mesenteric vascular bed of the pig, substance P infused in sequentially increasing doses from 0.6 ng/kg/min caused a dose-dependent increase in superior mesenteric artery blood flow. This response was not affected by tetrodotoxin or dihydroergotamine. Therefore, sodium or serotonergic-dependent neurons may not be involved (42). Intravenous infusion at 75 ng/kg/min for 50 min increased blood flow to the muscularis of the fundus, antrum, duodenum, and jejunum (50).

The preprandial plasma substance P concentration is 22 pg/ml and rises to 37 pg/min postprandially (1). Administering exogenous substance P usually raises plasma concentrations well beyond the maximum physiological level (89 pg/ml) (50). Furthermore, none of the effects of substance P are known to be produced by concentrations normally present in the blood

(22). Therefore, substance P may act physiologically as a modulator of neural transmission rather than as a circulating vasoactive hormone.

GASTRIC INHIBITORY POLYPEPTIDE

Scientific literature regarding the vascular effects of gastric inhibitory polypeptide (GIP) is almost nonexistent. One study, however, revealed that GIP is a vasodilator in the splanchnic vascular bed (3). Intravenous infusions of GIP (10 ng/kg/min) had no effect on blood flow to the splanchnic organs, but at 50 ng/kg/min, it increased blood flow to the duodenum, jejunum, and superior mesenteric artery by 64%, 45%, and 45%, respectively (3). Plasma levels of GIP rise after feeding (8). Fasting levels of GIP in serum are around 250 pg/ml, and postprandial levels rise to over 1,000 pg/ml 45 min after feeding (8). However, intravenous infusions of GIP (6.7 ng/kg/min) raise plasma concentrations to 1,400 to 2,300 pg/ml (2). Evidently, the vasodilation observed during GIP infusions (3) was a pharmacological event.

CONCLUSIONS

All the gastrointestinal hormones discussed in this chapter, except somatostatin, increase intestinal blood flow. For any given hormone, the vascular responses of the different layers of the gut wall and different sections of the small intestines may vary. In the case of several of these hormones, some of the vascular effects may be secondary to effects on intestinal functions. Only the vasodilator effect of CCK in the duodenum and jejunum and that of neurotensin in the ileum could be considered physiological. However, some hormones, such as VIP, substance P, and enkephalin, may act as neurotransmitters. Indeed, all 10 hormones may act as local tissue hormones, that is, may exert paracrine effects, rather than as circulating hormones to modulate local blood flow. Further studies are required to determine whether they act as local hormones that regulate intestinal blood flow under physiological conditions.

ACKNOWLEDGMENTS

Supported by Research Grant HL15231 from the National Institutes of Health and a grant from the Michigan Heart Association.

REFERENCES

1. Akande, B., Reilly, P., Modlin, I. M., and Jaffe, B. M. (1981): Radioimmunoassay measurements of substance P release following a meat meal. *Surgery*, 89:378–383.
2. Andersen, D. K. (1981): Physiological effects of GIP in man. In: *Gut Hormones*, 2nd ed., edited by S. R. Bloom and J. M. Polak, pp. 256–263. Churchill Livingstone, New York.
3. Andersen, D. K., Zenelmen, M. E., Denoy, D. J., Waldron, R. P., and Zinner, M. J. (1982): The effect of GIP on splanchnic and systemic blood flow. *Gastroenterology*, 82:1008.
4. Baca, I., Mittmann, V., Feurle, G. E., Haas, M., and Muller, T. H. (1981): The effect of neurotensin on regional intestinal blood flow in the dog. *Res. Exp. Med. (Berl.)*, 179:53–85.
5. Bayliss, W. M., and Starling, E. H. (1902): The mechanism of pancreatic secretion. *J. Physiol.*, 28:325–335.
6. Biber, B. (1973): Vasodilator mechanisms in the small intestine. *Acta Physiol. Scand.*, 89:449–458.
7. Bowen, J. C., Pawlik, W., Fang, W. F., and Jacobson, E. D. (1975): Pharmacological effects of gastrointestinal hormones on intestinal oxygen consumption and blood flow. *Surgery*, 78(4):515–519.
8. Brown, J. C., Dryburgh, J. R., Maccea, P., and Pederson, R. A. (1975): The current status of GIP. In: *Gastrointestinal Hormones*, edited by J. C. Thompson, pp. 537–547. University of Texas Press, Austin.
9. Chayvialle, J. A., Miyata, M., Rayford, P. L., and Thompson, J. C. (1980): Effects of test-meal, intragastric nutrients, and intraduodenal bile on plasma concentrations of immunoreactive somatostatin and vasoactive intestinal peptide in dogs. *Gastroenterology*, 79:844–852.
10. Chou, C. C., Hsieh, C. P., and Dabney, J. M. (1977): Comparison of vascular effects of gastrointestinal hormones on various organs. *Am. J. Physiol.*, 232(2):H103–H109.
11. Chou, C. C., Hsieh, C. P., Yu, Y. M., Kvietys, P., Yu, L. C., Pittman, R., and Dabney, J. M. (1976): Localization of mesenteric hyperemia during digestion in dogs. *Am. J. Physiol.*, 230:583–589.
12. Eklund, S., Jodal, M., Lundgren, O., and Sjoqvist, A. (1979): Effects of vasoactive intestinal polypeptide on blood flow, motility and fluid transport in the gastrointestinal tract of the cat. *Acta Physiol. Scand.*, 105:461–468.
13. Fahrenkrug, J., Haglund, V., Jodal, M., Lundgren, O., Olbe, L., and Schaffalitzky de Muchadell, O. B. (1978): Nervous release of vasoactive intestinal polypeptide in the gastrointestinal tract of cats: Possible physiological implications. *J. Physiol.*, 284:291–303.
14. Fara, J. W., and Madden, K. S. (1975): Effect of se-

cretin and cholecystokinin on small intestinal blood flow distribution. *Am. J. Physiol.*, 229:1365–1370.
15. Fara, J. W., Rubinstein, E. H., and Sonnenschein, R. R. (1972): Intestinal hormones in mesenteric vasodilation after introduodenal agents. *Am. J. Physiol.*, 223(5):1058–1067.
16. Fasth, S., Filipsson, S., Hulten, L., and Martinson, J. (1973): The effect of gastrointestinal hormones on small intestinal motility and blood flow. *Experientia*, 29:982–984.
17. Fasth, S., and Hulten, L. (1971): The effects of glucagon on intestinal motility and blood flow. *Acta Physiol. Scand.*, 83:169–173.
18. Houvenaghel, A., VanBeeck, L., and Wechsung, L. (1978): Effect of gastrointestinal hormones on blood flow through the superior mesenteric artery in the pig. *Zentralbl. Veterinarmed.*, 25(A):425–432.
19. Granger, D. N., Kvietys, P. R., Perry, M. A., and Taylor, A. E. (1982): Relationship between intestinal volume secretion and oxygen uptake. *Dig. Dis. Sci.*, 27:42–48.
20. Granger, D. N., Kvietys, P. R., Wilborn, W. H., Mortillaro, N. A., and Taylor, A. E. (1980): Mechanism of glucagon-induced intestinal secretion. *Am. J. Physiol.*, 239:G30–G38.
21. Hallberg, D., and Pernow, B. (1975): Effects of substance P on various vascular beds in the dog. *Acta Physiol. Scand.*, 93:277–285.
22. Hokfelt, T., Johansson, O., Ljungdahl, A., Lundberg, J. N., and Schultzberg, M. (1980): Peptidergic neurons. *Nature*, 283:391–393.
23. Jaspen, J., Polonsky, K., and Levis, M. (1979): Reduction in portal vein blood flow by somatostatin. *Diabetes*, 28:888–892.
24. Kock, N. G., Rading, B., Hahnloser, P., Tibblin, S., and Schenk, W. G. (1980): The effect of glucagon on hepatic blood flow. *Arch. Surg.*, 100:147–149.
25. Konturek, S. J., Jaworek, J., Cieszkowski, M., Pawlik, W., Kania, J., and Bloom, S. R. (1983): Comparison of effects of neurotensin and fat on pancreatic stimulation in dogs. *Am. J. Physiol.*, 244:G590–G598.
26. Mailman, D. (1978): Effects of vasoactive intestinal polypeptide on intestinal absorption and blood flow. *J. Physiol.*, 279:121–132.
27. Mailman, D. (1980): Effects of morphine on canine intestinal absorption and blood flow. *Br. J. Pharmacol.*, 68:617–624.
28. Mailman, D. (1980): Effects of pentagastrin on intestinal absorption and blood flow in the anesthetized dog. *J. Physiol.*, 307:429–442.
29. Matsup, Y., and Seki, A. (1978): The coordination of gastrointestinal hormones and the autonomic nervous system. *Am. J. Gastroenterol.*, 69:1043–1048.
30. Mitchell, S. J., and Bloom, S. R. (1978): Measurement of fasting and postprandial plasma VIP in man. *Gut*, 19:1043–1048.
31. Pawlik, W. W., Fondacaro, J. D., and Jacobson, E. D. (1980): Metabolic hyperemia in canine gut. *Am. J. Physiol.*, 239:G12–G17.
32. Pawlik, W., Walus, K. M., and Fondacaro, J. D. (1980): Effects of methionine enkephalin on intestinal circulation and oxygen consumption. *Proc. Soc. Exp. Biol. Med.*, 165:26–31.
33. Richardson, P. D. I. (1975): The effects of glucagon and pentagastrin on capillary filtration coefficient in the innervated jejunum of the anesthetized cat. *Br. J. Pharmacol.*, 54:225P.
34. Richardson, P. D. I. (1976): The actions of natural secretin on the small intestinal vasculature of the anesthetized cat. *Br. J. Pharmacol.*, 58:127–135.
35. Rosell, S., Burcher, E., Chang, D., and Folkers, K. (1976): Cardiovascular and metabolic actions of neurotensin and (Gln[4])-neurotensin. *Acta Physiol. Scand.*, 98:484–491.
36. Ross, G. (1970): Cardiovascular effects of secretin. *Am. J. Physiol.*, 218(4):1166–1170.
37. Ross, G. (1970): Regional circulatory effects of pancreatic glucagon. *Br. J. Pharmacol.*, 38:735–742.
38. Said, S. I., and Mutt, V. (1970): Potent peripheral and splanchnic vasodilator peptides from normal gut. *Nature*, 225:863–864.
39. Samnegard, H., Thulin, L., Andreen, M., Tyden, G., Hallberg, D., and Efendic, S. (1979): Circulatory effects of somatostatin in anesthetized dogs. *Acta Chir. Scand.*, 145:209–212.
40. Schaffalitzky de Muckadell, O. B., Fahrenkrug, J., Holst, J. J., and Lauritsen, K. B. (1977): Release of vasoactive intestinal polypeptide (VIP) by intraduodenal stimuli. *Scand. J. Gastroenterol.*, 12:793–799.
41. Schrauwen, E., and Houvenahgel, A. (1980): A comparison of the threshold doses of various vasodilators in the pig mesenteric vascular bed. *Physiology*, 8:107.
42. Schrauwen, E., and Houvenahgel, A. (1980): Substance P–A powerful intestinal vasodilator in the pig. *Pfluegers Arch.*, 386:281–284.
43. Tibblin, S., Kock, N. G., and Schenk, W. G. (1970): Splanchnic hemodynamic responses to glucagon. *Arch. Surg.*, 100:84–89.
44. Thulin, L. (1973): Effect of gastro-intestinal polypeptides on hepatic bile flow and splanchnic circulation. *Acta Chir. Scand. (Suppl.)*, 441:1–31.
45. Unger, R. H., and Orci, L. (1976): Physiology and pathophysiology of glucagon. *Physiol. Rev.*, 56:778–826.
46. Wahren, J., and Felig, P. (1976): Influence of somatostatin on carbohydrate disposal and absorption in diabetes mellitus. *Lancet*, 2:1213–1216.
47. Walsh, J. H. (1981): Endocrine cells of the digestive system. In: *Physiology of the Gastrointestinal Tract*, edited by L. R. Johnson, pp. 59–144. Raven Press, New York.
48. Walus, K. M., Fondacaro, J. D., and Jacobson, E. D. (1980): Hemodynamic and metabolic responses to increased intestinal motor activity. *Gastroenterology*, 78:1287.
49. Walus, K. M., Pawlik, W., Konturek, S. J., and Schally, A. V. (1981): Effect of Met-enkephalin and morphine on gastric secretion and blood flow. *Acta Physiol. Pol.*, 32:383–392.
50. Yeo, C. J., Zinner, M. J., Denoy, D., and Jaffe, B. M. (1982): Intravenous substance P (SP) infusion in conscious dogs: Its effects on hemodynamics, regional blood flow, glucose, insulin and cortisol. *Gastroenterology*, 82:1216.

Physiology, Pharmacology, and Pathology of the Colonic Circulation

Peter R. Kvietys and D. Neil Granger

Department of Physiology, College of Medicine, University of South Alabama, Mobile, Alabama 36688

The blood and lymph circulations of the colon differ both anatomically and physiologically from those of the small bowel. The aim of this chapter is to review briefly the anatomy, physiology, pharmacology, and pathophysiology of the colonic circulation and emphasize those features that differ significantly from the small intestine.

ANATOMICAL CONSIDERATIONS

Blood Circulation

The blood circulation of the large bowel has been extensively described in previous monographs (29,40,48). The arterial supply to the colon is derived from both the superior mesenteric artery (supplying primarily the proximal portion) and the inferior mesenteric artery (supplying primarily the distal portion). The venous drainage is via the superior (draining primarily the proximal portion) and inferior (draining primarily the distal portion) mesenteric veins. The characteristic extra- and intramural anastomoses between these vessels provide significant collateral circulation.

The most striking differences between the circulations of the small and large bowel are found in the mucosal layers (Fig. 1A). In the small intestine, the circulation of the villi is characterized by a vascular "hairpin loop," so that the arterial and venous vessels run in close proximity for a relatively long distance. This arrangement is the anatomical basis for the proposed countercurrent exchange system in the small intestine (see Chapter 7). By contrast, the colonic mucosa is devoid of villi. Hence, the vascular architecture does not favor countercurrent exchange. In the colonic mucosa, the arterioles and their capillary branches pass to the epithelial surface between the crypts (glands) forming an extensive network of capillary plexi around the glands (Fig. 1A). The mucosal capillaries are fenestrated. Their fenestral openings are most abundant in the upper third of the mucosa and are located exclusively on the side of the capillary wall facing the transporting epithelia. Colonic capillaries are situated much closer to the epithelial cells than their counterparts in the small intestine (36).

Lymphatic Circulation

The lymphatic system of the colon has also been extensively described (1,15,36). As with the blood circulations, the major difference between the lymphatic drainages of the small and large intestines is found in the mucosal region (Fig. 1B). In contrast to the prominent central lacteal in the villus of the small intestine, the initial lymphatics of the colonic mucosa are characteristically smaller in caliber and sparsely distributed (36). They originate near the bases of the glands in the lower third of the mucosa and are situated six to eight times further from the surface epithelium than their counterparts in the villi of the small intestine (15).

BLOOD FLOW

Hemodynamics

Available estimates of resting (preprandial) colonic blood flow range from 8 to 75 ml/min × 100 g (33). This large range of reported

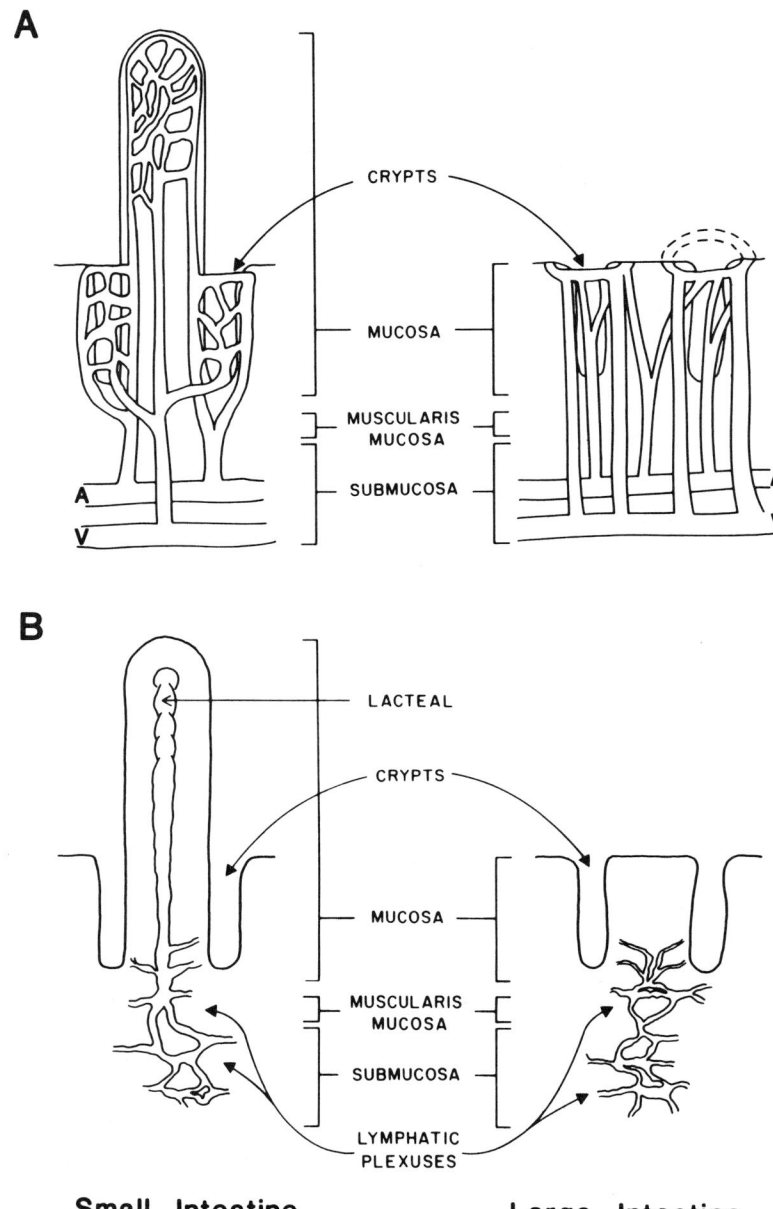

FIG. 1. A: Schematic representation of the mucosal-submucosal blood circulation of the small and large intestine. (Adapted from Boley et al. and Swan et al., refs. 3 and 6, with permission.) **B:** Schematic representation of the mucosal-submucosal lymphatic circulation of the small and large intestine. (Modified from Kvietys et al., ref. 36, with permission.)

blood flows can be attributed to species differences, anesthesia, and experimental techniques. Despite these influences, some generalizations concerning colonic blood flow can be made. The proximal colon receives a greater share of blood flow than the more distal portions (11), and total colonic blood flow is somewhat lower than total blood flow to the small intestine (33).

The colon wall is anatomically subdivided into mucosal, submucosal, and muscularis regions. Although it is generally accepted that blood vessels of the muscularis region are in parallel with those of the mucosal and submucosal regions, it is not known with certainty whether the vessels of the mucosa and submucosa are in parallel or in series (19). Because most estimates of blood flow to the submucosa suggest that it receives the smallest share of intramural blood flow (10% of total wall flow), most investigators have chosen to treat the mucosal and submucosal layers as a single compartment (see Table 1). The existing data suggest that the intramural distribution of colonic blood flow favors the more metabolically active mucosa-submucosa (33). Various physiologic, pathologic, and pharmacologic interventions that alter total colonic blood flow and its intramural distribution are listed in Table 1.

Intrinsic Regulation

Intrinsic regulation of colonic blood flow is evidenced by phenomena such as reactive hyperemia, pressure-flow autoregulation, and functional hyperemia (23,30,35). Both metabolic and myogenic factors are believed to play a major role in the regulation of colonic blood flow (29,33).

The metabolic theory of local blood flow control holds that tissue metabolism and vascular smooth muscle constitute a local control system that serves to match tissue perfusion to nutritional demands (20,21). Arteriolar and "precapillary sphincter" tone are modulated by either vasodilator metabolites released from parenchymal cells or interstitial Po_2, or both (20,21,45). One version of the metabolic model of local circulatory control (20,21) predicts that oxygen delivery to the tissue, not blood flow per se, is the controlled variable. The proponents of the oxygen delivery version of the metabolic theory maintain that this system is designed to prevent cell hypoxia.

The myogenic theory of local blood flow control holds that vascular smooth muscle tone is directly proportional to transmural pressure and that stretch (or tension) stimulates smooth muscle activity (26,27) (see Chapter 4). In this scheme, a decrease in vascular transmural pressure (reduction in arterial pressure) would lead to relaxation of arteriolar and precapillary sphincter smooth muscles. The proponents of the myogenic theory maintain that this control system serves to maintain capillary pressure and transcapillary fluid balance at a relatively constant level (26,27). However, the concept of myogenic autoregulation of capillary filtration rate in the small intestine has recently been challenged (17).

Reactive Hyperemia

The large intestine exhibits reactive hyperemia after brief periods of arterial occlusion; the magnitude and duration of the hyperemia are directly related to the duration of occlusion (35). Although both metabolic and myogenic hypotheses predict active dilation of resistance vessels during arterial occlusion, only metabolic factors can account for the direct relationship between the duration of occlusion and the magnitude of the reactive hyperemia.

Pressure-Flow Autoregulation

Autoregulation is defined as the ability of an organ to maintain a relatively constant blood flow in the face of a fluctuating arterial pressure. Under resting (nonabsorbing) conditions, the colon does not autoregulate its blood flow as well as the small intestine; the incidence of autoregulation is only 20% as compared to 70% in the small intestine (23,33). The autoregulatory ability of the colon improves substantially during periods of enhanced metabolic activity, that is, absorption (31). Furthermore, the autoregulatory ability of the more metabolically active absorptive region of the large intestine exceeds that of the whole organ (16).

When perfusion pressure is moderately reduced (i.e., to 60 mm Hg), the decrease in blood flow is accompanied by a sufficient increase in oxygen extraction to maintain colonic oxygen uptake within normal limits (35). Further reductions in perfusion pressure and blood flow

TABLE 1. *Physiologic, pathologic, and pharmocologic factors that alter colonic blood flow, capillary filtration coefficient, and oxygen uptake*

Factors	Blood flow			Capillary filtration coefficient[a]	Oxygen uptake	Ref.[b]
	Total	Mucosal-submucosal	Muscularis			
Physiologic						
Feeding						
30–45 min after meal	NC, ↓36	67, ↓30	NC			33
90 min after meal	NC	NC	NC			33
Intraluminal nutrients						
Tyrodes solution	NC				↑12–20	30
Volatile fatty acid (acetic, propionic, butyric; 135 mM)	↑24				↑20	30
Posterior hypothalamic stimulation (50 Hz, 3–8 V, 1 msec)	↓40	↓46	↓42			10
Mucosal stimulation (mechanical)	↑50					8
Sympathetic stimulation (4–8/sec, 5 msec, 8–12 V)						
Autoregulatory escape	↓25–30	↓50	↓50	↓30		24,33
Post-stimulation hyperemia	↑50–300	↑13	↑400			24,33
Parasympathetic stimulation (4–8/sec, 5 msec, 5–8 V)						
Pelvic nerves	↑170	↑200–300	↑100	NC		24
Pathologic						
Hemorrhage						
Arterial pressure not reduced	↓27				NC	9
Arterial pressure reduced to 40–60 mm Hg	↓50–67	↓50–67	↓50–67			33
Pericardial tamponade (1–18 mm Hg pericardial pressure)	↓5–85				NC—↓73	4
Carotid artery occlusion (increase in arterial pressure of 40 mm Hg)	↑34	↓5	↑40			33
Lumenal distention						
15 mm Hg	↓13	↓55	↓150			33
60 mm Hg	↓75	↓80	↓18			33
Elevated portal pressure (20 mm Hg)	↓26	↓26	↓26	↑31	↓8	11,35

Inflammatory bowel disease				
Ulcerative colitis				
Exudative stage	↑310	↑350	↑50	25
Fibrotic stage	↓34	↓25	↓34	25
Crohn's disease				
Exudative stage	↑430	↑600	↑68	25
Fibrotic stage	↓23			25
Pharmacologic[c]				
Catecholamines and related compounds				
Epinephrine (5 mg/kg)	↓85			24
Norepinephrine (40–1,000 ng/min)	↓18–59		NC–↓40	5
Isoproterenal (40–1,000 ng/min)	↑15–50		NC	5
Cholinergic agents and related compounds				
Physostigmine (0.15–0.19 µg/kg × min i.v.)	↓46	↓42		5
Acetylcholine	↑	NC		24
Autocoids and related compounds				
Histamine (100–1,000 ng × min)	NC, ↑20		NC	5
Bradykinin (0.004–1 µg/ml blood)	↑5–100			5
Serotonin (50–100 µg × min)	↓33			5
Dihydroergotamine (1 µg/kg i.v.)	↓33			8
Hormones				
Pentagastrin (64–4,000 ng/kg i.v.)	↓10–35			5
Cholecystokinin (64–4,000 ng/kg i.v.)	NC			5
Vasopressin (1–5 mU/min)	↑15–68		↓12–30	5
VIP (3.4–15.5 nmoles/min)	↑22–100			5
Glucagon (12.5 ng/min)	↑100	↑100		33
Miscellaneous drugs				
Papaverine (0.6 mg/min)	↑77			5
Acetic acid (0.82 mM/ml blood)	↑34		↑21	30
Adenosine (10–100 µg/min)	↑61–120		↑19	16,35
PGF$_2\alpha$ (50–100 µg/min)	↓70			5
Digoxin (10–1,000 ng/ml blood)	↓10–60		NC–↓40	4
Hydrocortisone (0.17 g%; i.l.)	NC		NC	2
Methylparaben (0.18 g%; i.l.)	↑42		NC	2
Polysorbate 80 (0.014 g %; i.l.)	NC		↓12	2
Carboxypolymethylene (0.17 g%; i.l.)	↑16.5		NC	2

[a] The capillary filtration coefficient ($K_{f,c}$) is a measure of the hydraulic conductance of the exchange vessels and is influenced by the density of perfused capillaries as well as the porosity of each capillary. Generally, the changes in $K_{f,c}$ listed in this table have been attributed to changes in capillary density. However, some agents (e.g., bradykinin) have been shown to alter intestinal capillary permeability, and therefore some of the changes in $K_{f,c}$ listed in the table may be, at least in part, attributed to changes in capillary porosity.

[b] The references listed represent either the original papers or review articles in which the original papers are quoted.

[c] Agents were administered intraarterially unless otherwise specified; i.v., intravenously; i.l., intraluminally.

are not accompanied by sufficient increases in oxygen extraction and colonic oxygenation is compromised.

Since both myogenic and metabolic theories predict decreases in vascular resistance during reductions in arterial pressure, it is evident that neither mechanism exerts sufficient influence over the colonic vasculature to maintain a constant blood flow during arterial pressure alterations. However, since the oxygen delivery version of the metabolic theory predicts that tissue oxygenation (not blood flow, per se) is the regulated variable (20,21), the ability of the colon to maintain its oxygen uptake during reductions in perfusion pressure to 60 mm Hg suggests that a metabolic mechanism may be operative in the colon, at least during moderate decreases in arterial pressure. The role of the microvasculature in maintaining tissue PO_2 above the critical level remains uncertain.

Venous Pressure Elevation

Acute venous hypertension decreases colonic blood flow and increases vascular resistance. These findings are consistent with the myogenic theory of local circulatory control (which predicts vasoconstriction in response to increased transmural pressure). As total blood flow decreases during acute venous hypertension, colonic oxygen extraction increases to minimize any reductions in colonic oxygen uptake (35). In the colon, the capillary filtration coefficient (an index of perfused capillary density) increases during venous pressure elevation (35), a response opposite to that observed in the small intestine (19). These findings suggest either a greater sensitivity of colonic precapillary "sphincters" to metabolic factors or a weaker myogenic influence.

The vascular response to venous pressure elevation can be affected by several factors. Intraarterial infusion of papavarine abolishes the myogenic resistance response to acute venous hypertension (23), suggesting that an active contraction of vascular smooth muscle is involved. The increase in vascular resistance during venous pressure elevation is also abolished if the colon is in an absorptive state (31), presumably reflecting an increased influence on the vasculature by metabolic factors.

Functional Hyperemia

The existence of a postprandial (functional) hyperemia in the small intestine is well documented (5,14,19). Convincing evidence for a functional hyperemic response in the colon is still lacking (Table 1). However, there is evidence that colonic blood flow is affected by absorption, secretion, and motility.

Colonic oxygen uptake increases after luminal instillation of solutions containing electrolytes (31) or volatile fatty acids (30). The increase in oxygen uptake in response to electrolytes is directly related to the net volume absorption rate and due solely to an increase in oxygen extraction. In contrast, volatile fatty acids increase colonic oxygen uptake solely through an increase in blood flow. Thus, during absorption of naturally occurring nutrients, the increase in colonic oxygen demand is met by either an increase in blood flow or oxygen extraction, responses consistent with the metabolic hypothesis.

No evidence is available for either myogenic or metabolic mechanisms operating during the circulatory adjustments to secretion or enhanced motor activity. The augmentation in flow accompanying mucus secretion (induced by pelvic nerve stimulation) can be abolished by cholinergic blockade, indicating that a neural mechanism is involved (24). Although a functional hyperemia in the small intestinal muscle layer during enchanced motor activity has been demonstrated (5), no information is available concerning this phenomenon in the colon. In general, during spontaneous motility, colonic blood flow is inversely related to intraluminal pressure (44). However, in many cases, augmentation of colonic venous outflow occurs after a contraction, the magnitude and duration of which are largely dependent on the strength and duration of the contraction.

Extrinsic Regulation

Extrinsic regulation of colonic blood flow is mediated by nervous and circulating factors.

Table 1 lists the effects of extrinsic factors on colonic blood flow, capillary filtration coefficient, and oxygen uptake.

Nervous Influences

Sympathetic control of colonic blood flow is mediated via the splanchnic and lumbar nerves. The vasoconstrictor fibers of the splanchnic nerves regulate the circulation in the proximal portion of the colon; those of the lumbar nerves regulate blood vessels of the distal colon (24). Stimulation of these sympathetic fibers results in a transient, intense vasoconstriction, which is followed by a partial recovery of blood flow despite continued stimulation (autoregulatory escape). Upon cessation of stimulation there is a hyperemia. The capillary filtration coefficient also decreases during sympathetic stimulation. Since the capillary filtration coefficient remains reduced during the entire period of stimulation, there appears to be no autoregulatory escape of precapillary sphincters (24). In general, the responses of resistance and exchange vessels to sympathetic stimulation appear to be less intense in the colon than in the small intestine.

The parasympathetic nerve supply to the colon is derived from the vagus and pelvic nerves. Subdiaphragmatic stimulation of the vagus nerve does not affect colonic blood flow. Pelvic nerve stimulation results in an intense, yet transient, hyperemia followed by a more prolonged period of rhythmic augmentation of flow. The vascular response to pelvic nerve stimulation is associated with enhanced colonic motility and mucus secretion, suggesting that the vasodilation is secondary to enhanced functional activity. Although cholinergic blockade abolishes the secretory effects and the rhythmic augmentation of blood flow, it does not affect the initial hyperemic response or the motor effects (24). The initial hyperemic response is abolished by ganglionic blocking agents, suggesting that another transmitter is released from the terminals of the fibers in the pelvic nerve. Several lines of evidence suggest that the kinin system (7) or vasoactive intestinal polypeptide (VIP) (6) may be involved in the vasodilation induced by pelvic nerve stimulation. Capillary exchange capacity does not appear to be affected by activation of the parasympathetic supply to the colon (24).

Circulating Factors

The effects of various circulating agents on colonic blood flow, capillary filtration coefficient, and oxygen uptake are listed in Table 1. In general, the effects of various drugs and hormones on colonic hemodynamics and oxgenation are qualitatively similar to those observed in the small intestine (5,12,32). Vasodilators tend to increase the capillary filtration coefficient, whereas vasoconstrictors tend to reduce the capillary filtration coefficient. These findings indicate that, as in the small intestine (12), vascular elements controlling perfused capillary density in the colon possess specific receptors for a wide variety of circulating agents. The effects of vasoactive agents on colonic oxygen uptake can be predicted from the relationship between colonic blood flow and oxygen uptake (Fig. 2). Vasoactive agents that alter colonic oxidative metabolism would be expected to shift the curve either upward (increased O_2 demand; pathway A or F) or downward (decreased O_2 demand; pathway C or D). Vasoactive agents that do not alter oxidative metabolism would follow the normal curve, as indicated by pathway B or E.

CAPILLARY FLUID AND SOLUTE EXCHANGE

Fluid Exchange

Capillary and Interstitial Forces

The exchange of fluid between capillaries and the interstitium is governed by the hydrostatic and oncotic pressure gradients across the capillary wall as well as the permeability and hydraulic conductivity of the capillaries. The factors determining capillary fluid exchange are generally related by the following expression of the Starling hypothesis (18,34,47):

$$J_{v,c} = K_{f,c} [(P_c - P_t) - \sigma_d (\pi_p - \pi_t)], \quad (1)$$

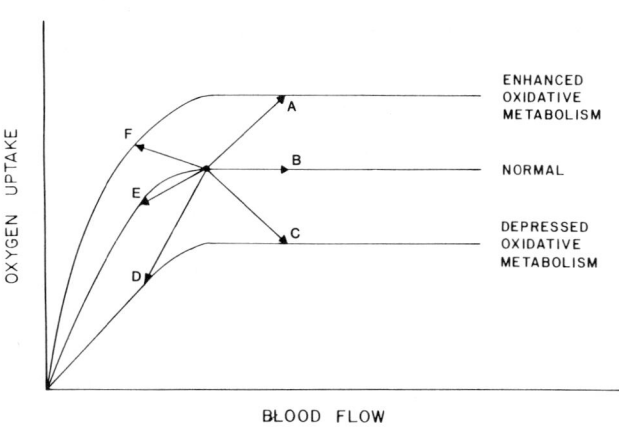

FIG. 2. Diagrammatic representation of the relationship between blood flow and oxygen uptake. Alterations in tissue oxidative metabolism shift the curve vertically. *(Dot)* Control blood flow under normal conditions. *Pathway A* is taken by vasodilator that increases oxidative metabolism. *Pathway B* is taken by vasodilator that does not affect metabolism. *Pathway C* is taken by vasodilator that decreases metabolism. *Pathway D* is taken by vasoconstrictor that decreases metabolism. *Pathway E* is taken by vasoconstrictor that does not affect metabolism. *Pathway F* is taken by vasoconstrictor that increases metabolism. (Modified from Bulkley et al. and Kvietys and Granger, refs. 4 and 32, with permission.)

where $J_{v,c}$ (ml/min × 100 g) is the net volume flow across the capillary, $K_{f,c}$ (ml/min/mm Hg × 100 g) is the capillary filtration coefficient, P_c (mm Hg) is the capillary hydrostatic pressure, P_t (mm Hg) is the interstitial fluid pressure, σ_d is the osmotic reflection coefficient, π_p (mm Hg) is the plasma oncotic pressure, and π_t (mm Hg) is the interstitial oncotic pressure. Using the above equation the following values were derived from data obtained in the canine colon (35,41): $0.015 = 0.204 \, [(11.0) - 0.85 \, (12.8 - 8.0)]$. Since colonic capillary or interstitial fluid pressure have not been measured, the value for the transcapillary hydrostatic pressure gradient (11.0 mm Hg) was calculated from the measured variables in the Starling equation.

Interaction of Capillary and Interstitial Forces

Increases in colonic capillary pressure enhance the rate of fluid filtration from the capillaries into the interstitium (41). As fluid enters the interstitium, interstitial fluid pressure rises and tissue oncotic pressure falls. These changes in interstitial forces oppose further filtration of fluid out of the capillaries. In addition, the increased tissue pressure provides the driving force for enhanced removal of interstitial fluid via the lymphatics. In general, for a small rise in capillary pressure the tissue forces are able to readjust sufficiently to resist edema formation, and a new steady state is achieved with a slightly more hydrated interstitium. The ability of interstitial forces and lymph flow to prevent edema formation is referred to as the "edema safety factors." The magnitude of the compensatory changes in each force can be estimated (47). Figure 3 compares the safety factors against edema in the small intestine and colon for a 12- to 13.2-mm Hg increment in capillary pressure. In both the small and the large intestine, the increased oncotic pressure gradient and interstitial fluid pressure are the major safety factors; lymph flow plays a minor role.

Stimulation of net fluid absorption does not alter colonic lymph flow (36). The absorbed fluid is apparently removed from the interstitium exclusively via the capillaries. By contrast, in the small intestine dramatic increases in lymph flow (up to 20-fold) accompany fluid absorption, and the absorbate leaves the interstitium via both the capillaries and lymphatics (12). These functional differences are in accord with the ultrastructure of the blood and lymphatic microcirculations within the mucosa of the small and large intestine (Fig. 1). The initial lym-

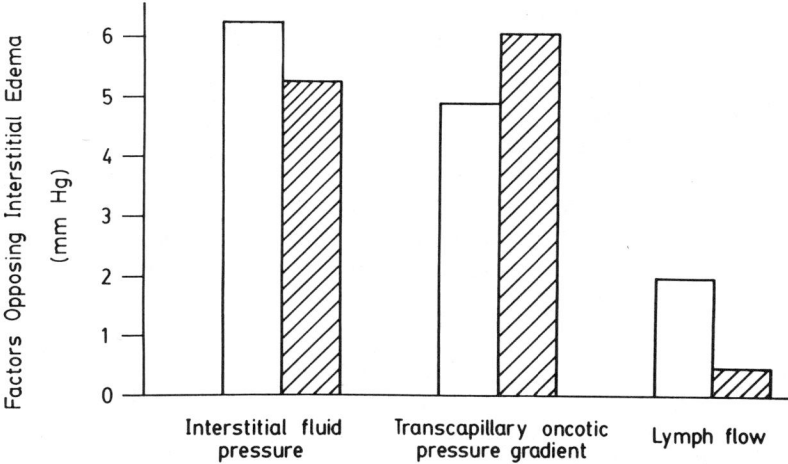

FIG. 3. Safety factors against interstitial edema in the small intestine *(open bars)* and the colon *(hatched bars)* for an increment in capillary pressure of 12–13.2 mm Hg. (Modified from Granger and Barrowman, ref. 12, with permission.)

phatics of the colonic mucosa are much smaller in caliber and more sparsely distributed than lymphatics in the mucosa of the small intestine. In addition, the fenestrated capillaries of the colonic mucosa are much closer to the absorptive epithelial cells than their counterparts in the small intestine (36), a situation that appears to be advantageous for the removal of absorbed fluid via the capillaries.

Stimulation of active fluid secretion also does not alter colonic lymph flow (36). This response contrasts with the reduction or cessation of lymph flow associated with active secretion in the small bowel (12). The interstitium at the level of the initial lymphatics of the colonic mucosa (Fig. 1B) is presumably unaffected by the secretory process.

Solute Exchange

The fluid continuously leaving the capillaries of the large intestine contains plasma proteins. The rate of protein leakage across the capillaries is about 50 mg $\times$ min^{-1} $\times$ 100 g^{-1}, a value one-third of that reported for the small intestine (12). Estimates of the osmotic reflection coefficient (σ_d) for plasma proteins of various molecular radii demonstrate selective restriction of proteins by the capillaries in accordance with their size. The σ_d is 0.75 for albumin (37 Å), and σ_d progressively increases with molecular size up to β-lipoprotein (120 Å), where σ_d is 0.98 (41). Irreversible thermodynamic and hydrodynamic principles have been applied to the reflection coefficient data to estimate the dimensions and the number of transport pathways for macromolecules. Two equivalent "pore" populations are predicted, namely, a population of small pores of 53 Å in radius and a population of large pores of 180 Å. The relative number of small pores compared to large pores is 550 to 1, and the area of small pores relative to large pores is 48 to 1. Although the sizes of the small and large pores of the small intestinal capillaries are similar to those of the colon, the relative number of small to large pores (6400:1) and the relative area of small to large pores (340:1) are much greater in the small intestine (39).

PATHOPHYSIOLOGY OF THE COLONIC CIRCULATION

The major vascular disorders of the large intestine are ischemia (e.g., necrotizing enterocolitis), venous hypertension (e.g., portal hypertension, vascular ectasias), and inflammatory bowel disease (e.g., ulcerative colitis,

Crohn's disease). All these pathologic conditions are characterized by interstitial edema, vascular dilation, and, in severe cases, frank bleeding with epithelial desquamation in the mucosa-submucosal layers of the large bowel. The pathologic changes in the colonic circulation that are associated with these disorders have been described in several comprehensive reviews (13,28,43). Only a brief description of the pathophysiology of these disorders is given here.

Ischemia

The colonic vascular supply, which is derived from the superior and inferior mesenteric arteries, is characterized by an extensive extra- and intramural plexus of collateral vessels. These vascular connections provide significant collateral perfusion in the event an arterial vessel is occluded. The point of junction between the superior and inferior mesenteric arteries (i.e., Griffith's point) is the most critical area of anastomotic supply and is the region of the colon most susceptible to ischemic attacks (43). Although ischemic injury is more difficult to induce in the colon than in the small intestine, recovery from ischemic injury is more prolonged in the colon (42).

Ischemic injury in the colon is characterized by a slight amount of epithelial desquamation and relatively mild dilation of blood vessels in the mucosa during the ischemic period (42). Massive desquamation of the epithelium, variable amounts of cell necrosis on the sides of the crypts, edema, and substantial vascular dilation are only observed after reperfusion (42). This series of events is similar to those observed in the small intestine during ischemia (37,38).

In the small intestine, two mechanisms appear to be involved in ischemic damage: hypoxia per se (22) and the production of oxygen free radicals (37,38). During the ischemic period, shunting of oxygen by the "countercurrent exchange" system in the villi during low flow states leads to hypoxic foci in the villus tips which subsequently are responsible for the minor mucosal damage during ischemia (22). The more substantial mucosal damage observed upon reperfusion is believed to be due to cytotoxic oxygen-derived free radicals produced by xanthine oxidase acting on hypoxanthine and the oxygen delivered to the cells during reperfusion (37,38). Although both mechanisms may also be involved in ischemic injury to the colon, there is reason to doubt their importance in this organ. The minor damage incurred during the ischemic period may well be due to hypoxic foci in the colonic mucosa, but the involvement of a countercurrent shunting of oxygen seems unlikely, since the colonic mucosa is devoid of villi and their associated hairpin vascular architecture (Fig. 1A). Although free radical-induced damage is also likely to occur in the colon during reperfusion, the enzyme systems involved may be different. Unlike the small intestine, which is a rich source of xanthine oxidase, the colon has relatively little activity of this enzyme (37). However, the colon is a rich source of aldehyde oxidase, another enzyme that can generate oxygen radicals.

Venous Hypertension

Portal hypertension (e.g., as a consequence of liver disease) does not affect the large intestine to the same extent as the small intestine. The dilated submucosal-mucosal vessels and interstitial edema are generally localized to the portion of the colon drained by the superior mesenteric vein, namely, the ascending colon; involvement of the transverse and descending colon is rare (13). The pattern of collateral colonic venous drainage during portal hypertension is believed to be responsible for this localization of the vascular abnormalities. The dilated vessels and interstitial edema are generally attributed to the enhanced capillary filtration resulting from increased vascular pressure.

Inflammatory Bowel Disease

The vascular disorders in early (exudative) stages of ulcerative colitis and Crohn's disease are characterized by dilated vessels in mucosal and submucosal layers of the large bowel with interstitial edema and mucosal exudation (13,25).

These vascular changes vary considerably and appear to be related to the severity of the inflammation. The major factors that have been implicated in edema formation in inflammatory bowel disease are increased capillary permeability and increased capillary hydrostatic pressure (13,25). Increased capillary permeability is believed to be caused by chemicals (e.g., kinins, histamine) released from inflamed tissue (28), bacterial endotoxins (28), and oxygen-derived free radicals produced by infiltrating leukocytes (13). An increase in capillary pressure in the early (exudative) stage of ulcerative colitis or Crohn's disease may also play a role in edema formation, because blood flow to the mucosa-submucosa is enhanced two- to sixfold (Table 1). Assuming that the decrease in colonic vascular resistance occurs predominantly at the arteriolar level, capillary pressure may increase by 20 to 40 mm Hg. The later (fibrotic) stage of either ulcerative colitis or Crohn's disease is characterized by fibrosis in the mucosal and submucosal areas, atrophied mucosa, and, in some cases, decreased vascularity and blood flow (25).

CONCLUSIONS

The significant anatomical and functional differences between the microcirculations of the small and large bowels suggest that data obtained in the small intestine cannot be readily extrapolated to the colon. Although major advances have been made in our understanding of the physiology and pathology of the colonic circulation, the significant gaps still remaining warrant attention.

REFERENCES

1. Barrowman, J. A. (1978): *Physiology of the Gastro-Intestinal Lymphatic System*. Cambridge University Press, London.
2. Barrowman, J. A., Kvietys, P. R., Granger, D. N., McElearney, P. M., and Perry, M. A. (1983): Effects of the constituents of a corticosteroid enema preparation on colonic blood flow and oxygen uptake in the dog. *J. Pharm. Exp. Ther.*, 226:217–221.
3. Boley, S. J., Sammortano, R., Adams, A., DiBiase, A., Kleinhaus, S., and Sprayregen, S. (1977): On the nature and etiology of vascular ectasias of the colon. Degenerative legions of aging. *Gastroenterology*, 72:650–660.
4. Bulkley, G. B., Kvietys, P. R., Perry, M. A., and Granger, D. N. (1983): Effects of cardiac tamponade on colonic hemodynamics and oxygen uptake in the anesthetized dog. *Am. J. Physiol.*, 244:G604–G612.
5. Chou, C. C., and Kvietys, P. R. (1981): Physiological and pharmacological alterations in gastointestinal blood flow. In: *Measurement of Blood Flow: Applications to the Splanchnic Circulation*, edited by D. N. Granger and G. B. Bulkley, pp. 475–509. Williams and Wilkins, Baltimore.
6. Fahrenkrug, J., Haglund, U., Jodal, M., Lundgren, O., Olbe, L., and Schaffalitzky de Muckadell, O. B. (1978): Nervous release of vasoactive intestinal polypeptide in the gastrointestinal tract of cats: possible physiological implications. *J. Physiol.*, 284:291–305.
7. Fasth, S., Hulten, L., Johnson, J., Nordgren, S., and Zeitlin, J. (1978): Mobilization of colonic kallikrein following pelvic nerve stimulation in the atropinized cat. *J. Physiol.*, 285:471–478.
8. Fasth, S., Hulten, L., Lundgren, O., and Nordgren, S. (1977): Vascular responses to mechanical stimulation of the mucosa of the cat colon. *Acta Physiol. Scand.*, 101:98–104.
9. Gilmour, D. G., Aitkenhead, A. R., Hothersall, A. P., and McA. Ledingham, I. (1980): The effect of hypovolemia on colonic blood flow in the dog. *Br. J. Surg.*, 67:82–84.
10. Gilsdorf, R. B., Urdaneta, L. F., Leonard, A. S., and Delaney, J. P. (1983): Posterior hypothalamic effect on gastrointestinal blood flow in the conscious cat. *Proc. Soc. Exp. Biol. Med.*, 143:329–334.
11. Grandison, A. S., Yates, J., and Shields, R. (1981): Capillary blood flow in the canine colon and other organs at normal and raised portal pressure. *Gut*, 22:223–227.
12. Granger, D. N., and Barrowman, J. A. (1983): Microcirculation of the alimentary tract. I. Physiology of transcapillary fluid and solute exchange. *Gastroenterology*, 84:846–868.
13. Granger, D. N., and Barrowman, J. A. (1983): Microcirculation of the alimentary tract. II. Pathophysiology of edema. *Gastroenterology*, 84:1035–1049.
14. Granger, D. N., and Kvietys, P. R. (1981): The splanchnic circulation: Intrinsic regulation. *Annu. Rev. Physiol.*, 43:409–418.
15. Granger, D. N., and Kvietys, P. R. (1984): Small and large intestines: Lymphatic circulation. In: *Blood Vessels and Lymphatics in Organ Systems*, edited by D. I. Abramson and P. B. Dobrin, pp. 450–458. Academic Press, New York.
16. Granger, D. N., Kvietys, P. R., Mailman, D., and Richardson, P. D. I. (1980): Intrinsic regulation of functional blood flow and water absorption in canine colon. *J. Physiol. (Lond.)*, 307:443–451.
17. Granger, D. N., Mortillaro, N. A., Perry, M. A., and Kvietys, P. R. (1982): Autoregulation of intestinal capillary filtration rate. *Am. J. Physiol.*, 242:G6475–G6584.
18. Granger, D. N., Perry, M. A., and Kvietys, P. R. (1983): The microcirculation and fluid transport in digestive organs. *Fed. Proc.*, 42:1667–1672.
19. Granger, D. N., Richardson, P. D. I., Kvietys, P. R.,

and Mortillaro, N. A. (1980): Intestinal blood flow. *Gastroenterology*, 78:837–863.
20. Granger, H. J., and Nyhof, R. A. (1982): Dynamics of intestinal oxygenation: Interactions between oxygen supply and uptake. *Am. J. Physiol.*, 243:G691–G696.
21. Granger, H. J., and Shepherd, A. P. (1979): Dynamics and control of the microcirculation. *Adv. Biomed. Eng.*, 7:1–61.
22. Haglund, U., and Lundgren, O. (1978): Intestinal ischemia and shock factors. *Fed. Proc.*, 37:2729–2733.
23. Hanson, K. M., and Johnson, P. C. (1967): Pressure-flow relationships in isolated dog colon. *Am. J. Physiol.*, 212:574–578.
24. Hulten, L. (1969): Extrinsic nervous control of colonic motility and blood flow. *Acta Physiol. Scand. (Suppl.)*, 335:1–116.
25. Hulten, L., Lindhagen, J., Lundgren, O., Fasth, S., and Ahren, C. (1977): Regional intestinal blood flow in ulcerative colitis and Crohn's disease. *Gastroenterology*, 72:388–396.
26. Johnson, P. C. (1978): Principles of peripheral circulatory control. In: *Peripheral Circulation*, edited by P. C. Johnson, pp. 111–139. John Wiley and Sons, Inc., New York.
27. Johnson, P. C. (1980): The myogenic response. In: *Handbook of Physiology, Section II, Cardiovascular System, Vol. II, Vascular Smooth Muscle*, edited by D. F. Bohr, A. T. Somlyo, and H. V. Sparks, pp. 409–442. American Physiological Society, Bethesda.
28. Kirsner, J. B. (1976): Observations on the etiology and pathogenesis of inflammatory bowel disease. In: *Gastroenterology*, edited by H. L. Bockus, pp. 521–539. Saunders, Philadelphia.
29. Kvietys, P. R. (1984): The microcirculation of the large intestine. In: *The Physiology and Pharmacology of the Microcirculation*, edited by N. A. Mortillaro, Vol. 2, Academic Press, New York.
30. Kvietys, P. R., and Granger, D. N. (1981): Effects of volatile fatty acids on blood flow and oxygen uptake by the dog colon. *Gastroenterology*, 80:962–969.
31. Kvietys, P. R., and Granger, D. N. (1980): Effects of solute-coupled fluid absorption on blood flow and oxygen uptake in the dog colon. *Gastroenterology*, 81:450–457.
32. Kvietys, P. R., and Granger, D. N. (1982): Vasoactive agents and splanchnic oxygen uptake. *Am. J. Physiol.*, 243:G1–G9.
33. Kvietys, P. R., and Granger, D. N. (1982): Regulation of colonic blood flow. *Fed. Proc.*, 41:2100–2110.
34. Kvietys, P. R., and Granger, D. N. (1983): The role of the microcirculation in intestinal transmucosal fluid transport. In: *Microcirculation of the Alimentary Tract—Physiology and Pathophysiology*, edited by A. Koo, pp. 241–252. World Scientific Publ., Singapore.
35. Kvietys, P. R., Miller, T., and Granger, D. N. (1980): Intrinsic control of colonic blood flow and oxygenation. *Am. J. Physiol.*, 238:G478–G484.
36. Kvietys, P. R., Wilborn, W. H., and Granger, D. N. (1981): Effects of net transmucosal volume flux on lymph flow in the canine colon. Structural-functional relationship. *Gastroenterology*, 81:1080–1090.
37. Parks, D. A., Bulkley, G. B., and Granger, D. N. (1983): Role of oxygen-derived free radicals in digestive tract pathology. *Surgery*, 94:428–432.
38. Parks, D. A., and Granger, D. N. (1983): Oxygen-derived radicals and ischemia-induced tissue injury. In: *Oxy Radicals and Their Scavenger Systems, Vol. II: Cellular and Medical Aspects*, edited by R. A. Greenwald and G. Cohen, pp. 135–144. Elsevier Science Publishing Co., New York.
39. Perry, M. A., Crook, W. J., and Granger, D. N. (1981): Permeability of gastric capillaries to small and large molecules. *Am. J. Physiol.*, 241:G478–G486.
40. Reynolds, D. G., and Kardon, R. H. (1981): Methods of studying the splanchnic microvascular architecture. In: *Measurement of Blood Flow: Applications to the Splanchnic Circulation*, edited by D. N. Granger and G. B. Bulkley, pp. 69–88. Williams and Wilkins, Baltimore.
41. Richardson, P. D. I., Granger, D. N., Mailman, D., and Kvietys, P. R. (1980): Permselectivity of colonic capillaries. *Am. J. Physiol.*, 239:G300–G305.
42. Robinson, J. W. L., Haroud, M., Winistorfer, B., and Mirkovitch, V. (1974): Recovery of function and structure of dog ileum and colon following two hours acute ischemia. *Eur. J. Clin. Invest.*, 4:443–452.
43. Saegesser, F., Roenspies, U., and Robinson, J. W. L. (1979): Ischemic diseases of the large intestine. In: *Pathobiology Annual*, edited by H. L. Ioachim, Vol. 9, pp. 303–337. Raven Press, New York.
44. Semba, T., and Fuju, Y. (1970): Relationship between venous flow and colonic peristalsis. *Jpn. J. Physiol.*, 20:408–416.
45. Sparks, H. V. (1980): Effects of local metabolic factors on vascular smooth muscle. In: *Handbook of Physiology, Section II, Cardiovascular System, Vol. II, Vascular Smooth Muscle*, edited by D. F. Bohr, A. T. Somlyo, and H. V. Sparks, pp. 475–513. American Physiological Society, Bethesda.
46. Swan, K. G., Spees, E. K., Reynolds, D. G., Kerr, J. C., and Zinnes, M. J. (1978): Microvascular architecture of anthropoid primate intestine. *Cir. Shock*, 5:375–382.
47. Taylor, A. E. (1981): Capillary fluid filtration. Starling forces and lymph flow. *Circ. Res.*, 49:557–575.
48. Wheaton, L. G., Sarr, M. G., Schlossberg, L., and Bulkley, G. B. (1981): Gross anatomy of the splanchnic vasculature. In: *Measurement of Blood Flow: Applications to the Splanchnic Circulation*, edited by D. N. Granger and G. B. Bulkley, pp. 9–45. Williams and Wilkins, Baltimore.

Tissue Oxygenation and Splanchnic Blood Flow

H. Glenn Bohlen

Department of Physiology, Indiana University School of Medicine, Indianapolis, Indiana 46223

The two major aspects of the interactions between oxygen and the splanchnic vasculature are that oxygen affects the splanchnic vasculature and, conversely, that vascular behavior influences tissue oxygenation. Equally important is that virtually no oxygen storage capability exists in splanchnic organs. Therefore, tissue oxygen demand must be accommodated on a second-to-second basis by vascular control of blood flow. This chapter explores the interaction of oxygen and the splanchnic vasculature in the contexts of oxygen controlling vascular behavior and vascular behavior altering tissue oxygenation.

TISSUE Po_2 AT REST

The Po_2 at any point within the tissue is a function of oxygen consumption, diffusion distances to nearby capillaries, and the blood-borne delivery of oxygen. The delivery of oxygen is a function not only of blood flow but also of the tissue's ability to extract oxygen from blood. At the typical tissue Po_2 and capillary blood Po_2 of the small intestine (1,2), the disassociation of oxygen and hemoglobin is within the "linear" portion of the oxygen-hemoglobin saturation curve. Therefore, the extraction of oxygen can be modeled mathematically using Renkin's (25) equation for extraction (E):

$$E = 1 - e^{(-PS/F)}, \qquad (1)$$

where P is capillary permeability, S defines capillary surface area, and F represents blood flow.

Permeability can be considered a constant because oxygen diffuses readily through cell membranes and is unlikely to be influenced by physiological or pathological events. Therefore, oxygen extraction at steady state is predominately a function of the capillary surface area to blood flow ratio (S/F) for any given blood to tissue oxygen diffusion gradient. Either an increase in the S/F ratio caused by increased surface area, that is, more capillaries actively perfused, or a decrease in flow would increase oxygen extraction. Conversely, a decreased S/F ratio, caused by reduced numbers of capillaries actively perfused or by increased flow, would depress extraction. The flow primarily determines the convective delivery of oxygen to the capillary bed and the red cell transit time in the capillary. During the transit time, oxygen is released from hemoglobin, and it diffuses from the interior of the red cell to the capillary wall. The number of perfused capillaries has the direct effect of determining surface area for exchange between blood and tissue. The number of perfused capillaries also has an indirect effect. For a given total flow through the tissue, the velocity of flow in each capillary is decreased as the number of perfused capillaries increases. Theoretically, as the velocity of capillary flow decreases, the time available for exchange is lengthened, thus potentially increasing oxygen extraction. However, whether or not the time available for extraction is of practical significance has yet to be investigated in the splanchnic vasculature.

The effect on tissue Po_2 of the diffusion distance from a capillary to a given point in the tissue was originally and elegantly modeled by Krogh (17). As the amount of tissue increases through which oxygen must diffuse, the tissue Po_2 decreases approximately as the square of the diffusion distance. Consequently, minor changes in the distance between perfused capillaries could potentially cause substantial effects on tissue Po_2.

The bulk exchange of oxygen is the product of the blood concentration of dissolved oxygen *[A]* (excluding hemoglobin-bound oxygen and assuming a very low Po_2 at some point in the tissue), the flow and extraction ratio. Because the bulk exchange depends on the extraction ratio, which is itself an exponential function of flow *(F)*, blood flow *(F)* changes do not have a simple linear effect on bulk exchange *(BE)* as shown in Eq. 2:

$$BE = [A] \, F \, (1 - e^{(-PS/F)}). \qquad (2)$$

At high flow rates, the bulk exchange of material approximates a linear relationship with flow. However, to reach this relationship, the formula predicts that blood flow must usually be two to three times higher than at rest. As flow is reduced from control, bulk exchange begins to fall precipitously at flows below about 60% to 70% of control.

The basic point of the preceding discussion is to make the reader aware that a particular tissue Po_2 value and changes in tissue Po_2 values should only be attributed with caution to changes in a given cardiovascular variable. Furthermore, studies of the effects of tissue Po_2 on vascular control seldom take into account that the only portions of the vasculature that are directly exposed to tissue Po_2 are the smallest arterioles, capillaries, and smallest venules. Indeed the walls of the majority of arterioles primarily work at nearly the Po_2 of the blood (6). Arteriolar blood Po_2 is usually much higher than tissue Po_2. Therefore, direct effects of oxygen on the vascular smooth muscle are probably better related to the Po_2 of blood in the vessel than the average tissue Po_2.

Although an extensive literature treats the interaction of oxygen with splanchnic blood vessels, direct measurements of tissue Po_2 are relatively uncommon. In the rat small intestine, both the muscle and superficial submucosal tissue typically operate at a tissue Po_2 of 20 to 30 mm Hg, with an average near 25 mm Hg in the muscle layer (1,2). By comparison, skeletal muscle in rats typically has a tissue Po_2 of 15 to 25 mm Hg, with an average below 20 mm Hg (9,23,24). The tissue Po_2 in the intestinal mucosa of rats depends on the point of measurement along the villus (1,2). As shown in Table 1, the average apical villus Po_2 of 13.2 ± 1.3 (SE) mm Hg is generally lower than that at the villus base of 23.6 ± 1.7 mm Hg by 10 to 12 mm Hg. Paired measurements in villi indicate that an extensive variation exists in both apical and base Po_2 as well as the difference between these two Po_2 values (1). The cause of the lower apical than basal villus Po_2 values may result from the countercurrent shunting of oxygen from arteriole to venule at the villus base as proposed by Kampp and co-workers (15,16). Alternatively, a higher rate of oxygen consumption by the more mature cells at the villus tip than at the base could explain the Po_2 difference between base and apex. (For a discussion of countercurrent exchange, see Chapters 7 and 24.) It would be reasonable to assume that both of these influences are present until more definite studies are available. Furthermore, recent studies by Gannon et al. (8) showed that some species, including man, may not have the countercurrent arrangement of blood vessels in villi reported in rats and cats (8). Therefore, extrapolation of mucosal tissue Po_2 measurements in rats to other species should be made with caution.

The major variations in villus tissue Po_2 along the villus shaft are in sharp contrast to the relatively homoegeneous tissue Po_2 in intestinal muscle. In Fig. 1, the tissue Po_2 values measured approximately 15 μm radially from the arterial, midpoint, and venous sections of the same capillary are presented (3). Normal and diabetic animals are included in the figure and further discussion of these data will be presented in Chapter 30. Under conditions in which the penetration by oxygen electrodes had no measurable effect on capillary blood flow, the drop in tissue Po_2 from the arterial to venous end of a capillary is remarkably small (2–4 mm Hg). These data indicate that tissue Po_2 is relatively homogeneous in the intestinal muscle layer at resting blood flow. If the electrode was

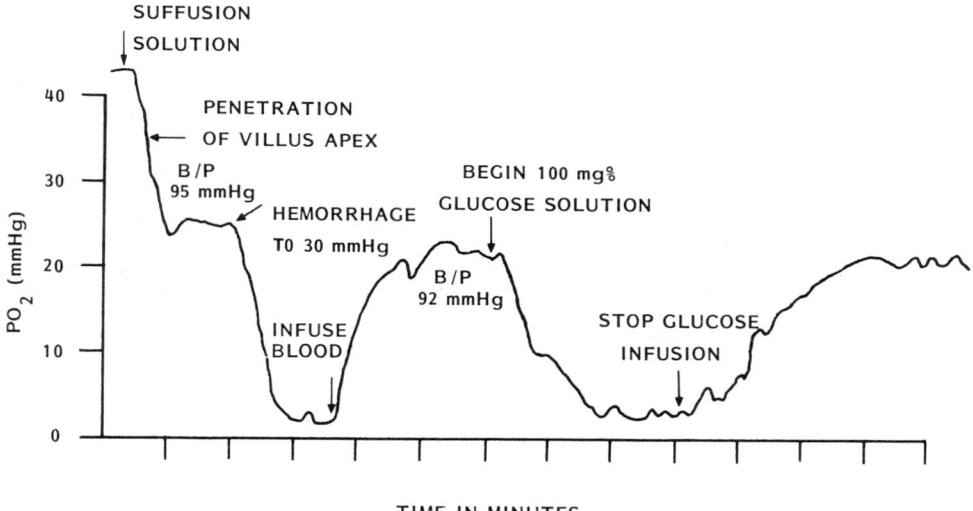

FIG. 1. Tissue P_{O_2} measured about 15 μm radially from the arterial, midpoint, and venous sections of the same capillary at rest and at the midpoint during maximum dilation. Normal and diabetic animals are included and further discussion is presented in Chapter 30. In both groups of animals, capillary blood flow during vasodilation was about twice that at rest. (From Bohlen, ref. 3, with permission.)

used to intentionally occlude the capillary, tissue P_{O_2} immediately decreased 3 to 7 mm Hg at the capillary wall. This small decrease in P_{O_2} probably reflects the overlap of diffusion fields for oxygen from adjacent capillaries. In effect, flow stoppage in a single capillary that is surrounded by several perfused capillaries would not cause localized hypoxia. Therefore, local adjustments of capillary surface area caused by flow stoppage in some fraction of the available capillaries could change fluid and solute exchange without undue risk to tissue P_{O_2} and, therefore, to oxidative metabolism. In contrast, a twofold increase in flow in normal and diabetic rats during maximum dilation caused the tissue P_{O_2} at the capillary-tissue midpoint to increase only 4 to 8 mm Hg as shown in Fig. 1. As previously stated, extraction is a negative exponential function of flow, and bulk exchange is a linear function of flow and extraction. Therefore, simply because flow doubles or triples does not mean that exchange between the tissue and blood is similarly increased unless extraction remains constant or increases. In the experiments being discussed, virtually all capillaries were perfused at rest even though red cell velocity in the capillaries was about half maximal. Therefore, maximum dilation primarily increases flow rather than both flow and capillary surface area (number of perfused capillaries). In this context, the magnitude of tissue P_{O_2} changes from rest to maximum hyperemia could be much greater in species that maintain a sizable population of unperfused capillaries during resting conditions.

TISSUE OXYGENATION DURING ABSORPTION

There is universal agreement in the literature that active absorption of sugars or amino acids is associated with increased oxygen consumption by the small intestine (27,28,30). Studies by Chou et al. (5), Fara et al. (7), and Kvietys et al. (21) also indicate that lipid absorption in the presence of bile salts increases oxygen usage. The hyperemia that accompanies absorption is generally thought to be related, in part, to the increased metabolism of the absorptive epithelium. However, it is debatable whether or not oxygen plays a specific role in the vasodilation associated with absorption. Bohlen (1) has shown that glucose absorption decreased mucosal tissue P_{O_2} from a resting value of 12 to 17 mm Hg to 4 to 7 mm Hg within less than 2 min (60%–70% of the transient occurred during the 1st min after glucose exposure). An example of the villus tissue P_{O_2} response to hypotension and then glucose exposure is shown in Fig. 2. The point to be made is that the P_{O_2} values in both circumstances are about equal but hypotension almost stops villus flow whereas absorption causes hyperemia. The decrease in villus tissue P_{O_2} during absorption despite the hyperemia emphasizes the major increase in mucosal oxygen consumption. Tissue P_{O_2} in the remainder of the bowel wall remained constant or increased slightly (1). Because normoxic and slightly hypoxic arterioles throughout the bowel wall dilated by about the same proportional amount as the relatively hypoxic villus arterioles, one would predict that tissue P_{O_2} per se is an unlikely cause of vasodilation at sites other than the mucosa. In subsequent studies, Bohlen (2) demonstrated that if the mucosal tissue P_{O_2} at rest was artificially reduced to near that during absorption, by lowering the suffusion solution P_{O_2}, total intestinal flow increased 25% to 30%. These data are presented in Figs. 3 and 4. The typical absorptive hyperemic response in the rat was an 80% to 110% increase in flow at a suffusion P_{O_2} of 40 to 45 mm Hg (Fig. 4). Therefore, oxygen lack might make a direct contribution equal to one-fourth to one-third of the overall absorptive hyperemic response. However, in species other than rats, the absorptive hyperemic response is predominately caused by vasodilation of the mucosal vasculature and to a lesser extent by the muscle vasculature (4,31). Therefore, the dependence of the hyperemic response on oxygenation in the villus may be greater in species other than the rat. Unfortunately, this possibility has not been explored.

Elevation of the mucosal suffusion solution P_{O_2} to 70 to 75 mm Hg (muscle layer fluid at P_{O_2} = 40–45 mm Hg) decreased resting blood flows by about 40% (2). During simultaneous glucose exposure (100 mg%) and elevation of mucosal suffusion P_{O_2} (70–75 mm Hg), the hyperemic response was a 15% to 20% increase in flow relative to the flow at rest in the presence

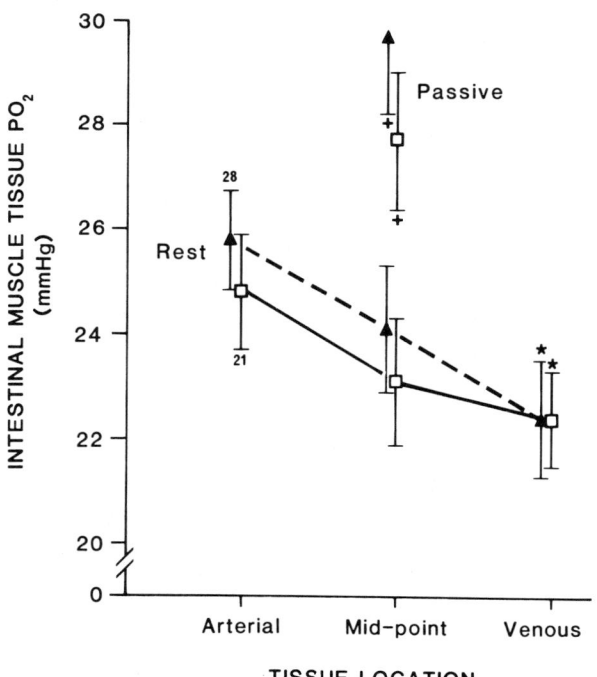

FIG. 2. Mid-shaft tissue P_{O_2} in a rat villus during hypotension and glucose exposure. The glucose-containing suffusion solution was rapidly washed into and out of the tissue chamber. However, the initial fall in tissue P_{O_2} and subsequent rise with glucose exposure and removal may reflect physiological and mechanical events. *(Squares)* Normal; *(triangles)* diabetic.

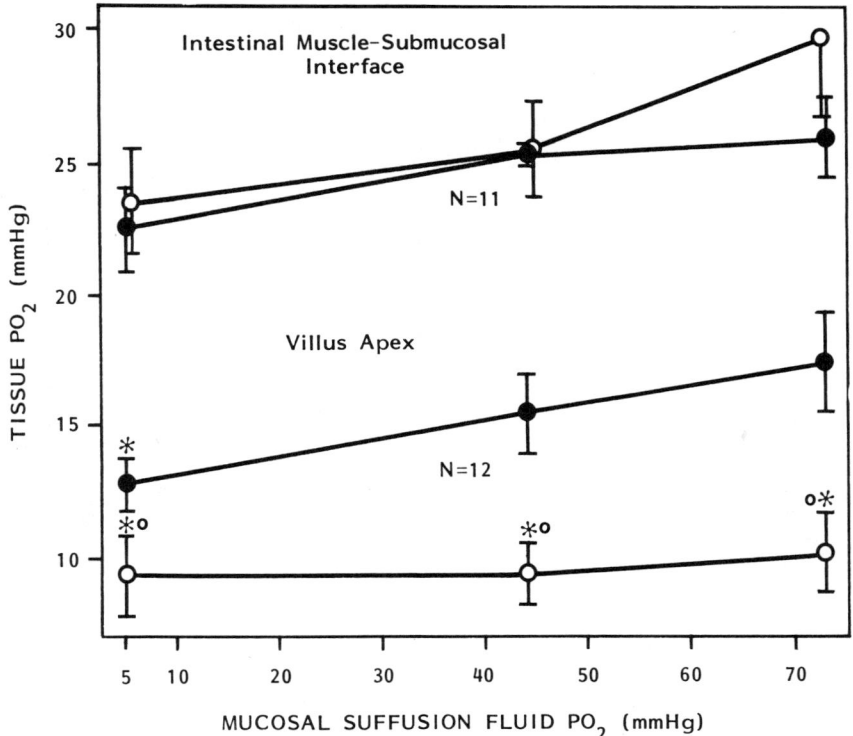

FIG. 3. Tissue Po_2 in the intestinal muscle layer and villi of rats at rest and during glucose exposure (100 mg%) at various mucosal solution Po_2 levels; muscle layer solution Po_2 was held constant at 40–45 mm Hg. *(Closed circles)* Saline; *(open circles)* saline-glucose. (From Bohlen, ref. 2, with permission.)

of a 40 to 45 mm Hg mucosal suffusion Po_2. However, if resting flow and absorptive flow are compared at the high suffusion Po_2, glucose absorption caused a 50% to 60% increase in flow. The major implications of these data and those presented in the preceding paragraph are that although an increased availability of oxygen can attenuate the magnitude of absorptive hyperemia, a decreased availability of oxygen does not augment the absorptive hyperemic response. This latter point is shown by the data presented in Fig. 4 in which a suffusion Po_2 of 5 to 45 mm Hg has a minimal effect on absorptive blood flow. The fact that at high suffusion Po_2 the absorptive hyperemic response is well developed compared to the resting blood flow at this high Po_2 indicates that one or more well-developed mechanisms other than oxygen contribute to regulation of intestinal blood flow during absorption.

Whether or not oxygen is an important factor in absorptive hyperemia, the overall process of absorptive hyperemia apparently sensitizes the vasculature to changes in blood flow or to intravascular pressure. Norris et al. (22), Shepherd (27), and Granger and Norris (12) have shown that autoregulation of intestinal blood flow is substantially improved during absorption. Whether the sensitization of the autoregulation mechanism involves oxygen, vasodilator metabolites, or a redistribution of blood flow in the bowel wall has not been determined. It is possible that the myogenic regulatory mechanism is better developed during absorptive hyperemia, as shown by Shepherd (27), and that increased myogenic sensitivity improves expression of the autoregulatory phenomena. However, in the same species, the dog, Granger and Norris (12) report an attenuation of myogenic vasoconstriction in response to venous pressure

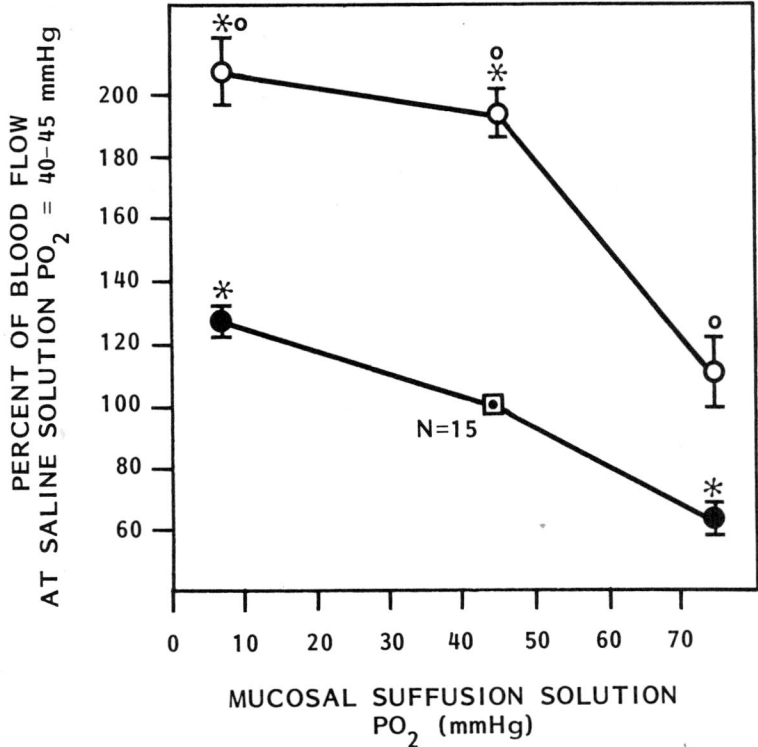

FIG. 4. Rat intestinal blood flow at rest and during glucose exposure (100 mg%) at various mucosal solution P_{O_2} levels; muscle layer solution P_{O_2} was held constant at 40–45 mm Hg. *(Closed circles)* Saline; *(open circles)* saline-glucose. (From Bohlen, ref. 2, with permission.)

elevation during absorption. Whatever the cause of the autoregulation potentiation during the increased metabolism of absorption, it is very interesting that some mechanism exists to protect the elevated blood flow during absorption from minor to moderate changes in arterial pressure. Yet in the nonabsorptive state, the quality of intestinal blood flow autoregulation is marginal.

OXYGEN CONSUMPTION REGULATION

Systematic studies of splanchnic organ oxygen consumption have revealed that these organs often "autoregulate" oxygen exchange and consumption better than blood flow. Studies by Shepherd (26,27) and Granger and Norris (12) on the intestine, Kvietys et al. (20) on the colon, Kvietys et al. (19) on the pancreas, and Holm-Rutilli et al. (13) on stomach all indicate better "autoregulation" of oxygen usage than blood flow at subnormal arterial pressures. In cases where blood flow is subnormal but oxygen uptake is normal or at least closer to normal than flow, the means by which oxygen usage is sustained is improved oxygen extraction (12,13,19,20,23,26). The improvement in extraction as blood flow decreases is generally considered to be evidence of a greater number of actively perfused capillaries (19–21). However, as previously mentioned, a reduction in flow would lengthen the time available for capillary exchange and thereby also improve extraction. Furthermore, if more capillaries are perfused, the red cell transit time in each capillary would be greater than normal whether flow remained at control or decreased. This effect occurs because capillary red cell transit time is related to the ratio of the number of perfused capillaries relative to the blood flow. Thus, improved extraction at subnormal blood flows, particularly for oxygen, is partly a passive phenomenon that can be actively augmented to various extents if the number of perfused capillaries is increased.

The whole question of the effects of blood flow and number of actively perfused capillaries on oxygen bulk exchange is important to the physiology of absorptive hyperemia. With the exception of rats (1,2), the magnitude of hyperemia during active absorption is typically 10% to 40% above control flow (12–14,17–20). However, oxygen usage typically increases by an average of 40% or more (12,26,27,30). Even if the increase in blood flow matched the percent increase in oxygen usage, the increased flow would probably not be totally capable of supplying the needed oxygen because extraction efficiency should fall as capillary flow velocity increases. Therefore, an increase in the number of perfused capillaries may be vitally important to gas exchange when the fractional increase in blood flow is small compared with the fractional increase in oxygen consumption.

The mechanics of increasing the number of perfused capillaries in splanchnic organs is not known; I will simply point out the possibilities. The microcirculation of the intestinal, colon, and gastric muscle layers closely resembles the skeletal muscle vasculature in that few precapillary sphincters exist and capillaries have relatively few interconnections (10,23,24). However, it is well established that in skeletal muscle the number of actively perfused capillaries can and does change owing to actions of the smallest arterioles (23). Something similar may occur in the vasculature of the intestinal muscularis, although direct evidence has not been obtained. In the mucosal vasculature, the basic pattern of mucosal capillary branching varies among species, but all animals appear to share the common characteristic of extensively interconnected capillaries (8,10). In fact, a network is the best way to describe the mucosal capillary branching pattern. Closing the origin of a given capillary does not necessarily mean that the remainder of the capillary is unperfused; interconnecting capillaries at branch points within the network can provide some perfusion even though the direction of flow may reverse. As a consequence, it is difficult to predict how mucosal capillary surface area is altered even though a number of studies indicate that the total intestinal perfused surface area can increase or decrease depending on whether constrictor or dilator stimuli are present. This topic has been recently reviewed by Shepherd (28). It is possible that when the origins of some fraction of the capillaries prevent flow, the collateral flow to these capillaries is so low and flow velocity so slow that exchangeable materials rapidly reach equilibrium. In effect, those capillaries with only collateral flow may not appreciably contribute to the physiologically active capillary exchange surface area. The proposed situation would appear during measurement of surface area with blood-borne tracers as if the perfused capillary surface area were less than maximum, when, in fact, virtually all capillaries are perfused, but some vessels are not necessarily perfused to an extent that contributes to capillary exchange. As stated at the beginning of this paragraph, the mechanisms that govern capillary surface area in the splanchnic organs are not precisely known. Therefore, the above proposals are offered as behavior patterns that are feasible but not necessarily extant.

RELATIONSHIP BETWEEN INTESTINAL BLOOD FLOW AND OXYGEN CONSUMPTION

In the previous discussion, we considered the regulation of intestinal oxygen consumption by a vasculature capable of actively changing perfused capillary density and vascular resistance. Kvietys et al. (11,18) reported that in the totally passive intestinal vasculature, oxygen consumption was essentially constant above some minimum blood flow; below this minimum flow, oxygen consumption decreased approximately linearly with flow. The term *minimum flow* is somewhat misleading because the flow at which oxygen consumption first becomes constant is about the same as the flow in the intestine when vascular control is present. Similar observations have also been made when vascular control is present (12,29). To explain the flow-independent and flow-dependent components of the oxygen consumption and flow relationship in the bowel, Jacobson et al. (14) have proposed that a tissue compartment exists that is underperfused relative to the oxygen needs of the tissue and that a second compartment has more than adequate flow to serve tissue oxygen requirements. This model predicts a flow-dependent component of oxygen consumption below some given flow, but, at greater flows, the flow-limited compartment would no longer have a flow that retards oxygen consumption. In effect, total oxygen use of both compartments would be flow-independent once the flow-limited compartment is properly perfused. The basic problem with this model is that essentially a permanent partially hypoxic tissue compartment would have to exist except when vasodilation is induced. One would expect local vascular control mechanisms sensitive to the direct and indirect effects of oxygen and tissue metabolites would tend to prevent a permanent state of hypoxia. A much simpler explanation for a range of flows in which oxygen consumption is flow-limited and flow-independent can be offered. For any given rate of metabolism, the tissue has a given oxygen demand. If delivery of oxygen is inadequate to meet the oxygen demand, oxygen consumption will be a function of blood flow. Once the blood flow is sufficiently increased to meet the oxygen requirement, further increases in blood flow will not increase oxygen consumption. Even if the distribution of flow between the muscle and mucosal layers is altered as blood flow is manipulated, each vasculature would follow the simpler model just proposed. Above some given total flow, oxygen consumption becomes constant because each vasculature would receive adequate or more than adequate flow for oxygen needs.

CONCLUSION

Maintenance of intestinal oxygenation appears to depend on the microvasculature's ability to change flow and to alter the number of actively perfused capillaries. It is difficult at this time to define a specific regulatory role for oxygen lack in terms of a direct cellular or indirect vasodilatory effect through tissue metabolites. However, there is ample evidence that the intestinal vasculature is sensitive to tissue oxygen demands and that it is capable of maintaining a constant or increased oxygen supply as the need warrants.

ACKNOWLEDGMENTS

Studies referenced to H. G. Bohlen were supported by NHLB7 NIH Grants HL-20605 and HL-25824. Dr. Bohlen is the recipient of NHLBI Research Career Development Award HL-01089. The author wishes to thank Miss Marsha Hunt for typing the manuscript.

REFERENCES

1. Bohlen, H. G. (1980): Intestinal tissue PO_2 and microvascular responses during glucose exposure. *Am. J. Physiol.*, 238:H164–H171.
2. Bohlen, H. G. (1980): Intestinal mucosal oxygenation influences absorptive hyperemia. *Am. J. Physiol.*, 239:H489–H493.
3. Bohlen, H. G. (1983): Tissue PO_2 in the intestinal muscle layer of rats during chronic diabetes. *Circ. Res.*, 52:677–682.
4. Chou, C. C., Hsieh, C. P., and Yu, Y. M. (1976): Localization of mesenteric hyperemia during digestion in dogs. *Am. J. Physiol.*, 230:583–589.
5. Chou, C. C., Kvietys, P. R., and Post, J. (1978): Constituents of chyme responsible for postprandial intestinal hyperemia. *Am. J. Physiol.*, 4:H677–H682.
6. Duling, B. R., and Berne, R. M. (1970): Longitudinal gradients in perivascular oxygen tension. *Cir. Res.*, 27:669–678.
7. Fara, J. W., Rubinstein, E. H., and Sonnenschein, R. R. (1972): Intestinal hormones in mesenteric vasodilation after intraduodenal agents. *Am. J. Physiol.*, 223:1058–1067.
8. Gannon, B. J., Gore, R. L., and Rogers, P. A. W. (1981): Is there an anatomical basis for a vascular counter-current mechanism in rabbit and human intestinal villi? *Biomed. Res. (Suppl.)*, 2:235–241.
9. Gorczyski, R. J., and Duling, B. R. (1978): Role of oxygen in arteriolar functional vasodilation in hamster striated muscle. *Am. J. Physiol.*, 235:505–515.
10. Gore, R. W., and Bohlen, H. G. (1977): Microvascular pressures in rat intestinal muscle and mucosal villi. *Am. J. Physiol.*, 233:H685–H693.
11. Granger, D. N., Kvietys, P. R., and Perry, M. A. (1982): Role of exchange vessels in the regulation of intestinal oxygenation. *Am. J. Physiol.*, 242:G570–G574.
12. Granger, H. J., and Norris, C. P. (1980): Intrinsic reg-

ulation of intestinal oxygenation in the anesthetized dog. *Am. J. Physiol.*, 238:H836–H843.
13. Holm-Rutilli, L., Perry, M. A., and Granger, D. N. (1981): Autoregulation of gastric blood flow and oxygen uptake. *Am. J. Physiol.*, 241:G143–G149.
14. Jacobson, E. D., Gallavan, R. H., and Fondacaro, J. D. (1982): A model of the mesenteric circulation. *Am. J. Physiol.*, 242:G541–G546.
15. Kampp, M., and Lundgren, O. (1968): Blood flow and flow distribution in the small intestine of the cat as analyzed by the Kr^{85} wash-out technique. *Acta Physiol. Scand.*, 72:282–297.
16. Kampp, J., Lundgren, O., and Sjostrand, J. (1968): The distribution of intravascularly administered lipid solute and lipid insoluble substances in the mucosa and submucosa of the small intestine of the cat. *Acta Physiol. Scand.*, 72:469–480.
17. Krogh, A. (1918): The number and distribution of capillaries in muscles with calculations of oxygen pressure head necessary for supplying the tissue. *J. Physiol. (Lond.)*, 52:409–415.
18. Kvietys, P. R., and Granger, D. N. (1982): Relation between intestinal blood flow and oxygen uptake. *Am. J. Physiol.*, 242:G202–G208.
19. Kvietys, P. R., McLendon, J. M., Bulkley, G. B., Perry, M. A., and Granger, D. N. (1982): Pancreatic circulation: Intrinsic regulation. *Am. J. Physiol.*, 242:G596–G602.
20. Kvietys, P. R., Miller, T., and Granger, D. N. (1980): Intrinsic control of colonic blood flow and oxygenation. *Am. J. Physiol.*, 238:G478–G484.
21. Kvietys, P. R., Wilborn, W. H., and Granger, D. N. (1981): Effect of atropine on bile-oleic acid-induced alterations in dog jejunal hemodynamics, oxygenation, and net transmucosal water movement. *Gastroenterology*, 80:31–38.
22. Norris, C. P., Barnes, G. E., Smith, E. E., and Granger, H. J. (1979): Autoregulation of superior mesenteric flow in fasted and fed dogs. *Am. J. Physiol.*, 237:H174–H177.
23. Prewitt, R. L., and Johnson, P. C. (1976): The effect of oxygen on arteriolar red cell velocity and capillary density in the rat cremaster muscle. *Microvasc. Res.*, 12:59–70.
24. Proctor, K. G., and Bohlen, H. G. (1981): Exercise hyperemia in the absence of a tissue PO_2 decrease. *Blood Vessels*, 18:58–66.
25. Renkin, E. M. (1968): Transcapillary exchange in relation to capillary circulation. *J. Gen. Physiol.*, 52:96S–102S.
26. Shepherd, A. P. (1979): Intestinal O_2 uptake during sympathetic stimulation and partial arterial occlusion. *Am. J. Physiol.*, 236:H731–H735.
27. Shepherd, A. P. (1980): Intestinal blood flow autoregulation during foodstuff absorption. *Am. J. Physiol.*, 239:H156–H162.
28. Shepherd, A. P. (1982): Role of capillary recruitment in the regulation of intestinal oxygenation. *Am. J. Physiol.*, 242:G435–G441.
29. Shepherd, A. P., and Riedel, G. L. (1982): Effect of pulsatile pressure and metabolic rate on intestinal autoregulation. *Am. J. Physiol.*, 242:H769–H775.
30. Valleau, J. D., Granger, D. N., and Taylor, A. E. (1979): Effect of solute-coupled volume absorption on oxygen consumption in cat ileum. *Am. J. Physiol.*, 236:E198–E203.
31. Yu, Y. M., Yu, L. C., and Chou, C. C. (1975): Distribution of blood flow in the intestine with hypertonic glucose in the lumen. *Surgery*, 78:S20–S25.

Role of the Splanchnic Circulation in Reflex Control of the Cardiovascular System

Loring B. Rowell and *John M. Johnson

*Departments of Physiology and Biophysics and Medicine, School of Medicine, University of Washington, Seattle, Washington 98195; and *Department of Physiology, University of Texas Health Science Center at San Antonio, San Antonio, Texas 78284*

In mammals, the splanchnic organs receive approximately 25% of the cardiac output at rest and contain 20% to 30% of total blood volume. The splanchnic region, the "venesector and blood giver of the circulation" (30), is thought to play a major role in the reflex control of the circulation, especially in humans. Therefore, much of this chapter focuses on splanchnic hemodynamics in humans.

The importance of the splanchnic circulation in overall circulatory regulation has been questioned because sustained vasoconstriction often does not occur in anesthetized cats and dogs in response to falling blood pressure (17,25,31)[1]. Also, the lack of a reduction in splanchnic blood flow (SBF) during stresses such as exercise in dogs has been taken as evidence against the importance of blood flow redistribution in humans (34,58). Some investigators (51,58) feel that apparent discrepancies result from differences in methodology. The indicator dilution technique developed by Bradley et al. (7) permits only discontinuous measurements of blood flow through the entire hepatic-portal system; hepatic arterial and portal venous blood flows cannot be measured separately. (For details, limitations, and validity of the method see refs. 6,26,50). Flowmeters make it possible to evaluate continuously changes in blood flow to portions of the splanchnic region. However, when simultaneously compared, the dye extraction methods used to measure SBF [and renal blood flow (53)] yield the same values as those derived from electromagnetic flow probes or made by actual direct measurements of flow (timed collections of effluent blood) (51). Therefore in our view, disparities in splanchnic vascular responses to various drives are attributable to species differences in the control of the peripheral circulation (49,53). These differences can be observed when the same methods are applied to different species (22,23,36,49,53).

Humans are faced with unique hemodynamic problems that require extensive redistribution of blood *flow* and blood *volume*. For example, when humans stand up, large volumes of blood are translocated to dependent veins (16). Blood volume and flow must be redistributed to maintain blood pressure and adequate cardiac output. Quantification of splanchnic blood volume (SBV) is difficult, especially in humans (6). Our discussion of SBV mobilization draws heavily from experiments with animals in which the basic relationships among SBV, SBF, and pressures within the region have been quantified. Our primary objective is to show how reflexly and locally induced changes in blood flow, vascular resistance, and vascular volume of the splanchnic region aid in the regulation of blood pressure, regional oxygen delivery, heat transport, and the distribution of total blood volume.

ROLE IN BLOOD PRESSURE REGULATION

Obviously, a region that comprises one-fourth of total vascular conductance is potentially im-

---

[1]In order to limit the length of the bibliography, we have sometimes cited only the review article in which the original work is cited.

portant to blood pressure regulation. Nevertheless, its actual importance has been unclear (17,21,31), partly because of the techniques used to alter blood pressure. For example, pressures have been manipulated by hemorrhage, by changing carotid sinus transmural pressure (with and without competing drives from aortic baroreceptors), and by electrical stimulation of the carotid sinus nerve (31). In addition, species differences and interactions of baroreflexes with other reflexes or with local influences have contributed to differences in experimental results (18,36,40).

Hemorrhage has directed attention to the splanchnic region as the "blood giver" of the circulation. However, results from anesthetized animals reveal great variability in splanchnic vasomotor responses to this stress. Splanchnic vasoconstriction may or may not accompany hemorrhage (17,21). The myriad of factors that might account for this variability is beyond the purview of this chapter (for a review, see Chapter 5). In short, reflex changes can be opposed or reinforced by metabolites or humoral agents released during hemorrhage. Of particular importance are the opposing effects of circulating epinephrine on SBF and SBV. The β-adrenergic effect of epinephrine on splanchnic arterioles is dilation (3,21). In contrast, epinephrine appears to cause splanchnic venoconstriction (18,19,21). A common conclusion is that the splanchnic circulation does not contribute much to compensatory changes in systemic vascular conductance during hemorrhage (17,21,35).

In most species, hemorrhage has major effects on SBV (35,43,46). In cats, for example, the splanchnic vasculature tends to release a volume of blood equivalent to 25% to 65% of the total volume lost in hemorrhage (20,37). Price et al. (43) removed 15% to 20% of estimated total blood volume from normal humans and found a 40% decrease in SBV to be the only significant response (SBF did not change). However, we do not understand how cardiac output, heart rate, mean arterial pressure, and "central" blood volume could all remain unaltered. These findings conflict with those made during lower-body negative pressure (LBNP), as discussed below. The mechanism of the decrease in SBV is unknown. Apparently, it is not a passive effect of decreased splanchnic venous pressure associated with reduced perfusion. One possibility is a splanchnic venoconstriction mediated by the sympathetic nervous system. Another possibility is that a decreased central venous pressure, which must have occurred (16), created a pressure gradient between the right atrium and hepatic veins thus reducing SBV. Finally, increased circulating epinephrine (not measured but probably increased) could oppose arteriolar constriction and, at the same time, cause venoconstriction (18,19).

In humans, hemorrhage can be simulated by applying LBNP at levels sufficient to draw as much as 750 ml into distended blood vessels of the legs (54). In contrast to the results of Price et al. (43), LBNP markedly reduced cardiac output, stroke volume, and central blood volume and raised heart rate and total vascular resistance. SBF fell by 34% and splanchnic vascular resistance (SVR) rose by 34%. Splanchnic vasoconstriction accounted for one-third of the decrease in total vascular conductance. Thus, the region played a major role in the maintenance of blood pressure. Although no measurements were made, we assume that SBV decreased during LBNP because central venous pressure and SBF both fell. These changes should passively reduce SBV (see section "Role in Blood Volume Distribution").

Reflexes originating at cardiopulmonary baroreceptors have their largest effects on splanchnic and renal resistance vessels in dogs (38,42). In humans, however, increments in SVR during LBNP appeared to be more closely associated with the fall in aortic pulse pressure (mean aortic pressure was unchanged) than with the fall in right atrial pressure at the onset of LBNP (54). This suggested to Johnson et al. (29) that arterial baroreflexes exert greater effects on the splanchnic region than do cardiopulmonary baroreflexes. LBNP was applied in a ramp that elicited a gradual decline in right atrial pressure with stable mean aortic pressure, pulse pressure, and maximal dP/dt. Later, both right atrial pressure and aortic pulse pressure were reduced

(Fig. 1). The reduction in right atrial pressure elicited only a 10% decrease in SBF in contrast to the 33% reduction in forearm blood flow. The major decrease in SBF accompanied falling aortic pulse pressure; the reduction was 30% before any change in mean pressure occurred. Abboud et al. (1) found that splanchnic vasoconstriction during LBNP could be reversed by raising carotid sinus transmural pressure when central venous pressure remained low and forearms were vasoconstricted. Thus, arterial baroreceptors appear to dominate in the control of SBF. If cardiopulmonary baroreflexes defend against thoracic blood volume depletion, vasoconstriction may not be an appropriate response. Vasoconstriction could augment the reduction in central venous volume and pressure unless it occurred in a capacious and compliant region such as the splanchnic bed where a reduction in flow would mobilize volume centrally and serve to reduce the stimulus (this point is discussed later). We were surprised that splanchnic vasoconstriction was not more pronounced.

Does the splanchnic region reflexly vasodilate in response to elevated blood pressure? Such a response implies that there be vasoconstrictor tone that can be withdrawn, as active vasodilator reflexes are not usually involved in baroreflexes (8). Lautt (36) concluded that the splanchnic region in dogs and cats receives no tonic vasoconstrictor outflow (cf. 21). Yet, Donald (13) observed increases in SBF when carotid sinus pressure was raised. The reasons for this discrepancy are unclear. Although the presence of some vasoconstrictor tone in splanchnic organs is suggested by the increased levels of SBF after sympathectomy in hypertensive humans (62), normotensive humans appear to lack such tone. For example, SBF does not increase during high spinal anesthesia (39) and SVR does not fall when carotid sinus transmural pressure is increased by applying suction to the neck (L. B. Rowell et al., *unpublished observations*). Finally, Tyden et al. (57) applied electromagnetic flowmeters to the common hepatic, gastroduodenal, ileocolic, colic, and external iliac arteries in anesthetized patients undergoing abdominal surgery. Carotid sinus stimulation caused release of vasoconstriction only in the iliac artery, which supplies a region with high vasoconstrictor tone. The conclusion

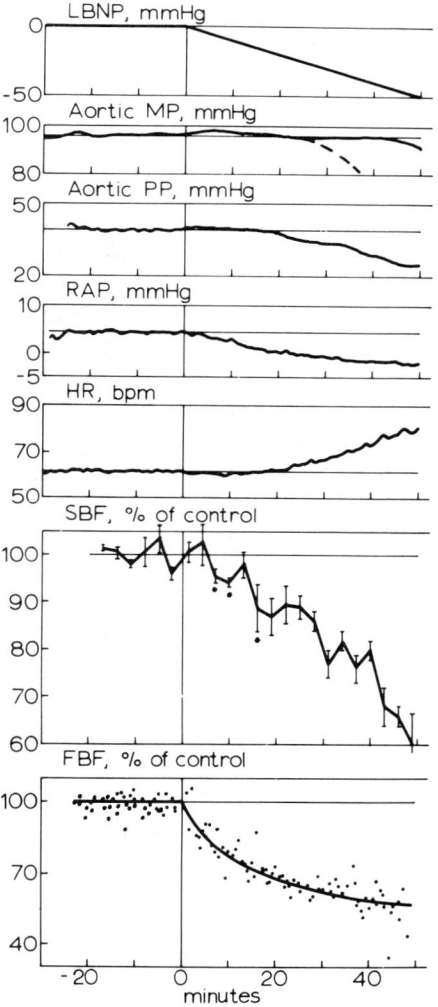

FIG. 1. Circulatory responses to a slow ramp (−1 Torr/min) of lower-body negative pressure (LBNP) (9 subjects). During the first 20 min of LBNP, no change in aortic mean pressure (MP), pulse pressure (PP), or heart rate (HR) occurred (aortic dP/dt was also constant). There was a progressive fall in right atrial pressure (RAP). Splanchnic blood flow (SBF) significantly (*) decreased by 10% and forearm blood flow (FBF) fell by 35%. After 20 min, note the association among falling aortic PP, falling SBF, and rising HR. (From Johnson et al., ref. 29, with permission.)

is that SVR does not fall in response to acute hypertension.

Role in Orthostatic Adjustments

Humans spend a substantial portion of their lives in the upright posture with the heart situated above a compliant venous system containing a major fraction of the total blood volume. When humans stand up, approximately 600 to 700 ml of blood move into dependent veins, causing large reductions in central venous pressure, thoracic blood volume, stroke volume, and cardiac output (16). Mean arterial pressure, however, is well maintained by vasoconstriction. The 45% increase in SVR (12) makes a major contribution to the total change in systemic vascular conductance. This was revealed when hypertensive patients experienced severe postural hypotension after splanchnic sympathectomy (61). In addition, the 40% decrease in SBF should also exert a major influence on the distribution of blood volume.

ROLE IN SYSTEMIC BLOOD FLOW REGULATION

Diseases that reduce cardiac output during rest or exercise are associated with a marked redistribution of blood flow away from splanchnic organs when normal vasomotor control mechanisms are present. This response is thought to optimize the distribution of cardiac output so that adequate perfusion of the heart and brain is secured (59).

Regional Oxygen Transport in Exercise

Humans redistribute blood flow away from nonworking regions, especially splanchnic organs and kidneys, during exercise (49,59); SBF is reduced in proportion to the increase in total oxygen consumption ($\dot{V}O_2$), heart rate, and plasma norepinephrine (NE) concentration (49,53). The rise in NE concentration appears to reflect changes in sympathetic nervous activity so long as mechanisms for release and reuptake are normal (11). During severe exercise, the distribution of cardiac output in normal subjects is similar to that seen at rest or mild exercise in cardiac patients (5). The falls in SBF and renal blood flow during exercise are inversely related to the percent of maximal $\dot{V}O_2$ required by that level of work (49). Maximal $\dot{V}O_2$ is a measure of the circulatory capacity to transport oxygen to the tissues and is usually limited by the maximal cardiac output (49).

Although striking differences exist between individuals compared at the same absolute $\dot{V}O_2$, when examined in relative terms (percent of maximal $\dot{V}O_2$), changes in plasma NE concentration, SBF, heart rate, and systemic arteriovenous O_2 difference during exercise are virtually identical (11,24,53). An example of the close inverse relationship between SBF and relative metabolic demands is shown in Fig. 2. Rowell et al. *(unpublished observations)* had the rare opportunity to alter acutely maximal $\dot{V}O_2$ in a 46-year-old man with heart block by controlling his pacemaker. (The subject was otherwise healthy and physically active.) Responses to graded exercise up to the maximal $\dot{V}O_2$ with heart rate fixed at 70 and at 110 bpm are shown; maximal $\dot{V}O_2$ was 2.1 liter/min and 3.2 liter/min at the two heart rates, respectively. The relationship between SBF and the percent of maximal $\dot{V}O_2$ required for each level of work remained constant.

It is this redistribution of blood flow away from regions that extract little oxygen to working skeletal muscle that makes it possible for 85% of the available oxygen to be extracted from blood at maximal $\dot{V}O_2$. The importance of cardiac output redistribution increases as the ability to increase cardiac output declines. Quantitative aspects have been reviewed in detail elsewhere (49). A redistribution of 3 liter/min (or 600 ml O_2/min) from the splanchnic, renal, and other nonworking regions to working muscle at maximal $\dot{V}O_2$ is of major significance to total oxygen transport in subjects with abnormally low maximal cardiac outputs. In addition, loss of regional vasoconstriction would cause a substantial fall in blood pressure in these individuals. These effects would be small in the athlete because the splanchnic region represents such a small fraction of total flow and

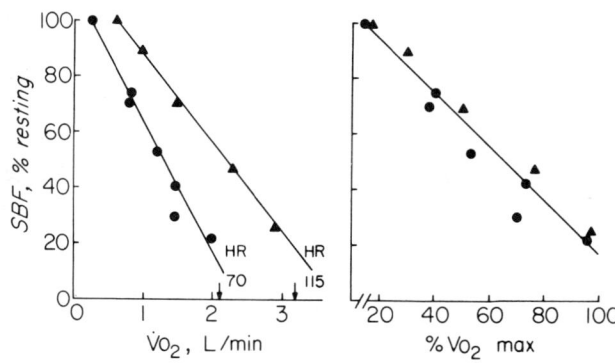

FIG. 2. Splanchnic blood flow (SBF) as percent of resting (100%) vs total oxygen consumption ($\dot{V}_{O_2}$) during graded exercise up to maximal $\dot{V}_{O_2}$ with the heart paced at 70 bpm and at 115 bpm (maximal $\dot{V}_{O_2}$, 2.1 and 3.2 liter/min, respectively). The subject had heart block and an implanted pacemaker. Changes in SBF estimated from changes in indocyanine green clearance. Note in *right panel* the close relationship of responses to percent of $\dot{V}_{O_2}$ max required. (Rowell et al., *unpublished observations*.)

conductance during heavy exercise. The nature of the reflexes causing splanchnic vasoconstriction in exercise is still unknown (55).

In contrast to humans, normal dogs do not reduce SBF or renal blood flow even during severe exercise (58). However, SVR increases along with blood pressure (the importance of this adjustment is discussed later). If the ability to raise cardiac output in dogs is compromised, human-like vasomotor responses, which can be eliminated by α-adrenergic blockade, are observed (58).

Regional Oxygen Transport in Hypoxia

Hypoxia also causes a redistribution of cardiac output but with marked variation in regional vasomotor responses, even within the hepatic-portal circulation (32). Variation is due, in part, to the complex interaction among local, humoral, and reflex effects of hypoxia and to the nonuniformity of these effects in different organs. Although hypoxia increases splanchnic nerve activity (27), other factors such as circulating epinephrine may override or alter neural influences (32). Limited evidence from resting humans suggests SBF does not fall and may even increase (10,45).

The combined stresses of hypoxia and exercise cause large increments in plasma NE and epinephrine concentrations and in heart rate (15). Maximal $\dot{V}_{O_2}$ falls in proportion to the reduction in arterial oxygen content. The close relationship between the percent of maximal $\dot{V}_{O_2}$ required and the heart rate or plasma NE concentration observed during exercise in normoxic conditions is unaffected by hypoxia. However, hypoxia does drastically alter the relationship between SBF and these variables (15). SBF did not decrease further during hypoxia, as would be predicted from the rise in heart rate and NE concentration. In some cases, SBF even rose markedly as SVR fell. The high plasma epinephrine concentrations during hypoxia could cause splanchnic vasodilation. If so, splanchnic *venoconstriction* would also be expected (18,19), and it would oppose any flow-induced volume displacement into this region. Local effects of hypoxia may also contribute to the fall in SVR. (See Chapters 3 and 12.)

Heat Transport

Human skin has a dense network of capacious veins and a high blood-flow capacity. Because of these features, heat stress causes two major regulatory problems: (a) maintenance of adequate cardiac filling pressures when a large volume of blood has been transferred into cutaneous veins and (b) maintenance of adequate cutaneous perfusion in conditions where demands for flow by other regions are high (e.g., skeletal muscle during exercise). Thus volume shifts associated with cutaneous vasodilation decrease the ability of the heart to meet increased demands for flow (52,53). Splanchnic compensation for blood volume shifts is discussed in the next section.

Splanchnic and renal vasoconstriction in response to heat stress are well established in many species (22,23,53,56) and are particularly pronounced in humans and other primates (23,44). The increases in SVR, heart rate, cardiac output, and plasma NE concentrations all parallel the rise in core temperature (14,53). Alpha blockade prevents mesenteric vasoconstriction in heat-stressed baboons (44). Prevention of heat-induced increases in renin release did not block splanchnic vasoconstriction (14). Increased vasoconstrictor activity to the splanchnic system is triggered by thermal stimulation of receptors in the hypothalamus and spinal cord (56). Baroreflexes appear not to be involved (52,53). Because the rise in cardiac output is so great, the reduction in SBF makes only a 10% to 20% contribution to the increase in skin blood flow in supine, resting humans (49). The splanchnic circulation is, however, important to volume distribution as discussed in the next section.

When resting humans are upright, heat stress imposes severe regulatory problems; the ability to adjust to cutaneous vasodilation without syncope is quite limited (53). During exercise, compression of veins by active muscle improves the situation, but the rise in cardiac output is still limited by reductions in filling pressure and stroke volume caused by the transfer of blood volume to cutaneous veins. As a result, cardiac output cannot meet the combined demands of skeletal muscle and skin for blood flow. The relationship between SBF (or renal blood flow) and total $\dot{V}O_2$ during exercise is changed so that SBF is substantially lower at a given $\dot{V}O_2$. The added vasoconstriction redistributes 600 to 800 ml of blood to skin each minute at moderate intensities of exercise (49). However, the close inverse relationship between SBF and heart rate or plasma NE concentration is preserved (see Summary). Again, these variables appear to reflect a rise in sympathetic nervous activity.

ROLE IN BLOOD VOLUME DISTRIBUTION

There is little doubt that the splanchnic circulation is the blood giver of the circulation. With 20% to 30% of the blood volume in a region of high compliance (e.g., hepatic compliance is 10 times that of the systemic circulation), small changes in transmural pressure will have large effects on SBV (4,13). Blood volume can be mobilized from splanchnic veins by either active or passive mechanisms (see Chapter 6). Volume is mobilized *actively* by constriction of splanchnic veins and *passively* by effects of reduced flow on venous pressure and volume. For conflicting views concerning the importance of these processes, see refs. 19 and 37.

Measurements of SBV in humans are scarce. Qualitative estimates of SBV from X-ray dimensions of the liver show that its volume is reduced during heat stress and hemorrhage (53). Studies in other species show that reductions in SBV accompany reductions in SBF (e.g., 4,13). The quantitative aspects of this relationship are discussed by Rothe in Chapter 6. However, as mentioned previously, SBV can decrease without a change in SBF. Nevertheless, under many conditions, control of SBF is an essential factor in the regulation of SBV and systemic blood volume distribution, which, especially in humans, determines cardiac filling pressure and thus the performance of the heart.

Krogh's Model

Krogh (33) suggested how the distribution of blood flow could determine the distribution of blood volume. He conceptually divided the cardiovascular system into a compliant and a noncompliant circuit and proposed that the distribution of blood flow between these two circuits determines the volume of blood available for cardiac filling. Krogh's ideas have recently been applied to explain effects of vasoactive drugs on the distribution of blood volume (9). The ideas also apply to situations in which *reflexes* control the distribution of flow between different circuits.

The response to heat stress provides a good illustration; a rise in blood flow to one compliant region (skin) is compensated for by a reduction in flow to another (the splanchnic region). Initially, release of blood from splanchnic veins probably attends the marked fall in right atrial pressure accompanying heating. The pressure gradient established between the right atrium and hepatic veins favors a passive reduction in SBV. Subsequent splanchnic vasoconstriction will further reduce splanchnic venous pressure and SBV. Inasmuch as these adjustments occur when the splanchnic veins are near their maximal compliance, the release of volume must be substantial, minimizing depletion of central sumps. This concept is illustrated in Figure 3.

The response to upright exercise also illustrates Krogh's thinking. Muscular compression of veins transfers blood volume toward the heart, reversing the reduction in cardiac filling pressure that accompanies stationary upright posture. The venous compliance of active skeletal muscle must approach zero during exercise so that even the highest muscle blood flows are without effect on systemic volume distribution (53). As exercise continues, skin blood flow increases with rising body temperature (28). The progressive rise in cutaneous blood volume is partially counteracted by a rise in SVR that roughly parallels the increase in skin blood flow (49). Even during mild supine exercise SBV can fall by nearly 40% (60), with greater decrements anticipated during more strenuous work when SBF is lower.

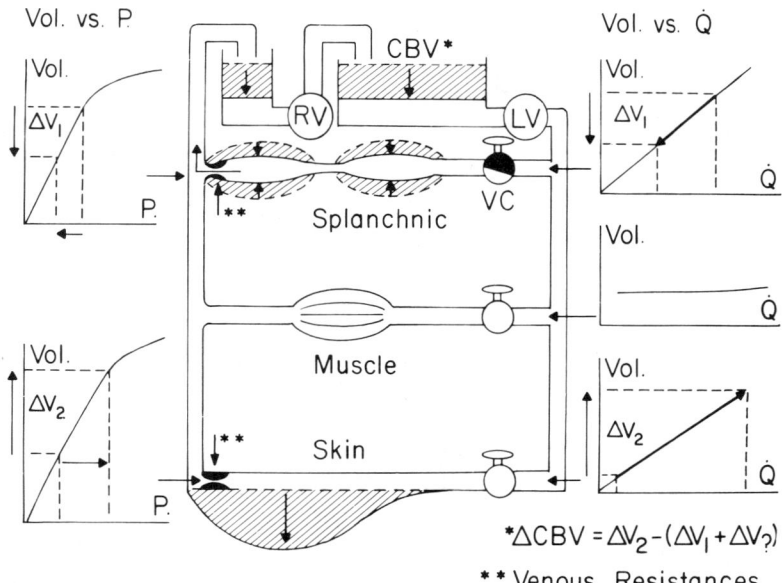

FIG. 3. Compensation for skin vasodilation by splanchnic vasoconstriction: an illustration of Krogh's hypothesis. Splanchnic and skin circuits are highly compliant as shown by the volume (Vol) vs pressure (P) curves (left). As skin vessels dilate, the volume vs flow ($\dot{Q}$) panel (right) (and the shaded area in the skin circuit) shows the increase in skin venous volume (ΔV_2). This reduces pre-right ventricular (RV) and pre-left ventricular (LV) or pulmonary (CBV) volume sumps causing a fall in ventricular filling pressures and stroke volume. Partial compensation is achieved by vasoconstriction (VC) of the splanchnic region, which passively reduces splanchnic venous volume (shaded region) by reducing splanchnic pressure (Vol vs P, upper left) and flow (Vol vs $\dot{Q}$, upper right). This minimizes the reduction in CBV (*ΔCBV, lower right), which equals the difference between ΔV_2 and ΔV_1, and any other constricted compliant regions ($\Delta V_?$). Vasodilation of active noncompliant muscle does not influence distribution (Vol. vs $\dot{Q}$ is flat). Passive volume shift from peripheral to central veins requires a venous pressure gradient and thus a resistance to venous flow, as schematically indicated by the resistors (two asterisks). (From Rowell, ref. 52, with permission.)

We pointed out earlier that dogs maintain a constant SBF during exercise by raising SVR and SBV as blood pressure rises. Ashkar (2) revealed the importance of this adjustment when he eliminated nervous control of splanchnic blood vessels and the adrenal medulla by thoracic sympathectomy. After surgery, the dogs showed a deficit in the cardiovascular response to exercise (Fig. 4) similar to that caused in humans by vasodilation of skin. We assume that this deficit was caused by passively increasing SBF and SBV, with accompanying falls in cardiac filling pressures. A curious feature of Ashkar's studies is that loss of sympathetic control of the splanchnic vasculature had no effect on the responses so long as adrenal medullary function was intact. Once again, the importance of epinephrine as an agent that actively reduces SBV is suggested.

Finally, the splanchnic region serves as a pre-right ventricular volume sump that smoothes out respiratory oscillations in venous return (41). These are mechanical (rather than reflex) changes caused by diaphragmatic compression of hepatic veins.

SUMMARY

In humans undergoing a variety of stresses, there is a close negative correlation between SBF and both heart rate (Fig. 5) and plasma NE concentration. The similarity of the regression equations from different laboratories is noteworthy. During exercise, SBF starts to decrease at higher heart rates than when stresses are applied during rest, probably because the contribution of vagal withdrawal to the initial rise in heart rate is greater during exercise (47). Increments in plasma NE concentration (11) are inversely proportional to SBF during exercise (24) and heat stress (14). Also, the relationships of plasma NE concentration to heart rate during rest and exercise differ in the same manner as those relating SBF to heart rate. In exercise NE starts to rise at a higher heart rate (11). Thus, it appears that increased sympathetic nervous

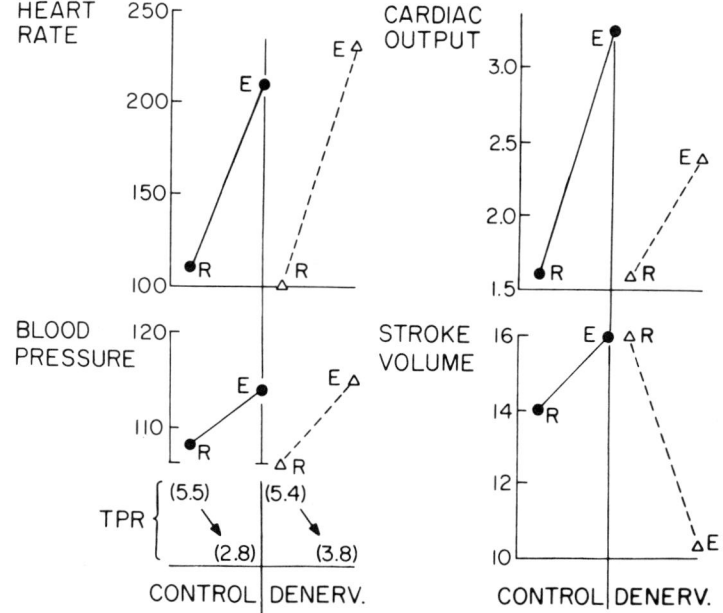

FIG. 4. Circulatory responses to exercise (E) (R is rest) in dogs before *(solid lines)* and after *(dashed lines)* denervation (Denerv.) of the splanchnic organs and adrenal medulla by thoracic sympathectomy. Denervation reduced the rise in cardiac output through a reduction in stroke volume. (Adapted from Ashkar, ref. 2, with permission.)

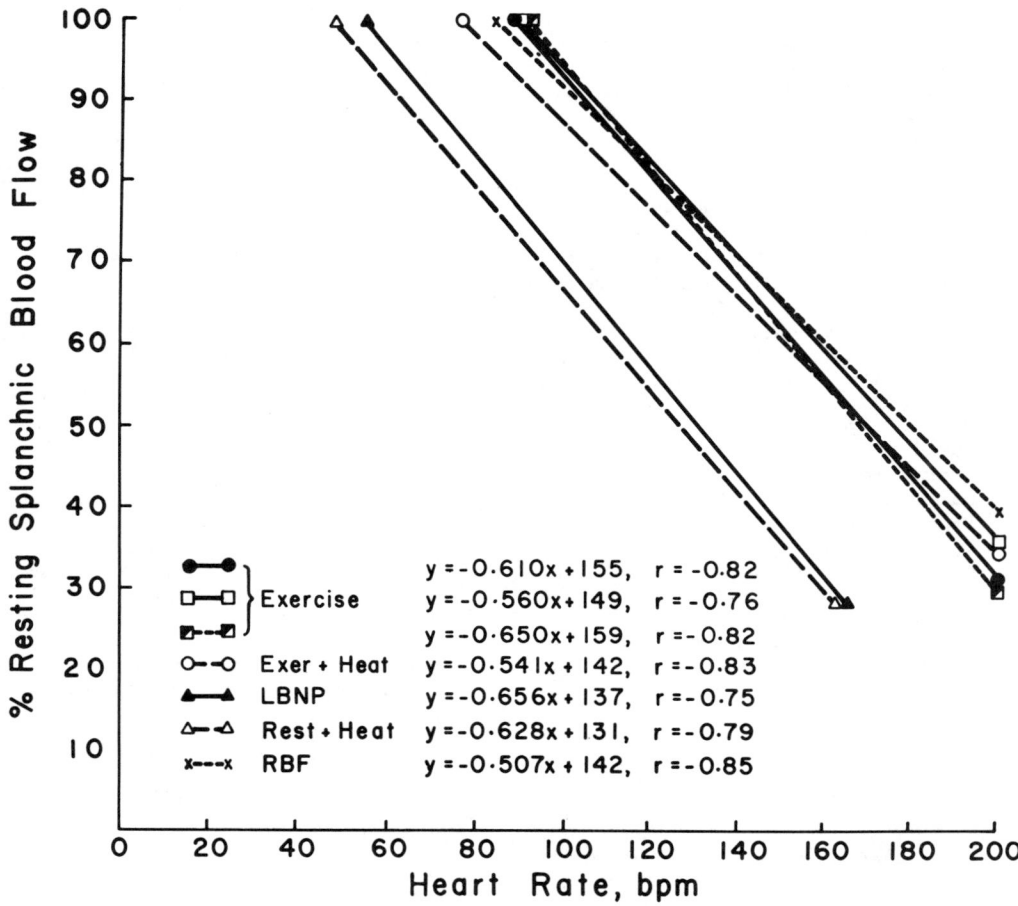

FIG. 5. Relationship between splanchnic blood flow as percent of resting and heart rate during exercise *(five curves on right)* and rest *(two curves on left)*. Despite the fact that exercise was carried out in neutral and hot environments, before and after physical conditioning, or with different muscle groups (see ref. 49), all regression lines (from four different laboratories) were virtually the same, including one study of renal blood flow during exercise *(X's and dashed lines)*. Regression lines for data collected in supine resting subjects stressed by heat or lower-body negative pressure (LBNP) are displaced to the left, as are the data for plasma norepinephrine concentration vs heart rate (see text and ref. 11). (From Rowell, ref. 48, with permission.)

activity to the heart to increase its rate is accompanied by proportional increases in vasoconstrictor outflow to splanchnic organs. The close correlation between SBF and each of these variables during exercise is abolished by hypoxia and possibly during certain degrees of hemorrhage. In such conditions, a marked rise in plasma epinephrine concentration (or local influences) could override vasoconstriction. The magnitude of the splanchnic vascular contribution to the distribution of blood flow and blood volume gives this region a pivotal role in the reflex control of the cardiovascular system.

ACKNOWLEDGMENTS

The authors' research was supported by NHLBI Grant 16910.

REFERENCES

1. Abboud, F. M., Eckberg, D. L., Johannsen, U. J., and Mark, A. L. (1979): Carotid and cardiopulmonary

baroreceptor control of splanchnic and forearm vascular resistance during venous pooling in man. *J. Physiol. (Lond.)*, 286:173–184.
2. Ashkar, E. (1982): Effects of bilateral splanchnicectomy on circulation during exercise in dogs. *Acta Physiol. Lat. Am.*, 23:171–177.
3. Bearn, A. G., Billing, B., and Sherlock, S. (1951): The effect of adrenaline and noradrenaline on hepatic blood flow and splanchnic carbohydrate metabolism in man. *J. Physiol. (Lond.)*, 115:430–441.
4. Bennett, T. D., and Rothe, C. F. (1981): Hepatic capacitance responses to changes in flow and hepatic venous pressure in dogs. *Am. J. Physiol.*, 240 *(Heart and Circ. Physiol.)* 9:H18–H28.
5. Blackmon, J. R., Rowell, L. B., Kennedy, J. W., Twiss, R. D., and Conn, R. D. (1967): Physiological significance of maximal oxygen intake in pure mitral stenosis. *Circulation*, 36:497–510.
6. Bradley, S. E. (1963): The hepatic circulation. In: *Handbook of Physiology. Circulation*, edited by W. F. Hamilton and P. Dow, sect. 2, vol. II, chapt. 41, pp. 1387–1438. American Physiological Society, Washington, D.C.
7. Bradley, S. E., Ingelfinger, F. J., Bradley, G. P., and Curry, J. J. (1945): The estimation of hepatic blood flow in man. *J. Clin. Invest.*, 24:890–897.
8. Brodie, M. J. (1978): Histaminergic and cholinergic vasodilator systems. In: *Mechanisms of Vasodilation*, edited by P. M. Vanhoutte and I. Leusen, pp. 255–277. Karger, Basel.
9. Caldini, P., Permutt, S., Waddell, J. A., and Riley, R. L. (1974): Effect of epinephrine on pressure, flow, and volume relationships in the systemic circulation of dogs. *Cir. Res.*, 34:606–623.
10. Capderou, A., Polianski, J., Mensch-Dechene, J., Drouet, L., Antezana, G., Zelter, M., and Lockhart, A. (1977): Splanchnic blood flow, O_2 consumption, removal of lactate, and output of glucose in highlanders. *J. Appl. Physiol.: Respir. Environ. Exercise Physiol.*, 43:204–210.
11. Christensen, N. J., and Galbo, H. (1983): Sympathetic nervous activity during exercise. *Annu. Rev. Physiol.*, 45:139–153.
12. Culbertson, J. W., Wilkins, R. W., Ingelfinger, F. J., and Bradley, S. E. (1951): The effect of the upright posture upon hepatic blood flow in normotensive and hypertensive subjects. *J. Clin. Invest.*, 30:305–311.
13. Donald, D. E. (1981): Mobilization of blood from the splanchnic circulation. In: *Hepatic Circulation in Health and Disease*, edited by W. W. Lautt, pp. 193–202. Raven Press, New York.
14. Escourrou, P., Freund, P. R., Rowell, L. B., and Johnson, D. G. (1982): Splanchnic vasoconstriction in heat-stressed man—role of the renin-angiotensin system. *J. Appl Physiol.: Respir. Environ. Exercise Physiol.*, 52:1438–1443.
15. Escourrou, P., Rowell, L. B., Johnson, D. G., and Blackmon, J. R. (1983): Plasma catecholamines, hepatic function and blood flow during hypoxia and exercise in humans. *Fed. Proc.*, 42:1097.
16. Gauer, O. H., and Thron, H. L. (1965): Postural changes in the circulation. In: *Handbook of Physiology. Circulation*, edited by W. F. Hamilton and P. Dow, sect. 2, vol. III, chapt. 67, pp. 2409–2439. American Physiological Society, Washington, D.C.
17. Grayson, J., and Mendel, D. (1965): *Physiology of the Splanchnic Circulation*. Williams and Wilkins, Baltimore.
18. Greenway, C. V. (1982): Mechanisms and quantitative assessment of drug effects on cardiac output with a new model of the circulation. *Pharmacol. Rev.*, 33:213–251.
19. Greenway, C. V. (1983): Role of splanchnic venous system in overall cardiovascular homeostasis. *Fed. Proc.*, 42:1678–1684.
20. Greenway, C. V., and Lister, G. E. (1974): Capacitance effects and blood reservoir function in the splanchnic vascular bed during non-hypotensive hemorrhage and blood volume expansion in anesthetized cats. *J. Physiol. (Lond.)*, 237:279–294.
21. Greenway, C. V., and Stark, R. D. (1971): Hepatic vascular bed. *Physiol. Rev.*, 51:23–65.
22. Hales, J. R. S., and Dampney, R. A. L. (1975): The redistribution of cardiac output in the dog during heat stress. *J. Thermal Biol.*, 1:29–34.
23. Hales, J. R. S., Rowell, L. B., and King, R. B. (1979): Regional distribution of blood flow in awake heat-stressed baboons. *Am. J. Physiol.*, 237:H705–H712.
24. Hansen, J. F., Hesse, B., and Christensen, N. J. (1978): Enhanced sympathetic nervous activity after intravenous propranolol in ischaemic heart disease: Plasma noradrenaline, splanchnic blood flow and mixed venous oxygen saturation at rest and during exercise. *Eur. J. Clin. Invest.*, 8:31–36.
25. Hanson, K. M. (1978): Liver. In: *Peripheral Circulation*, edited by P. C. Johnson, pp. 285–314. John Wiley and Sons, New York.
26. Hultman, E. (1966): Blood circulation in the liver under physiological and pathological conditions. *Scand. J. Clin. Lab. Invest. (Suppl.)*, 18(92):27–41.
27. Iriki, M., Riedel, W., and Simon, E. (1972): Patterns of differentiation in various sympathetic efferents induced by changes of blood gas composition and by central thermal stimulation in anesthetized rabbits. *Jpn. J. Physiol.*, 22:585–602.
28. Johnson, J. M., and Rowell, L. B. (1975): Forearm skin and muscle vascular responses to prolonged leg exercise in man. *J. Appl. Physiol.*, 39:920–924.
29. Johnson, J. M., Rowell, L. B., Niederberger, M., and Eisman, M. M. (1974): Human splanchnic and forearm vasoconstrictor responses to reductions of right atrial and aortic pressure. *Circ. Res.*, 34:515–524.
30. Katz, L. N., and Robdard, S. (1939): The integration of the vasomotor responses in the liver with those in other systemic vessels. *J. Pharmacol. Exp. Ther.*, 67:407–422.
31. Kirchheim, H. R. (1976): Systemic arterial baroreceptor reflexes. *Physiol. Rev.*, 56:100–176.
32. Korner, P. I., Chalmers, J. P., and White, S. W. (1967): Some mechanisms of reflex control of the circulation by the sympatho-adrenal system. *Circ. Res. (Suppl.)*, 20,21 (II):157–172.
33. Krogh, A. (1912): The regulation of the supply of blood to the right heart. *Scand. Arch. Physiol.*, 27:227–248.
34. Lacroix, E., and Leusen, I. (1966): Splanchnic hemodynamics during induced muscular exercise in the

anesthetized dog. *Arch. Intern. Physiol. Biochem.*, 74:235–250.
35. Lacroix, E., and Leusen, I. (1967): Splanchnic and general hemodynamics after acute hemorrhage in the anesthetized dog. *Arch. Intern. Physiol. Biochem.*, 75:12–26.
36. Lautt, W. W. (1980): Hepatic nerves: A review of their functions and effects. *Can. J. Physiol. Pharmacol.*, 58:105–123.
37. Lautt, W. W., Brown, L. C., and Durham, J. S. (1980): Active and passive control of hepatic blood volume responses to hemorrhage at normal and raised hepatic venous pressure in cats. *Can. J. Physiol. Pharmacol.*, 58:1049–1057.
38. Lundgren, O. (1983): Role of splanchnic resistance vessels in overall cardiovascular homeostasis. *Fed. Proc.*, 42:1673–1677.
39. Lynn, R. B., Sancetta, S. M., Simeone, F. A., and Scott, R. W. (1952): Observations on the circulation in high spinal anesthesia. *Surgery*, 32:195–213.
40. Mellander, S., and Johansson, B. (1968): Control of resistance, exchange and capacitance functions in the peripheral circulation. *Pharmacol. Rev.*, 20:117–196.
41. Moreno, A. H., and Burchell, A. R. (1982): Respiratory regulation of splanchnic and systemic venous return in normal subjects and in patients with hepatic cirrhosis. *Surg. Gynecol. Obstet.*, 154:257–267.
42. Pelletier, C. L., Edis, A. J., and Shepherd, J. T. (1971): Circulatory reflex from vagal afferents in response to hemorrhage in the dog. *Circ. Res.*, 29:626–634.
43. Price, H. L., Deutsch, S., Marshall, B. E., Stephen, G. W., Behar, M. G., and Neufeld, G. R. (1966): Hemodynamic and metabolic effects of hemorrhage in man, with particular reference to splanchnic circulation. *Circ. Res.*, 18:469–474.
44. Proppe, D. W. (1980): α-Adrenergic control of intestinal circulation in heat-stressed baboons. *J. Appl. Physiol.: Respir. Environ. Exercise Physiol.*, 48:759–764.
45. Ramsøe, K., Jarnum, S., Preisig, R., Tauber, T., Tygstrup, N., and Westergaard, H. (1970): Liver function and blood flow at high altitude. *J. Appl. Physiol.*, 28:725–727.
46. Reynell, P. C., Marks, P. A., Chidsey, C., and Bradley, S. E. (1955): Changes in splanchnic blood volume and splanchnic blood flow in dogs after haemorrhage. *Clin. Sci.*, 14:407–419.
47. Robinson, B. F., Epstein, S. E., Beiser, G. D., and Braunwald, E. (1966): Control of heart rate by the autonomic baroreceptor mechanisms and exercise. *Circulation Res.*, 19:400–411.
48. Rowell, L. B. (1973): Regulation of splanchnic blood flow in man. *Physiologist*, 16:127–142.
49. Rowell, L. B. (1974): Human cardiovascular adjustments to exercise and thermal stress. *Physiol. Rev.*, 54:75–159.
50. Rowell, L. B. (1974): Measurement of hepatic-splanchnic blood flow in man by dye techniques. In: *Dye Curves: The Theory and Practice of Indicator Dilution*, edited by D. A. Bloomfield, chapt. 12, pp. 209–229. University Park, Baltimore.
51. Rowell, L. B. (1975): The splanchnic circulation. In: *The Peripheral Circulations*, edited by R. Zelis, chapt. 8, pp. 163–192. Grune and Stratton, New York.
52. Rowell, L. B. (1983): Cardiovascular aspects of human thermoregulation. *Circulation Res.*, 52:367–379.
53. Rowell, L. B. (in press). Cardiovascular adjustments to thermal stress. In: *Handbook of Physiology. Peripheral Circulation and Organ Blood Flow*, edited by J. T. Shepherd and F. M. Abboud. American Physiological Society, Bethesda.
54. Rowell, L. B., Detry, J.-M. R., Blackmon, J. R., and Wyss, C. (1972): Importance of the splanchnic vascular bed in human blood pressure regulation. *J. Appl. Physiol.*, 32:213–220.
55. Shepherd, J. T., Blomqvist, C. G., Lind, A. R., Mitchell, J. H., and Saltin, B. (1981): Static (isometric) exercise. Retrospection and introspection. *Circ. Res. (Suppl.)*, 48(1):I179–I188.
56. Simon, E., and Riedel, W. (1975): Diversity of regional sympathetic outflow in integrative cardiovascular control: patterns and mechanisms. *Brain Res.*, 87:323–333.
57. Tyden, G., Samnegård, H., and Thulin, L. (1979): The effects of changes in the carotid sinus baroreceptor activity on splanchnic blood flow in anesthetized man. *Acta Physiol. Scand.*, 106:187–189.
58. Vatner, S. F. (1975): Effects of exercise on distribution of regional blood flows and resistances. In: *The Peripheral Circulations*, edited by R. Zelis, chapt. 10, pp. 211–233. Grune and Stratton, New York.
59. Wade, O. L., and Bishop, J. M. (1962): *Cardiac Output and Regional Blood Flow.* Blackwell, Oxford.
60. Wade, O. L., Combes, B., Childs, A. W., Wheeler, H. O., Cournand, A., and Bradley, S. E. (1956): The effect of exercise on the splanchnic blood flow and splanchnic blood volume in normal man. *Clin. Sci.*, 15:457–463.
61. Wilkins, R. W., Culbertson, J. W., and Ingelfinger, F. J. (1951): The effect of splanchnic sympathectomy in hypertensive patients upon estimated hepatic blood flow in the upright as contrasted with the horizontal position. *J. Clin. Invest.*, 30:312–317.
62. Wilkins, R. W., Culbertson, J. W., and Rymut, A. A. (1952): The hepatic blood flow in resting hypertensive patients before and after splanchnicectomy. *J. Clin. Invest.*, 31:529–531.

Cardiovascular Reflexes of Gastrointestinal Origin

John C. Longhurst

Cardiology Division, Department of Medicine, School of Medicine, University of California, San Diego, La Jolla, California 92093

For over a century scientists have realized that stimulating the abdominal viscera reflexly affects the cardiovascular system and that reflexes from the abdominal visceral region are important in establishing a continuous, correct, and accurately balanced interaction between different parts of the body as well as between the body and its environment (72). The suggestion that stimulation of abdominal visceral organs, for example, distension of the gallbladder or bile duct, could cause cardiovascular reflexes in association with pain can be traced back to Sherrington (83). In fact, Sherrington (18) developed the classification of exteroceptors (cutaneous receptors) and interoceptors (depth receptors located in muscle and visceral regions).

ELECTROPHYSIOLOGICAL STUDIES

Nerve endings or receptors in abdominal visceral organs that are innervated by either vagal or sympathetic (spinal) afferent nerve fibers have been studied with electrophysiological recording techniques (Table 1). The sympathetic nerves constitute the more important afferent pathway for reflex cardiovascular effects.

The ratio of afferent to efferent nerves located within the splanchnic nerve, which contains the largest number of spinal afferent fibers from the abdominal visceral region, is 3:1 (54). In fact, in the cat (63) there are as many sensory fibers in the splanchnic nerves (28,000) as there are in the lower thoracic vagus nerves (28,100). A major difference between populations of afferents located in these two nerves is the ratio of myelinated to unmyelinated axons. The lower thoracic vagus contains mostly unmyelinated axons (99%), whereas the splanchnic nerves contain approximately equal numbers of myelinated and unmyelinated axons, 54% vs. 46% (33,75). Splanchnic afferents lose their investment of myelin in the peripheral portions of the nerves (76). Thus, depending on the location of stimulating and recording electrodes, there may be variations in the calculated conduction velocity for an axon.

The terminal structure of the endings of myelinated spinal afferents innervating abdominal visceral organs is either a Pacinian corpuscle or a free nerve ending (82). Unmyelinated nerve fibers characteristically terminate as free nerve endings. Afferent fibers innervating Pacinian corpuscles constitute approximately 5% of the total number of afferent fibers (33,75). The Pacinian corpuscle senses high-frequency vibration (37,38). Many Pacinian corpuscles are present in the mesentery, but some are located in other visceral organs, such as stomach, small intestine, liver, and pancreas (25,38,58). They frequently are located in close proximity to vessels (37). Thus, they often discharge with a cardiac rhythm that is related to local mechanical deformation of the receptor by the arterial pulse (Fig. 1). It is uncertain if stimulation of Pacinian corpuscles causes cardiovascular reflex adjustments, although this possibility has been suggested (37).

Free nerve endings can be classified into receptors that are mechanically or chemically sensitive and those that are polymodal, that is, sensitive to both forms of stimuli. Afferent fibers that innervate mechanically sensitive receptors may or may not branch and innervate several (up to seven) separate receptive fields

TABLE 1. *Classification of afferent fibers from abdominal viscera*

Fiber type	Cross-sectional diameter (μm)	Conduction velocity (m/sec)	Terminal ending	Effective stimulus
Aβ (myelinated)	6–12	20–84	Pacinian corpuscle	Vibration
Aδ (finely myelinated)	2–6	3–30	Unknown, bare nerve endings	Vibration, pulse pressure, contraction, distension, chemicals, noxious stimuli
C (unmyelinated)	0.3–1.5	0.3–2.5	Unknown, bare nerve endings	Strong mechanical stimuli, chemicals, noxious stimuli

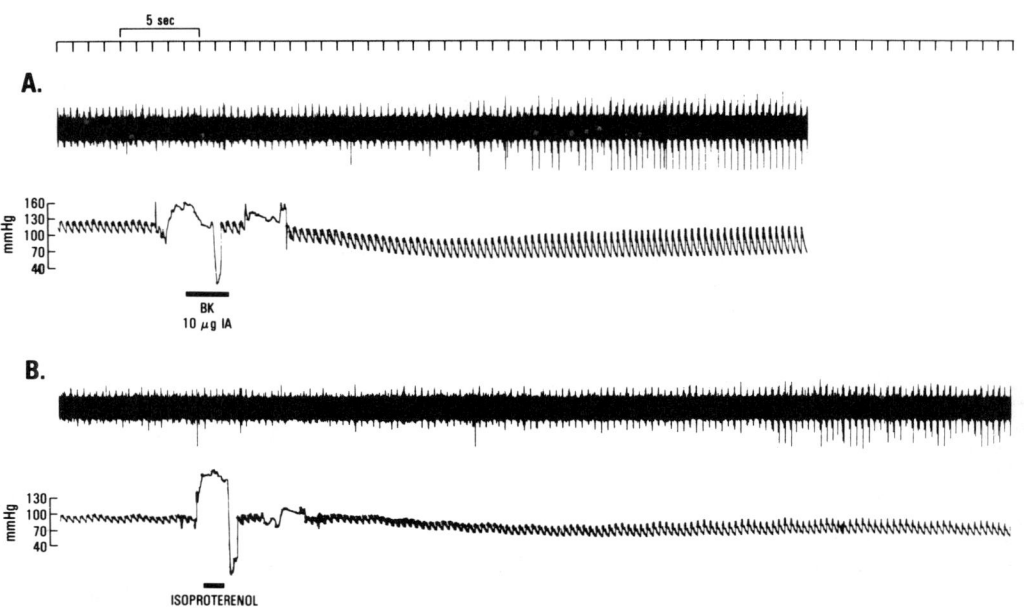

FIG. 1. Response of a group A afferent splanchnic nerve fiber (cv = 46 m/sec) to stimulation by bradykinin and isoproterenol. The fiber was very sensitive but adapted rapidly with an on/off discharge to sustained pressure on its single receptive field located in the serosa of the duodenum. Before stimulation **(A)**, the fiber was silent, but the recording electrode situated near the heart picked up an ECG artifact *(top panel)*. Nineteen seconds after injection of bradykinin into the thoracic aorta and coincident with an increase in pulse pressure, the fiber discharged with a cardiac rhythm. A similar cardiac rhythm of fiber discharge occurred following injection of isoproterenol coincident with the increased pulse pressure **(B)**. Thus the fiber was stimulated by local mechanical compression by the adjacent artery rather than by the chemicals.

(58,63). The endings frequently are found near vessels, particularly at branch points (58,63). However, they also are located deeper in organs. If an ending is located in the bowel or stomach wall, generally it is in the serosa or muscularis layer but not in the muscosa, which is where endings of vagal afferents are located (63,74). Like afferents innervating Pacinian corpuscles, those innervating mechanosensitive receptors frequently discharge with a cardiovascular or a respiratory rhythm (11,74). For the most part, these receptors adapt slowly to a maintained mechanical stimulus. They respond to distension with an initial phasic discharge followed by a slower tonic discharge (11,63,74). However, unlike vagal mechanosensitive receptors, the discharge of splanchnic receptors does not directly correlate with the degree of distension (63). Thus, these receptors do not reliably transduce volume within the gastrointestinal tract. In addition to distension, these receptors respond to contraction of the smooth muscle of the bowel wall (54,63). Because distension is an effective stimulus of abdominal visceral cardiovascular reflexes, sensory fibers innervating slowly adapting mechanoreceptors probably form part of the afferent limb of these reflexes.

The existence of spinal afferent fibers that innervate chemosensitive receptors is not accepted by all investigators (54,63). Thus, some have suggested that chemicals such as bradykinin primarily stimulate slowly adapting mechanoreceptors (31,32,63). However, other studies have been able to locate chemosensitive refjceptors in abdominal organs (58,81). For instance, bradykinin stimulates mechanically sensitive receptors in the pancreas (58). Because the pancreas does not contain smooth muscle, bradykinin probably stimulates a polymodal receptor that responds both to chemical and to external mechanical stimuli. That other chemical substances stimulate chemosensitive receptors in abdominal visceral organs is quite likely because a number of substances are capable of eliciting reflex cardiovascular adjustments when they are applied or injected into visceral organs.

REFLEX STUDIES

Stimulation of mechanosensitive and chemosensitive receptors in the abdominal visceral organs reflexly affects the cardiovascular, respiratory, somatic, and even other abdominal visceral organs. This review is limited to discussion of reflex effects on the cardiovascular system.

Reflexes from Mechanosensitive Receptors

Altering perfusion pressure in splanchnic arteries and veins causes reflex cardiovascular adjustments. Thus, increasing the perfusion pressure in mesenteric veins either increases or decreases blood pressure (18). Afferent unit recordings have demonstrated that the threshold pressure required for stimulation is 5 to 10 mm Hg (65). Associated with stimulation of mesenteric and portal venous afferents is a strong discharge of intestinal and hepatic efferent nerve fibers (3). Slowly adapting mechanoreceptors probably are responsible for these effects (3).

Lowering the perfusion pressure in mesenteric, gastric, and splanchnic arteries also increases blood pressure. Some investigators believe that this response is a direct hemodynamic effect caused by a passive shift of blood out of low resistance and into high resistance vascular circuits (45,80,87). However, other investigators have shown a reflex component to the pressor response (18,84,85). This so-called splanchnic baroreceptor reflex is weak in dogs but is more prominent in cats.

Much information is currently available regarding reflex cardiovascular effects caused by traction on the mesentery or distension of hollow organs such as the stomach, intestines, gallbladder, or biliary tract. For instance, gentle movement of the intestine stretches the mesentery and in some animals, particularly cats, this maneuver reflexly increases blood pressure, heart rate, and myocardial contractility (Fig. 2). It is likely that these responses are caused by stimulation of slowly adapting stretch receptors located throughout the mesentery and innervated by spinal afferent nerve fibers.

Several older studies demonstrated that pinching or distending the stomach of dogs increases blood pressure (18,61). Recently, investigators have noted both pressor and depressor responses (18). These studies indicate that passive distension of the stomach of cats causes an increase in blood pressure, heart rate, and left ventricular contractility (57,60). The response begins at a pressure of 11 mm Hg across the wall of the stomach. This pressure corresponds to a volume of 35 ml (Fig. 3). As pressure and volume in the stomach are increased, the reflex blood pressure response increases. Because cardiac output is unchanged during distension, calculated systemic vascular resistance is increased. Studies that have used radioactive microspheres

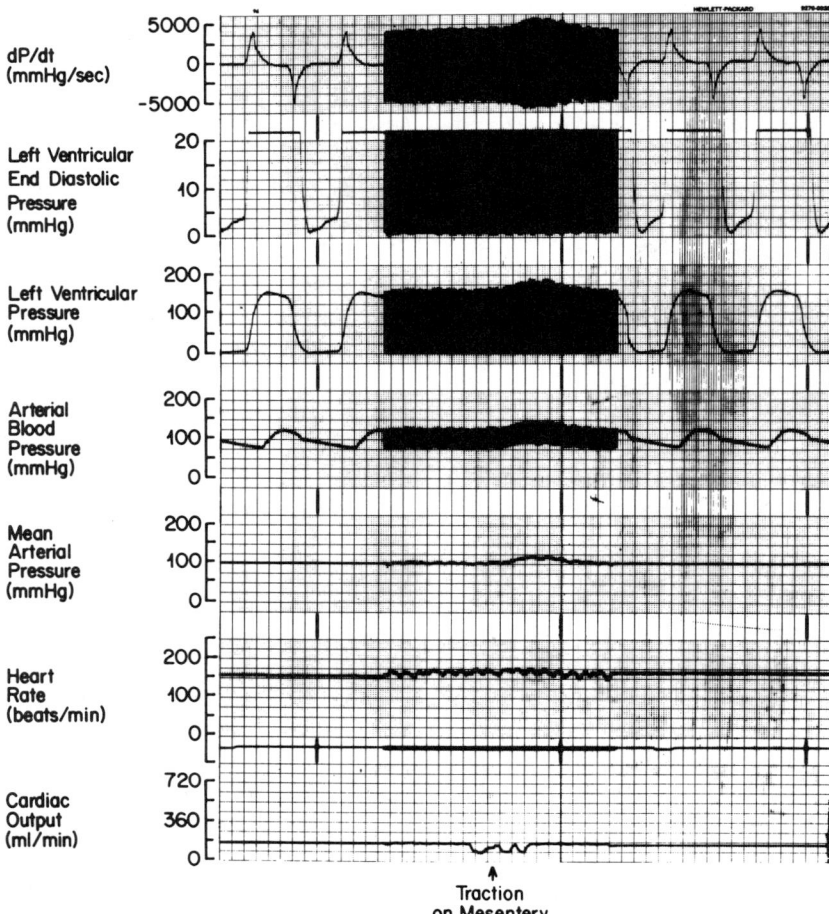

FIG. 2. Response of the cardiovascular system to traction placed on the cat's mesentery by gently lifting up and shifting the position of a loop of the bowel by a few centimeters. A similar response could not be evoked by placing a similar amount of pressure on the bowel wall without shifting its position. The rate of left ventricular pressure development, an index of cardiac contractility, is denoted as dP/dt.

and constant flow perfusion of vascularly isolated regional circulations have demonstrated vasoconstriction in mesenteric, renal, and skeletal muscle circulations (48,56).

With regard to efferent mechanisms, stimulation of β-adrenergic receptors causes the tachycardia and inotropic responses, and α-adrenergic receptors mediate the systemic and regional vasoconstriction during distension of the stomach (57). In addition, the adrenal medulla plays an important role in heart rate and contractility responses. Thus, distension of the cat's stomach causes a generalized sympathoadrenal activation of the cardiovascular system.

The reflex nature of the cardiovascular response to distension of the stomach has been demonstrated by transecting the afferent neural pathways (60). Although the vagi are not important afferent pathways, transecting the greater splanchnic nerves abolishes these reflexes. The only exception to these findings occurs in rats. When their stomachs are distended, the cardiovascular responses are transmitted solely by afferents contained within the vagus nerves (42).

Distension of other areas including the esophagus, small intestine, colon, and rectum either increases or decreases blood pressure (18,73). Although many studies have shown an increase

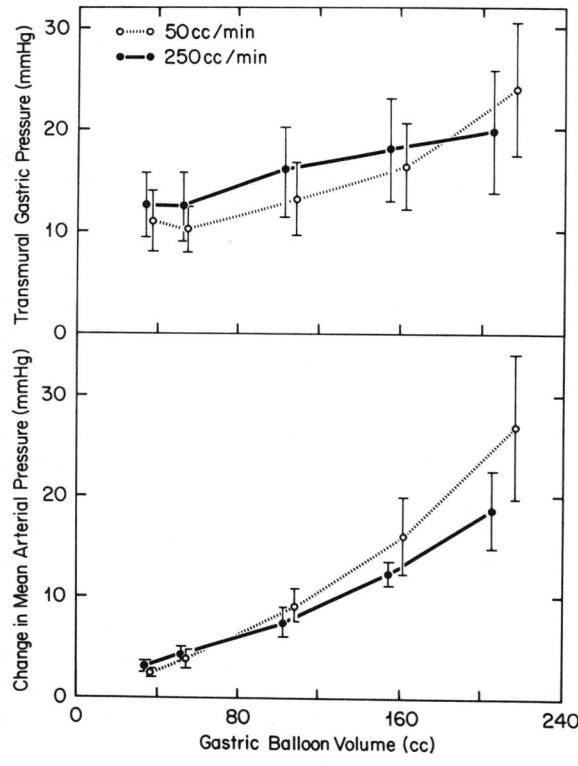

FIG. 3. Relation between balloon volume and transmural pressure in the stomachs of 8 cats *(top panel). (Dots)* Mean values; *(vertical brackets)* the standard errors. Relation between balloon volume in the cats' stomachs and change in mean arterial pressure in the same animals *(bottom panel).* During both rapid and slow rates of distension the threshold of initial cardiovascular response occurred at similar gastric pressures (11–13 mm Hg). The blood pressure responses were progressive and similar increases occurred with both rates of distension beyond threshold. (From Longhurst et al., ref. 60, with permission).

in heart rate, a baroreceptor-induced bradycardia will occur if there is a large pressor response to passive distension. In this regard, most studies have used anesthetized animals, a situation that frequently leads to significant parasympatholysis and high heart rates. Therefore, mechanical stimulation of abdominal visceral organs in anesthetized animals produces only a small increase in heart rate, an effect that is mediated largely by neurohumoral stimulation of adrenergic receptors in the heart. In unanesthetized animals and in humans, withdrawal of parasympathetic tone probably plays a more important role in the chronotropic response to distension of the stomach.

Stimulating splanchnic mechanosensitive receptors by squeezing or pinching the intestine or by putting traction on the mesentery reflexly elicits increases in blood pressure that are smaller in spinal than in intact animals (26,27). In decerebrate preparations there is an exaggerated response (26). Thus, abdominal visceral cardiovascular responses are mediated, in part, by spinal reflexes. In addition, supratentorial or higher cerebral centers inhibit the full manifestation of abdominal visceral cardiovascular reflexes.

Stimulating mechanosensitive abdominal visceral receptors reduces coronary blood flow (18, 47). However, it is not certain whether myocardial oxygen demands and coronary perfusion pressures were increased or decreased in these studies. In addition, recent results suggest that distension of the cat's stomach does not alter coronary vascular resistance (56). Because myocardial oxygen demands were increased, the coronary vessels would be expected to vasodilate in this situation. A lack of vasodilation could result from competition between metabolic vasodilation and neurogenic vasoconstriction (7).

Early studies suggested that manipulation of the gallbladder and biliary tract reflexly activated the cardiovascular system (18,64,83). However, recent studies suggested that compared to distension of the stomach, distension of the gallbladder is a less effective stimulus of reflex cardiovascular responses (60,69).

Reflexes from Chemosensitive Receptors

Studies of cardiovascular responses to stimulation of abdominal visceral chemosensitive receptors have used both foreign or exogenous chemical stimuli and endogenous substances. Foreign chemical agents include capsaicin, nicotine, lobeline, potassium carbonate, cyanide, carbachol, eserine, methacholine, pilocarpine, mustard, hypertonic sodium iodide, mercuric chloride, sodium nitrate, and phenyldiguanide. Endogenous substances include bradykinin, acetylcholine, 5-hydroxytryptamine, histamine; as well as acidic, alkaline, peptone, hypertonic, and hypotonic solutions; and hypoxia, hypercapnea, epinephrine, prostaglandins, potassium chloride, calcium chloride, cysteine, glutamic acid, and tryptophan.

It is useful to study the cardiovascular responses to stimulation by foreign chemical substances for two reasons. First, they demonstrate that abdominal visceral organs can potentially affect the cardiovascular system through a reflex mechanism. Second, some substances stimulate a certain class of receptors or afferent fiber types.

When injected into mesenteric arteries or directly into the small intestine or stomach, *nicotine* usually increases blood pressure, heart rate, myocardial contractility, and respiration (14,18,34,79). *Cyanide*, like nicotine, causes reflex activation of the cardiovascular system when it is injected into vessels supplying abdominal visceral organs (18,79). Nicotine and cyanide demonstrate that many abdominal visceral organs are capable of eliciting profound cardiovascular responses.

Capsaicin, an extract of paprika, in very small concentrations causes pain. It is particularly useful because it stimulates endings of abdominal visceral C fiber splanchnic nerve afferents much more frequently than it stimulates endings of A fiber afferents (58). Therefore, capsaicin allows one to determine if a particular organ is reflexogenic, particularly in regard to C fiber afferents. When it is applied to the serosal surface or injected into vessels supplying the stomach, intestine, gallbladder, or pancreas, cardiovascular reflexes are manifested by increases in blood pressure, heart rate, myocardial contractility, and systemic vascular resistance (9,10,55,68,69). However, capsaicin does not cause a reflex pressor response from all abdominal visceral organs. When it is injected into the liver, for instance, a depressor cardiovascular response that is transmitted by spinal afferents frequently occurs (6). This observation is interesting because, as noted previously, stimulation of spinal afferent pathways from visceral organs generally causes reflex excitation of the cardiovascular system.

Bradykinin, a naturally occurring peptide, stimulates receptors in the stomach, gallbladder, pancreas, small intestine, spleen, and urinary bladder to cause reflex activation of the cardiovascular system (18,28,43,59,68,69). For most organs, except the liver (5), the pattern of cardiovascular response is similar to that caused by capsaicin (Fig. 4). However, the latency of cardiovascular response is much longer for bradykinin (13–20 sec) than for capsaicin (3–7 sec). This may be due to formation of prostaglandin intermediates that act in concert with bradykinin to stimulate sensory endings in visceral organs (28). Part of the bradykinin-induced reflex excitation of the cardiovascular system is caused by stimulation of the adrenal medulla (24).

Bradykinin and kallikrein, the enzyme that catalyzes the formation of bradykinin, are found diffusely throughout the gastrointestinal tract, in the pancreas, and in bile (2,46). Because the threshold concentration of bradykinin necessary to produce a cardiovascular response is in the nanogram and picogram range (Fig. 5) (59,69), this peptide may cause reflex cardiovascular responses in certain physiological or pathophysiological conditions.

Acetylcholine stimulates abdominal visceral organs such as the stomach, intestine, liver, and spleen, thus evoking reflex cardiovascular responses (4,17,18,29,34,43,51,78). Acetylcholine generally excites the cardiovascular and

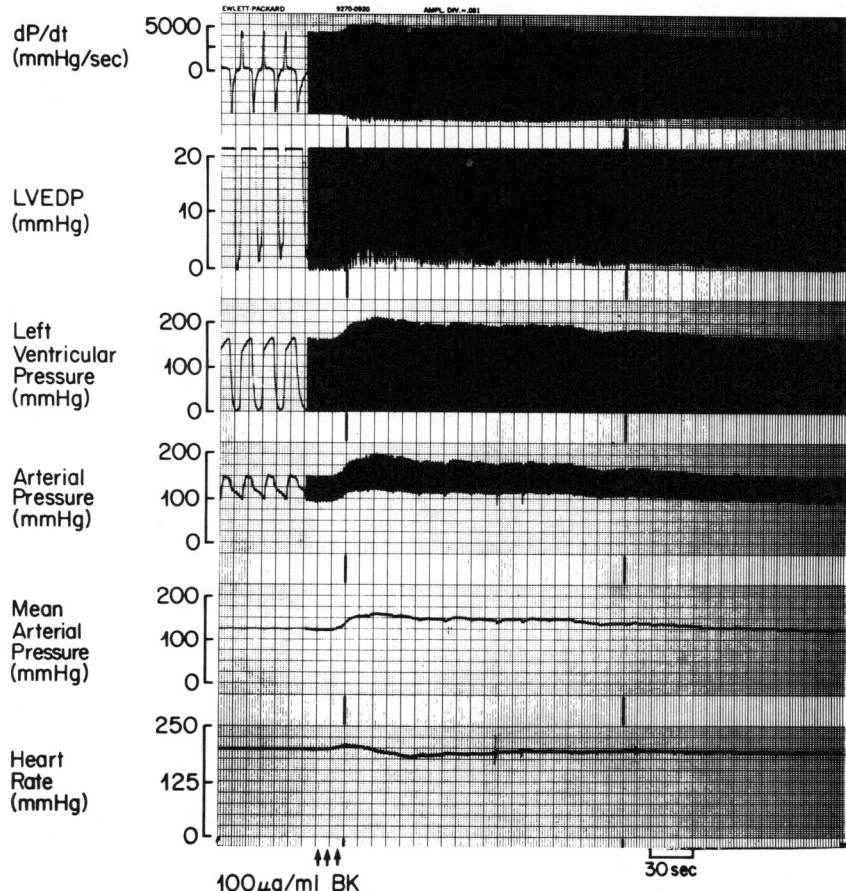

FIG. 4. Cardiovascular responses evoked by application of bradykinin (100 μg/ml, total dose = 5 μg) to the gallbladder of a cat. Note that approximately 13 sec after the initial application of bradykinin that dP/dt, left ventricular systolic pressure, arterial systolic, diastolic and mean pressures, and heart rate increased. The total duration of the response was 5.4 min. (From Ordway and Longhurst, ref. 69, with permission.)

respiratory systems through stimulation of spinal afferents with muscarinic receptors (14,17,34). It stimulates mechanosensitive and chemosensitive receptors. Because there is no relationship between the degree of contraction of visceral smooth muscle and the cardiovascular response and because preventing contraction does not alter the cardiovascular response, the reflex effects of acetylcholine probably are caused by stimulation of chemosensitive or polymodal receptors in abdominal visceral organs (17,18). The concentration of acetylcholine required to provoke cardiovascular reflexes far exceeds the local concentrations of acetylcholine that occur naturally. Therefore, acetylcholine probably does not play an important role in initiating reflex responses from abdominal visceral organs.

Several other naturally occurring chemical substances or solutions cause abdominal visceral cardiovascular reflexes. These include hypercapnea (14,18), venous blood (79), hypertonic solutions (18), peptone solutions (14), lactic or hydrochloric acid (18,43,53), histamine (9,43), potassium (8,10,45,52), tryptophan (51), as well as solutions that, relative to body temperature, are either hot or cold (18). Despite the fact that blood pressure is increased reflexly, large or pharmacological concentrations of these sub-

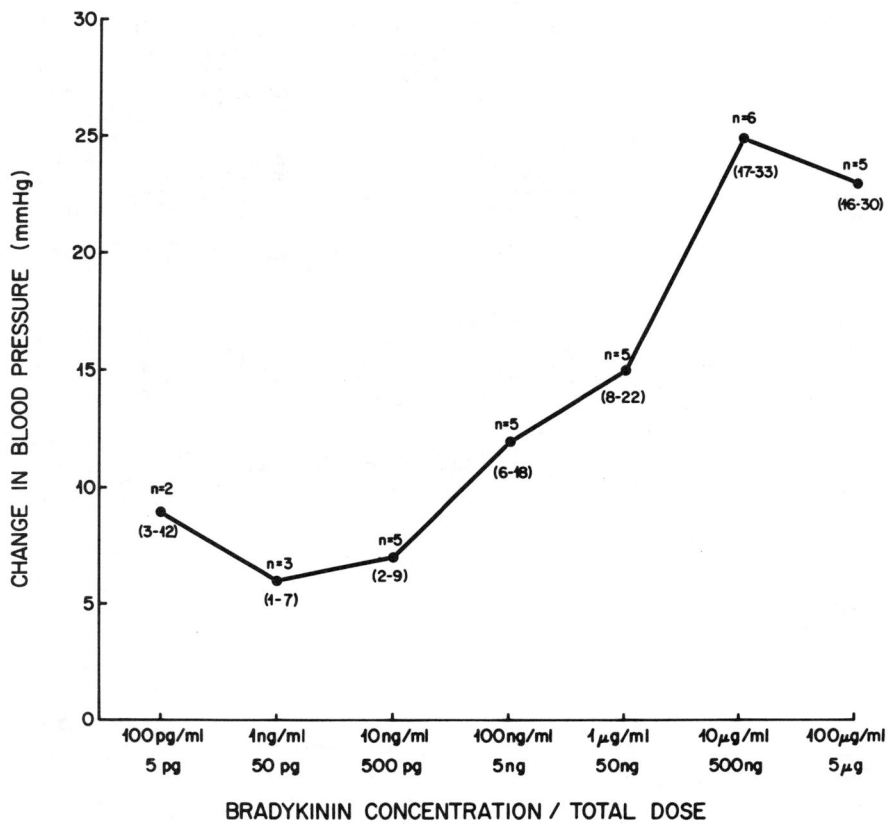

FIG. 5. Relationship between average change in mean arterial pressure and increasing concentrations (or total dose) of bradykinin applied to the serosal surface of the gallbladder of six cats. The number of cats (n) studied at each concentration is indicated as is the range of changes in blood pressure (numbers in parentheses). Note that a cardiovascular response can be detected with concentrations as low as 100 pg/ml, that it increases sharply between 10 ng/ml and 10 µg/ml, and that it does not further increase above 10 µg/ml. (From Ordway and Longhurst, ref. 69, with permission.)

stances usually must be used (45). Substances such as 5-hydroxytryptamine may stimulate visceral receptors by causing contraction of the intestine rather than by a direct chemical effect. Some substances, such as potassium, can directly depolarize afferent nerves so that they may exert their effects in a nonspecific manner. Finally, several studies have not clearly demonstrated that the cardiovascular responses are reflex in nature and have not localized the responses to organs in the abdominal visceral region. Thus, the importance of many naturally occurring substances in stimulating abdominal visceral cardiovascular reflexes in physiological or pathophysiological conditions presently is not known.

SIGNIFICANCE OF ABDOMINAL VISCERAL CARDIOVASCULAR REFLEXES

Normal Conditions

Vagal and sympathetic afferents from abdominal visceral organs may normally serve different functions. Vagal afferents exert important reflex control over the gastrointestinal system (54). Thus, these afferents are concerned with control of digestion and with sending hunger and satiety signals to the central nervous system. In most species, other than the rat, vagal afferents from abdominal visceral organs have little to do with reflex control of the cardiovascular system. Conversely, sympathetic or spinal afferents likely play an important role in the control of cardiovascular function, both in normal and in certain pathological situations. With regard to normal conditions, afferents from the intestine may tonically activate the cardiovascular system (18). Overall, however, the importance of abdominal visceral afferents in the reflex control of cardiovascular function under normal situations still remains to be identified. In fact, some investigators have suggested that only small changes in cardiovascular function are caused by stimulation of gastrointestinal organs in healthy subjects (18). On the other hand, gastric endoscopy causes changes in heart rate and blood pressure, effects that can be abolished with atropine or propranolol (36,71). Such responses could be caused by an anxiety reaction or, alternatively, by reflexes originating in the stomach or esophagus. Another observation is that hunger contractions can be associated with an increased heart rate and vasodilation of vessels in the forearms of some patients (15). The ingestion of food also can be associated with transient increases in heart rate, blood pressure, and cardiac output in animals and man (1,23, 35,41,86). Finally, distension of the duodenum in man to volumes that do not produce pain causes vasoconstriction in the extremities (16). Such reports not not prove cardiovascular reflexes of gastrointestinal origin but certainly are compatible with their existence.

Pathological Conditions

Substantial evidence indicates that stimulation of abdominal visceral organs causes reflex cardiovascular responses in pathological conditions. Also, it is well accepted that abdominal visceral spinal afferents transmit the sensation of pain; stimulation of these nerves with the algesic agents, capsaicin and bradykinin, elicits profound cardiovascular alterations. Bradykinin is produced in certain inflammatory conditions (67,77). Such situations frequently are associated with activation of the cardiovascular system. Thus, acute pancreatitis, peptic ulcer disease, and acute cholecystitis are some of the more common conditions associated with activation of the cardiovascular system and with electrocardiographic abnormalities (12,13,19,20, 22,44,62,69,88). Although the association of abdominal visceral pain and cardiovascular changes is well recognized, it is less clear whether or not pain is necessary to produce the cardiovascular responses. A variety of algesic agents that stimulate abdominal visceral afferents in man have been studied (50,51). Threshold concentrations that produce a nociceptive reflex response have been determined, but subthreshold concentrations of these substances can cause reflex cardiovascular effects (Table 2). Cardiovascular responses to subalgesic concentrations of these chemicals are weaker than those associated with algesic concentrations (51). However, it appears that pain is not a necessary factor in the production of cardiovascular responses during chemical stimulation of abdominal visceral organs. In addition, some chemicals such as methacholine, pilocarpine, and histamine are not associated with pain, yet they elicit reflex cardiovascular responses. Thus, specific cardiovascular reflexes of gastrointestinal origin occur in the absence of pain.

A commonly observed clinical condition is postprandial angina pectoris. Several possible mechanisms including reflex effects from the gastrointestinal tract could produce this syndrome. Animals or patients with heart disease and particularly those with both heart and gastrointestinal abnormalities develop cardiovascular alterations in response to stimulation of the gastrointestinal tract (18,70). If reflexes from abdominal visceral organs are etiologically important in postprandial angina, they could exert their effects by two mechanisms. The first is a supply-demand imbalance in which reflex excitation of the cardiovascular system causes myocardial oxygen demand to exceed supply at

TABLE 2. *Thresholds of cardiovascular pressor and nociceptive reflexes from stomach and small intestine of cats as compared with cutaneous pain thresholds in man*

Substance	Threshold concentrations		
	Cardiovascular pressor reflex in cats (ng/ml)	Nociceptive reflex in cats (μg/ml)	Nociceptive reflex in humans[a] (μg/ml)
Acetylcholine	1–10	10–50	10–50
Methacholine	1–10	None up to 1000	None up to 1000
Pilocarpine	1–10	None up to 1000	None up to 1000
Carbachol	1–10	500	250–750
Nicotine	50–500	5–10	100–500
5-hydroxytryptamine	0.1	1–100	0.1–1
Bradykinin	1	0.5	0.1–1
Histamine	1–10	10–1000	10–1000
Capsaicin	0.001	0.01–0.1	0.4[b]
		mEq/L	
Potassium chloride	2–4	30–40	15–30
Ammonium chloride	<15	125–150	150[c]
Sodium chloride	185	350–400	300[c]

[a]Application to blister base (Keele and Armstrong, 1964).
[b]Application to conjunctiva (Heubner, 1925).
[c]Intradermal injection (Lindahl, 1961).
Modified from Khayutin et al. (1976).

rest and possibly even more so during exercise (23,30,40,49). The second mechanism is reflex coronary vasoconstriction that would cause a primary reduction in coronary blood flow (39). Stimulation of abdominal visceral organs has been claimed to be a cause of coronary vasoconstriction (22). However, reflex coronary vasoconstriction and even reflex activation of the cardiovascular system have not been proven unequivocally to be important causative events in postprandial angina.

Other conditions that may be associated with reflex activation of the cardiovascular system through stimulation of abdominal visceral afferent nerves are the carcinoid and dumping syndromes. In both conditions, large amounts of bradykinin are produced in the gastrointestinal system (21,66,89). The concentrations of bradykinin produced are greater than the threshold concentrations necessary to produce cardiovascular reflexes. Thus, it is possible that reflex cardiovascular excitation, particularly an increase in blood pressure, is caused by stimulation of abdominal visceral afferents. This vasoconstrictor response may offset the direct relaxation of vascular smooth muscle caused by bradykinin in these syndromes.

CONCLUSIONS

Stimulation of chemosensitive or mechanosensitive nerve endings in any of several abdominal visceral organs causes strong reflex cardiovascular effects. The response frequently, but not always, consists of cardiovascular excitation manifested by increases in heart rate, blood pressure, myocardial contractility, and systemic vascular resistance. The major afferent pathways are in the splanchnic nerves that ascend through the spinal cord. The major efferent pathways consist of the sympathetic nerves and the adrenal medulla. Although these reflex effects are well documented, the specific physiological, mechanical, and chemical stimuli that initiate them are not as clearly understood.

ACKNOWLEDGMENT

Ms. Gabriele Drumm and Ms. Lynne Keith are to be thanked for their secretarial assistance. Work cited in this chapter was partially supported by AHA grants #80-784 and #83-758, NHLBI HL 30222, and NINCDS NS 30165.

REFERENCES

1. Abramson, D. I., and Fierst, S. M. (1941): Peripheral vascular responses in man during digestion. *Am. J. Physiol.*, 133:686–693.
2. Amundsen, E., and Nustad, K. (1965): Kinin forming and destroying activities of cell homogenates. *J. Physiol. (Lond.)*, 179:479–488.
3. Andrews, C. J. H., Andrews, W. H. H., and Orbach, J. (1972): A sympathetic reflex elicited by distension of the mesenteric venous bed. *J. Physiol. (Lond.)*, 226:119–131.
4. Andrews, W. H. H., and Palmer, J. F. (1976): Afferent nervous discharge from the canine liver. *Q. J. Exp. Physiol.*, 62:269–276.
5. Ashton, J. H., Iwamoto, G. A., Longhurst, J. C., and Mitchell, J. H. (1980): Cardiovascular changes during bradykinin injection into the liver of the dog. *Physiologist*, 23:43. (Abstract)
6. Ashton, J. H., Iwamoto, G. A., Longhurst, J. C., and Mitchell, J. H. (1982): Reflex cardiovascular depression induced by capsaicin injection into canine liver. *Am. J. Physiol.*, 242:H955–H960.
7. Aung-Din, R., Mitchell, J. H., and Longhurst, J. C. (1981): Reflex α-adrenergic coronary vasoconstriction during hindlimb static exercise in dogs. *Circ. Res.*, 48:502–509.
8. Baraz, L. A. (1961): On the sensitivity of small intestine receptors to K ions. *Dokl. Acad. Nauk. SSSR Otd. Biol.*, 140:1213–1216.
9. Baraz, L. A., and Khayutin, V. M. (1965): Serotonin and histamine as excitors of self-regulatory and nociceptive vasomotor reflexes. In: *Physiology and Pathology of the Cardiovascular System*, pp. 82–85. Institute of the Normal and Path. Physiol. Acad. Med. USSR, Moscow.
10. Baraz, L. A., Khayutin, V. M., and Molnar, J. (1968): Analysis of the stimulatory action of capsaicin on receptors and sensory fibers of the small intestine in the cat. *Acta Physiol. Acad. Sci. Hung.*, 33:225–235.
11. Bessou, P., and Perl, E. R. (1966): A movement receptor of the small intestine. *J. Physiol. (Lond.)*, 182:404–426.
12. Bettman, R. B., and Rubinfeld, S. H. (1935): Gallbladder-heart reflexes in man under spinal anesthesia. *Am. Heart J.*, 10:550–552.
13. Buch, J., Buch, A., and Schmidt, A. (1980): Transient EKG changes during acute pancreatitis. *Acta Cardiol.*, 35:381–390.
14. Bykov, K. M., and Chernigovskiy, V. N. (1947): Interoceptors of the stomach. *J. Physiol. USSR*, 33:3–15.
15. Carlson, A. J. (1912): Contributions to the physiology of the stomach. IV. The influence of the contractions of the empty stomach in man on the vasomotor center, on the rate of the heart beat, and on the reflex excitability of the spinal cord. *Am. J. Physiol.*, 31:318–326.
16. Carmichael, E. A., Doupe, J., Harper, A. A., and McSwiney, B. A. (1939): Vasomotor reflexes in man following distension. *J. Physiol. (Lond.)*, 95:276–281.
17. Chernigovskiy, V. N. (1940): Investigation of the receptors of some of the internal organs. Report III. Effect of acetylcholine, nicotine, histamine, and KCL on the receptors of the spleen. *Physiol. J. USSR*, 29:526–535.
18. Chernigovskiy, V. N. (1960): In: *Interoceptors*, edited by D. B. Lindsley. American Psychological Association, Washington, D.C.
19. Clark, W. E. (1945): Gastrointestinal conditions stimulating or aggravating cardiovascular disease. *J. Am. Med. Assoc.*, 128:352–356.
20. Cohen, M. H., Rolsztain, A., Bowen, P. J., and Shugoll, G. I. (1971): Electrocardiographic changes in acute pancreatitis resembling acute myocardial infarction. *Am. Heart J.*, 82:672–677.
21. Colman, R. W., and Wong, P. Y. (1980): Kallikrein-kinin system in pathologic conditions. *Pharmacol. Rev.*, 32:569–607.
22. Cullen, M. L., and Reese, H. L. (1952): Myocardial circulatory changes measured by clearance of Na^{24}: Effect of common duct distension on myocardial circulation. *J. Appl. Physiol.*, 5:281–284.
23. Degenais, G. R., Oriol, A., and McGregor, M. (1966): Hemodynamic effects of carbohydrate and protein meals in man: Rest and exercise. *J. Appl. Physiol.*, 21:1157–1162.
24. DellaBella, D., Benelli, G., and DePooli, A. M. (1972): Indirect nervous mechanism in some effects of bradykinin. *Arch. Int. Pharmacodyn.*, 196:50–63.
25. Downman, C. B. B., and Evans, M. H. (1957): The distribution of splanchnic afferents in the spinal cord of the cat. *J. Physiol. (Lond.)*, 137:66–79.
26. Downman, C. B. B., and McSwiney, B. A. (1946): Reflexes elicited by visceral stimulation in the acute spinal animal. *J. Physiol. (Lond.)*, 105:80–94.
27. Downman, C. B. B., McSwiney, B. A., and Voss, C. C. N. (1948): Sensitivity of the small intestine. *J. Physiol. (Lond.)*, 107:97–106.
28. Ferreira, S. H., Moncada, S., and Vane, J. R. (1973): Prostaglandins and the mechanism of analgesia produced by aspirin like drugs. *Br. J. Pharmacol.*, 49:86–97.
29. Ferry, C. B. (1963): The sympathomimetic effect of acetylcholine on the spleen of the cat. *J. Physiol. (Lond.)*, 167:487–504.
30. Figueras, J., Singh, B. N., Ganz, W., and Swan, H. J. C. (1979): Hemodynamic and electrocardiographic accompaniments of resting postprandial angina. *Br. Heart J.*, 42:402–409.
31. Floyd, K., Hick, V. E., Koley, J., and Morrison, J. F. B. (1977): Effects of bradykinin mediated by autonomic efferent nerves. *Q. J. Exp. Physiol.*, 62:11–17.
32. Floyd, K., Hick, V. E., Koley, J., and Morrison, J. F. B. (1977): The effects of bradykinin on afferent units in intra-abdominal sympathetic nerve trunks. *Q. J. Exp. Physiol.*, 62:19–25.
33. Foley, J. O. (1948): The functional types of nerve fibers and their numbers in the great splanchnic nerve. *Anat. Rec.*, 100:766–777.
34. Frank, M. H. (1975): Cardiovascular chemoreflexes from the perfused innervated ileum of the cat. *Am. J. Physiol.*, 228:944–953.

35. Fronek, K., and Stahlgren, L. H. (1968): Systemic and regional hemodynamic changes during food intake and digestion in nonanesthetized dogs. *Circ. Res.*, 23:687–692.
36. Fujita, R., and Kumura, F. (1975): Arrhythmias and ischemic changes of the heart induced by gastric endoscopic procedures. *Am. J. Gastroenterol.*, 64:45–48.
37. Gammon, G. D., and Bronk, D. M. (1935): The discharge of impulses from Pacinian corpuscles in the mesentery and its relation to vascular changes. *Am. J. Physiol.*, 114:77–84.
38. Gernandt, B., and Zotterman, Y. (1946): Intestinal pain: An electrophysiological investigation on mesenteric nerves. *Acta Physiol. Scand.*, 12:56–72.
39. Gilbert, N. C., Fenn, G. K., and LeRoy, G. V. (1940): The effect of distension of abdominal visceral on the coronary blood flow and on angina pectoris. *J. Am. Med. Assoc.*, 115:1962–1967.
40. Goldstein, R. E., Redwood, D. R., Rosing, D. R., Beiser, G. D., and Epstein, S. E. (1971): Alterations in the circulatory response in exercise following a meal and their relationship to postprandial angina pectoris. *Circulation*, 44:90–100.
41. Grollman, A. (1929): Physiological variations in the cardiac output of man. III. The effect of the ingestion of food on the cardiac output, pulse rate, blood pressure and oxygen consumption of man. *Am. J. Physiol.*, 89:366–370.
42. Grundy, D., and Davison, J. S. (1981): Cardiovascular changes elicited by vagal gastric afferents in the rat. *Q. J. Exp. Physiol.*, 66:307–310.
43. Guzman, F., Braun, C., and Lim, R. K. S. (1962): Visceral pain and the pseudoaffective response to intra arterial injection of bradykinin and other algesic agents. *Arch. Int. Pharm.*, 136:353–384.
44. Hampton, A. G., Beckwith, J. R., and Wood, E. J., Jr. (1959): The relationship between heart disease and gallbladder disease. *Ann. Intern. Med.*, 50:1135–1148.
45. Heymans, C., Dmitrenko, A. M., Schaepdryver, A. F. De, and Vleeschhouwer, G. R. De (1960): Abdominal baro- and chemosensitivity in dogs. *Circ. Res.*, 8:347–352.
46. Hilton, S. M., and Jones, M. (1968): The role of plasma kinin in functional vasodilation in the pancreas. *J. Physiol. (Lond.)*, 195:521–533.
47. Hinrichsen, I., and Ivy, A. C. (1933): Effect of stimulation of visceral nerves on coronary flow in dogs. *Arch. Intern. Med.*, 51:932–937.
48. Johansson, B., and Langston, J. B. (1964): Reflex influence of mesenteric afferents on renal, intestinal and muscle blood flow and on intestinal motility. *Acta Physiol. Scand.*, 6:400–412.
49. Jones, W. B., Thomas, H. D., and Reeves, T. J. (1965): Circulatory and ventrilatory responses to postprandial exercise. *Am. Heart J.*, 69:668–676.
50. Keele, C. A., and Armstrong, D. (1964): In: *Substances Producing Pain and Itch*. Arnold, London.
51. Khayutin, V. M., Baraz, L. A., Lukoshkova, E. V., Sonina, R. S., and Chernilovskoya, P. E. (1976): Chemosensitive spinal afferents: Threshold of specific and nociceptive reflexes as compared with thresholds of excitation for receptors and axons. *Prog. Brain Res.*, 43:293–306.
52. Khayutin, V. M., Mitsanyi, A., Sonina, R. S., and Erdelyi, A. (1969): Reflex responses of the vascular system and renal sympathetic efferents induced by potassium ions injected into the superior mesenteric artery and the effect of tonic baroreceptor inflow thereon. *Arch. Int. Physiol. Biochem.*, 77:829–854.
53. Lebedeva, V. A., and Chernigovskiy, V. N. (1951): Investigation into the mechanisms of chemoreception. Report II. Effect of acid and alkali compounds on the chemoreceptors of the intestine. *Bull. Exp. Biol. Med.*, 31:153–158.
54. Leek, B. F. (1977): Abdominal and pelvic visceral receptors. *Br. Med. Bull.*, 33:163–168.
55. Longhurst, J. C., Aston, J. H., and Iwamoto, G. A. (1980): Cardiovascular reflexes resulting from capsaicin stimulated gastric receptors in anesthetized cats. *Circ. Res.*, 46:780–788.
56. Longhurst, J. C., and Ibarra, J. (1984): Reflex regional vascular responses during passive gastric distension in cats. *Am. J. Physiol.*, 247, in press.
57. Longhurst, J. C., and Ibarra, J. (1982): Sympathoadrenal mechanisms in hemodynamic responses to gastric distension in cats. *Am. J. Physiol.*, 243:H748–H753.
58. Longhurst, J. C., Kaufman, M. P., Ordway, G. A., and Musch, T. I. (1984): Effects of capsaicin and bradykinin on endings of afferent fibers from visceral organs in cats. *Am. J. Physiol.*, in press.
59. Ordway, G. A., Longhurst, J. C., and Mitchell, J. H. (1984): Stimulation of noncreatic afferents reflexly activates the cardiovascular system in cats. *Am. J. Physiol.*, 245:R820–R826.
60. Longhurst, J. C., Spilker, H. L., and Ordway, G. A. (1981): Cardiovascular reflexes elicited by passive gastric distension in anesthetized cats. *Am. J. Physiol.*, 240:H539–H545.
61. Mayer, S., and Pribram, A. (1872): Studien zur Physiologie des Herzens und der Blutgefässe II. Abt. Über refektiorische Beziehungen des Magens zu den Innervationscentren für die Kreislauforgane. *Sitzungesber. Mathem-Naturwiss Akad der Wiss*, 66 (III):102–115. Abt. S.
62. McLemore, G. A., and Levine, S. A. (1955): The possible therapeutic value of cholecystectomy in Adams-Stokes disease. *Am. J. Med. Sci.*, 229:386–391.
63. Morrison, J. F. B. (1977): The afferent innervation of the gastrointestinal tract. In: *Nerves and the Gut*, edited by P. W. Evers, pp. 297–326. Charles B. Slack, Inc., New Jersey.
64. Newman, P. P. (1974): In: *Visceral Afferent Functions of the Nervous System*, pp. 35–37. Edward Arnold, London.
65. Niijima, A. (1977): Afferent discharges from venous pressoceptors in liver. *Am. J. Physiol.*, 232:C76–C81.
66. Oates, J. A., Pettinger, W. A., and Doctor, R. B. (1966): Evidence for the release of bradykinin in carcinoid syndrome. *J. Clin. Invest.*, 45:173–178.
67. Ofstad, E. (1970): Formation and destruction of plasma kinins during experimental hemorrhagic pancreatitis in dogs. *Scand. J. Gastroenterol. (Suppl.)*, 5:1–44.
68. Ordway, G. A., Mitchell, J. H., and Longhurst, J. C. (1982): Bradykinin stimulates pancreatic afferents to activate the cardiovascular system. *Trans. Assoc. Am. Physicians*, 95:229–236.

69. Ordway, G. A., and Longhurst, J. C. (1983): Cardiovascular reflexes arising from the gallbladder of the cat, effects of capsaicin, bradykinin and distension. *Circ. Res.*, 52:26–35.
70. Owen, S. W. (1933): A study of viscerocardiac reflexes: I. The experimental production of cardiac irregularities by visceral stimulation. *Am. Heart J.*, 8:496–506.
71. Palmer, E. D. (1976): The abnormal upper gastrointestinal vagovagal reflexes that effect the heart. *Am. J. Gastroenterol.*, 66:513–522.
72. Pavlov, I. P. (1963): On the imperfection of contemporary physiological analysis of drug action. In: *Readings in Pharmacology*, edited by B. Holmstedt and G. Liljestrand, pp. 216–218. Raven Press, New York.
73. Popova, T. V. (1953): Interoceptive reflexes of dogs in hypoxemia. *Bull. Exp. Biol.*, 39:32–44.
74. Ranieri, F., Crousillat, J., and Mei, N. (1970): Activite unitaire des mecano-recepteurs splanchniques de l'estomac. *CR Soc. Biol.*, 164:2578–2583.
75. Ranieri, F., Crousillat, J., and Mei, N. (1975): Etude electrophysiologique et histologique des fibres afferentes splanchniques. *Arch. Ital. Biol.*, 113:354–373.
76. Ranson, S. W., and Billingsley, P. R. (1918): The thoracic truncus sympathicus, renal communicantes and splanchnic nerves in the cat. *J. Comp. Neurol.*, 29:405–438.
77. Regoli, D., and Barabe, J. (1980): Pharmacology of bradykinin and related kinins. *Pharmacol. Rev.*, 32:1–46.
78. Riker, W. K. (1958): Reflexes from the intestinal mesentery elicited by veratidine, acetylcholine and nicotine. *J. Pharmacol. Exp. Ther.*, 124:120–126.
79. Saphir, R., and Rapaport, E. (1969): Cardiovascular responses of the cat to mesenteric intra-arterial administration of nicotine, cyanide and venous blood. *Circ. Res.*, 25:713–724.
80. Selkurt, E. E., and Rothe, C. F. (1960): Splanchnic baroreceptors in the dog. *Am. J. Physiol.*, 199:335–340.
81. Sharma, K. N., and Nasset, E. S. (1962): Electrical activity in mesenteric nerves after perfusion of the gut lumen. *Am. J. Physiol.*, 202:725–730.
82. Sheehan, D. (1932): The afferent nerve supply of the mesentery and its significance in the causation of abdominal pain. *J. Anat. (Lond.)*, 67:233–249.
83. Sherrington, C. S. (1906): *The Integrative Action of the Nervous System*. Scribners, New York.
84. Tuttle, R. S., and McCleary, M. (1975): Mesenteric baroreceptors. *Am. J. Physiol.*, 229:1514–1519.
85. Tuttle, R. S., and McCleary, M. (1979): Inferior cardiac nerve activity in the cat during occlusion of the mesenteric artery. *Am. J. Physiol.*, 236:H286–H290.
86. Vatner, S. F., Franklin, D., and Citters, R. L. Van (1970): Coronary and visceral vasoactivity associated with eating and digestion in the conscious dog. *Am. J. Physiol.*, 219:1380–1385.
87. Vyden, J. K., Nagasawa, K., and Corday, E. (1974): Hemodynamic consequences of acute occlusion of the superior mesenteric artery. *Am. J. Cardiol.*, 34:687–691.
88. Werner, M. H., Hayes, D. F., Lucas, C. E., and Rosenberg, I. K. (1974): Renal vasoconstriction in association with acute pancreatitis. *Am. J. Surg.*, 127:185–190.
89. Zeitlin, I. J., and Smith, A. N. (1966): 5-Hydroxyindoles and kinin in the carcinoid and dumping syndromes. *Lancet*, 2:986–991.

Fetal and Neonatal Intestinal Circulations

Daniel I. Edelstone and Ian R. Holzman

Departments of Obstetrics and Gynecology and Pediatrics, Magee-Women's Hospital, University of Pittsburgh School of Medicine, Pittsburgh, Pennsylvania 15213

During development, intestinal processes such as absorption, secretion, motility, and, in particular, growth consume energy and thus require a satisfactory circulation and sufficient quantities of oxygen for optimum aerobic metabolism. In the fetus, intestinal weight doubles approximately every 3 weeks (4), whereas, in the neonate, the intestinal tract doubles its weight approximately every 2 weeks (10). This rapid intestinal growth makes it likely that the perfusion and oxidative demands necessary for satisfactory function of the fetal and neonatal intestines differ from those of the adult. Furthermore, because intestinal function in the fetus differs fundamentally from that of the neonate, the intestinal circulation before and after birth may respond differently to factors that affect perfusion or oxygen supply. Only over the past few years have research efforts focused on measuring the basal requirements for blood flow and oxygen in the intestines of the fetus and neonate. Studies are now being conducted to determine how alterations in oxygen supply and oxygen demand affect intestinal metabolism and how neurohumoral systems modulate these relationships. In this chapter, we discuss the regulation of intestinal blood flow and oxygenation during the perinatal period. Because the methods used to study the fetus and neonate differ from those generally used to investigate the intestine of the adult, we begin with a discussion of the methodologies generally employed.

METHODOLOGY

In adult animals, the regulation of the intestinal circulation has primarily been studied in isolated segments of perfused intestine. This approach has the advantage that local control mechanisms can be studied separately from extrinsic neurohumoral influences, but its major disadvantage is that studies must be performed on anesthetized animals that have recently been surgically prepared. In contrast, most experiments on fetuses and neonates have been done in chronically catheterized, unanesthetized animals. With this approach investigators have sought to eliminate the confounding acute influences of anesthetics and surgery, factors that in the fetus or neonate can adversely affect the results (7,9). Thus, the intestinal circulatory responses that have been observed in perinatal animals represent the sum of local and extrinsic mechanisms. This technique allows us to determine how the fetal and neonatal intestinal circulations respond when the intact organism is subjected to factors that affect perfusion or oxygenation.

Much of the experimental work done on the intestines of the fetus and neonate has been performed in three species: the sheep, the pig, and the rabbit. Because approximately 80% of all research has been done on sheep, we briefly describe how fetal and neonatal lambs are prepared for chronic study. For fetal studies (9), pregnant sheep are given anesthesia, after which the maternal abdomen and pregnant uterus are incised. Polyvinyl catheters are then inserted via peripheral blood vessels into the fetal descending aorta, inferior vena cava, and mesenteric vein. In sheep, the mesenteric vein drains the entire small intestine and colon, with the exception of a small portion of proximal duodenum and distal rectum (5,9). Thus, a blood sample obtained from the mesenteric vein represents the mixed venous drainage of the whole intestinal tract, rather than that of the small intestine only. All catheters are brought out subcutaneously to the sheep's flank where they are stored in a pouch. The mother is allowed several days to recover from surgical and anethestic stresses. In neonatal lambs, similar blood vessels are catheterized with two additions: catheters are inserted retrograde into the left atrium via the right carotid artery and into the portal vein via the umbilical vein (7,8,10).

After the animals have recovered from surgery, they are brought to the laboratory and allowed to adjust to the environment before studies are begun. Our experience has shown that considerable patience is necessary to obtain a stable physiologic state at the time measurements are made. Several methods for measuring blood flow are available for assessing the intestinal circulation. Because of the small size of the mesenteric arteries in fetal and neonatal sheep, the radionuclide labeled microsphere technique, rather than the flow transducer method, has been more widely used in studies of intestinal blood flow. With the microsphere technique, microspheres labeled with various gamma emitters are injected into the inferior vena cava for fetal studies (9) or into the left atrium for neonatal studies (7). In both cases, a reference blood sample is withdrawn from the descending aorta. Intestinal blood flow (Q_i) is calculated as follows:

$$Q_i = (cpm_i/cpm_{ref}) \cdot Q_{ref},$$

where cpm_i = radioactive counts/minute in the intestines, cpm_{ref} = radioactive counts/minute in the aortic reference blood sample, and Q_{ref} = reference blood flow as determined by calibration of the withdrawal pump. Several variables of intestinal oxygenation can be determined simultaneously if modifications of the Fick principle are used:

$$\text{intestinal } O_2 \text{ delivery } (Do_{2i}) = Q_i \cdot Cao_2,$$
$$\text{intestinal } O_2 \text{ consumption } (Vo_{2i}) = Q_i \cdot (Cao_2 - C\bar{v}o_2),$$
$$\text{intestinal } O_2 \text{ extraction} = Vo_{2i}/Do_{2i} = (Cao_2 - C\bar{v}o_2)/Cao_2,$$

where $Cao_2 = O_2$ concentration in arterial blood and $C\bar{v}o_2 = O_2$ concentration in mesenteric venous blood. Cao_2 and $C\bar{v}o_2$ are both complex functions of several variables (e.g., Po_2 and hemoglobin type), the values of which differ substantially among fetus, neonate, and adult.

REGULATION OF INTESTINAL BLOOD FLOW AND OXYGENATION

Intestinal Circulation During Perinatal Growth and Development

During embryogenesis in most mammals (21), the small intestine develops from the midgut and is characterized by rapid elongation, particularly of the cephalic end (duodenum, jejunum, and proximal ileum). During fetal development, intestinal growth continues at an accelerated rate. As a proportion of body weight, the intestines of the fetal lamb increase from about 1% at the midpoint of gestation to about 3% to 4% at term (4). In absolute terms, intestinal weight increases about 30-fold during the second half of gestation. In the last third of the sheep pregnancy, the fetal intestine doubles its weight every 3 weeks (4). Intestinal tract blood flow increases from about 40 ml/min/100 g (3% of cardiac output) at midgestation (27) to 100 ml/min/100 g (6% of cardiac output) near term gestation (9,27). It is not clear what the oxidative requirements of the fetal intestinal tract are early in development because the only measurements of intestinal tract oxygen consumption have been made in near-term fetal lambs. Near term, fetal intestinal O_2 consumption averages 2 ml/min/100 g and intestinal O_2 extraction averages 25% (9).

After birth, the intestines of the neonate continue to grow rapidly. Intestinal weight doubles approximately every 2 weeks during the first 6 weeks of life in the lamb (10). In the pig, the growth spurt is even greater, with intestinal and body weight increasing three- to fourfold during the first 10 days of life (34). Thus it is easy to understand why basal intestinal blood flow in the neonatal sheep (10) and pig (1) averages about 200 ml/min/100 g, or twice that of the fetal lamb. Furthermore, intestinal O_2 consumption (10) in the fasted newborn lamb (at 5.6 ml O_2/min/100 g) is also substantially greater than that of the fetal lamb (see Table 1), yet the intestinal O_2 extraction ratio is about 20%, a value similar to that found in the fetus. In both the fetus and neonate, intestinal O_2 supply in the basal state exceeds O_2 demand by four- to fivefold.

Effects of Changes in O_2 Supply and O_2 Demand on Perinatal Intestinal Oxygenation

An organ's ability to satisfy its oxygen requirements is due to two characteristics common to most tissues (16): (a) the rate of oxidative metabolism is independent of the partial pressure of oxygen (Po_2) so long as cellular Po_2 is kept above a critical minimum; and (b) when cellular Po_2 falls below this critical minimum as O_2 supply or O_2 demand changes, tissues vasoregulate their circulations to return cell Po_2 to values greater than the critical level.

The metabolic theory of blood flow regulation predicts that O_2 supply and O_2 demand are carefully balanced by the interplay between changes in blood flow and alterations in oxygen extraction (15,16). The O_2 flux to cells, rather than blood flow per se, is postulated (16) to be the controlled variable (see Chapter 3). Adjustments in blood flow (which serve to minimize fluctuations in capillary Po_2) result from increases or decreases in arteriolar vascular resistance, whereas alterations in oxygen extraction are produced by constriction or relaxation of precapillary sphincters (which influence O_2 extraction by controlling diffusion variables such as the capillary-to-cell diffusion distance or the capillary surface area available for O_2 exchange). In the fetus and neonate, effects of changes in O_2 supply or O_2 demand have been studied primarily in sheep. The principal effects studied to date are those of reduced O_2 supply or increased O_2 demand.

Reduced O_2 Supply

Investigators have used several methods to reduce O_2 supply to the fetal and neonatal intes-

TABLE 1. *Variables of intestinal circulation in the basal state in fetal and neonatal lambs*

	Fetus	Neonate
Body weight (kg)	2.9	4.8
Age (days)	127 (term = 147)	7
Intestinal weight (g)	57	131
Arterial blood values		
Mean pressure (mm Hg)	46	60
O_2 content (Cao_2, ml O_2/dl)	8.2	12.6
O_2 tension (Pao_2, mm Hg)	20	83
Hematocrit (%)	30	27
Mesenteric venous blood values		
Mean pressure (mm Hg)	5	3
O_2 content ($C\bar{v}o_2$, ml O_2/dl)	6.1	10.3
O_2 tension (Pvo_2, mm Hg)	16	46
Intestinal blood flow		
(ml/min/100 g intestine)	100	214
(ml/min/kg body)	19	59
Intestinal vascular resistance		
(mm Hg/ml/min/100 g intestine)	0.40	0.27
(mm Hg/ml/min/kg body)	2.2	1.0
Intestinal O_2 delivery		
(ml/min/100 g intestine)	7.9	27.0
(ml/min/kg body)	1.6	7.4
Intestinal O_2 extraction (%)	26	21
Intestinal O_2 consumption		
(ml/min/100 g intestine)	2.1	5.6
(ml/min/kg body)	0.4	1.5

Only mean values are given; fetal data are from Edelstone and Holzman (9); neonatal data are from Edelstone and Holzman (7,10); some calculations also were made from the raw data of Edelstone et al. (7,9,10) and have not been reported previously. Intestinal O_2 delivery = intestinal blood flow · Cao_2; intestinal O_2 extraction = ($Cao_2 - C\bar{v}o_2$)/Cao_2; and intestinal O_2 consumption = intestinal blood flow · ($Cao_2 - C\bar{v}o_2$).

tines. These techniques include hypoxic hypoxemia, anemic hypoxemia, and hemorrhagic hypotension. Most of the studies to date have focused on the circulatory effects of hypoxic hypoxemia.

The intestinal responses to *hypoxic hypoxemia* have been investigated both in fetal and in neonatal lambs. In the fetus, hypoxic hypoxemia is induced by administering to the mother a gas mixture low in oxygen. Hypoxic hypoxemia (3,9,23,26) generally does not affect intestinal blood flow until the degree of hypoxemia is severe, at which point vascular resistance increases and intestinal blood flow declines (Fig. 1). Thus, if aerobic metabolism is to be maintained in the intestines during hypoxemia, O_2 extraction, rather than blood flow, must increase. In the fetal lamb, we (9) found that intestinal O_2 consumption remained stable during moderate degrees of hypoxemia (O_2 supply reduced up to about 45%), because O_2 extraction increased sufficiently to compensate for the reduced O_2 supply (Fig. 1). In contrast, as hypoxemia became more severe (O_2 supply reduced more than 45%), intestinal oxygen delivery was so profoundly decreased that, even though oxygen extraction increased further, the increase was insufficient to maintain oxygen consumption. Mesenteric acidemia developed, indicating that intestinal oxygenation was inadequate and that anaerobic metabolism had ensued. These data indicate that the fetal intestines are able to maintain aerobic metabolism so long as the oxygen supply is above a critical minimum. The primary tissue response to reduction in oxygen supply was an increase in oxygen extraction rather than a change in perfusion. This observation is consistent with those made in adult animals. If O_2 supply is reduced when the prevailing O_2-availability-to-demand ratio is high (as in the fetal intestines), increases in oxygen extraction are the primary means by which aerobic metabolism is maintained (15).

In the neonatal intestines, hypoxic hypoxemia evoked responses that were qualitatively similar to those seen in the fetal intestines (Fig. 2). Despite differences in basal O_2 demands at the two developmental ages, the circulatory responses to hypoxemia were the same; comparable increases in O_2 extraction occurred during hypoxemia (10). As long as O_2 supply remained above a critical minimum, aerobic metabolism was maintained. However, the specific intestinal responses to hypoxemia differed before and after birth. In the fetus (9), intestinal blood flow was linearly related to O_2 consumption (Fig. 3, *top*). At normal or near normal intestinal blood flows, O_2 consumption was stable. When intestinal blood flow fell during hypoxemia, intestinal O_2 consumption decreased, indicating that fetal intestinal metabolism may be limited by perfusion. In contrast, in the intestines of the neonate (Fig. 3, *bottom*), blood flow varied over a wide range without O_2 consumption or aerobic metabolism being affected (10). The specific factors responsible for the age-related differences in the relationship of intestinal perfusion to O_2 consumption are unknown but may be due to differences in vascular tone or reactivity of mesenteric blood vessels during the perinatal period.

The effect of isovolemic *anemia* on the intestinal circulation has received little attention. In adult animals, anemia results in a generalized hyperemia as the primary compensation for reduced O_2 capacity of the blood. In the fetal lamb, we (12) have preliminary data indicating that intestinal blood flow increases only slightly during anemic hypoxemia. Because of this, intestinal O_2 delivery decreases, although the decrease is not as great as that which occurs during a comparable degree of hypoxic hypoxemia. In our preliminary studies, O_2 extraction and O_2 consumption were not measured. In the neonatal lamb (29), preliminary data show that the intestinal circulatory responses are similar to those seen in the anemic fetus. We also found that reduced O_2 supply to the intestines in the neonate resulted in increases in oxygen extraction of sufficient magnitude for intestinal O_2 consumption to remain stable at hematocrits as low as 10%.

The effect of reduced perfusion pressure on the intestines of the fetus and neonate has also received limited attention. In fetal lambs, hemorrhage of approximately 10% to 15% of blood

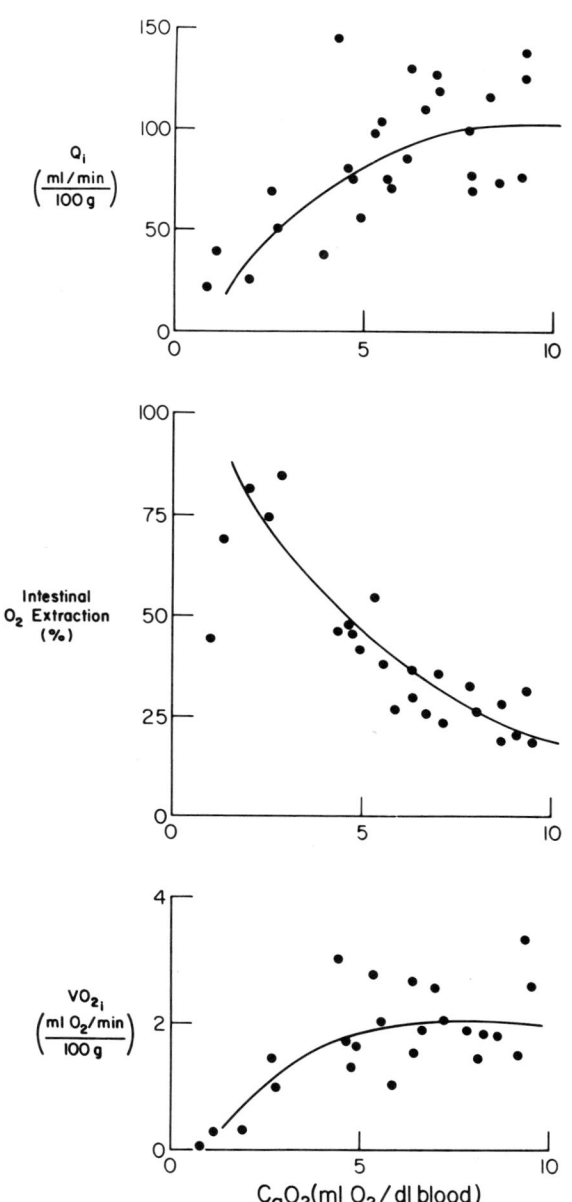

FIG. 1. Fetal intestinal blood flow (Q_i), O_2 extraction, and O_2 consumption (Vo_{2i}) as functions of arterial blood O_2 content (Cao_2) in lambs ($n = 7$). Curves drawn in this figure (and in Figs. 2 and 3) are derived from covariance analysis. (From Edelstone and Holzman, ref. 9, with permission.)

volume causes reductions in blood pressure and blood flow that are approximately equal (13,31). Fetal intestinal vascular resistance did not change during hypotension. These data indicate the absence of active flow autoregulation, but tissue oxygenation was not assessed simultaneously. Therefore, it is impossible to determine whether O_2 supply to cells was maintained by increases in O_2 extraction. Comparable studies on the neonatal intestinal response to hypotension have not been done.

Increased O_2 Demand

Whether nutrient administration to the fetal intestinal tract can increase oxygen demand by intestinal tissues is unclear. In fetal lambs (5), infusion of nutrients into the stomach had no effect on intestinal blood flow or oxygen con-

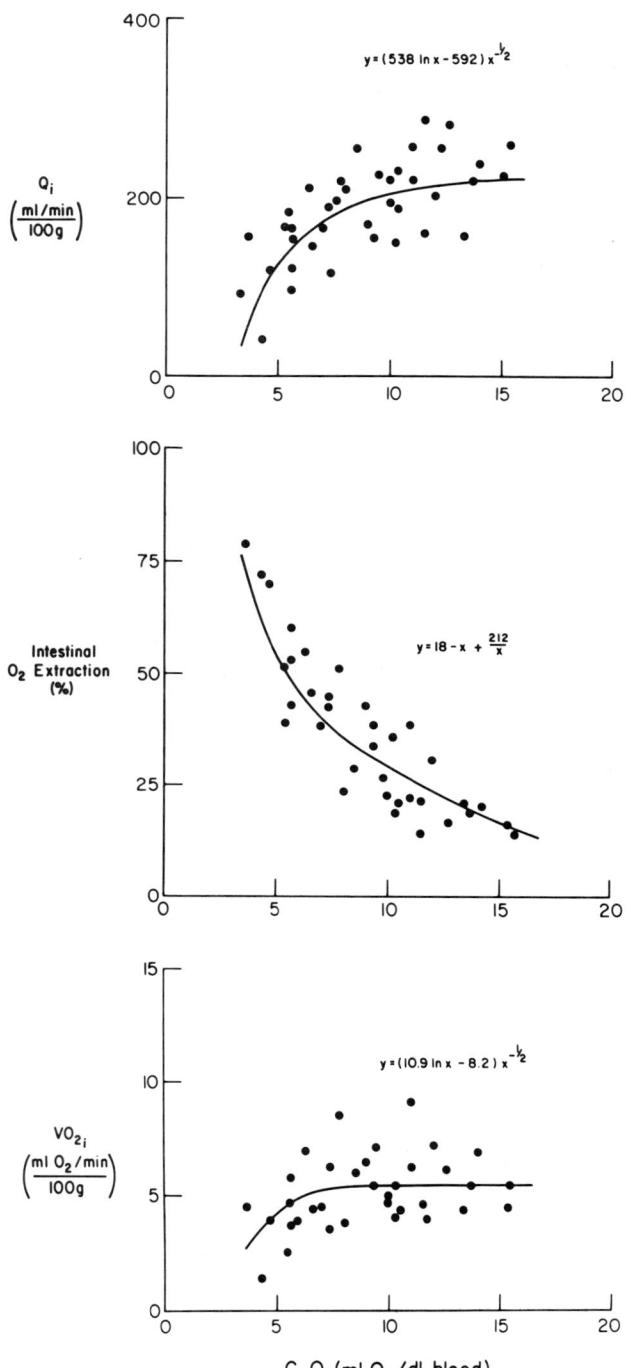

FIG. 2. Neonatal intestinal blood flow (Q_i), O_2 extraction, and O_2 consumption ($V_{O_{2i}}$) as a function of arterial blood O_2 content (Ca_{O_2}) (data from 12 lambs). (From Edelstone et al., ref. 10, with permission.)

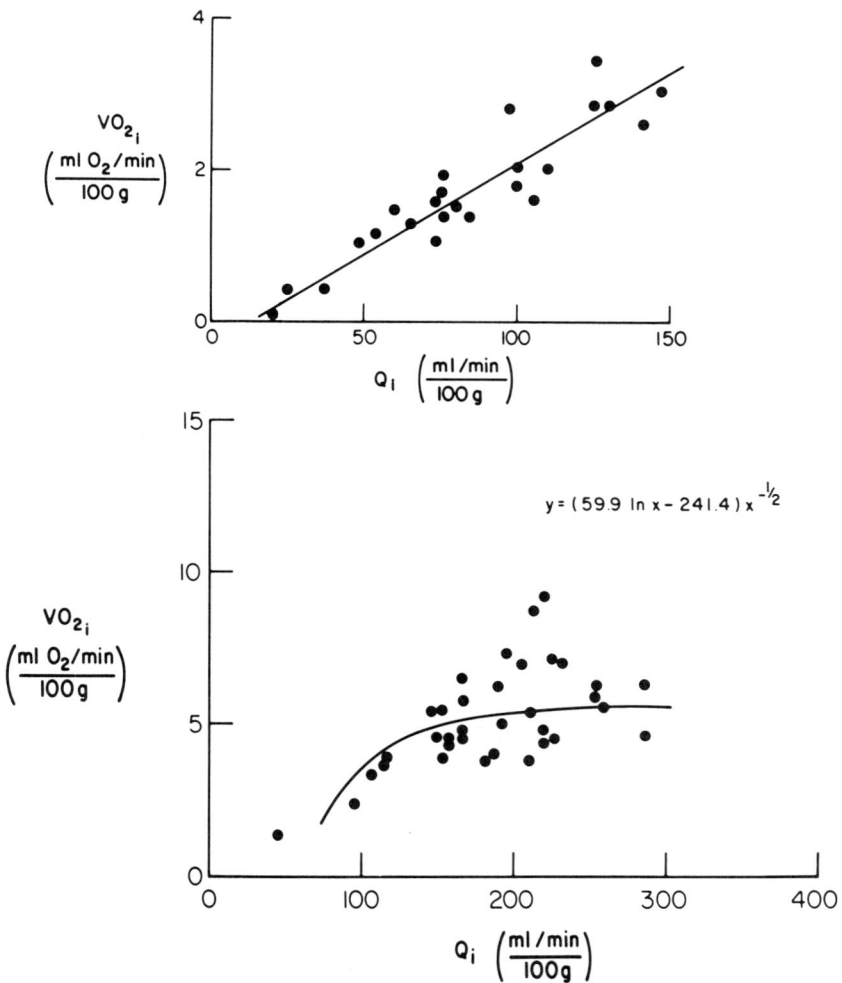

FIG. 3. Top: Relationship of fetal intestinal O_2 consumption ($V_{O_{2i}}$) to blood flow (Q_i). [Redrawn from the raw data (19) and printed with permission.] **Bottom:** Relationship of neonatal intestinal O_2 consumption ($V_{O_{2i}}$) to blood flow (Q_i). (From Edelstone et al., ref. 10, with permission.)

sumption even though these nutrients were absorbed across the intestinal mucosa at such a rate that about 40% of the entire fetal uptake of nutrients was derived from fetal intestinal absorption of nutrients. (In the normal state, 5 to 10% of the total uptake of nutrients by the fetal organism is via the gastrointestinal tract with the balance coming from the placenta.) It is not clear why fetal intestinal oxygen consumption did not increase even though absorption increased substantially. Further studies are necessary to clarify this observation.

In neonatal lambs, we (8) measured blood flow and oxygen consumption by the entire gastrointestinal tract before, and hourly for 6 hr following, the ingestion of milk. During digestion, intestinal blood flow did not change (Fig. 4), whereas gastrointestinal oxygen consumption increased 30% to 60% over the first 3 hr post-prandially (Fig. 5). This increase in oxygen demand was met entirely by increases in oxygen extraction. (The only gastrointestinal organ to exhibit a hyperemia during digestion was the stomach and that was observed only at

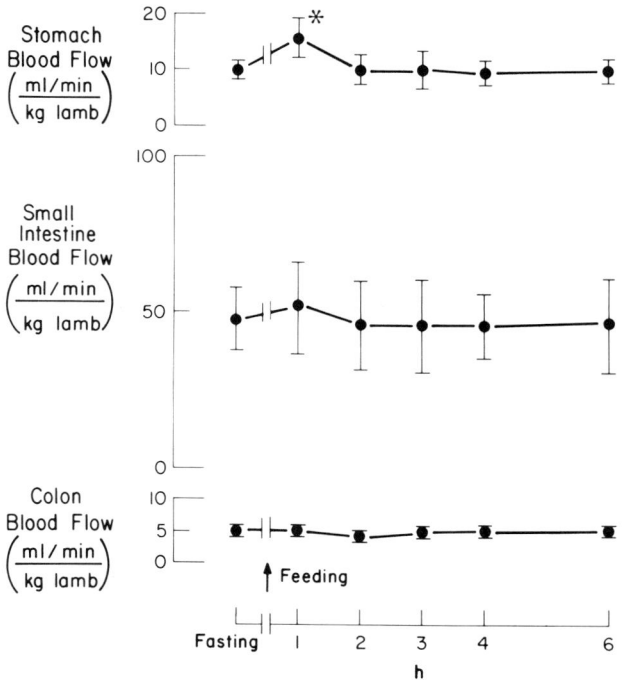

FIG. 4. Effects of digestion on blood flow to neonatal stomach, small intestine, and colon. Values are means ± SD for 7 lambs. *(Asterisk)* $p < 0.05$ when compared with values obtained in fasted lambs. (Redrawn from Edelstone and Holzman, ref. 8, with permission.)

1 hr post-prandially.) The lack of a small intestinal hyperemia in the lamb post-prandially may be due to its ruminant digestive system or it may be a feature common to all neonatal animals. Future experiments should allow us to make this distinction.

Neural and Neurohumoral Control of the Intestinal Circulation in the Fetus and Neonate

The nervous and endocrine systems are important in the overall regulation of intestinal blood flow and oxygen consumption. These systems have their effects at the tissue or the cellular level, either by directly influencing the microcirculation or by indirectly affecting systemic cardiovascular function. For the fetus and neonate, these regulatory systems undergo a maturation process. Thus, the absence of a response to a particular neural or chemohumoral stimulus in the immature fetus does not necessarily imply that the response will be absent in a mature fetus or a neonate. This maturational factor must be considered in the design of studies of neural or endocrine control of the intestinal circulation during perinatal life.

Neural Reflex Control

The activity of the baroreceptor reflex has been assessed in fetal and neonatal animals. Most of the studies have been performed on fetal lambs in which baroreceptor activity has been demonstrated as early as the two-thirds point of gestation (14). In other species, including the human, this reflex matures post-natally. The interrelationship of the splanchnic circulation with the overall control of blood pressure and heart rate in the fetus and newborn has not been adequately studied. In fetal lambs, relatively acute reductions in blood volume and blood pressure reduce gastrointestinal tract blood flows, but the specific role of the baroreflex in these adjustments has not been determined (13). The possibility of the fetal mesenteric circulation having functioning baroreceptors (17) also has not been examined. For a discussion of splanchnic baroreceptors in the adult, see Chapter 14.

The functions of the peripheral chemoreceptor reflexes, as they relate to overall cardiovascular regulation, have been studied in fetal and newborn animals. The human fetus during the

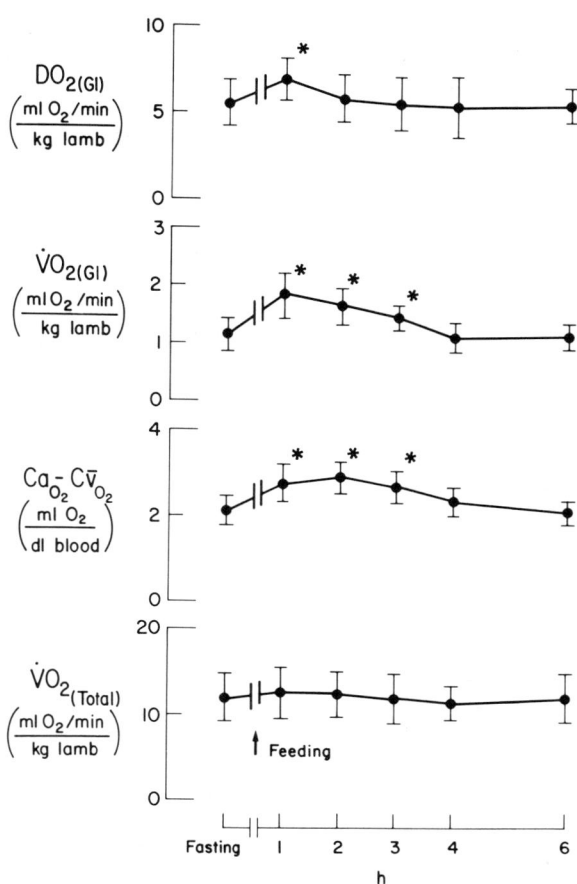

FIG. 5. Effects of digestion on neonatal gastrointestinal O_2 delivery ($\dot{D}O_{2GI}$) and O_2 uptake ($\dot{V}O_{2GI}$), O_2 concentration difference between arterial and portal venous blood ($Ca_{O_2} - C\bar{v}_{O_2}$), and whole-body O_2 uptake ($\dot{V}O_{2total}$). Values are means ± SD for 10 lambs. *(Asterisk)* $p<0.05$ when compared with values obtained in fasted lambs. (From Edelstone and Holzman, ref. 8, with permission.)

second trimester has an anatomically mature carotid body (19). In the lamb fetus, stimulation of the arterial chemoreceptors produces fetal bradycardia and hypertension (20). The threshold for peripheral chemoreceptor activity is relatively low in the fetus (6). After birth, as neuroreflex maturation continues, the threshold for activation of chemoreceptors increases in most species, including the human. The way in which the peripheral chemoreceptors affect the splanchnic circulation during fetal and neonatal life, however, is unknown.

The effects of autonomic neural control of the general circulation of the fetus and neonate have been relatively well studied. Vapaavouri et al. (32) noted that basal autonomic activity, rather than end-organ responsiveness, changes during fetal life. They detected autonomic neural activity by 85 days of gestation in the sheep (full term = 147 days); parasympathetic and alpha-adrenergic activity increased from 101 to 120 days, and beta-adrenergic activity increased after 120 days. In contrast, however, both Woods et al. (35) and Nuwayhid et al. (24) found in the lamb that the sympathetic nervous system preceded the parasympathetic system in fetal cardiovascular maturation and control. Furthermore, their studies showed that changes in end-organ responsiveness were primarily responsible for the observed changes in autonomic neural activity. After birth, neurohumoral tone declines progressively whereas responsiveness to autonomic agonists increases (2,30). The rat and rabbit are born with scant autonomic control of cardiovascular function, but the guinea pig, lamb, and human are more mature at birth (25).

Neuro- and Chemohumoral Control of the Intestinal Circulation

Few studies have been done on neurohumoral or chemohumoral control of the intestinal vasculatures during development. In near-term fetal lambs, Zink and Van Petten (36) compared the vascular effects of norepinephrine with those of tyramine, a releaser of norepinephrine from sympathetic nerve endings. Their results indicated that the gastrointestinal tract (studied as a single vasculature) was vasoconstricted equally by both substances. McCuskey et al. (23) found that the mesenteric blood vessels of fetal rabbits in the latter portion of gestation constricted equally to epinephrine and norepinephrine administered topically. These responses were blocked by phentolamine, but not by propranolol. Fehn and McCuskey (11) also showed that catecholamines produced more of a response in intestinal arterioles than in mesenteric arterioles of the rabbit fetus. In all splanchnic arterioles, beta-adrenergic responsiveness developed post-natally. Catecholamines had no effects on mesenteric venules. Su et al. (28) noted an increased vasoconstrictive response of mesenteric arteries of the fetal lamb to norepinephrine and 5-hydroxytryptamine as gestation progressed. Avner and Yabek (3) suggested that prostaglandin E modulates the fetal mesenteric vascular reactivity to catecholamines.

A number of other substances released systemically or locally may also play an as yet undefined part in the control of intestinal blood flow. The activity of the renin-angiotensin-aldosterone system is increased in newborn lambs when compared with that of adults. Although inhibition of antiotensin-converting enzyme has no effect on ileal and jejunal blood flows, this inhibition blunts the vasoconstrictive effects of hypoxemia (33). The contribution of the renin-angiotensin-aldosterone system to the control of intestinal blood flow in the fetus and newborn is unknown. The same can be said for the role of enkephalins or adenosine. The entire series of gastrointestinal peptides are presently the focus of investigations in the newborn. Many are found in higher concentrations in the blood of neonates than at any other time of life (22). Although these peptides have obvious vascular effects in adults (18), their effects on the intestinal circulation during the perinatal period have not been studied.

CLINICAL CORRELATIONS

A number of important clinical questions are directly related to the regulation of fetal and neonatal intestinal blood flow and oxygenation. The impact of intrauterine and perinatal asphyxia on the integrity of the newborn intestine is of critical importance for the practice of neonatal medicine. One disease in which asphyxia may play a pathogenic role is necrotizing enterocolitis, a condition seen primarily in premature infants whose intestines develop focal areas of necrosis. In these infants, intestinal oxygen supply may be reduced below the critical level necessary for aerobic metabolism. Might other factors, such as an inappropriate neural or chemohumoral response or failure of capillary regulation, play a role in the disease process in these infants? Also, a number of infants are born with alterations in red blood cell mass. Infants of diabetic mothers and infants who have suffered intrauterine malnutrition are often polycythemic. Unless clinical intervention occurs, these infants must perfuse their intestines with hyperviscous blood that might reduce intestinal O_2 supply. Similarly, a decreased red cell mass, due either to perinatal blood loss (often compounded by hypotension) or to hemolysis, occurs clinically and requires further investigation. The possibility of utilizing the gastrointestinal tract for nutritional supplementation in the fetus has been shown to be feasible in the lamb (5). The implication of this finding for clinical care is exciting, and it underscores the importance of understanding the control of fetal intestinal oxygenation.

CONCLUSION

The regulation of the intestinal circulation during development provides a unique topic for investigation. The concept of tissue growth adds a difficult-to-measure, yet vital, component to the study of the basic physiology of this circulation. Additionally, the transition from fetal to newborn life introduces a sudden change in function for the intestinal tract at a time when the metabolic demands of growth continue to be large. Therefore, it is not surprising that intestinal blood flow and oxygen consumption more than double after birth, and that the interrelationships between O_2 consumption and blood flows differ pre- and post-natally. Clearly, much research remains to be done on the regulation of the intestinal circulation during fetal and neonatal life.

ACKNOWLEDGMENTS

We gratefully acknowledge the excellent secretarial assistance of Lynn Heddinger and Marge Guzik in the preparation of this manuscript.

Most of the authors's work reported in this chapter was supported by the March of Dimes Birth Defects Foundation (Basil O'Connor Grant #5-225) and by the National Institute of Child Health and Human Development (Grant #HD-16368).

REFERENCES

1. Alwood, C. T., Hook, J. B., Helmrath, T. A., Mattson, J. C., and Bailie, M. D. (1978): Effects of asphyxia on cardiac output and organ blood flow in the newborn piglet. *Pediatr. Res.*, 12:824–827.
2. Assali, N. S., Brinkman, C. R., III, Woods, J. R., Jr., Dandavino, A., and Nuwayhid, B. (1977): Development of neurohumoral control of fetal, neonatal, and adult cardiovascular functions. *Am. J. Obstet. Gynecol.*, 129:748–759.
3. Avner, B. P., and Yabek, S. M. (1978): The effects of hypoxia and indomethacin on the responsiveness of fetal and neonatal mesenteric arteries to epinephrine. *Proc. West. Pharmacol. Soc.*, 21:189–195.
4. Barcroft, Sir Joseph (1946): *Researches on Pre-Natal Life*. Blackwell Scientific Publications, Ltd., Oxford.
5. Charlton, V. E., and Reis, B. L. (1981): Effects of gastric nutritional supplementation on fetal umbilical uptake of nutrients. *Am. J. Physiol.*, 241 (*Endocrinol. Metab.* 4):E178–E185.
6. Dawes, G. S., Duncan, S. L. B., Lewis, B. V., Merlet, C. L., Owen-Thomas, J. B., and Reeves, J. T. (1969): Cyanide stimulation of the systemic arterial chemoreceptors in foetal lambs. *J. Physiol.*, 201:117–128.
7. Edelstone, D. I., and Holzman, I. R. (1981): Oxygen consumption by the gastrointestinal tract and liver in conscious newborn lambs. *Am. J. Physiol.*, 240 (*Gastrointest. Liver Physiol.* 3):G297–G304.
8. Edelstone, D. I., and Holzman, I. R. (1981): Gastrointestinal tract O_2 uptake and regional blood flows during digestion in conscious newborn lambs. *Am. J. Physiol.*, 241 (*Gastrointest. Liver Physiol.* 4):G289–G293.
9. Edelstone, D. I., and Holzman, I. R. (1982): Fetal intestinal oxygen consumption at various levels of oxygenation. *Am. J. Physiol.*, 242 (*Heart Circ. Physiol.* 11):H50–H54.
10. Edelstone, D. I., Lattanzi, D. R., Paulone, M. E., and Holzman, I. R. (1983): Neonatal intestinal oxygen consumption during arterial hypoxemia. *Am. J. Physiol.*, 244 (*Gastrointest. Liver Physiol.* 7):G278–G283.
11. Fehn, P. A., and McCuskey, R. S. (1971): Response of the fetal mesenteric microvascular system to catecholamines. *Microvasc. Res.*, 3:104–109.
12. Fumia, F. D., Edelstone, D. I., and Holzman, I. R. (1982): Blood flow and O_2 delivery to fetal gastrointestinal organs as a function of arterial hematocrit. *Physiologist*, 25:290.
13. Gilbert, R. D. (1980): Control of fetal cardiac output during changes in blood volume. *Am. J. Physiol.* 238 (*Heart Circ. Physiol.* 7):H80–H86.
14. Gootman, P. M., Buckley, N. M., and Gootman, N. (1979): Postnatal maturation of neural control of the circulation. In: *Reviews in Perinatal Medicine*, edited by E. M. Scarpelli and E. V. Cosmi, pp. 1–72. Raven Press, New York.
15. Granger, H. J., and Norris, C. P. (1980): Intrinsic regulation of intestinal oxygenation in the anesthetized dog. *Am. J. Physiol.*, 238 (*Heart Circ. Physiol.* 7):H836–H843.
16. Granger, H. J., and Shepherd, A. P., Jr. (1973): Intrinsic microvascular control of tissue oxygen delivery. *Microvasc. Res.*, 5:49–72.
17. Grayson, J., and Mendel, D. (1965): *Physiology of the Splanchnic Circulation*, pp. 32–55. Edward Arnold Ltd., London.
18. Grossman, M. I. (1979): Chemical messengers: A view from the gut. *Fed. Proc.*, 38:2341–2343.
19. Hervonen, A., and Korkala, O. (1972): Fine structure of the carotid body of the midterm human fetus. *Z. Anat. Entwickl.-Gesch.*, 138:135–144.
20. Itskovitz, J., and Rudolph, A. M. (1982): Denervation of arterial chemoreceptors and baroreceptors in fetal lambs in utero. *Am. J. Physiol.*, 242 (*Heart Circ. Physiol.* 11):H916–H920.
21. Langman, J. (1975): *Medical Embryology*. Williams & Wilkins Company, Baltimore, Maryland.
22. Lucas, A., Aynsley-Green, A., and Bloom, S. R. (1981): Gut hormones and the first meals. *Clin. Sci.*, 60:349–353.
23. McCuskey, R. S., McClugage, S. G., Jr., Moore, T. J., and Miller, M. L. (1969): Response of the fetal mesenteric microvascular system to maternal hypoxia. *Proc. Soc. Exp. Biol. Med.*, 132:636–639.
24. Nuwayhid, B., Brinkman, C. R., III, Su, C., Bevan, J. A., and Assali, N. S. (1975): Development of autonomic control of fetal circulation. *Am. J. Physiol.*, 228:337–344.
25. Pappano, A. J. (1977): Ontogenetic development of autonomic neuroeffector transmission and transmitter reactivity in embryonic and fetal hearts. *Pharmacol. Rev.*, 29:3–33.
26. Peeters, L. L. H., Sheldon, R. E., Jones, M. D., Jr.,

Makowski, E. L., and Meschia, G. (1979): Blood flow to fetal organs as a function of arterial oxygen content. *Am. J. Obstet. Gynecol.*, 135:637–646.
27. Rudolph, A. M., and Heymann, M. A. (1970): Circulatory changes during growth in the fetal lamb. *Circ. Res.*, 26:289–299.
28. Su, C., Bevan, J. A., Assali, N. S., and Brinkman, C. R., III (1977): Regional variation of lamb blood vessel responsiveness to vasoactive agents during fetal development. *Circ. Res.*, 41:844–848.
29. Tabata, B. K., Holzman, I. R., and Edelstone, D. I. (1983): Gastrointestinal oxygenation during isovolemic anemia in neonatal lambs. *Fed. Proc.*, 42:341.
30. Tabsh, K., Nuwayhid, B., Murad, S., Ushioda, E., Erkkola, R., Brinkman, C. R., III, and Assali, N. S. (1982): Circulatory effects of chemical sympathectomy in fetal, neonatal, and adult sheep. *Am. J. Physiol.*, 243 (*Heart Circ. Physiol.* 12):H113–H122.
31. Toubas, P. L., Silverman, N. H., Heyman, M. A., and Rudolph, A. M. (1981): Cardiovascular effects of acute hemorrhage in fetal lambs. *Am. J. Physiol.*, 240 (*Heart Circ. Physiol.* 9):H45–H48.
32. Vapaavouri, E. K., Shinebourne, E. A., Williams, R. L., Heymann, M. A., and Rudolph, A. M. (1973): Development of cardiovascular responses to autonomic blockade in intact fetal and neonatal lambs. *Biol. Neonate*, 22:177–188.
33. Weismann, D. N., Herrig, J. E., McWeeny, O. J., and Robillard, J. E. (1983): Organ tissue blood flow responses to hypoxemia in lambs: Effect of angiotensin converting enzyme inhibitor. *Pediatr. Res.*, 17:195–199.
34. Widdowson, E. M., Colombo, V. E., and Artavanis, C. A. (1976): Changes in the organs of pigs in response to feeding for the first 24 h after birth. *Biol. Neonate*, 28:272–281.
35. Woods, J. R., Jr., Dandavino, A., Murayama, K., Brinkman, C. R., III, and Assali, N. S. (1977): Autonomic control of cardiovascular functions during neonatal development and in adult sheep. *Circ. Res.*, 40:401–407.
36. Zink, J., and Van Petten, G. R. (1981): Noradrenergic control of blood vessels in the premature lamb fetus. *Biol. Neonate*, 39:61–69.

Intestinal Lymph Formation

J. A. Barrowman

Faculty of Medicine, Memorial University of Newfoundland, St. John's, Newfoundland, Canada, A1B 3V6

The notion that intestinal lymph participates in the absorptive function of the gastrointestinal tract preceded an appreciation of the general absorptive role of lymphatics. Asellius' historic demonstration of lymphatics in the small intestine required a fed dog rather than a fasting animal. It was more than a century later that William Hunter and his colleagues recognized the general absorptive function of lymphatics, but a full understanding of the crucial role of the lymphatics in returning fluid and protein to the blood awaited the formulation by E. H. Starling of the balance of hydrostatic and oncotic pressures across the capillary wall and the recognition that a small but significant amount of plasma protein leaves the bloodstream and enters the interstitial space. This chapter examines the formation of intestinal lymph and its relationship to the function of the alimentary tract. Although intestinal lymphatics, like those of other areas, are involved in the recirculation of lymphocytes, this aspect of lymphatic function will not be considered.

THE ANATOMY OF INTESTINAL LYMPH FORMATION

Intestinal lymph is derived from the interstitial fluid of the mucosa, submucosa, and muscularis. Interstitial fluid is, in turn, derived from capillary filtrate and also from absorbed fluid in the case of the mucosa. Therefore, it is necessary to consider the anatomical structure of the absorbing epithelium, the microvasculature, the interstitium, and the initial lymphatics. Most attention is given to the mucosal layer of the intestine because a large proportion of total intestinal blood flow passes through this layer and because large volumes of absorbed and secreted fluid pass through the mucosa.

The ultrastructure of blood capillaries and initial lymphatics is treated in Chapter 2. This chapter describes only the anatomical disposition of the microvessels in the intestine and their functional significance. The intestinal epithelium, through which absorbed and secreted fluid passes, lies on a basement membrane. Fenestrated capillaries lie about 2 μm below the basement membrane in the case of the small intestine and 1 μm in the large intestine (45). The fenestrae of the capillaries are found on the portion of the vessel wall that faces the epithelium. Yablonski and Lifson (87) have proposed that a distinct juxta-capillary compartment exists between the epithelium and these subepithelial capillaries. This compartment, by virtue of its small volume, would be very sensitive to hydrostatic or oncotic pressure changes that could serve to direct incoming fluid from the intestinal lumen to these microvessels. On the other hand, the central lacteal of the small intestinal villus lies approximately 50 μm from the absorbing epithelium (23). If functional compartments of the interstitium do exist in the mucosa, the lymphatic is in contact with a much larger compartment than the subepithelial capillaries. The anatomy of colonic mucosal lymphatics is discussed in Chapter 11.

THE INTERSTITIUM

Although it is most readily characterized in terms of its biochemical, physical, and functional characteristics (38), the interstitium must be considered anatomically because it lies between the exchange vessels, the blood capillaries, and the initial lymphatics. The interstitial compartment comprises three components—fibers, ground substance, and fluid. Total interstitial fluid amounts to three times the plasma volume. In some areas the ground substance is denser than in others. Thus, regions of the interstitium can be designated "colloid-rich" or "water-rich." There are three main types of fibers, namely, collagenous and reticular forms with a few elastic fibers. The reticular fibers that form fine networks around the cells are closely related to basement membranes. A mechanical support system is provided by fibrous interstitial structures. Collagen fibers range from a few to several hundred microns in diameter. Among various tissues the collagen content is quite variable, with little in the normal liver and much larger amounts in the skin. The ground substance of the interstitium is a gel-like matrix consisting of glycosaminoglycans of which the most ubiquitous is hyaluronic acid, a linear polymer of glucuronic acid and N-acetyl glucosamine. At physiological pH, glycosaminoglycans are polyanions. The chains of the glycosaminoglycans are tangled around the collagen fibers, and in areas where these chains are densely packed, there is a high concentration of negative charge. The ability of other macromolecules, notably proteins, to penetrate the mesh is limited probably by their size and shape. Thus, proteins are excluded from a portion of the interstitium. Increasing hydration of the interstitial gel, by opening the mesh, reduces the extent of macromolecular exclusion in this compartment. For example, in the cat small intestine, the excluded volume fraction for albumin is 0.37. During net volume absorption from the gut lumen, this value falls sharply with increasing interstitial fluid volume and matrix hydration (28). Under these circumstances, the hydraulic conductivity of the interstitium is greatly enhanced; this facilitates the passage of fluid and solutes into blood and lymphatic vessels. When absorbed fluid enters the interstitium, a fall in protein exclusion amplifies the transcapillary oncotic pressure gradient and facilitates the uptake of fluid by the blood capillaries. The simultaneous rise in interstitial fluid hydrostatic pressure enhances fluid dispersal by both capillaries and lymphatics.

Although the overall hydraulic conductivity of the interstitium is low, the "water-rich" zones may provide fluid channels that allow relatively free movement of water and small molecules. Dyes escaping from capillaries have been observed to follow such preferential channels. In some tissues, these channels are associated with collagen fibers, and free-fluid channels may possibly be found as gaps between the fibrils that make up a collagen fiber (88). In the rat mesentery, Fox and Wayland (19) concluded from diffusion studies that the interstitium behaves as if it were a system of pores about 50 Å in radius. This system can be compared to the gels used for molecular exclusion chromatography. When one compares the rates at which lymph-to-plasma ratios for albumin and fibrinogen approach steady state levels in the dog hind paw, one finds that the larger molecule approaches the steady state level more rapidly than the smaller one just as it does in a gel filtration column (84). However, in the frequently studied model of the interstitium, Wharton's jelly of the umbilical cord, this phenomenon is not observed (38).

An important unanswered question is what part does the interstitium play in restricting the movement of fluid and solutes from blood to the lymph? Traditionally, the capillary endothelium and its basement membrane have been considered the major filter. Although this may be true in continuous and possibly in fenestrated capillaries, the interstitium may offer the major restriction in sinusoidal beds such as the liver where morphological appearances suggest a highly permeable microvascular wall.

LYMPH FORMATION, FLOW, AND COMPOSITION

Under isovolumetric or isogravimetric conditions, lymph flow from an organ represents the net capillary filtration rate that is governed by the hydrostatic and oncotic forces operating across the capillary wall (72). Net capillary filtration, $J_{v,c}$, is given by the following:

$$J_{v,c} = K_{f,c}[(P_c - P_t) - \sigma_d(\pi_p - \pi_t)],$$

where $K_{f,c}$ is the capillary filtration coefficient, P_c is the capillary hydrostatic pressure, P_t is the interstitial fluid pressure, σ_d is the osmotic reflection coefficient, π_p is the plasma oncotic pressure, and π_t is the interstitial oncotic pressure. Capillary filtrate accumulates in the interstitium and the lymphatics appear to play a homeostatic role in regulating the volume of this compartment. Because the intestinal interstitium is concerned with transepithelial transport of fluids and solutes, lymph flow changes are closely related to absorption and secretion (see below). Under "resting" conditions at a portal venous pressure of 0 mm Hg and with minimal mucosal fluid transport, lymph flows from the small intestine and colon are 0.045 and 0.015 ml/min/100 g, respectively (24).

Most investigators agree that the hydrostatic pressure gradient from interstitium to initial lymphatic is responsible for driving interstitial fluid into these vessels. In the intestine, this view is supported by the relationship between lymph flow and interstitial fluid volume or pressure (24).

Other than net transmucosal fluid movement, a number of physiological and pharmacological factors influence small intestinal lymph flow. These are summarized in Table 1.

The composition of intestinal lymph is chiefly determined by contributions from the plasma, that is, the capillary filtrate, together with the absorbate from the intestine. Some substances of local origin are also found in high concentration in intestinal lymph. These include immunoglobulin A derived from mucosal plasma cells (64,80,81) and alkaline phosphatase derived from the brush border of enterocytes. In both rat and man, this enzyme is released into the gut lumen and intestinal lymph during fat absorption, and its release is closely linked to the process of lipid absorption (43,46,52).

Intestinal lymph from resting conscious rats in a nonabsorptive state has a protein concentration of approximately 1 to 2 g% (5), and similar values are obtained in other species (4). All plasma proteins are found in intestinal lymph,

TABLE 1. *Factors altering small intestinal lymph flow*

Flow	Ref.
Increased flow	
Elevated portal venous pressure	56,87
Plasma dilution	30,31
Histamine	55
Bradykinin	34
Isoproterenol	34
Glucagon	27
Cholecystokinin (and analogs)	33,77
Secretin	33,47
Prostaglandin E_1	35
Diuretics	74
Intestinal distension	26
Decreased flow	
Arterial hypotension	29
Hypertonic glucose	51
Vasopressin	63
Theophylline	25
Vasoactive intestinal polypeptide	25

indicating that each of these molecules can leave the vascular compartment and enter the interstitium and lymph. The protein lymph-to-plasma ratios (C_L/C_P) fall with increasing molecular size, reflecting the restrictive properties of the blood-lymph barrier to these macromolecules. The permeability characteristics of the intestinal blood-lymph barrier to macromolecules (37) are discussed in detail in Chapter 18.

INTESTINAL FLUID ABSORPTION AND LYMPH FLOW

In tissues such as the small intestine that are concerned with solute-coupled fluid absorption, the lymphatics have to play an agile role in maintaining the homeostasis of the interstitium. During net fluid absorption from the intestine, there is an increase in intestinal lymph flow, the extent of which is rather variable and dependent on multiple factors. An influx of fluid into the interstitium increases the interstitial hydrostatic pressure (48) and reduces the colloid osmotic pressure of interstitial fluid. Both dilution and a fall in plasma protein exclusion in the hydrated interstitium contribute to reducing π_t. The rise in interstitial fluid hydrostatic pressure provides a driving force for lymphatic filling and converts filtering capillaries into absorbing vessels (24).

As fluid absorption rate increases, there is a rise in interstitial fluid pressure at low absorption rates with relatively little change in interstitial fluid oncotic pressure. As absorption rates rise further, interstitial compliance increases so that further hydrostatic pressure changes are minimal. Finally at high rates of fluid absorption, the fall in interstitial fluid oncotic pressure becomes more important in the alteration of Starling forces opposing capillary filtration (23).

Lymph flow in the thoracic duct or cisterna chyli increases during intestinal fluid absorption, but attempts to quantify the proportion of absorbed fluid transported by the lymphatics have yielded variable results ranging from less than 1% to 85% (5,6,12,15,49,57,58,69). These conflicting results have been attributed to differing experimental conditions, such as variable portal venous pressure, intraluminal pressures, or composition of the mucosal fluid. In cat ileum, in which these variables are held fairly constant, the rate of absorption of fluid from the intestinal lumen is a major determinant of intestinal lymph flow. At absorption rates greater than 0.15 ml/min/100 g, approximately 80% to 85% of absorbed fluid is transported by blood capillaries and the remainder by the lymphatics (36). By contrast, Lee (49) was unable to demonstrate any correlation between fluid absorption rate and intestinal lymph flow in rat jejunum. At high lymph flows, a maximum rate for lymphatic removal of absorbed flow is probably reached because of the transport capacity of the draining lymph trunks. Reaching maximum lymph flow may affect the partition of absorbed fluid between capillaries and lymphatics.

In both the small bowel and the colon, small, readily diffusible water-soluble molecules such as glucose and amino acids are probably partitioned between the portal venous and lymphatic routes in parallel with concurrently absorbed fluid.

INTESTINAL SECRETION AND LYMPH FLOW

The intestine has secretory functions in addition to its normally predominant absorptive role. Interest in secretion has greatly increased recently along with our understanding of the mechanisms of active fluid and electrolyte secretion by the enterocyte. Four established mechanisms for net fluid and electrolyte secretion are recognized: increased luminal osmolality, active electrolyte secretion, decreased electrolyte absorption, and increased hydrostatic pressure in the mucosal interstitium. Clinical examples of these four would be lactase deficiency, cholera, celiac disease, and volume expansion, respectively. The secretion by an active process such as the cyclic AMP-mediated response to cholera toxin can be compared with passive filtration secretion induced by an increase in hydrostatic pressure in the mucosal interstitium due to fluid accumulation. In the former case, the secreted fluid is devoid of protein, whereas in the latter, the interstitial fluid that enters the lumen contains appreciable amounts of protein (30).

In both forms of secretion, disturbances in the interstitium of the mucosa will ultimately alter lymph flow. In the case of active secretion, one would anticipate a water-depletion in the mucosal interstitium, a fall in interstitial hydrostatic pressure, and a rise in tissue fluid oncotic pressure. The fall in tissue fluid hydrostatic pressure would reduce lymphatic filling, and lymph flow would decrease. This prediction is borne out by the effects on intestinal lymph flow of active secretagogues such as cholera toxin, theophylline, vasoactive intestinal polypeptide, and human carcinoid serum (25,30). Similarly, cholera toxin reduces villus lacteal pressure and, presumably, villus interstitial hydrostatic pressure (50). It is interesting that colonic lymph flow does not respond in a similar way to stimulation of active secretion by theophylline (45).

On the other hand, the filtration secretion that can be produced by portal hypertension, plasma dilution, or agents that alter capillary permeability, is caused by enhanced formation of interstitial fluid in the mucosa. It appears that an imbalance in Starling forces in excess of 12 mm Hg is required to induce filtration secretion (17,56). When mucosal fluid pressure increases by 4 to 5 mm Hg, channels in the mucosal membrane open at the villus tips allowing passage of interstitial fluid containing solutes as large as albumin, and mucosal conductance increases (16,87). The effects on the mucosal membrane can be visualized with electron microscopy. For example, in plasma volume expansion, dilation of the intercellular spaces is observed (16), and infusions of prostaglandin E_1 (35) and glucagon (27) lead to villus tip erosions. These erosions would be expected to allow the passage of all macromolecules into the intestinal lumen. During both elevation of portal venous pressure and plasma dilution, lymph flow initially rises markedly, but with the onset of filtration secretion, lymph flow falls rapidly. The secondary fall in lymph flow suggests that when a low-resistance channel through the mucosal epithelium opens, interstitial fluid pressure falls and reduces the driving force for lymphatic filling (31).

INTESTINAL LYMPH AND LIPID TRANSPORT

Absorption and Transport of Ingested Lipids

The intestinal lymphatics play a special role in lipid absorption. This is strikingly demonstrated by the "milky" lymph vessels in the mesentery of a recently fed animal. The milky appearance is due to particulate fat derived from mucosal synthesis of absorbed products of fat digestion. Chylomicra are particles of fat (diameter 0.075–0.6 μm) composed mainly of triglyceride. In addition to chylomicra, large amounts of very low density lipoproteins (VLDL) are transported in intestinal lymph. Dietary triglyceride is efficiently hydrolyzed in the lumen by pancreatic lipase to monoglycerides and fatty acids (61). These are passively absorbed, and (76) triglyceride is resynthesized. A polar coat of phospholipid and lipoprotein is added, and the completed chylomicron leaves the enterocyte by reverse pinocytosis through the basolateral cell membrane (65). Microtubules may participate in the process (22). From the lateral intercellular space, the chylomicra make their way to the central lacteal of the villus, a distance of approximately 50 μm. Details of intracellular translocation of chylomicra are not well understood; even less is known of this extracellular journey. The only information is morphological. The chylomicra must first cross the basement membrane of the epithelial cells. Although gaps in the basement membrane admit the chylomicra to the lamina propria of the villus, these gaps are infrequently seen on ultrastructural examination. Furthermore, accumulations of chylomicra are often seen on either side of an apparently intact membrane (65). From consideration of the "structure" of the interstitium, one would anticipate that the relatively large chylomicra would encounter considerable resistance to flow through the lamina propria. It seems possible that they would follow some free fluid preferential channels in the interstitium *en route* to the lacteal, but pertinent morphological evidence is not available. Entry of chylomicra to the lacteal is a matter of debate because electron micrographs show both membrane-bound vesicular transport of chylomicra across the lymphatic endothelium and passage of the particles in bulk through open interendothelial gaps (13). The greater frequency of the latter appearance, however, favors this as the major route. Another route proposed by Azzali (2) involves the creation of transient channels by cytoplasmic processes arising from lymphatic endothelial cells. These channels, 8 to 14 μm in length, are arranged along the long axis of the intestinal villus. They are open at their apical end to the abluminal surface and at their basal end to the lymphatic lumen. The driving force for lymphatic uptake of chylomicra from the interstitium is unknown.

Lipid Transport During Fasting

During fasting, intestinal lymph also transports lipid mainly as VLDL from the mucosal epithelium, and the small intestine contributes approximately 30% of the circulating VLDL (68). However, chylomicra or similar particles are found in intestinal lymph of diabetic dogs (73). The source of lymph lipids in the fasting state is controversial; biliary lipids have been considered the main source. This conclusion is based on the effects of biliary diversion or cholestyramine administration on small intestinal VLDL synthesis and lymphatic transport of lipid (59). However, recent studies suggest that pancreatico-biliary secretions contain factors that stimulate intestinal triglyceride synthesis. Thus, plasma substrates may form a major source of the triglyceride of VLDL during fasting (44).

The Partition of Absorbed Lipids Between Portal Venous Blood and Intestinal Lymph

The concept that absorbed fatty acids of chain lengths greater than 12 carbon atoms are destined for transport in intestinal lymph as resynthesized chylomicron triglyceride and fatty acids of shorter chain lengths are transported in the unesterified form via the portal venous route has been faithfully preserved since the original studies (8,9). This principle, though essentially correct, requires substantial qualification. Only minor amounts of medium-chain fatty acid appear in intestinal lymph. However, Blomstrand (7) found up to 16% of absorbed decanoic acid appeared in thoracic duct lymph of rats, and it was esterified in triglycerides and phospholipids. With lauric acid, between 15% and 55% can be found in intestinal lymph. The concomitant feeding of long-chain triglyceride with medium-chain triglyceride may enhance the proportion of medium-chain fatty acids that appears in lymph (3). With respect to long-chain fatty acids longer than 14 carbon atoms, only minor proportions were transported in portal venous blood in early studies. However, a recent investigation has shown that a substantial proportion of long-chain fatty acids is transported from the rat intestine by portal venous blood (54). At low rates of delivery of fatty acid to the intestine, as much as 58% of linoleic and 69% of linolenic acid bypass the lymphatic route while only 28% of stearic acid is not carried by lymph. At higher rates of fat absorption, proportionally more of a fatty acid species is carried by lymph. Thus, both the rate of absorption and the degree of saturation of the fatty acid play a part in determining the partition.

The proportion of long-chain fatty acid transported by the portal venous route seems to increase in abnormal situations where mucosal handling of the fatty acid is impaired. Thus in puromycin-treated animals, presumed to have defective mucosal synthesis of lipoproteins, absorbed oleic acid seems to be diverted to the portal vein (42). Bile-salt deficiency also appears to divert long-chain fatty acids to the portal vein (10). In rats with bile fistulae, Saunders and Dawson (66) demonstrated that oleic acid absorption is depressed; the major proportion is transported by the portal vein. This effect, which can be reversed by supplying taurocholate, is probably due to defective mucosal esterification of the fatty acid with bile-salt deficiency (20).

Minor lipid species such as cholesterol and the fat-soluble vitamins are largely transported in lymph (4). Lipophilic xenobiotics (certain drugs and environmental pollutants) also appear to be transported as components of chylomicra in intestinal lymph (62). However, the more polar subspecies of the fat-soluble vitamins enter the portal venous blood. For example, 25-hydroxyvitamin D_3 is transported in both portal venous blood and lymph (40) whereas 1,25-dihydroxyvitamin D_3 is mainly carried in portal blood (71) as is some retinol (39). Metabolism of compounds in the enterocyte such as vitamin A produces more polar derivatives that favor portal venous transport (18). This principle may apply to a number of substances, including xenobiotics. The rate of delivery of these substances to the absorbing epithelium may determine the proportion metabolized and, hence, the principal route of transport.

Another factor determining partition of absorbed lipids between lymph and blood may be the nature of other lipid substances concurrently absorbed. For example, absorption of polyunsaturated long-chain fatty acids appears to divert concurrently absorbed retinol from the lymphatic to the portal venous route (39).

Intestinal Lymph Flow and Fat Absorption

Fat feeding has a marked intestinal lymphagogic effect (11,70,75). This enhanced lymph flow is associated with a pronounced increase in lymphatic protein flux due to a substantial escape of plasma protein from the intestinal microcirculation (85). The increase in plasma protein flux via the intestinal lymph is apparently independent of the route of transport of the absorbed lipid, since a similar effect is observed during absorption of medium-chain triglyceride (78). The effect is abolished if triglyceride in the intestine is protected from hydrolysis by pancreatic exclusion which also abolishes absorption and lymphatic transport of the triglyceride. Infusion of long-chain or medium-chain fatty acids into the duodenum enhances intestinal lymph flow and protein flux (79). Neither the changes in the intestinal microcirculation responsible for the increased fluid and protein flux nor the mechanisms bringing them about have been fully established. The enhanced capillary exchange capacity might be due to increased surface area (capillary recruitment), increased capillary permeability, or a combination of these. Using the osmotic reflection coefficient as an estimate of permeability independent of surface area, Granger et al. (33) demonstrated that cream or a bile-oleic acid mixture infused into the cat ileum increases capillary permeability. A pore size analysis suggested that the permeability change is largely due to an increase in the size of "large pores," the apparent radius increasing from approximately 200 Å to 300 Å. The morphological equivalent of "large pores" in the intestinal capillaries may be the open fenestrae (60). Neither antihistamines nor prostaglandin inhibitors affect the fat-induced change in capillary permeability, nor does local intraarterial infusion of cholecystokinin or secretin alter the capillary reflection coefficient under basal conditions (33). The lack of effect of antihistamines on capillary permeability in these studies contrasts with observations of Wollin and Jacques (86), who were able to block the capillary permeability changes in response to fat feeding in rats with a combination of H_1 and H_2 receptor antagonists. Thus, the mediators of the change in permeability are not yet clearly identified. Increased capillary surface area may contribute to intestinal lymph flow during fat absorption. There is a well-recognized rise in blood flow to the digestive organs in the postprandial period (14), and there is evidence for capillary recruitment (see Chapter 3). Moreover, the advantages of capillary recruitment during fat absorption are worthy of speculation. During absorption large quantities of plasma protein move between the blood and the mucosal interstitium. During fat absorption these proteins, while in the interstitium, could serve as vehicles for transport of unesterified fatty acids. The degree of hydration and the porosity of the mucosal interstitium may also be substantially increased during fat absorption, facilitating the movement of chylomicra to the initial lymphatic vessels.

Lymphatic Transport of Protein from the Intestine

The intestinal mucosal interstitium serves as a mixing pool for proteins derived from several sources: plasma proteins filtered from the blood, proteins synthesized in the enterocyte (notably lipoproteins and enzymes), and immunoglobulin A derived from plasma cells of the lamina propria. In addition, very small amounts of intact protein can be absorbed from the intestinal lumen. Compounds shown to be absorbed include egg albumin, various toxins (including those of *Clostridium botulinum* and *Escherichia coli*) horseradish peroxidase, ^{131}I-labeled elastase, and ^{3}H-labeled bovine serum albumin (1,21,41,53,82,83). For each of these compounds, a significant amount of the absorbed material is transported in intestinal lymph. In contrast to the adult animal, the newborn of various species are able to absorb substantial amounts of intact protein for a variable period of neonatal life. Most studies have concentrated on the physiologically important absorption of colostrum-derived immunoglobulins. Here, also, there is evidence of an important role for intestinal lymph in the transport of the absorbed protein (67).

However, in most of these studies of macromolecular absorption and transport, there is evidence for portal venous transport in addition to lymphatic transport. The proportion of a protein entering the mucosal capillaries or lymphatics is likely to depend on conditions in the interstitium during absorption. In the nonabsorbing intestine, mucosal capillaries are in filtering state. Plasma protein tends to move from the blood to the interstitium by both convection and diffusion and to be removed to a large extent by the lymphatics. However, during net fluid absorption, there may be a convective flux of protein from the interstitium to the blood (32). If this is so, the lymphatic protein flux during absorption (5,36) probably underestimates the increased escape of plasma protein. The route taken by other proteins in the interstitium, either synthesized locally or absorbed intact from the intestine, probably depends on the magnitude of concurrent fluid absorption and the concentration of the protein in the interstitium, because the oncotic pressure of the interstitial fluid tends to reduce the convective flux of proteins into the capillaries and channel them toward the lymphatics.

REFERENCES

1. Alexander, H. L., Shirley, K., and Allen, D. (1936): The route of ingested egg white to the systemic circulation. *J. Clin. Invest.*, 15:163–167.
2. Azzali, G. (1982): The ultrastructural basis of lipid transport in the absorbing lymphatic vessel. *J. Submicrosc. Cytol.*, 14:45–54.
3. Bach, A., and Métais, P. (1970): Graisses à chaines courtes et moyennes: Aspects physiologiques, biochimiques, nutritionels et thérapeutiques. *Ann. Nutr. Aliment.*, 24:75–144.
4. Barrowman, J. A. (1978): *Physiology of the Gastro-Intestinal Lymphatic System.* Monographs of the Physiological Society, Cambridge University Press, Cambridge, England.
5. Barrowman, J. A., and Roberts, K. B. (1967): The role of the lymphatic system in the absorption of water from the intestine of the rat. *Q. J. Exp. Physiol.*, 52:19–30.
6. Benson, J. A., Lee, P. R., Scholer, J. F., Kim, K. S., and Bollman, J. L. (1956): Water absorption from the intestine via portal and lymphatic pathways. *Am. J. Physiol.*, 184:441–444.
7. Blomstrand, R. (1955): Transport form of decanoic acid-1-^{14}C in the lymph during intestinal absorption in the rat. *Acta Physiol. Scand.*, 34:67–70.
8. Bloom, B., Chaikoff, I. L., and Reinhardt, W. O. (1951): Intestinal lymph as pathway for transport of absorbed fatty acids of different chain lengths. *Am. J. Physiol.*, 166:451–455.
9. Bloom, B., Chaikoff, I. L., Reinhardt, W. O., Entenman, C., and Dauben, W. G. (1950): The quantitative significance of the lymphatic pathway in transport of absorbed fatty acids. *J. Biol. Chem.*, 184:1–8.
10. Borgstrom, B. (1953): On the mechanism of intestinal fat absorption. 5. The effect of bile diversion on fat absorption in the rat. *Acta Physiol. Scand.*, 28:279–286.
11. Borgstrom, B., and Laurell, C. B. (1963): Studies on lymph and lymph-proteins during absorption of fat and saline by rats. *Acta Physiol. Scand.*, 29:264–280.
12. Brunsson, I., Eklund, S., Jodal, M., Lundgren, O., and Sjovall, H. (1979): The effect of vasodilation and sympathetic nerve activation on net water absorption in the cat's small intestine. *Acta Physiol. Scand.*, 106:61–68.
13. Casley-Smith, J. R. (1962): The identification of chylomicra and lipoproteins in tissue sections and their passage into jejunal lacteals. *J. Cell Biol.*, 15:259–277.
14. Chou, C. C., and Kvietys, P. R. (1981): Physiological and pharmacological alterations in gastrointestinal blood flow. In: *The Measurement of Splanchnic Blood Flow*, edited by G. B. Bulkley and D. N. Granger, pp. 475–509. Williams & Wilkins Co., Baltimore.
15. Code, C. F., and Pickard, D. W. (1973): The importance of the lymphatic system in the absorption of water from the intestine. *J. Physiol.*, 231:40P.
16. Dibona, D. R., Chen, L. C., and Sharp, G. W. G. (1974): A study of intercellular spaces in the rabbit jejunum during acute volume expansion and after treatment with cholera toxin. *J. Clin. Invest.*, 53:1300–1307.
17. Duffy, P. A., Granger, D. N., and Taylor, A. E. (1978): Intestinal secretion induced by volume expansion in the dog. *Gastroenterology*, 75:413–418.
18. Fidge, N. H., Shiratori, T., Ganguly, J., and Goodman, D. S. (1968): Pathways of absorption of retinal and retinoic acid in the rat. *J. Lipid Res.*, 9:103–109.
19. Fox, J. R., and Wayland, H. (1979): Interstitial diffusion of macromolecules in the rat mesentery. *Microvasc. Res.*, 18:255–276.
20. Gallagher, N., Webb, J., and Dawson, A. M. (1965): The absorption of ^{14}C oleic acid and ^{14}C triolein in bile fistula rats. *Clin. Sci.*, 29:73–82.
21. Gans, H., and Matsumoto, K. (1974): Are enteric endotoxins able to escape from the intestine? *Proc. Soc. Exp. Biol. Med.*, 147:736–739.
22. Glickman, R. M., Perrotto, J. L., and Kirsch, K. (1976): Intestinal lipoprotein formation: Effect of colchicine. *Gastroenterology*, 70:347–352.
23. Granger, D. N. (1981): Intestinal microcirculation and transmucosal fluid transport. *Am. J. Physiol.*, 240:G343–G349.
24. Granger, D. N., and Barrowman, J. A. (1983): Microcirculation of alimentary tract. I. Physiology of transcapillary fluid and solute exchange. *Gastroenterology*, 84:846–868.
25. Granger, D. N., Cross, R., and Barrowman, J. A. (1982): Effects of various secretagogues and human carcinoid serum on lymph flow in the cat ileum. *Gastroenterology*, 83:896–901.

26. Granger, D. N., Kvietys, P. R., Mortillaro, N. A., and Taylor, A. E. (1980): Effect of luminal distension on intestinal transcapillary fluid exchange. *Am. J. Physiol.*, 23:G516–G523.
27. Granger, D. N., Kvietys, P. R., Wilborn, W. H., Mortillaro, N. A., and Taylor, A. E. (1980): Mechanisms of glucagon-induced intestinal secretion. *Am. J. Physiol.*, 239:G30–G38.
28. Granger, D. N., Mortillaro, N. A., Kvietys, P. R., Rutili, G., Parker, J. C., and Taylor, A. E. (1980): Role of the interstitial matrix during intestinal volume absorption. *Am. J. Physiol.*, 238:G183–G189.
29. Granger, D. N., Mortillaro, N. A., Perry, M. A., and Kvietys, P. R. (1982): Autoregulation of intestinal capillary filtration rate. *Am. J. Physiol.*, 243:G475–G483.
30. Granger, D. N., Mortillaro, N. A., and Taylor, A. E. (1977): Interactions of intestinal lymph flow and secretion. *Am. J. Physiol.*, 232:E13–E18.
31. Granger, D. N., Parker, R. E., Quillen, E. W., Brace, R. A., and Taylor, A. E. (1977): Lymph flow transients. In: *Lymphology*, edited by P. Malek, V. Bartos, H. Weissleder, and M. H. Witte, G. Thieme, Stuttgart.
32. Granger, D. N., Perry, M. A., Kvietys, P. R., and Taylor, A. E. (1981): Interstitium-to-blood movement of macromolecules in the absorbing small intestine. *Am. J. Physiol.*, 241:G31–G36.
33. Granger, D. N., Perry, M. A., Kvietys, P. R., and Taylor, A. E. (1982): Permeability of intestinal capillaries: Effects of fat absorption and gastrointestinal hormones. *Am. J. Physiol.*, 242:G194–G201.
34. Granger, D. N., Richardson, P. D. I., and Taylor, A. E. (1979): Effects of isoprenaline and bradykinin on capillary filtration in the cat ileum. *Br. J. Pharmacol.*, 67:361–366.
35. Granger, D. N., Shackleford, J. S., and Taylor, A. E. (1979): Prostaglandin E_1-induced filtration secretion in the feline ileum. *Am. J. Physiol.*, 236:E788–E798.
36. Granger, D. N., and Taylor, A. E. (1978): Effects of solute-coupled transport on lymph flow and oncotic pressures in cat ileum. *Am. J. Physiol.*, 235:E429–E436.
37. Granger, D. N., and Taylor, A. E. (1980): Permeability of intestinal capillaries to endogenous macromolecules. *Am. J. Physiol.*, 238:H457–H464.
38. Granger, H. J. (1981): Physicochemical properties of the extracellular matrix. In: *Tissue Fluid Pressure and Composition*, edited by A. R. Hargens, Williams & Wilkins, Baltimore.
39. Hollander, D. (1980): Retinol lymphatic and portal transport: Influence of pH bile and fatty acids. *Am. J. Physiol.*, 239:G210–G214.
40. Hollander, D., Rim, E., and Morgan, D. (1979): Intestinal absorption of 25-hydroxyvitamin D_3 in unanesthetized rat. *Am. J. Physiol.*, 236:E441–E445.
41. Katayama, K., and Fujita, T. (1972): Studies on biotransformation of elastase. II. Intestinal absorption of ^{131}I-labelled elastase *in vivo*. *Biochim. Biophys. Acta*, 288:181–189.
42. Kayden, H. J., and Medick, M. (1969): The absorption and metabolism of short and long chain fatty acids in puromycin-treated rats. *Biochim. Biophys. Acta*, 176:37–43.
43. Keiding, R. (1966): Intestinal alkaline phosphatase in human lymph and serum. *Scand. J. Clin. Lab. Invest.*, 18:134–140.
44. Kotler, D. P., Shiau, Y. F., and Levine, G. M. (1980): Effects of luminal contents on jejunal fatty acid esterification in the rat. *Am. J. Physiol.*, 238:G414–G418.
45. Kvietys, P. R., Wilborn, W. H., and Granger, D. N. (1981): Effects of net transmucosal volume flux on lymph flow in the canine colon. Structural-functional relationship. *Gastroenterology*, 81:1080–1090.
46. Lam, K. Ch., and Mistilis, S. P. (1973): Role of intestinal alkaline phosphatase in fat transport. *Aust. J. Exp. Biol. Med. Sci.*, 51:411–416.
47. Lawrence, J. A., Bryant, D., Roberts, K. B., and Barrowman, J. A. (1981): Effect of secretin on intestinal lymph flow in the rat. *Q. J. Exp. Physiol.*, 66:297–305.
48. Lee, J. S. (1979): Lymph capillary pressure of rat intestinal villi during fluid absorption. *Am. J. Physiol.*, 237:E301–E307.
49. Lee, J. S. (1981): Lymph flow during fluid absorption from rat jejunum. *Am. J. Physiol.*, 240:G312–G316.
50. Lee, J. S., and Silverberg, J. W. (1973): Effect of cholera toxin on fluid absorption and villus lymph pressure in dog jejunal mucosa. *Gastroenterology*, 62:993–1000.
51. Levine, S. E., Granger, D. N., Brace, R. A., and Taylor, A. E. (1978): Effect of hyperosmolality on vascular resistance and lymph flow in the cat ileum. *Am. J. Physiol.*, 234:H14–H20.
52. Madsen, N. B., and Tuba, J. (1952): One source of alkaline phosphatase in rat serum. *J. Biol. Chem.*, 195:741–750.
53. May, A. J., and Whaler, B. C. (1958): The absorption of *Clostridium botulinum* type A toxin from the alimentary canal. *Br. J. Exp. Pathol.*, 39:307–316.
54. McDonald, G. B., Saunders, D. R., Weidman, M., and Fisher, L. (1980): Portal venous transport of long-chain fatty acids absorbed from rat intestine. *Am. J. Physiol.*, 239:G141–G150.
55. Mortillaro, N. A., Granger, D. N., Kvietys, P. R., Rutili, G., and Taylor, A. E. (1981): Effects of histamine and histamine antagonists on intestinal capillary permeability. *Am. J. Physiol.*, 240:G381–G386.
56. Mortillaro, N. A., and Taylor, A. E. (1976): Interaction of capillary and tissue forces in the cat intestine. *Circ. Res.*, 39:348–358.
57. Nelson, R. A., and Code, C. F. (1969): Absorbed water and intestinal lymph flow. *Fed. Proc.*, 28:462.
58. Noyan, A. (1964): Water absorption from the intestine via portal and lymphatic pathways in rats. *Proc. Soc. Exp. Biol. Med.*, 117:317–320.
59. Ockner, R. K., Hughes, F. B., and Isselbacher, K. J. (1969): Very low density lipoproteins in intestinal lymph: Origin, composition and role in lipid transport in the fasting state. *J. Clin. Invest.*, 48:2079–2088.
60. Palade, G. E., Simionescu, M., and Simionescu, N. (1979): Structural aspects of the permeability of the microvascular endothelium. *Acta Physiol. Scand.*, 463:11–32.
61. Patton, J. S. (1981): Gastrointestinal lipid digestion. In: *Physiology of the Gastrointestinal Tract*, Vol. 2,

edited by L. R. Johnson, pp. 1123–1146. Raven Press, New York.
62. Pocock, D. M. E., and Vost, A. (1974): DDT absorption and chylomicron transport in the rat. *Lipids*, 9:374–381.
63. Quillen, E. W., Granger, D. N., and Taylor, A. E. (1977): The effects of arginine vasopressin on capillary filtration in the cat ileum. *Gastroenterology*, 72:474–478.
64. Quin, J. W., Husband, A. J., and Lascelles, A. K. (1975): The origin of the immunoglobulins in intestinal lymph of sheep. *Aust. J. Exp. Biol. Med. Sci.*, 53:1–9.
65. Sabesin, S. M., and Frase, S. (1977): Electron microscopic studies of the assembly intracellular transport and secretion of chylomicrons by rat intestine. *J. Lipid Res.*, 18:496–511.
66. Saunders, D. R., and Dawson, A. M. (1963): The absorption of oleic acid in the bile fistula rat. *Gut*, 4:254–260.
67. Shannon, A. D., and Lascelles, A. K. (1968): Lymph flow and protein composition of thoracic duct lymph in the newborn calf. *Q. J. Exp. Physiol.*, 53:415–421.
68. Shiau, Y. F. (1981): Mechanisms of intestinal fat absorption. *Am. J. Physiol.*, 240:G1–G9.
69. Simmonds, W. J. (1954): The effect of fluid, electrolyte and food intake on thoracic duct lymph flow in unanesthetized rats. *Aust. J. Exp. Biol. Med. Sci.*, 32:285–300.
70. Simmonds, W. J. (1955): Some observations on the increase of thoracic duct lymph flow during intestinal absorption of fat in unanaesthetized rats. *Aust. J. Exp. Biol. Med. Sci.*, 33:305–313.
71. Sitrin, M. D., Pollack, K. L., and Rosenberg, I. H. (1981): Intestinal absorption of 1,25-(OH)$_2$ vitamin D$_3$ (1,25-D$_3$) in the rat. *Gastroenterology*, 80:1288.
72. Starling, E. H. (1896): On the absorption of fluid from the connective tissue spaces. *J. Physiol.*, 19:312–326.
73. Steiner, G., Poapst, M., and Davidson, J. K. (1975): Production of chylomicronlike lipoprotein from endogenous lipid by the intestine and liver of diabetic dog. *Diabetes*, 24:263–271.
74. Szwed, J. J., Maxwell, D. R., Elliott, R., and Redlich, L. R. (1977): Diuretics and small intestinal lymph flow in the dog. *J. Pharmacol. Exp. Ther.*, 200:88–94.
75. Tasker, R. R. (1951): The collection of intestinal lymph from normally active rats. *J. Physiol.*, 115:292–295.
76. Thomson, A. B. R., and Dietschy, J. M. (1981): Intestinal lipid absorption: Major extracellular and intracellular events. In: *Physiology of the Gastrointestinal Tract*, edited by L. R. Johnson, vol. 2, pp. 1147–1220. Raven Press, New York.
77. Turner, S. G., and Barrowman, J. A. (1977): The effects of cholecystokinin and cholecystokinin-octapeptide on intestinal lymph flow in the rat. *Can. J. Physiol. Pharmacol.*, 55:1391–1396.
78. Turner, S. G., and Barrowman, J. A. (1977): Intestinal lymph flow and lymphatic transport of protein during fat absorption. *Q. J. Exp. Physiol.*, 62:175–180.
79. Turner, S. G., and Barrowman, J. A. (1978): Enhanced intestinal lymph formation during fat absorption: The importance of triglyceride hydrolysis. *Q. J. Exp. Physiol.*, 63:255–264.
80. Vaerman, J. P., André, C., Bazin, H., and Heremans, J. F. (1973): Mesenteric lymph as a major source of serum IgA in guinea pigs and rats. *Eur. J. Immunol.*, 3:580–584.
81. Vaerman, J. P., and Heremans, J. R. (1970): Origin and molecular size of immunoglobulin A in the mesenteric lymph of the dog. *Immunology*, 18:27–38.
82. Warshaw, A. L., and Walker, W. A. (1974): Intestinal absorption of intake antigenic protein. *Surgery*, 76:495–499.
83. Warshaw, A. L., Walker, W. A., Cornell, R., and Isselbacher, K. J. (1971): Small intestinal permeability to macromolecules. Transmission of horse radish peroxidase into mesenteric lymph and portal blood. *Lab. Invest.*, 25:675–684.
84. Watson, P. D., Bell, D. R., and Renkin, E. M. (1980): Early kinetics of large molecule transport between plasma and lymph in dogs. *Am. J. Physiol.*, 239:H525–H531.
85. Wollin, A., and Jaques, L. B. (1973): Plasma protein escape from the intestinal circulation to the lymphatics during fat absorption. *Proc. Soc. Exp. Biol. Med.*, 142:1114–1117.
86. Wollin, A., and Jaques, L. B. (1976): Blocking of olive oil induced plasma protein escape from the intestinal circulation by histamine antagonists and by a diamine oxidase releasing agent. *Agents Actions*, 6:589–592.
87. Yablonski, M. E., and Lifson, N. (1976): Mechanism of production of intestinal secretion by elevated venous pressure. *J. Clin. Invest.*, 57:904–915.
88. Zweifach, B. W., and Silverberg, A. (1979): The interstitial-lymphatic flow system. In: *International Review of Physiology, Cardiovascular Physiology III*, edited by A. C. Guyton and D. B. Young, vol. 18, pp. 215–260. University Park Press, Baltimore.

Lymphatic Contractility

Jui S. Lee

Department of Physiology, University of Minnesota Medical School, Minneapolis, Minnesota 55455

The lymphatic system returns excess tissue fluid to the systemic circulation and is important in the maintenance of a constant plasma volume. In the small intestine, the lymphatic system also plays an important role in the absorption of fluid from the lumen. In fact, intestinal lymph flow accounts for 20% to 40% of the absorbed volume in rats and cats (6,12,18). The lymph capillaries (initial lymphatics, terminal lymphatics, or central lacteals) begin in the intestinal villi. These vessels converge to form submucosal collecting vessels, which emerge from the mesenteric border as mesenteric lymphatic ducts. These ducts were discovered by Asellius in 1622 (2) in a well-fed dog. During fat absorption, they appear as fine white threads containing milky lymph, and they are usually referred to as lacteal ducts. They run along the mesenteric arteries or veins and enter the mesenteric pedicle, which is composed of a chain of lymph glands. From the pedicle, the main intestinal lymph duct emerges and enters the thoracic duct that transports lymph to the systemic circulation.

The propulsion of lymph from its site of formation (lymph capillaries) to the systemic circulation depends on a number of factors, such as pressure gradients, arterial pulsations, muscular contractions, respiratory movements, and rhythmical contractions of the collecting lymphatic ducts. Because of one-way valves in most larger lymphatic ducts, any of these factors may promote lymph flow, as fully discussed by Drinker and Yoffey (8). The importance of intrinsic lymphatic contractions in propelling lymph from various organs has long been known; the literature has been reviewed by Yoffey and Courtice (34) and Barrowman (5). This chapter considers various aspects of mesenteric lymphatic contractility in promoting intestinal lymph flow.

HISTOLOGY OF MESENTERIC LYMPHATICS

In feline mesenteric lymphatic ducts, Carleton and Florey (7) have observed an inner endothelial layer similar to those in veins, except that the arrangement of the endothelial cells is more irregular. In a fairly large duct (150–450 μm in diameter), the wall is composed of collagen fibers, and the outermost fibers merge with those of the mesentery. Intimately mingled with the collagen fibers are smooth muscle cells. In the smaller lymphatics (~30 μm in diameter), no smooth muscle fibers are found, but these small lymphatics may still contract in response to strong electrical stimulation. In the lymphatics of most species, such as guinea pig, rat, mouse, dog, hedgehog, rabbit, and pig, smooth muscle fibers are abundant. Recently, by electron microscopy, Ohhashi et al. (28) found three layers of smooth muscle in bovine mesenteric lymphatic ducts: internal longitudinal, intermediate circumferential, and external longitudinal layers. The outermost layer is much thicker than the other two. Although there are abundant smooth muscle fibers in the larger mesenteric lymphatics of most species, spontaneous rhythmic contractions are seen only in rats and guinea pigs, but not in dog, cat, rabbit, squirrel, hedgehog, pig, mouse, or man (11). Bovine, rat, and guinea pig mesenteric lymphatics exhibit rhythmic contractions *in vitro*. Thus, they have been frequently used for studies of lymphatic contractility.

The innervation of the mesenteric lymphatics was examined by Carleton and Florey (7) in the guinea pig and squirrel. Intravital staining with methylene blue administered intraperitoneally showed that in the guinea pig the nerves run a longitudinal course along the lymphatic wall and that they are finely varicose and amyelinated. In the squirrel, the nerve fibers around larger lymphatics (~200 μm in diameter) anastomose freely and form a network. Ohhashi et al. (30) studied the innervation of bovine mesenteric lymphatics with histochemical methods. Adrenergic fibers were visualized by ths emission of a green catecholamine fluorescence induced by glyoxylic acid. Most of the varicose adrenergic fibers are distributed circularly although some run spirally or longitudinally. Some of the thick fluorescent fibers are in the adventitia; others run obliquely through the muscular coat. Some fine fibers among the smooth muscles reach the subendothelial layer. The distribution and density of these nerve fibers seem to be more dense near valves. Most of the cholinesterase-positive fibers or cholinergic fibers stained by the copper thiocholine method are oriented longitudinally. The pattern of their distribution is similar to that of the adrenergic fibers, but they are few in number.

METHODS OF STUDY

For physiological studies of the mesenteric lymphatics, several models are described below. As described by Hargens and Zweifach (14), the rat is under anesthesia; the *exteriorized mesentery* and intestine are placed on a warm stage. The area under observation is continuously superfused with physiological salt solution at body temperature. Other portions of the tissues are covered with cotton soaked with the superfusion fluid and enclosed in a plastic wrap to prevent evaporation.

An *exteriorized rat intestine preparation* as employed by Lee (17) for lymph capillary pressure studies may be also used for observing mesenteric lymphatics. The exteriorized intestine and its mesentery are placed in a warm chamber containing physiological salt solution. The test drugs and chemicals may be added to the bathing solution or given by a parenteral route. When the bathing fluid is temporarily removed, drugs may be applied topically to the lymphatics under study.

Lee (15) described an *in vitro rat intestine* preparation in which a short segment of intestine (~20 cm in length) is removed from the body with its intact mesentery and mesenteric pedicle. The preparation is placed in a warm chamber containing Krebs-Ringer solution. The lumen of the intestine is also perfused with Krebs-Ringer solution. The perfusion solution is placed in a reservoir with the fluid level about 7 cm above the intestine to set the intraluminal distension pressure at about 5 mm Hg. A pump continuously circulates the solution at a rate of ~30 ml/min. The main intestinal lymph duct is cannulated for the determination of lymph flow. Under these conditions the intestine absorbs fluid, and lymph flow is high for more than 1 hr. The segment is supported by a stainless steel screen to keep the mesentery in a horizontal position for microscopic observations of the mesenteric lymphatics. The mesenteric lymphatics exhibited spontaneous rhythmic contractions, and their behavior was found to be essentially the same as *in vivo*.

More recently, the *isolated bovine lymphatic duct* was extensively used for investigating various aspects of lymphatic contractility. Figure 1 shows the preparation of McHale and Roddie (21). A segment of lymph duct (28 mm long, 1–3 mm in diameter) is cannulated at both ends with glass cannulas. The vessel is placed in an open horizontal organ bath containing Krebs-Ringer solution gassed with 5% CO_2 in O_2 and maintained at a constant temperature (30–37°C). The inflow cannula is connected via heat exchangers to a reservoir. The height of the reservoir above the duct determines the perfusion pressure. Lymph flow is measured by a drop counter. The height of the reservoir and drop counter outflow are adjusted for zero flow when the vessel is not contracting. Ten minutes after a length of bovine lymphatic is prepared, spontaneous contractions may stabilize at a fairly constant frequency, but frequencies vary greatly

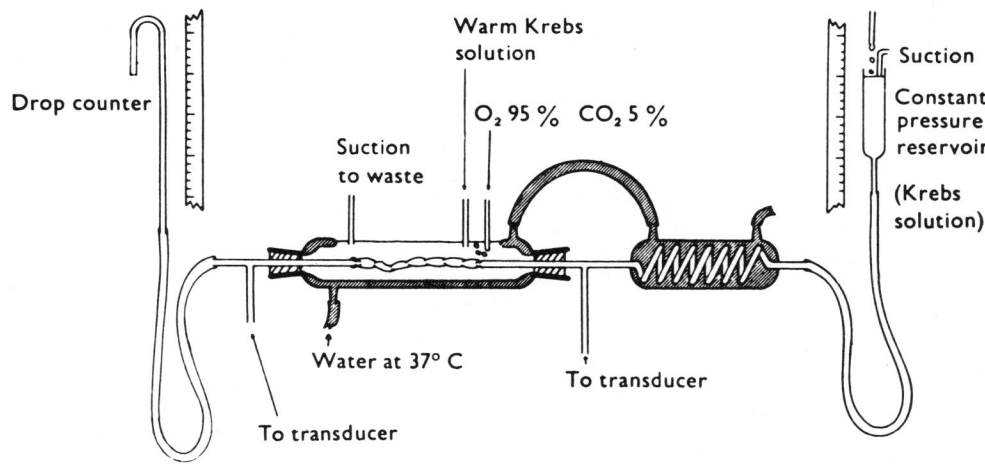

FIG. 1. A setup for perfusing isolated bovine lymphatic ducts. (From McHale and Roddie, ref. 21, with permission.)

among different lymphatics with a mean value of 2.6 beats/min (range 0.5–5.2). A similar model was described by Mislin and Schipp (25) for small guinea pig lymphatics.

Ohhashi et al. (29) have described a *bovine lymphatic strip*. Longitudinal strips (15 mm long) are prepared from mesenteric lymphatic ducts (2–5 mm in outer diameter). Each strip is placed in an organ bath containing physiological salt solution. The upper end of the strip is connected to the lever of an isotonic displacement transducer, and lower end is fixed to the bath bottom. A resting load between 100 and 200 dynes is applied to the strip. Isotonic contractions and relaxations are recorded by an electronic recorder.

EFFECT OF DRUGS OR CHEMICALS ON LYMPHATIC CONTRACTILITY

Epinephrine

Florey (11) has shown that topical applications of epinephrine increase the frequency of spontaneous contractions of cat, rat, and guinea pig lymphatics *in vivo*. Epinephrine also increases the frequency of lymphatic contractions in rats (15) and guinea pigs (25) *in vitro*. Baez (4) found that during hemorrhagic shock, spontaneous contractions of rat mesenteric lymphatics increase in frequency and become 4 to 5 times more sensitive to epinephrine. He also observed that the lymphatic reactivity to epinephrine is 15 to 20 times lower than the adjacent arteriolar reactivity. The frequency of normal spontaneous contractions, whether *in vivo* or *in vitro*, was found in the range of 2 to 19/min in the rat (4,13–15,33) or 8 to 22/min in the guinea pig (10,14,25).

Norepinephrine

Norepinephrine increases lymphatic contractility in the isolated bovine lymphatic duct (1,20,22,29). McHale and Roddie (22) also found that although norepinephrine increases the frequency of spontaneous contractions, lymph flow increases only in lymphatics with low resting flow but decreases in those with high resting flow because of a decrease in "stroke volume." However, when the drug is added to the fluid perfusing the lumen of the lymphatic, a profound depressant effect is obtained; both lymph flow and rhythmic contractions cease.

Isoproterenol

Isoproterenol is known to relax smooth muscles in the body such as vascular and intestinal muscles. It also relaxes the lymphatic musculature (20,22,29). At a dose of 50 ng/ml in an *in vitro* perfused bovine lymphatic, isoproterenol abolishes contractions within 3 min after being added to the bathing fluid (22).

Histamine

Histamine increases the frequency of spontaneous lymphatic contractions in guinea pigs (25) and in cattle (29). Its effect may be prevented by antihistamines.

Acetylcholine

Acetylcholine inhibits lymphatic contractions in guinea pigs, and its effect is not prevented by atropine (25). In bovine lymphatics, this drug may either exert no significant effect or some stimulation (3,20,29).

Anesthetics

Pentobarbital and inactin exert no effect on the frequency of lymphatic contractions in the rats and guinea pigs when these drugs are given up to 15 mg/kg body weight above their anesthetic level (14). Under *in vitro* conditions when pentobarbital sodium is added to the bathing fluid at a concentration of 15 mg/100 ml, it abolishes intestinal motility but has no effect on lymphatic contractility (16).

RESPONSE OF LYMPHATIC STRIPS TO VASOACTIVE SUBSTANCES

Ohhashi et al. (29) have carried out an extensive study of the response of bovine mesenteric lymphatic strips to various vasoactive substances. Dose-response curves to various vasoactive substances are shown in Fig. 2. Contractions of the lymphatic strips are induced by serotonin (5-HT), prostaglandin $F_{2\alpha}$ ($PGF_{2\alpha}$), norepinephrine (NA), histamine, dopamine, and acetylcholine (ACH). Serotonin and $PGE_{2\alpha}$ exert the greatest and ACh the least stimulatory effect on the lymphatic muscles. The contractile response to ACh was observed only in the valvular regions of lymphatics. Since the responses to 5-HT and histamine are completely suppressed by an antiserotonin agent (methylsergide) but are not affected by an α-adrenergic blocking agent (phentolamine), the contractions induced by these agents are apparently due to a direct stimulating action on the lymphatic muscles. Isoproterenol (ISP) is most potent in causing relaxation of lymphatic muscle. In decreasing order the relaxant effects are as follows: ISP > adenosine > ATP > ADP > cyclic AMP > AMP.

INTRALYMPHATIC PRESSURES

The pressures at various regions of the intestinal lymphatic system have been determined. In rat villi, lymph capillary pressure is about 1.4 cm H_2O, but at a high rate of absorption of hypotonic luminal fluid, it may increase to more than 5 cm H_2O (17). Lymph capillary pressure in the mesentery of cats and rats or in the omentum of rabbits (35) was found to be close to atmospheric, and it may vary between -1.0 and 3.5 cm H_2O. Pressure increases progressively in the collecting channels until the largest collecting ducts are reached. There pressures of 12 to 28 cm H_2O may be recorded. An increment in pressure as small as 1.0 to 1.5 cm H_2O is sufficient to open a closed lymphatic valve. This is, in general, the pressure differential across successive valves of the lymphatic ducts. The valve leaflets can withstand a retrograde pressure up to 27 cm H_2O without becoming incompetent. The valves of the larger bovine lymphatics (~ 3 mm O.D.) may withstand a pressure of about 70 cm H_2O without leakage (26). Thus, no reflux could occur under normal physiological conditions. Figure 3 shows a photomicrograph of a lymphatic valve.

RELATION BETWEEN INTRALYMPHATIC PRESSURE AND LYMPHATIC CONTRACTILITY

In an exteriorized mesentery of the rat under anesthesia, Hargens and Zweifach (14) have undertaken a micromanipulative study of the relation between intralymphatic pressure and lymphatic contractility. The flow of lymph is associated with an increase in lymph pressure in the segment and a progressive widening of the lymph vessel. Upon attaining a threshold pressure (5–17 cm H_2O) the vessel contracts. Obstructing lymph flow in a collecting lymphatic by an upstream microocclusion lowers both

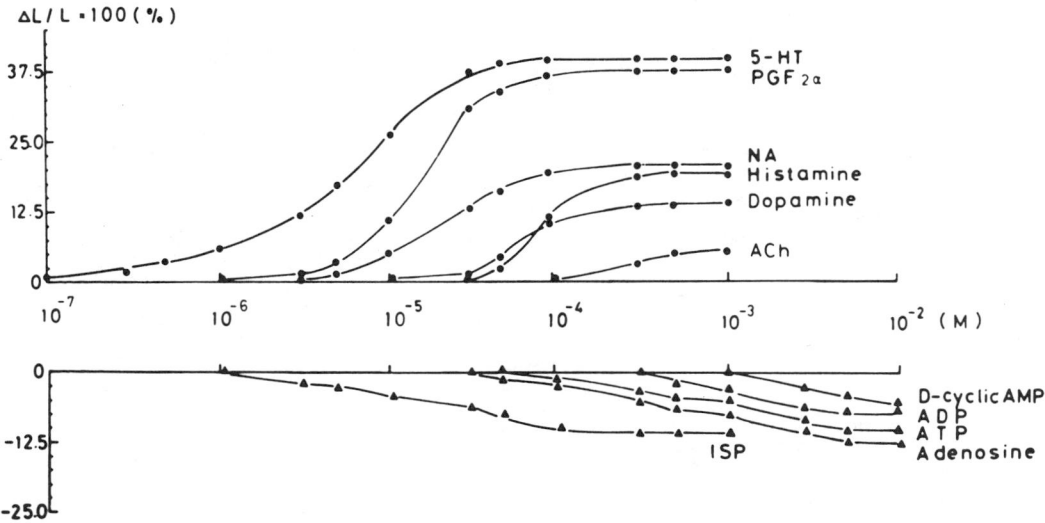

FIG. 2. Dose-response curves to vasoactive substances in bovine mesenteric lymphatics. ΔL, induced decrement (+) or increment (−) of duct length; L, resting length; 5-HT, serotonin; $PGF_{2\alpha}$, prostaglandin $F_{2\alpha}$; NA, norepinephrine; ACh, acetylcholine. (From Ohhashi et al., ref. 29, with permission.)

lymph pressure and the frequency of contraction. During total occlusion with cessation of lymph flow, lymphatics no longer contract. By inserting a micropipette (5–10 μm in diameter) into a collecting vessel, the intralymphatic pressure may be artificially increased or decreased by microinjection or withdrawal of fluid. When lymph pressure is artificially reduced to −1 cm H_2O by withdrawing lymph, spontaneous contractions cease. During the microinjection of saline to increase lymph pressure, the frequency of contractions could be increased by more than 100%. During extracellular volume loading or at spontaneously high lymph flows in the rat, lymphatic frequency always increases as reported by Granger and Zweifach (13). This is most likely due to increased intralymphatic pressure. Because a rise of lymph pressure should stretch the lymphatic wall, these observations strongly suggest that increased tension in the smooth muscle initiates contractions.

The relation between intralymphatic pressure and spontaneous lymphatic contractility has also been studied in lymphatics *in vitro*. In freshly isolated guinea pig mesenteric lymphatics (24,25), rhythmic contractile activity can be evoked by an increase in lymph pressure of 2 to 4 cm H_2O. Isolated bovine mesenteric lymphatics showed spontaneous contractions when intralymphatic pressure was maintained at 4 cm H_2O, as observed by McHale and Roddie (21). An increase in lymph pressure always increases frequency and vice versa.

Pressure-volume and pressure-radius relations in isolated bovine lymphatic segments are similar to those in the veins. The curves are nonlinear and convex toward the volume or radius axis, indicating a higher distensibility at lower pressure (26). Contractile force increases with increasing distension pressure until an optimal pressure is reached. With further increases in pressure, the contractile force decreases, but the frequency of contraction continues to increase.

NERVOUS REGULATION OF LYMPHATIC CONTRACTILITY

Florey (11) demonstrated that the mesenteric lymphatic ducts of the cat contract in response to splanchnic sympathetic nerve stimulation as well as to topically applied epinephrine. Recently, the effect of nervous factors on lymphatic contractility was examined in the isolated bovine lymphatic duct (31). A short segment of

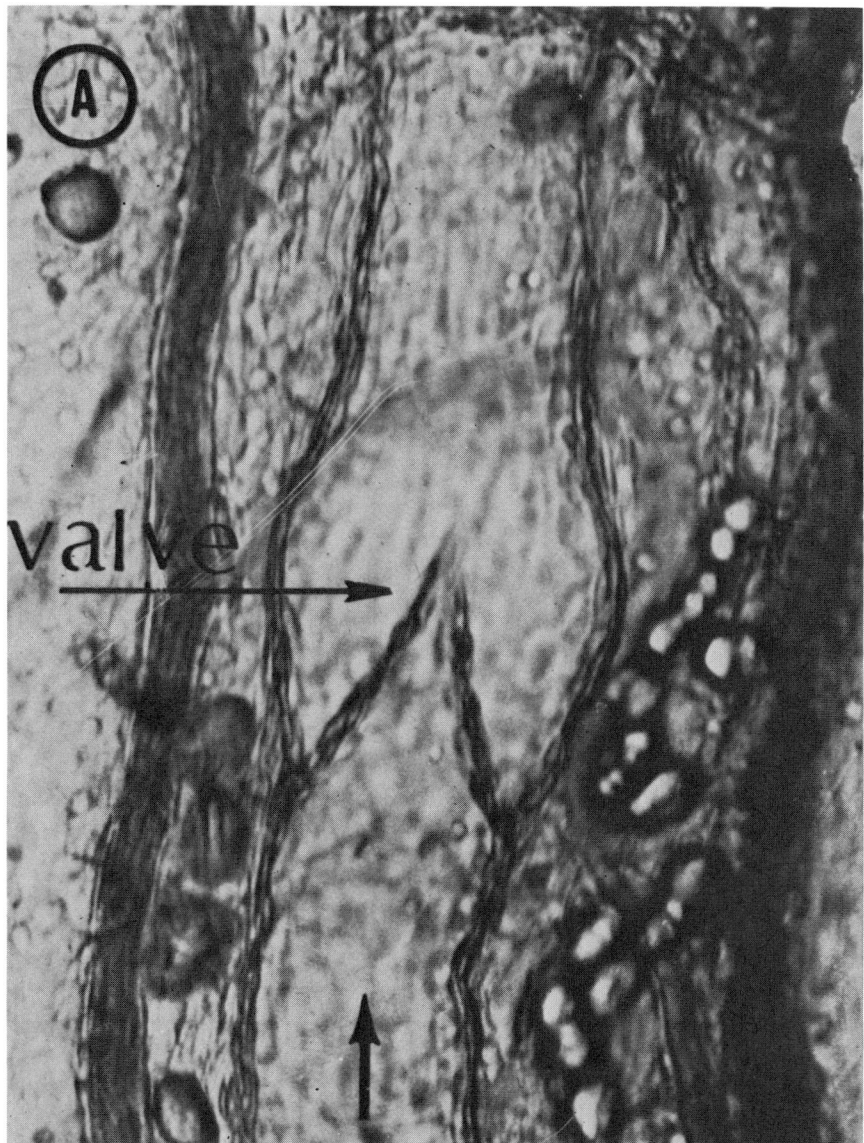

FIG. 3. Photomicrographs of valve leaflets of a collecting lymph duct in rat mesentery. **A:** During partial contraction. **B:** 3 sec later, duct is in relaxed state. (From Zweifach and Prather, ref. 35, with permission.)

the lymphatic vessel is placed in an organ bath containing physiological salt solution. Stimulating electrodes are placed in the bathing solution (not in contact with the vessel) for field stimulation of the nerves. The optimal stimuli are square wave impulses (0.1–0.4 ms in pulse width and 20–50 V) at various frequencies. Larger pulse width or voltage should not be used to avoid possible direct stimulation of the muscle. Field stimulation may elicit isometric contractions in quiescent vessels (32) or increase the frequency of contraction in those with spontaneous contractions (23). In the presence of tetrodotoxin, which paralyzes the nervous elements, these effects were not obtained. Phenoxybenzamine (an α-adrenoceptor antagonist) and propranolol

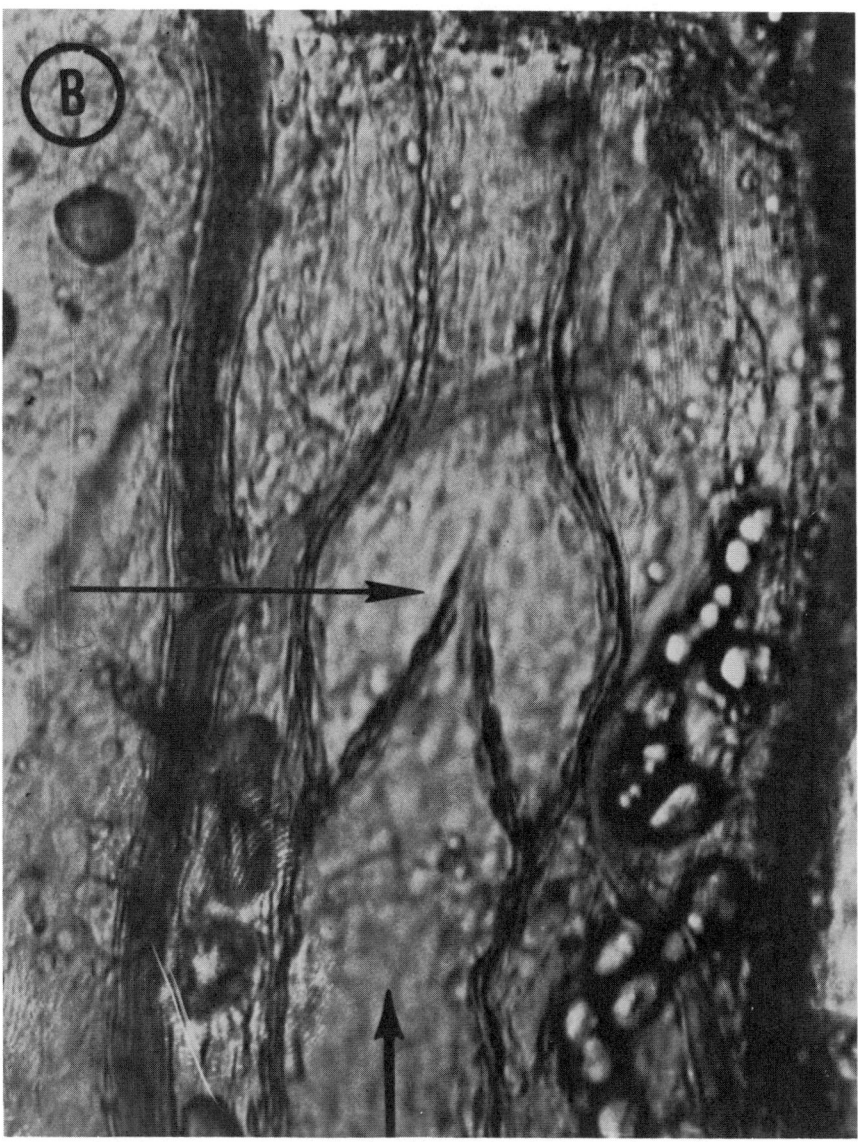

FIG. 3. *(Continued)*

(a β-adrenergic blocker) abolish and potentiate the effects of field stimulation, respectively. As shown in Fig. 4, the increased frequency of spontaneous contractions during field stimulation is more pronounced in the presence of propranolol. When both propranolol and phenoxybenzamine are present, no effect is obtained with field stimulation. These effects are expected if norepinephrine were being released during electrical stimulation of the sympathetic nerves, and they indicate clearly the existence of both α- and β-adrenoceptors in the lymphatic smooth muscle. The α excitatory effect normally predominates over a weaker β inhibitory effect. Inhibitory responses of the bovine mesenteric lymphatics were observed by Ohhashi and Roddie (32). In response to a 10-sec train of electric pulses (50 V for 0.3-ms pulse width at 2 Hz), the contraction of a lymphatic vessel is sometimes followed by a relaxation of either short or long duration. Both types of relaxation are abolished by tetrodotoxin. Propranolol re-

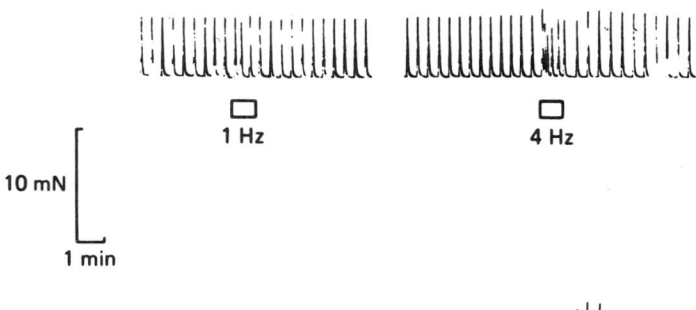
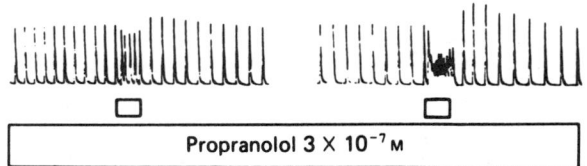
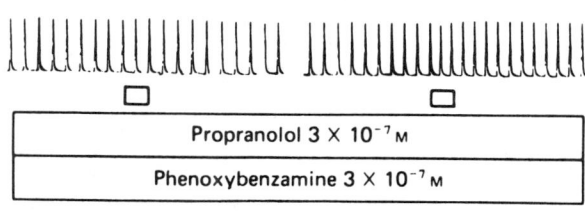

FIG. 4. Effect of field stimulation at 1 and 4 Hz *(upper record)* after addition of propranolol *(middle record)* and in the presence of both propranolol and phenoxybenzamine *(lower record)*. (From McHale et al., ref. 23, with permission.)

duces both types of relaxation but suppresses the short type more. Hexamethonium and atropine have no effect on either type of relaxation. Thus, relaxation occurs mainly in response to β-adrenergic inhibitory stimulation.

ELECTRICAL ACTIVITY OF LYMPHATIC MUSCLES

In bovine lymphatic strips, spontaneous action potentials, similar in appearance to the pacemaker potentials recorded from some other smooth muscle, have a one-to-one correspondence with the contraction waves (3). A similar relationship between action potentials and lymphatic contractility was observed in perfused bovine lymphatics (1). Each spontaneous contraction was preceded by a single action potential approximately 19 mV in amplitude. Employing intracellular electrodes, Ohhashi et al. (27) also determined the transmembrane potential in bovine lymphatic smooth muscle. The resting potential ranges from -41 to -57 mV.

ROLE OF LYMPHATIC CONTRACTILITY IN FLUID ABSORPTION FROM THE INTESTINE

One major function of the small intestine is to absorb fluid from its lumen, and a considerable fraction of the absorbed fluid is transported to the systemic circulation via the lymphatic system (5,34). In the absence of a blood supply, fluid transport in the rat is almost entirely via the lymphatic system. When the mesentery of the *in vitro* intestine is cut off, the rate of fluid absorption is significantly lower (by about 40%) than in the intestine with an intact mesentery. Segments with mesentery, mesenteric pedicle, and main intestinal lymph duct all intact have higher fluid absorption rates (by about 30%) than those with only the mesentery (15). These findings suggest that the increased rate of fluid absorption from the *in vitro* intestine with an intact lymphatic system may be mainly due to rhythmic lymphatic contractions promoting lymph flow. However, when an *in vitro* intestinal preparation was perfused at a high intraluminal distension pressure (20 mm Hg or above) as described by Fisher and Parsons (9), fluid transport no longer depended on the lymphatic system, but mostly on serosal transudation due apparently to disruption of the lymphatic system.

CONTRACTILITY OF MESENTERIC PEDICLE

The mesenteric pedicle or root of the mesentery is composed chiefly of a chain of lymph glands. The main intestinal lymph duct emerges therefrom to transport the postnodal or efferent intestinal lymph to the systemic circulation. Lee (15) has reported that in an *in vitro* rat mesentery preparation, lymph pressure in this duct was about 1.5 mm Hg, and it increased by 10% to 20% after addition of epinephrine to the bathing fluid. The amplitudes of the pressure waves increased by almost 100%. This was apparently mainly due to the increased mesenteric lymphatic contractility. However, under *in vivo* conditions when most abdominal organs (spleen, stomach, small and large intestine, omentum, and pancreas) including the mesentery were surgically removed in the rat under anesthesia, similar pressure waves were recorded from the main intestinal lymph duct *(unpublished observation)*. Therefore, these pressure waves must be the result of rhythmic contractions of the pedicle tissue or, most probably, the lymph glands. Epinephrine-induced contractions of canine intestinal lymph glands have been observed by Martin (19). Such contractions are considered to play a role in the expulsion of leukocytes. Whether or not glandular contractions could influence intestinal lymph flow remains to be studied.

REFERENCES

1. Allen, J. M., McHale, N. G., and Rooney, B. M. (1983): Effect of norepinephrine on contractility of isolated mesenteric lymphatics. *Am. J. Physiol.*, 244 (*Heart Circ. Physiol.*):H479–H486.
2. Asellius, G. (1627): *De lactibus sine lacteis venis quarto vasorum Mesarai corum genere novo invento.* Apud. Jo. Baptistam Bidellium, Mediolani.
3. Azuma, T., Ohhashi, T., and Sakaguchi, M. (1977): Electrical activity of lymphatic smooth muscle. *Proc. Soc. Exp. Biol. Med.*, 155:270–273.
4. Baez, S. (1957): Lymphatic adjustment in hemorrhagenic shock in rat. *Anat. Rec.*, 127:491.
5. Barrowman, J. A. (1978): *Physiology of the Gastrointestinal Lymphatic System.* Cambridge University Press, Cambridge.
6. Brunsson, I., Eklund, S., Jodal, M., Lundgren, O., and Sjovall, H. (1979): The effect of vasodilation and sympathetic nerve activation on net water absorption in the cat's small intestine. *Acta Physiol. Scand.*, 106:61–68.
7. Carleton, H. M., and Florey, H. (1927): The mammalian lacteal: Its histological structure in relation to its physiological properties. *Proc. R. Soc. London B*, 102:110–118.
8. Drinker, C. K., and Yoffey, J. M. (1941): *Lymphatics, Lymph and Lymphoid Tissue.* Harvard University Press, Cambridge.
9. Fisher, R. B., and Parsons, D. S. (1949): A preparation of surviving rat small intestine for the study of absorption. *J. Physiol. (Lond.)*, 110:36–46.
10. Florey, H. (1927): Observations on the contractility of lacteals, Part I. *J. Physiol. (Lond.)*, 62:267–272.
11. Florey, H. (1927): Observations on the contractility of lacteals, Part II. *J. Physiol. (Lond.)*, 63:1–18.
12. Granger, D. N., and Taylor, A. E. (1978): Effects of solute-coupled transport on lymph flow and oncotic pressure in cat ileum. *Am. J. Physiol.*, 235:E429–E436.
13. Granger, H. J., and Zweifach, B. W. (1976): Mechanics of active lymphatic pumping in rat mesentery. *Fed. Proc.*, 35:851.
14. Hargens, A. R., and Zweifach, B. W. (1977): Contractile stimuli in collecting lymph vessels. *Am. J. Physiol.*, 233:H57–65.
15. Lee, J. S. (1963): Role of mesenteric lymphatic systems in water absorption from rat intestine in vitro. *Am. J. Physiol.*, 204:92–96.
16. Lee, J. S. (1965): Motility, lymphatic contractility, and distention pressure in intestinal absorption. *Am. J. Physiol.*, 208:621–627.
17. Lee, J. S. (1979): Lymph capillary pressure of rat intestinal villi during fluid absorption. *Am. J. Physiol.*, 237:E301–E307.
18. Lee, J. S. (1981): Lymph flow during fluid absorption from rat jejunum. *Am. J. Physiol.*, 240:G312–G316.
19. Martin, H. E. (1932): Physiological leucocytosis. *J. Physiol. (Lond.)*, 75:113–129.
20. Mawhinney, H. J. D., and Roddie, I. C. (1973): Spontaneous activity in isolated bovine mesenteric lymphatics. *J. Physiol. (Lond.)*, 229:339–348.
21. McHale, N. G., and Roddie, I. C. (1976): The effect of transmural pressure on pumping activity in isolated

bovine lymphatic vessels. *J. Physiol. (Lond.)*, 261:255–269.
22. McHale, N. G., and Roddie, I. C. (1983): The effect of catecholamines on pumping activity in isolated bovine mesenteric lymphatics. *J. Physiol. (Lond.)*, 338:527–536.
23. McHale, N. G., Roddie, I. C., and Thornbury, K. D. (1980): Nervous modulation of spontaneous contractions in bovine mesenteric lymphatics. *J. Physiol. (Lond.)*, 309:461–472.
24. Mislin, H. (1976): Active contractility of the lymphangion and coordination of lymphangion chains. *Experimentia*, 32:820–822.
25. Mislin, H., and Schipp, R. (1967): Structural and functional relations of the mesenteric lymph vessels. In: *Progress in Lymphology. (Proc. Intern. Symp. on Lymphology, Zurich, Switzerland, July 19–23, 1966)*, edited by A. Ruttiman, pp. 360–365. Georg Thieme Verlag., Stuttgart.
26. Ohhashi, T., Azuma, T., and Sakaguchi, M. (1980): Active and passive mechanical characteristics. *Am. J. Physiol.*, 239:H88–H95.
27. Ohhashi, T., Azuma, T., and Sakaguchi, M. (1978): Transmembrane potentials in bovine lymphatic smooth muscle. *Proc. Soc. Exp. Biol. Med.*, 159:350–352.
28. Ohhashi, T., Fukushima, S., and Azuma, T. (1977): Vasa vasorum within the media of bovine mesenteric lymphatics. *Proc. Soc. Exp. Biol. Med.*, 154:582–586.
29. Ohhashi, T., Kawai, Y., and Azuma, T. (1978): The responses of lymphatic smooth muscles to vasoactive substances. *Pfluegers Arch.*, 375:183–188.
30. Ohhashi, T., Kobayashi, S., Tsukahara, S., and Azuma, T. (1982): Innervation of bovine mesenteric lymphatics: From the histochemical point of view. *Microvasc. Res.*, 24:377–385.
31. Ohhashi, T., McHale, N. G., Roddie, I. C., and Thornbury, K. D. (1980): Electrical field stimulation as a method of stimulating nerve or smooth muscle in isolated bovine mesenteric lymphatics. *Pfluegers Arch.*, 388:221–226.
32. Ohhashi, T., and Roddie, I. C. (1981): Relaxation of bovine mesenteric lymphatics in response to transmural stimulations. *Am. J. Physiol.*, 240:(Heart Circ. Physiol.), H498–H504.
33. Webb, R. L. (1933): Observations on the propulsion of lymph through the mesenteric lymphatic vessels of the living rat. *Anat. Rec.*, 57:345–350.
34. Yoffey, J. M., and Courtice, F. C. (1970): *Lymphatics, Lymph and the Lymphomyeloid Complex.* Academic Press, London.
35. Zweifach, B. W., and Prather, J. W. (1975): Micromanipulation of pressure in terminal lymphatics. *Am. J. Physiol.*, 228:1326–1335.

Transcapillary Exchange During Intestinal Fluid Absorption

D. Neil Granger, Michele Ulrich, Dale A. Parks, and Scot L. Harper

Department of Physiology, College of Medicine, University of South Alabama, Mobile, Alabama 36688

In most tissues (e.g., skeletal muscle) the hydrostatic and oncotic forces governing capillary fluid exchange always favor fluid movement in the direction of blood to interstitium. To maintain a constant interstitial volume, the rate of capillary filtration is balanced by an equal outflow of fluid via the lymphatics. Such an interaction between filtering capillaries and lymphatics does not occur in all capillary beds. The peritubular capillary plexus in the kidney is an absorptive vascular bed because the balance of forces governing capillary exchange favors fluid movement in the direction of interstitium to blood. Lymph (cortical) in this tissue is derived entirely from tubular reabsorbate not taken up by the peritubular capillaries (34,40).

The interaction between transcapillary and lymphatic fluid fluxes in the small bowel is unique in that intestinal capillaries alternate between periods of net fluid filtration and absorption. In the absence of solute-coupled fluid absorption by the mucosal membrane, intestinal capillaries are in a state of net fluid filtration. However, after ingestion of water or a meal, the capillaries are converted to an absorptive state. The ability of intestinal capillaries to convert from filtering to absorptive states has been attributed to alterations in the hydrostatic and oncotic pressures and the membrane parameters governing capillary fluid exchange (9,10,12,13). The aim of this chapter is to describe the series of events that occur in the intestinal interstitium, lymphatics, and capillaries when the nonabsorbing intestine is made to absorb water and electrolytes.

ROLE OF THE INTERSTITIUM

The first compartment exposed to absorbed water in the intestine is the interstitium. Accumulation of absorbed water in the interstitial spaces of the lamina propria initiates in the interstitial matrix a series of physical changes that ultimately facilitate the removal of absorbed fluid via blood and lymph capillaries. A description of the chemical composition and some of the physical properties of the interstitial matrix is presented in Chapter 16. Therefore, our discussion of this topic is limited to the physical properties that play a role in the absorptive process.

Whole organ studies using different extracellular markers (e.g., sucrose) indicate that interstitial volume in the nonabsorbing small bowel is 18 to 27 ml/100 g tissue (8,11,22,25). *In vitro* estimates of the extracellular space (ECS) in the mucosal and serosal layers of everted rat jejunum indicate that the mucosal ECS is four times smaller than that of serosa (8). The effect of net water absorption on total wall interstitial volume has been examined in autoperfused segments of cat ileum (11). As illustrated in Fig. 1, there is a positive linear correlation between interstitial volume and net fluid absorption rate. On the basis of this relationship, a doubling of interstitial volume is predicted at absorption rates greater than 1.80 ml/min × 100 g. If one assumes that the increment in interstitial volume occurs exclusively in the mucosal layer of the bowel wall and that this compartment comprises one-fourth to one-fifth the total organ interstitial volume (8), substantially larger increments

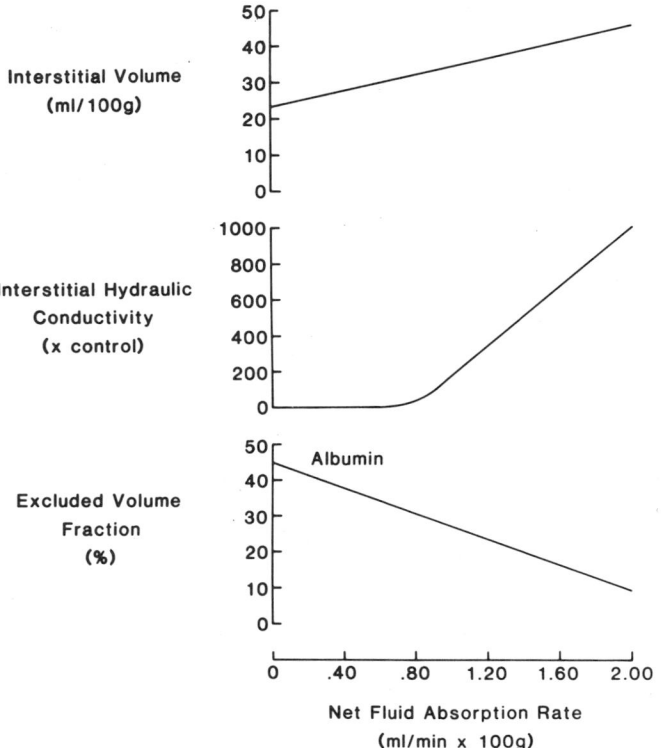

FIG. 1. Effects of net fluid absorption rate on intestinal interstitial volume, interstitial hydraulic conductivity, and the excluded volume fraction of albumin. (Data derived from Granger et al., ref. 11, and Kvietys and Granger, ref. 23, with permission.)

in interstitial volume may occur in the mucosa during absorption.

There are several physiologic consequences of the interstitial volume expansion that occurs during net fluid absorption in the intestine. These include (a) an increased hydraulic conductivity of the interstitial matrix, (b) a reduction in the ability of the interstitium to retard the diffusive and convective migration of solutes, (c) an increased interstitial hydrostatic pressure, and (d) a reduction of interstitial oncotic pressure. Because mucopolysaccharides tend to immobilize interstitial fluid, the hydraulic conductivity of the normally hydrated interstitium is quite low (11,18–20,31). *In vitro* and *in vivo* studies have clearly demonstrated that interstitial hydraulic conductivity increases greatly as matrix hydration increases. Figure 1 illustrates the effects of interstitial volume expansion caused by net fluid absorption on tissue hydraulic conductivity predicted from the aforementioned studies. This relationship indicates that interstitial hydraulic conductivity increases to approximately 200 times the nonabsorptive value at an absorption rate of 1.0 ml/min × 100 g and increases 1000-fold at a rate of 2.0 ml/min × 100 g. Such profound changes in hydraulic conductivity should allow small hydrostatic pressure gradients within the mucosal interstitium to move large amounts of fluid between the epithelia and microvessels (blood and lymph).

The effects of the interstitial matrix on solute diffusion is nearly as dramatic as its impact on the hydraulic flow of water (7,19,20). The restricted diffusion of solutes (e.g., albumin) through the normally hydrated interstitium results from the exclusion phenomenon and the frictional interaction of solutes with the matrix. The exclusion phenomenon describes the ability of a gel (e.g., the interstitium) to exclude solutes from a portion of the available intra-gel water. Macromolecules such as albumin normally distribute in only a fraction of the total matrix water volume because they cannot fit into certain parts of the meshwork with a high matrix density. In the nonabsorptive bowel, approximately 40% of the interstitial space accessible to water is not accessible to albumin (11). The interstitial volume expansion associated with fluid absorption leads to a reduction in the extent of albumin exclusion within the intestinal interstitium (Fig. 1). On the basis of albumin exclusion estimates in the nonabsorptive state, one can predict that the rate of diffusion of albumin in the interstitium is reduced by at least one-third its velocity in water because the volume or effective surface area for diffusion is limited by the exclusion effect. A further reduction of albumin movement (both diffusive and convective) through the interstitium occurs as a result of the steric interaction between the solute and that portion of the matrix that it can penetrate. A dramatic rise in the diffusive and convective movement of albumin in the matrix should occur during absorption. The degree of albumin exclusion falls to less than 10% at high absorption rates. Therefore, the area available for diffusive exchange should increase significantly. A more substantial increment in interstitial solute mobility would result from the diminished steric interaction between the solute and matrix associated with interstitial volume expansion. In fact, the equivalent pore radius of the matrix should rise from approximately 190 Å in the nonabsorptive state to over 1,000 Å in the absorptive state (11).

The most important physiologic consequence of the interstitial volume expansion associated with intestinal fluid absorption is the alteration of interstitial hydrostatic and oncotic pressures. Mathematical analyses (see Chapter 23) and results from capillary filtration studies in the intestine (33) suggest that the magnitude of the increment in interstitial volume during fluid absorption should significantly alter the interstitial forces, that is, increase interstitial hydrostatic pressure and decrease interstitial oncotic pressure. These changes enhance the removal of absorbed fluid from the lamina propria by (a) opposing further capillary filtration and converting filtering capillaries to absorbing capillaries, and (b) providing an increased hydrostatic pressure gradient for lymphatic filling.

There are relatively few estimates of interstitial hydrostatic pressure during absorption (15). The technical difficulty of directly measuring pressure within the interstitial spaces has necessitated the use of indirect approaches. Although the capsule technique has been used to measure interstitial fluid pressure in the nonabsorbing intestine (32), attempts to obtain pressures during absorption have not been reported. The size of the capsules are generally too large to be implanted into a single layer of the bowel wall (e.g., mucosa); therefore, these devices may not respond to processes that are confined to a single tissue layer, that is, fluid absorption. Two other indirect approaches have been used to estimate interstitial hydrostatic pressure during absorption—micropuncture measurements of central lacteal pressure (28) and calculation of interstitial pressure from Starling force measurements (15). Because of the highly permeable nature of the lymphatic wall, it can be assumed that central lacteal pressure should approximate interstitial hydrostatic pressure under steady state conditions. The relation between interstitial (lacteal) hydrostatic pressure and net fluid absorption rate is presented in Fig. 2. Although pressure was measured over a narrow range of absorption rates, it appears that interstitial hydrostatic pressure increases significantly as absorption rate increases, presumably owing to progressive interstitial volume expansion. Also shown in Fig. 2 are the interstitial hydrostatic pressure estimates calculated from Starling force measurements in the nonabsorptive and absorptive states (15). The values obtained using this approach also predict a significant rise in interstitial hydrostatic pressure during net fluid absorption. On the basis of this data and the reported changes in interstitial volume during fluid absorption (Fig. 1), an interstitial compliance of 3.5 ml/mm Hg is predicted. This value agrees favorably with the interstitial compliance (4.0 ml/mm Hg) reported for the same preparation during periods of enhanced capillary filtration (33).

Direct measurements of interstitial oncotic pressure changes induced by net fluid absorption have not been performed to date because

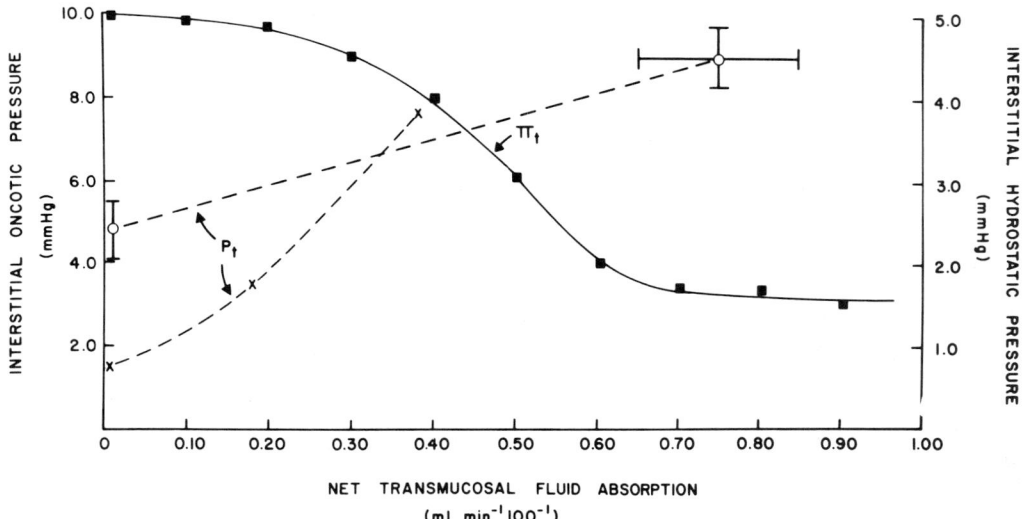

FIG. 2. Influence of net fluid absorption rate on intestinal interstitial oncotic (π_t) and hydrostatic (P_t) pressures. (X) micropuncture data obtained in rats (28); *(open circles)* whole-organ estimates (15).

of the limited size of the interstitial spaces. However, the indirect approach of using lymph oncotic pressure as an estimate of interstitial fluid oncotic pressure is widely accepted (see Chapter 16) and has been extensively applied to the small bowel (10). There are several studies that describe the influence of net fluid absorption on intestinal lymph protein concentration or lymph oncotic pressure (1–3,5,17,29,30,39,41). The results obtained from these studies indicate that interstitial (lymph) oncotic pressure is reduced by 2 to 7 mm Hg (from a normal value of 10 mm Hg) during fluid absorption. Furthermore, the results indicate that the magnitude of the reduction in interstitial oncotic pressure is dependent on net fluid absorption rate (Fig. 2). At absorption rates less than 0.30 ml/min × 100 g interstitial oncotic pressure is minimally reduced (when interstitial hydrostatic pressure is increasing). However, with higher rates of fluid absorption, interstitial oncotic pressure decreases by as much as 6 to 7 mm Hg.

The dependence of the interstitial (hydrostatic and oncotic) pressures on net fluid absorption rate has been attributed to differences in interstitial compliance at normal and increased interstitial volumes. Mortillaro and Taylor (33) have demonstrated a significant increase (0.40–4.00 ml/mm Hg) in interstitial compliance when interstitial volume is increased by more than 3.0 ml/100 g intestine due to enhanced capillary filtration. Increments in interstitial volume less than 3.0 ml/100 g produce a dramatic increase in interstitial hydrostatic pressure, yet tissue oncotic pressure is minimally altered. This contrasts with the large reductions in tissue oncotic pressure and the slight changes in interstitial hydrostatic pressure observed when interstitial volume increases by more than 3.0 ml/100 g. With net fluid absorption interstitial volume does not increase by 3.0 ml/100 g until absorption rates exceed 0.30 ml/min × 100 g, the point at which tissue oncotic pressure is significantly influenced by absorption rate. Therefore, the interstitial hydrostatic and oncotic pressure changes induced by varying absorption rates are consistent with the capillary filtration studies of Mortillaro and Taylor (33) and the hypothesis that the compliance of the interstitium increases when it is sufficiently expanded.

Yablonski and Lifson (42) have suggested that the fluid absorption-induced changes in interstitial oncotic pressure predicted from lymph measurements may underestimate the changes occurring in the pericapillary portion of the mucosal interstitium because of fluid compartmentation. Anatomically, the thin (2 μm) portion of the interstitial fluid lying between the capillary wall and basement membrane of the transporting epithelium is isolated from the bulk of the lamina propria and is approximately 50 μm from the lacteal (9,21). Therefore, estimates of hydrostatic and oncotic pressures using whole-organ approaches may not be entirely representative of the changes occurring in the juxtacapillary compartment. Compartmentation of the mucosal interstitium would provide a very sensitive mechanism for vascular removal of absorbed fluid. Because the volume of the juxtacapillary space is small, hydrostatic and oncotic pressures within this compartment would be expected to change dramatically with small increments in fluid absorption rate. Thus, compartmentation of the mucosal interstitium would allow the interstitial pressures in the juxtacapillary space to provide a larger net driving force for passive flow of water into the capillaries for a smaller change in interstitial volume than without compartmentation. Despite its attractiveness, there is no direct evidence supporting the compartmentation hypothesis.

ROLE OF THE LYMPHATICS

According to the classical view of lymph formation, the interstitial-to-initial lymphatic hydrostatic pressure gradient is the major driving force for lymphatic filling. Therefore, interstitial hydrostatic pressure is a major determinant of lymph flow. This view is supported by capillary filtration studies that indicate that intestinal lymph flow is related to interstitial hydrostatic pressure (33). The rise in interstitial pressure required for enhanced lymphatic filling is generally considered to result from interstitial volume expansion. However, intrinsic effects (e.g., active lymphatic contractility) and extrinsic influences (e.g., villus contraction and motility) can produce an occasional lacteal pressure decrease which also enhances lymph formation (26,27) (see Chapter 17).

The rise in interstitial hydrostatic pressure produced by net fluid absorption should lead to an increased rate of intestinal lymph formation. Indeed, there are numerous reports describing an increased intestinal or thoracic duct lymph flow following a meal or fluid ingestion (1–5,9). Intestinal lymph flow in the nonabsorptive state generally ranges between 0.02 and 0.06 ml/min $\times$ 100 g (10). During net fluid absorption, lymph flow can increase to as high as 0.45 ml/min $\times$ 100 g (11). The magnitude of the increase in lymph flow during fluid absorption appears to be quite variable. This variability has been attributed to factors such as tonicity of fluid placed into the lumen, portal vein pressure, intraenteric pressure, motility, and the use of lymph contaminated by contributions from other tissues (e.g., liver). If these factors are held constant or eliminated, the rate of fluid absorption becomes a major determinant of the intestinal lymph flow. The dependence of lymph flow on fluid absorption rate presumably results from the fact that interstitial volume and hydrostatic pressure are directly related to absorption rate.

The relative fraction of absorbed fluid that is removed from the mucosal interstitium by the lymphatics and capillaries has been studied by numerous investigators (1–5,9). In 1684 Leeuwenhoek (31) concluded, based on microscopic observations of the blood and lymph circulations of intestinal villi, that capillaries are the primary conduits for removal of absorbed nutrients and water. Although twentieth century estimates of the fraction of water leaving the intestine via lymph vessels range between 1% and 85% (9), most of the recent studies support Leeuwenhoek's assertion. Only at low absorption rates does the lymphatic contribution exceed 50% (see Fig. 3). At absorption rates greater than 0.20 ml/min $\times$ 100 g, the capillaries are the major route for removal of absorbed fluid from the interstitium, accounting for up to 85% of the total volume removed.

The differential role of capillaries and lymphatics in removing absorbed fluid when absorption rate is altered is consistent with the concept of a change in interstitial compliance at a low absorption rate. At low absorption rates, interstitial hydrostatic pressure increases

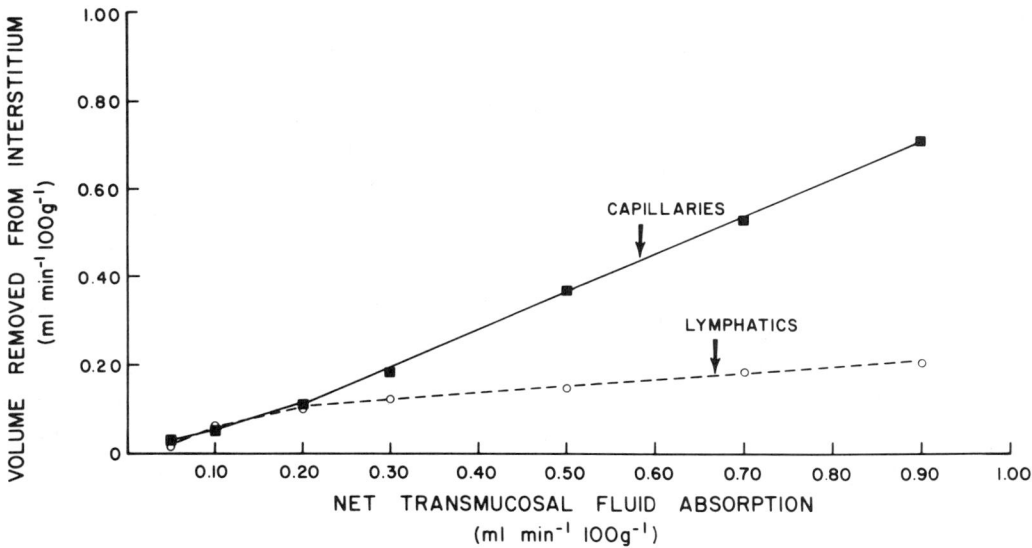

FIG. 3. Steady state relations between rate of removal of absorbed fluid by intestinal capillaries and lymphatics and net fluid absorption rate. (From Granger, ref. 9, with permission.)

but tissue oncotic pressure is virtually unaltered (Fig. 2). The increased hydrostatic pressure should preferentially drive fluid into the lymphatics because the hydraulic conductance of these vessels is greater than that of the capillaries (21). As fluid absorption rate is increased, tissue oncotic pressure falls and the driving force for capillary fluid absorption increases disproportionately to the driving force for lymphatic filling (because both interstitial forces act across the capillary wall but only the hydrostatic pressure is involved in lymphatic filling). Thus, absorbed fluid is preferentially removed via the capillaries at high absorption rates.

ROLE OF THE CAPILLARIES

Although the available evidence indicates that the change in interstitial forces induced by interstitial volume expansion is the primary event leading to vascular removal of absorbed fluid, alterations in capillary forces, surface area, and permeability appear to modify this response.

Capillary Pressure

Capillary pressure may increase during net fluid absorption because of the well-documented intestinal hyperemia associated with food ingestion or placement of nutrients into the bowel lumen (6,16). The postprandial intestinal hyperemia usually involves an increase in blood flow ranging between 10% and 60%, the magnitude of which depends on the nutrients placed in the lumen. If the reduction in vascular resistance during absorption occurs exclusively in the mucosal layer (6) and it is limited to the precapillary (arteriolar) segment of the vasculature, one might expect an increment in capillary pressure ranging between 0.5 and 3.0 mm Hg. The only available estimate of capillary pressure during absorption was derived from whole-organ gravimetric procedures and involved luminal perfusion with a glucose-electrolyte solution (15). The 16% increase in blood flow induced by glucose absorption produced a 1.1 mm Hg increase in intestinal capillary pressure. Although this increment in capillary pressure appears small and inconsequential, the fact that it is approximately one-half the net capillary absorptive force indicates that it significantly reduces the driving force for movement of absorbed fluid from the interstitium into the capillaries. The physiologic advantage of the "braking effect" of capillary pressure on capillary fluid exchange during absorption remains uncertain. However, there is evidence that large increases in capillary pressure induced by local intraarterial infusion of a selective mucosal vasodilator do not alter the absolute or relative amount of absorbed fluid removed by intestinal capillaries (5).

Plasma Oncotic Pressure

Another important intracapillary force that may influence the rate of entry of absorbed fluid into the capillary is plasma oncotic pressure. One might expect capillary oncotic pressure to be reduced if absorbed fluid enters the capillary at a rate sufficient to dilute plasma proteins, as occurs in the peritubular capillaries of the kidney. Because net fluid absorption rate is usually less than 5% of total intestinal plasma flow, it is not surprising that arteriovenous oncotic pressure differences cannot be detected in whole organ preparations. However, if estimates of villus or "absorptive site" blood flow are considered, then the extent of plasma dilution in those subepithelial capillaries involved in the absorptive process may be large. Estimates of absorptive site flow, based on inert gas clearance, indicator dilution or microsphere techniques, generally range between 5 and 8 ml/min × 100 g intestine (36). On the basis of a net water absorption rate of 1.0 ml/min × 100 g, plasma oncotic pressure is predicted to fall by 3 to 4 mm Hg owing to dilution of blood at the absorptive site. If capillary oncotic pressure is indeed reduced by this amount, the net driving force for movement of absorbed fluid from the interstitium into the capillaries will be greatly diminished along the length of the capillaries. Experimentation directly addressing this interesting possibility is warranted.

Capillary Filtration Coefficient

This membrane coefficient is a measure of the hydraulic conductance of a capillary bed and is influenced by the size and number of pores in each capillary as well as the number of perfused capillaries (10,37). Despite the potential influence of vascular permeability changes on the measurement of capillary filtration coefficients ($K_{f,c}$), changes in this parameter are usually attributed to alterations in the number of perfused (filtering) capillaries. There are several studies that demonstrate an effect of glucose-electrolyte absorption on the intestinal capillary filtration coefficient (15,24,38). $K_{f,c}$ increases by 43% to 300% during glucose absorption. The increment in $K_{f,c}$ induced by absorption is well correlated with the oxygen delivery-to-demand ratio (24). Therefore, the $K_{f,c}$ changes are likely to reflect capillary recruitment induced by metabolic factors, the concentrations of which are altered during absorption (35,38). The contention that capillary recruitment is responsible for the rise in $K_{f,c}$ associated with absorption is supported by reports that the permeability-surface area product (PS) for rubidium is also increased during absorption (35,38). Regardless of whether the absorption-induced increase in $K_{f,c}$ is entirely due to capillary recruitment or is a combination of increased vascular permeability and recruitment, the fact that capillary hydraulic conductance increases during absorption is of great physiologic importance because $K_{f,c}$ determines the imbalance in transcapillary forces that is required to move a given volume of absorbed fluid from the interstitium to blood. For example, a net absorptive force of only 2.0 mm Hg is required to move 0.60 ml/min × 100 g of fluid into the capillaries when $K_{f,c}$ is 0.30 ml/min/mm Hg/100 g (double normal), whereas a force of 4.0 mm Hg is required if $K_{f,c}$ is unchanged from control.

Vascular Permeability

Since the early studies of Borgstrom and Laurell (4) and Simmonds (39), an increased protein output in intestinal lymph has been consistently observed following food ingestion or intraluminal placement of nutrients. The effect of absorption on lymphatic protein transport is particularly pronounced during the absorption of fats. Most investigators have attributed the increased lymph protein flux to increased vascular permeability (1,17) because the magnitude of the increase (up to sevenfold) is too great to be explained by capillary recruitment. However, recent studies from our laboratory (23) demonstrate that the capillary osmotic reflection coefficient, a measure of vascular permeability, is unaltered by the absorption of glucose or electrolytes. If vascular permeability is not increased during glucose absorption, what accounts for the six- to sevenfold increments in lymph protein flux? An explanation may lie in the recent observation that $K_{f,c}$ can increase by three times normal during glucose absorption (24). A threefold increase in capillary surface area, coupled to a doubling of the diffusional gradient caused by dilution of interstitial proteins with absorbed fluid, could produce the large increments in capillary and lymph protein fluxes.

Although intestinal vascular permeability is not altered during the absorption of glucose or electrolytes, fat absorption is associated with a pronounced increase in vascular permeability (14). Estimates of the capillary osmotic reflection coefficient reveal a reduction from a normal value of 0.92 to 0.70 during fat absorption. The mechanism(s) involved in the fat absorption-induced increase in vascular permeability remain unknown. Nonetheless, it is clear that such a dramatic reduction in the reflection coefficient should modify the rate of removal of absorbed fluid via the capillaries. The osmotic reflection coefficient (σ_d) describes the fraction of the total oncotic pressure generated across the capillaries (impermeant proteins generate 100% of their maximum oncotic pressure and $\sigma_d = 1$, whereas freely permeable proteins do not generate an oncotic pressure and $\sigma_d = O$). A reduction in σ_d from 0.92 to 0.70 could decrease the effective absorptive force due to the transcapillary oncotic pressure gradient by as much as 3.0 mm Hg. A decrement in the net absorptive force of this magnitude would dramatically reduce the effectiveness of capillaries in removing absorbed fluid, provided $K_{f,c}$ remains unchanged. Since an increased vascular permeability should lead to a rise in $K_{f,c}$, it is possible that the resulting small absorptive force is still sufficient to drive fluid into the capillaries. Experiments in which $K_{f,c}$ is measured during fat absorption are warranted to test this possibility.

INTERACTIONS OF THE INTERSTITIUM, LYMPHATICS, AND CAPILLARIES DURING ABSORPTION

Our knowledge of the reactions initiated within the interstitial spaces, capillaries, and lymphatics during absorption is now sufficient to quantitatively describe the process by which absorbed fluid is removed from the intestinal interstitium. Figure 4 summarizes the changes in capillary filtration forces produced by glucose-coupled fluid absorption in the cat ileum (15). For the nonabsorptive state, there is a small (0.30 mm Hg) imbalance of forces across the capillary wall that favors net fluid filtration into the interstitium. To maintain the normal interstitial volume, the rate of capillary filtration is balanced by an equal outflow of fluid via the lymphatics. The latter assumption is confirmed experimentally by measuring lymph flow under conditions where the tissue is neither gaining nor losing weight.

Perfusion of the intestinal lumen with a glucose-electrolyte solution leads to net transmucosal fluid absorption (at a rate of 0.74 ml/min × 100 g) and a rise in interstitial volume (31%). Interstitial volume expansion produces an increase in interstitial hydrostatic pressure (2.0 mm Hg) and a reduction in interstitial oncotic pressure (1.8 mm Hg). Associated with the changes in interstitial forces are an increase in capillary pressure (1.1 mm Hg) and a doubling of capillary hydraulic conductance. Since vascular permeability is not altered by glucose absorption, the capillary reflection coefficient remains the same. The absorption-induced changes in capillary and interstitial forces modify the balance of pressures across intestinal capillaries to produce a net absorptive force of 2.3 mm Hg. This force, coupled to the elevated capillary hydraulic conductance, drives 82% of the absorbed fluid into the capillaries. Intestinal lymph flow also increases during absorption because of the increased lymphatic filling caused

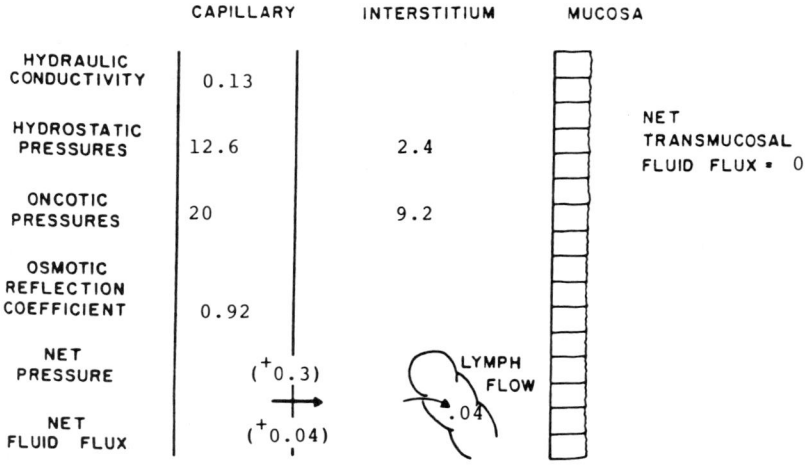

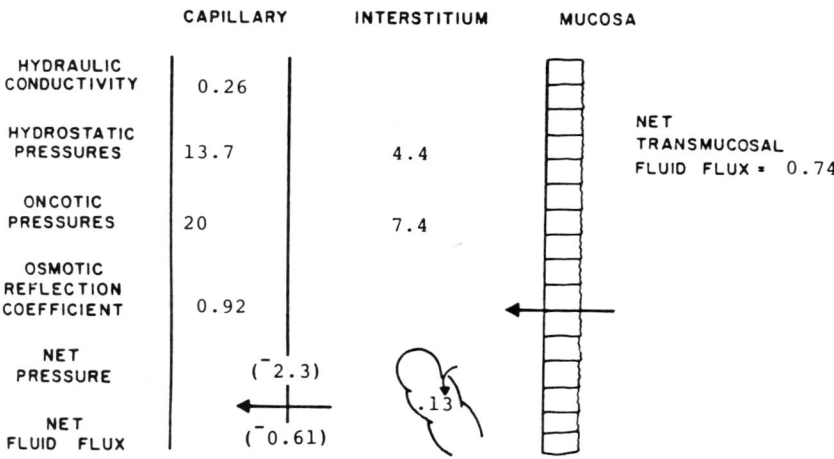

FIG. 4. Summary of capillary and interstitial forces, capillary, lymphatic, and mucosal fluid fluxes, and membrane coefficients in the nonabsorbing and absorbing small bowel. (Modified from Granger, ref. 9, with permission.)

by the rise in interstitial hydrostatic pressure. The enhanced lymph flow removes the remaining 18% of absorbed fluid from the mucosal interstitium.

It remains uncertain whether the aforementioned sequence of events, which describe glucose-electrolyte absorption, can be extrapolated to food ingestion or the absorption of other nutrients (e.g., amino acids, fats). Data in the literature indicate that fat absorption may involve different quantitative changes in capillary and interstitial forces since fat absorption increases vascular permeability and produces a greater intestinal hyperemia than glucose absorption. Complete steady state analyses of the forces governing capillary fluid exchange during the absorption of other nutrients, such as fats, are warranted. Furthermore, an attempt should be made to measure capillary and interstitial forces in the villi during absorption using microcirculatory techniques. Such studies would allow testing the concept of fluid compartmentation within the absorptive region of the bowel.

REFERENCES

1. Barrowman, J. A. (1978): *Physiology of the Gastrointestinal Lymphatic System*. Cambridge University Press, Cambridge.
2. Barrowman, J. A., and Roberts, K. B. (1967): The role of the lymphatic system in the absorption of water from the intestine of the rat. *Q. J. Exp. Physiol.*, 52:19–30.
3. Benson, J. A., Lee, P. R., Scholer, J. F., Kim, K. S., and Bollman, J. L. (1956): Water absorption from the intestine via portal and lymphatic pathways. *Am. J. Physiol.*, 184:441–444.
4. Borgstrom, B., and Laurell, C. B. (1953): Studies on lymph and lymph-protein during absorption of fat and saline by rats. *Acta Physiol. Scand.*, 29:264–280.
5. Brunsson, I., Eklund, S., Jodal, M., Lundgren, O., and Sjovall, H. (1979): The effect of vasodilation and sympathetic nerve activation on net water absorption in the cat's small intestine. *Acta Physiol. Scand.*, 106:61–68.
6. Chou, C. C., and Kvietys, P. R. (1981): Physiological and pharmacological alterations in gastrointestinal blood flow. In: *Measurements of Blood Flow. Applications to the Splanchnic Circulation*, edited by D. N. Granger and G. B. Bulkley, pp. 477–507. Williams and Wilkins, Baltimore.
7. Comper, W. D., and Laurent, T. C. (1978): Physiologic function of connective tissue polysaccharides. *Physiol. Rev.*, 58:255–315.
8. Esposito, G., Faelli, A., Tosco, M., Burlini, N., and Capraro, V. (1980): Extracellular space determination in rat small intestine by using markers of different molecular weights. *Pfluegers Arch.*, 382:67–71.
9. Granger, D. N. (1981): Intestinal microcirculation and transmucosal fluid transport. *Am. J. Physiol.*, 240:G343–G349.
10. Granger, D. N., and Barrowman, J. A. (1983): Microcirculation of the alimentary tract. I. Physiology of transcapillary fluid and solute exchange. *Gastroenterology*, 84:846–868.
11. Granger, D. N., Mortillaro, N. A., Kvietys, P. R., Rutili, G., Parker, J. C., and Taylor, A. E. (1980): Role of the interstitial matrix during intestinal volume absorption. *Am. J. Physiol.*, 238:G183–G189.
12. Granger, D. N., Mortillaro, N. A., Kvietys, P. R., and Taylor, A. E. (1980): Regulation of interstitial fluid volume in the small bowel. In: *Tissue Fluid Pressure and Composition*, edited by A. R. Hargens, pp. 173–183. Williams and Wilkins, Baltimore.
13. Granger, D. N., Perry, M. A., and Kvietys, P. R. (1983): The microcirculation and fluid transport in digestive organs. *Fed. Proc.*, 42:1667–1672.
14. Granger, D. N., Perry, M. A., Kvietys, P. R., and Taylor, A. E. (1982): Permeability of intestinal capillaries: Effects of fat absorption and gastrointestinal hormones. *Am. J. Physiol.*, 242:G194–G201.
15. Granger, D. N., Perry, M. A., Kvietys, P. R., and Taylor, A. E. (1984): Capillary and interstitial forces during absorption in the cat small intestine. *Gastroenterology*, 8:267–273.
16. Granger, D. N., Kvietys, P. R., Parks, D. A., and Benoit, J. N. (1984): Intestinal blood flow: Relations to function. *Surv. Dig. Dis.*
17. Granger, D. N., and Taylor, A. E. (1978): Effects of solute-coupled transport on lymph flow and oncotic pressures in cat ileum. *Am. J. Physiol.*, 233(*Endocrinol. Metab. Gastrointest. Physiol.* 2):E429–E436.
18. Granger, H. J. (1979): Role of the interstitial matrix and lymphatic pump in regulation of transcapillary fluid balance. *Microvasc. Res.*, 18:209–216.
19. Granger, H. J. (1980): Physicochemical properties of the extracellular matrix. In: *Tissue Fluid Pressure and Composition*, edited by A. R. Hargens, pp. 51–61. Williams and Wilkins, Baltimore.
20. Granger, H. J., and Shepherd, A. P. (1979): Dynamics and control of the microcirculation. In: *Advances in Biomedical Engineering*, edited by J. Brown, vol. 7, pp. 1–63. Academic Press, New York.
21. Kalima, T. V. (1973): Ultrastructure of the intestinal lymphatics in regard to absorption. *Scand. J. Gastroenterol.*, 8:193–196.
22. Katz, J. A., Sellers, L., Banoris, G., and Golden, S. (1970): Studies on the extravascular albumin of rats. In: *Plasma Protein Metabolism*, edited by M. Rothschild and P. Waldmonn, chapt. 8, pp. 129–154. Academic, New York.
23. Kvietys, P. R., and Granger, D. N. (1983): Role of the microcirculation in intestinal transmucosal fluid transport. In: *Microcirculation of the Alimentary Tract—Physiology and Pathophysiology*, edited by A. Koo, pp. 241–252. World Scientific Publishing Co., Singapore.
24. Kvietys, P. R., Perry, M. A., and Granger, D. N. (1983): Intestinal capillary exchange capacity and oxygen delivery-to-demand ratio. *Am. J. Physiol.*, 245:G635–G640.
25. Larsson, M., Johnson, L., Nylander, G., and Ohman, U. (1979): Plasma water and ^{51}Cr EDTA equilibration volume of different tissues in the rat. *Acta Physiol. Scand.*, 110:53–57.
26. Lee, J. S. (1969): A micropuncture study of water transport by dog jejunal villi *in vitro*. *Am. J. Physiol.*, 217:1528–1533.
27. Lee, J. S. (1971): Contraction of villi and fluid transport in dog jejunal mucosa *in vitro*. *Am. J. Physiol.*, 221:488–495.
28. Lee, J. S. (1979): Lymph capillary pressure of rat intestinal villi during fluid absorption. *Am. J. Physiol.*, 237:E301–307.
29. Lee, J. S. (1981): Lymph flow during fluid absorption from rat jejunum. *Am. J. Physiol.*, 240:G312–G316.
30. Lee, J. S., and Duncan, K. M. (1968): Lymphatic and

venous transport of water from rat jejunum: a vascular perfusion study. *Gastroenterology*, 54:559–567.
31. Leeuwenhoek, A. V. (1684): Anatomy of the slime within the guts and the use thereof. *Philos. Trans. R. Soc. London*.
32. Mortillaro, N. A. (1977): Intestinal interstitial fluid pressure and its relationship to intestinal volume. *Physiologist*, 20:66 (abstract).
33. Mortillaro, N. A., and Taylor, A. E. (1976): Interaction of capillary and tissue forces in the cat small intestine. *Circ. Res.*, 39:348–358.
34. Navar, L. G., Evan, A. P., and Rosivall, L. (1983): Microcirculation of the kidneys. In: *The Physiology and Pharmacology of the Microcirculation*, edited by N. A. Mortillaro, vol. 1, pp. 397–488. Academic Press, New York.
35. Pawlik, W. W., Fondacaro, J. D., and Jacobson, E. D. (1980): Metabolic hyperemia in canine gut. *Am. J. Physiol.*, 239(*Gastrointest. Liver Physiol.* 2):G12–G17.
36. Redfors, S., Sjovall, H., Jodal, M., and Lundgren, O. (1983): Intramural blood flow distribution in the small intestine of the cat studied by carbon monoxide uptake and [85]Krypton elimination. *Acta Physiol. Scand.*, 118:97–107.
37. Richardson, P. D. I., and Granger, D. N. (1981): Capillary filtration coefficient as a measure of perfused capillary density. In: *Measurement of Blood Flow: Application to the Splanchnic Circulation*, edited by D. N. Granger and G. B. Bulkley, pp. 319–336. Williams and Wilkins, Baltimore.
38. Shepherd, A. P. (1979): Intestinal capillary blood flow during metabolic hyperemia. *Am. J. Physiol.*, 237(*Endocrinol. Metab. Gastrointest. Physiol.* 6):E548–E554.
39. Simmonds, W. J. (1955): Some observations on the increase in thoracic duct lymph flow during intestinal absorption of fat in unanesthetized rats. *Aust. J. Exp. Biol. Med. Sci.*, 33:305–313.
40. Taylor, A. E. (1981): Capillary fluid filtration. Starling forces and lymph flow. *Circ. Res.*, 49:557–571.
41. Turner, S. G., and Barrowman, J. A. (1977): Intestinal lymph flow and lymphatic transport of protein during fat absorption. *Q. J. Exp. Physiol.*, 62:175–180.
42. Yablonski, M. E., and Lifson, N. (1976): Mechanism of production of intestinal secretion by elevated venous pressure. *J. Clin. Invest.*, 57:904–915.

Capillary Fluid Exchange and Intestinal Secretion

David Mailman

Biology Department, University of Houston, Houston, Texas 77004

Intestinal secretion is frequently considered a pathologic condition. An example is the diarrhea of cholera. Secretion is also a normal physiological response; secretions dilute a hypertonic meal in the jejunum (36). Secretion can be either active or passive. Active secretion is a transcellular, energy-requiring process that is associated with certain pathological events such as bacterial enterotoxins or increased plasma levels of certain hormones. Passive secretion is primarily a paracellular process that depends on cardiovascular parameters in the intestinal mucosa and that may be associated with pathological or normal stimuli. However, active secretion is indirectly affected by the same factors that directly determine passive secretion.

The source of fluid for both active and passive secretion *in vivo* is obviously the blood. Thus, the rate of secretion can be no greater than plasma flow past the secretory site. However, Starling forces in the blood and tissues can greatly affect the net rate of secretion. The magnitude of these forces depends, in part, on regional capillary blood flow and pressure. Moreover, blood flow provides the O_2 and nutrients to support active secretion and absorption.

PASSIVE SECRETORY MECHANISMS

Capillary Exchange Processes

Blood flow and pressure influence fluid movement across the intestinal mucosa. There is continuous and significant movement of most small molecules, up to approximately the size of glucose, in both a secretory and absorptive direction between the gut lumen and the blood with the smaller molecules exchanging faster than the larger ones. The difference between the two unidirectional fluxes determines the net flux. Alterations in mucosal blood flow and pressure can change both unidirectional fluxes equally, resulting in no change in net flux, or can change one unidirectional flux more than the other, resulting in an increase in net absorption or secretion (55,56). In general, the rate of blood flow per se alters diffusive exchange. Diffusive exchange does not alter net transport because the absorptive and secretory fluxes are affected equally unless a concentration difference of the substance exists between the blood and the lumen or interstitial space (37,55). An additional effect of blood flow is related to the delivery of O_2 to the intestinal epithelial cells (24) for the support of active transport. Frequently, changes in blood flow are associated with capillary pressure changes that affect the rate of ultrafiltration between blood and the lumen. The rate of both ultrafiltration and diffusive exchange are also partially determined by the permeability and conductivity of the mucosal tissues (15,38,39).

Diffusion Exchange

The magnitude of blood flow partly determines the rate of delivery or "washout" of solutes and H_2O from the interstitial space by altering the concentration gradients between the plasma and lumen (55,56). The diffusion rate of a substance to which capillary and tissue barriers are relatively impermeable is almost completely determined by the permeability of the mucosa. Thus, its fluxes are independent of blood flow. At the other extreme, a very diffusible substance can reach near-equilibrium between the plasma and lumen. Thus, its fluxes will be determined almost completely by the rate of blood flow. The magnitude of the solute flux relative to blood flow is determined by the number and permeability of the significant barriers to diffusion and the sizes of the compartments between the lumen and blood (55). The absorption of substances with intermediate degrees of permeability will vary between blood-flow dependence at low blood flows and blood-flow independence (diffusion-limited) at high blood flows.

Net Transport

The net movement of a substance between the blood and lumen implies either a diffusional process with a concentration gradient or a process dependent on other forces such as active transport or blood pressure. If active absorption is reduced enough, net secretion may occur if there is a concurrent secretory force such as active secretion or pressure-driven ultrafiltration. These forces are superimposed on the diffusional exchange. Given a certain magnitude of forces creating net transport, the rate of transport will depend on the conductances of the compartments through which the transport is occurring. The magnitude of the conductances themselves can vary depending on the rate and direction of net fluid movement because fluid fluxes alter the degree of hydration of the interstitial matrix, the width of the lateral intercellular spaces, and the integrity of tight junctions (15,23,36).

Net fluid transfer across capillaries is controlled by the interaction of Starling forces (tissue and plasma colloid osmotic and hydrostatic pressures) and the hydraulic conductance of the capillaries. Net fluid loss from capillaries into the interstitium tends to increase when capillary pressure or tissue colloid pressure increases and when tissue hydrostatic or plasma colloid pressure decreases. Capillary conductance influences net flux only when the Starling forces are not balanced. Estimating these forces from whole-gut studies is difficult because of the possibility of heterogeneity. Gore and Bohlen (14) found that capillary pressure in the rat villus averaged 14 mm Hg but was 24 mm Hg in the muscularis.

Interstitial Space

In a manner analogous to the capillary, hydrostatic and colloid osmotic pressures in the interstitial compartment alter net fluid movement across the mucosa. The magnitudes of these tissue forces and the tissue conductance are uncertain. In addition, the conductance of the interstitial matrix varies with its degree of hydration. The fibers of the intercellular matrix during nonabsorptive conditions are packed closely enough to exclude proteins from a large fraction of the total extracellular volume (15,20). During entry of fluid into the interstitial space, interstitial fluid volume increases from about 25% to 45%. The excluded volume for albumin decreases from about 40% to 10% of interstitial space when net fluid absorption increases from 0 to about 2 ml/min·100 g (20). As the degree of hydration of the interstitium increases, the spacing of the matrix increases, thus increasing its conductance 1,000-fold. The hydration state of the interstitial matrix can be changed by any factor that alters the rate of entry of fluid from either the plasma or the lumen, provided readjustments of the other forces do not remove the excess fluid. An additional complication is that the colloids interact with the mucopolysaccharides of the interstitial matrix, so that the effective colloid osmotic pressure is greater than their sum (7). Precise quantitative estimates of the tissue colloid osmotic pressures are difficult, but recent attempts are described in Chapter 18.

One estimate of tissue colloid osmotic pressure can be obtained by collecting lymph. However, lymph collected from the gut is a mixture from the various layers of the gut. The volume of lymph that comes from the absorptive portion of the mucosa is unknown. An upper level (20–40%) of the volume of absorbed fluid that enters the lymph has been estimated from the increase in lymph flow when absorption and blood flow are varied over a wide range (4). An estimate of 1% to 2% is obtained by determining the amount of ^3H_2O in the lumen that equilibrates with the lymph (39,56). The increased absorption of solutes may raise lymph flow by stimulating lymph production in nonmucosal areas. If so, lymph colloid osmotic pressure may not represent the mucosal interstitium. If mucosal lymph flow is a small fraction of the total, colloids in lymph will not be representative of mucosal colloids. There may also be sufficient resistance to flow and sieving within the interstitial matrix so that lymph pressure and protein concentration represent minimal values; the average interstitial values may be greater. Lymphatic pressure varies from about 1 cm H_2O during both nonabsorptive conditions and during absorption of Ringer solution up to about 5 cm H_2O during rapid absorption of hypotonic solutions (15). Lymph flow initially increases during procedures that cause passive secretion, for instance, saline infusion or venous pressure elevation, but decreases as intestinal secretion continues (21). This could reflect an increase in mucosal permeability, which drains off the increased interstitial fluid that was entering the lymph.

As tissue hydration increases, tissue pressure also increases. Tissue compliance increases in two stages. At low levels of hydration, compliance is low and a small increase in hydration causes a marked increase in pressure. With further hydration, the increase in pressure is less and pressure approaches a maximum. Therefore, the hydrostatic pressure of the interstitial space would be most sensitive to hydration changes in its nonabsorptive condition. The resting level of tissue pressure is still uncertain, but is probably between -2 and $+2$ mm Hg. The small amount of vascular filtration that takes place during nonabsorptive conditions is carried out of the tissue spaces by lymph flow. When the Starling forces favor net secretion, tissue pressure rises inducing increased lymph flow that removes the fluid and thus moderates the rise in tissue pressure. The tissue colloid osmotic pressure, which is about 10 mm Hg under nonabsorbing conditions, falls about 5 mm Hg as lymph flow increases to a maximum (15).

Mucosal Capillaries

The relative contribution of colloid osmotic pressure in either the blood plasma or tissue requires a measure of the reflection coefficient of the capillary membrane. If the capillaries are relatively impermeable to colloids, they will have a reflection coefficient near 1.0, and the theoretical maximum colloid osmotic pressure will be exerted across the capillary membrane. The value of the reflection coefficient can be estimated from the lymph (L) to plasma (P) protein concentration ratio at high lymph flow rates where the ratio becomes independent of lymph flow (see Chapter 18). The L/P ratio is about 0.92, indicating that about 90% of the theoretical colloid osmotic pressure is expressed across the capillary wall. However, it is not certain what fraction of the lymph comes from the absorptive site. Therefore, the specific reflection coefficient of capillaries at the absorptive site is unknown.

Capillary filtration is also a function of both the number of perfused capillaries and the hydraulic conductance of the capillary wall. Capillary filtration coefficient (K_f), a measure of both effective capillary surface area and conductance, decreases when venous pressure is elevated (29), during α-adrenergic stimulation and during angiotensin or serotonin infusion (47). K_f is increased by ischemia (18) or β-adrenergic stimulation (47). The increased filtration during ischemia is due both to increased numbers of perfused capillaries, based on increased lymphatic protein flux (18), and increased ^{86}Rb clearance from the plasma (50), and to increased capillary conductance, based on decreases in the colloid osmotic reflection coefficient (22).

Movement of fluid into or out of the plasma will alter the concentration of plasma proteins. The change in colloid osmotic pressure is disproportionate to the change in protein concentration. For example, increasing the protein concentration by 50% causes a 100% increase in colloid osmotic pressure. Thus, this increase acts as a mechanism for slowing the loss of fluid from the plasma; a similar effect may also occur in the interstitial space (7).

One significant problem in quantitating the various forces involved is that the effective mucosal blood flow to the absorptive site is not known with certainty (37). Estimates based on microsphere distribution, washout curves, and clearances of highly permeable compounds from the blood or lumen yield values of 5% to 60% of total blood flow. Part of the problem may be in determining what portion of the mucosa is involved with net and unidirectional movement between the lumen and the blood. Is it all or part of the villus, and are the crypts involved (8)? Another factor is a possible villus countercurrent exchange mechanism that "shunts" substances across the base of the villus between entering arterioles and draining capillaries or veins (2). Oxygen would be shunted across from arteriole to venule thus reducing the effective O_2 delivery to the absorptive cells of the villus. Absorbed solutes may be shunted from venule to arterioles and thus be sequestered in the villus. Thus, anatomical and functional mucosal blood flow may not be identical.

Passive Secretion

Perhaps the most direct method of inducing passive secretion across the intestinal mucosa is by infusing saline intravenously, which raises capillary pressure and dilutes out plasma colloids. Several studies have shown that the net secretion during volume expansion is due primarily to an increase in the unidirectional secretory flux into the lumen. Absorptive site blood flow remains nearly constant, but blood flow to the remainder of the gut increases by about 300% (10,41). The major cause of increased capillary pressure is increased venous pressure. Interstitial fluid volume and pressure increase, and the fractional excluded volume for tissue protein decreases (20).

Another direct method for inducing passive secretion is to increase capillary pressure by raising mesenteric *venous pressure*. Passive secretion begins to occur at a venous pressure above about 35 cm H_2O (57). Lymph flow and mucosal hydration also begin to increase above this threshold venous pressure value, suggesting that net entry of fluid into the interstitial space has increased. Hydration of nonmucosal regions of the gut increases in direct proportion to venous pressure without a threshold. This suggests there is a mucosal autoregulatory mechanism that reduces net plasma fluid loss into the tissue spaces as capillary pressure increases to a threshold value, but that this mechanism is not present in nonmucosal tissue.

A possible complication in interpreting the results of certain experiments is that the absorptive or secretory exchange compartment may be highly restricted within the mucosa (57). The villous capillaries lie within a few micrometers of the base of the epithelial cells, and their fenestrae face the epithelium. Local changes within the volume between the capillaries and epithelium may be the initial response to external perturbations of Starling forces and to changes in epithelial absorption or secretion. Small changes in fluid entry or loss from this restricted compartment could make this a very sensitive region for controlling transcapillary and mucosal fluxes.

Wells and Johnson (54) directly observed the intestinal mucosa and measured absorption during several experimental conditions. The resting, absorbing gut had a low, intermittent blood flow. Following feeding or local irritation, the gut became engorged with blood with varying degrees of reduced blood flow and venous congestion, and either arteriolar dilation or constriction. These conditions were associated with lower absorption or net secretion. The secretion was attributed to passive ultrafiltration caused by increased capillary pressure. Atropine reduced secretion in association with reduced portal venous pressure. It was pointed out in these studies that absorption of other substances such as glucose could still occur in the face of net volume secretion of salt and water.

Generally, changes in blood flow and Starling forces occur concomitantly, so it is difficult to separate effects of blood flow from those of driving forces (17). Changes in blood flow could affect secretion by limiting the volume that can be secreted or by limiting the O_2 supply that supports active secretion or absorption. The

Starling forces could modify transepithelial fluxes as previously described. Mailman (40) attempted to separate the individual contributions of blood flow and Starling forces by measuring unidirectional Na and H_2O fluxes and absorptive site blood flow (the clearance of ^3H_2O). Blood flow was altered by mesenteric artery or vein occlusion and by intraarterial infusion of the vasodilator Na nitroprusside. The absorptive fluxes of Na and H_2O were primarily dependent on absorptive site blood flow. The secretory flux of Na was mainly affected by capillary pressure, but the secretory flux of H_2O was affected by both absorptive site blood flow and capillary pressure. The effect of blood flow on the absorptive Na fluxes was mainly determined by O_2 delivery because the absorptive Na flux was much more dependent on blood flow than the secretory Na flux. Water fluxes were primarily dependent on flow-limited delivery and exchange and thus were largely passive.

ACTIVE SECRETORY RESPONSES

Active Secretion

Active intestinal secretion is generally but not always associated with stimuli that increase mucosal cyclic AMP. Certain bacterial enterotoxins, in particular cholera, and the gut hormone vasoactive intestinal polypeptide (VIP) increase both cyclic AMP and active secretion. The site of active secretion is not known with certainty. Cells in the crypts, or in both crypts and villi, are possible sources (8). During active secretion *in vitro*, the lateral spaces between the epithelial cells are closed and electrical resistance increases, indicating that mucosal conductivity is reduced. There is little agreement concerning the effect on effective mucosal blood flow during active secretion. Increased, decreased, and unchanged blood flows have been observed using several different techniques, different stimuli for active secretion and different species (39). Active secretion, *in vivo*, would initially draw fluid from the interstitial space thus reducing interstitial pressure and increasing tissue colloid osmotic pressure. This effect would tend to reduce net secretion by increasing the forces promoting passive absorptive fluxes during active secretion. At the same time, however, these changes in the interstitial forces will increase the rate of net transcapillary filtration, which will, in turn, partially support continued net secretion by moderating the forces promoting passive absorption. A similar response would be expected from passive secretion into hypertonic luminal fluid.

Donowitz et al. (9), using microspheres, studied the effects of both active (cholera toxin and serotonin) and passive (hypertonic mannitol) secretagogues on ileal mucosal plus submucosal blood flow. Secretion was not associated with significant changes in blood flow. However, increased absorption following methylprednisolone was associated with increased mucosal plus submucosal blood flow as well as increased flow to other abdominal organs. The authors concluded that changes in mucosal-submucosal blood flow were not necessarily correlated with net fluid secretion.

Hexamethonium (a ganglionic blocker), tetrodotoxin, and luminal lidocaine prevent the secretion induced by cholera toxin. In addition, hexamethonium prevents secretion following sodium deoxycholate. These findings suggest that a neural component is involved in the effects of both agents (5,30). Loperamide and propranalol block cholera toxin-induced secretion but not the increase in cyclic AMP. The secretory effect, but not the cyclic AMP increase, caused by cholera toxin is decreased by somatostatin and both are reduced by morphine (12). Cholera toxin and sodium deoxycholate increase active secretion through an increase in mucosal cyclic AMP. The inhibition of secretion by agents that inhibit neural action with or without changes in cyclic AMP suggests that other processes in the gut may override secretion. These processes may have direct effects on the secreting cell to inhibit active secretion. Alternatively, since there is neural control over the intestinal vasculature, passive secretory mechanisms may be altered and indirectly reduce secretion.

Drug and Hormone Effects

Because various drugs or hormones affect blood flow, motility, and cell function, it is difficult to determine the direct and indirect effects of such agents on transport and secretion. Directly altering motility or active transport can indirectly alter blood flow because of changes in metabolic O_2 demand. Conversely, changes in blood flow can indirectly affect oxygen-requiring gut functions. These interactions make analysis of the regulation of secretion difficult.

Small intestinal secretion is normal in several species of mammals and, in the upper intestine of many animals, secretion causes isotonic dilution of hypertonic meals (36). It is not well known what proportion of these secretions are active or passive, or whether changes in effective mucosal blood flow support or restrict net volume flow.

Several hormones or neurotransmitters are known to increase secretion *in vitro* apparently by increasing active secretion. If these agents affect blood flow or pressure *in vivo*, they could potentiate or reduce their own effects on transcellular secretion. *Cholinergic*, muscarinic agents, or adrenergic antagonists increase secretion both *in vivo* and *in vitro* (26,27,42,43), but the effect on total blood flow is variable because of variable effects on visceral smooth muscle tension (6,53). *Sympathectomy* causes increased secretion and the villi become engorged from vasodilatation as judged by direct microscopic observation (54). *Vagotomy* causes vasoconstriction in the villi and a decrease in total mesenteric blood flow (44) and increased absorption (54). Total blood flow during neural stimulation is not correlated with absorption since β-adrenergic stimuli do not alter absorption but increase total blood flow. However, α-adrenergic stimuli increase absorption but reduce total blood flow (4). In other experiments, sympathetic nerve stimulation did not affect villous blood flow, as judged by isotope dilution analysis, but total blood flow fell (51). There is an apparent conflict between sympathetic stimulation not changing villous blood flow and sympathectomy causing engorged villi, which may be due to technical differences or local muscosal regulatory mechanisms.

Atropine prevents the secretion following cholinergic stimuli and, by itself, can increase gut absorption in humans and rats *in vivo* and *in vitro* (26,27,42). In the dog, intravenous atropine can increase effective mucosal blood flow. Both the unidirectional secretory and absorptive water fluxes increase equally following intravenous atropine in the dog and thus net absorption is not changed (37) in contrast to the human and rat response. Atropine also prevents the secretory effect of luminal bile-oleic acid but not the disrupted villi and the increases in total gut blood flow and O_2 consumption. These were caused by luminal bile-oleic acid both before and after atropine (31). The reversal of secretion by atropine, even with injured villi, allows the possibility that local passive vascular absorption may be as significant as active transcellular absorption. Perhaps, under these conditions, excess leakage of proteins from the interstitial space into the lumen further lowers tissue colloid osmotic pressure and enhances passive absorption into the capillaries.

Neural interactions with hormone effects also occur. *Glucagon* generally increases secretion or reduces absorption, although this response is partly dependent on the dose, species, and region of the gut (39). Glucagon does not affect absorption *in vitro* and thus probably does not affect transcellular secretion (28). Glucagon increases total blood flow, but this response is potentiated by atropine (3), allowing the possibility that muscarinic neural compensation reduces the direct effects of glucagon. The major effect of glucagon on absorption appears to be mediated through cardiovascular changes. Pawlik et al. (45) measured total blood flow and the fractional distribution to the mucosa-submucosal beds with microspheres. Glucagon apparently increases blood flow, pressure, and ultrafiltration across the mucosa. Direct microscopic observation showed similar effects (25). Granger et al. (19) measured increases in total blood and lymph flow, capillary filtration coefficient, and protein concentration in lymph and secreted fluid during glucagon infusion. They concluded that glucagon increased mucosal capillary pressure and capillary permeability. The capillary reflection coefficient decreased, as judged by an increase in the lymph-to-plasma protein concentration ratio, which was further evidence that capillary permeability as well as the number of perfused capillaries increased. Glucagon also increased mucosal permeability as judged by the appearance of gaps in the villous epithelium observed with scanning electron microscopy. MacFerran and Mailman (33) also concluded that close intraarterial glucagon infusion increased absorptive site blood flow (estimated ^3H_2O clearance), and the calculated capillary pressure. However, glucagon infused intraarterially into an adjacent gut segment, vascularly isolated from the test segment, had generally opposite effects, as compared to the direct intraarterial infusion. Thus, the indirect systemic effects following recirculation of glucagon and the local direct vasodilating effect of glucagon were apparently opposite. The indirect effects may be related to the muscarinic compensation mentioned above or to the observation that α-adrenergic antagonists reverse the effect of intraarterial glucagon to increase the capillary filtration coefficient (48). The autonomic involvement may be stimulated by the fall in blood pressure.

Prostaglandins increase cyclic AMP levels and fluid secretion both *in vivo* and *in vitro*. Thus, the secretion has been considered active like that of cholera toxin (1). However, the presence of protein in the luminal secretion induced by prostaglandin is anomolous; active secretion is protein-free. Granger et al. (23) studied hemodynamic changes, lymph flow, and protein fluxes during prostaglandin-induced secretion. Lymph flow increased and then decreased during intestinal secretion (changes characteristic of passive secretion), and proteins entered the lumen. Ultrastructural analysis by scanning and transmission electron microscopy showed marked disruption of the villous tips and desmosomal disruption, which suggested erosion due to increased intercellular pressure. Intraluminal PGE_1 increases both the unidirectional absorptive and secretory ^3H_2O fluxes (1), which suggests increasing absorptive site blood flow (13) and pressure (37,40). Intraluminal $PGF_{2\alpha}$ increased the secretory H_2O flux but decreased the absorptive fluxes; this may reflect decreased effective mucosal blood flow but increased mucosal capillary pressure. Increased capillary pressure is consistent with the villous damage mentioned above. Thus, even agents that increase cyclic-AMP-mediated active secretion may have significant, if not primary, effects of causing passive secretion *in vivo*.

VIP is another gut hormone thought to cause active secretion through a cyclic-AMP-mediated process both *in vivo* and *in vitro*. VIP infused intravenously in the dog decreased absorptive site blood flow measured as ^3H_2O clearance (34), but it did not change villous blood flow in the rat as determined by direct microscopic observation (25). As with glucagon, some of the effects of VIP may be related to systemic hypotension because both atropine and guanethidine reduce the vascular effects of intravenous VIP (34), but atropine did not block the effect of intraarterial VIP (11). There was a negative correlation between estimated capillary pressure and the secretory Na fluxes, suggesting that passive ultrafiltration under the influence of Starling forces was not a significant factor in VIP-induced secretion (34). This view is reinforced by the observation that VIP reduces lymph flow (16).

Intestinal *ischemia* causes secretion that is associated with loss of villous epithelial cells and villous capillary congestion (49). Ischemia-induced ultrafiltration may, therefore, be responsible for the secretion. However, in ischemia, small solutes and India ink do not pass beyond the crypts or enter the lumen because of obstruction of the villous capillaries. Damage to the villi created by luminal agents reduces absorption but does not cause secretion. Because ischemia reduces active organic transport and the absorptive Na flux, but not the secretory flux, Robinson et al. (49) felt that the secretion was due to the loss of absorptive villous tip cells and, in addition, active secretion by crypt cells.

Most gastrointestinal hormones reduce intestinal absorption or cause secretion. A combination of gastrin, secretin, cholecystokinin, glucagon, and gastric inhibitory peptide, at levels that are present post-prandially, caused net secretion (46).

In both fed and fasted dogs (35), *pentagastrin*, intravenously, reduced absorption, owing primarily to increases in the secretory fluxes of Na and H_2O, and secondarily to decreases in the absorptive fluxes. Absorptive site blood flow decreased in fasted but not in fed dogs. There were proportional changes in mucosal blood flow and the absorptive fluxes. A proportional decrease in blood flow and absorptive fluxes could be due to pentagastrin decreasing active absorption, which, in turn, reduced oxygen utilization and, consequently, blood flow. Alternatively, if pentagastrin reduced blood flow and oxygen delivery, then active absorption could in turn be limited. Pentagastrin also reduced the proportionality between the secretory fluxes of Na and H_2O and the estimated capillary pressure. This suggests that passive ultrafiltration was not responsible for the increased secretion, but that either active secretion could have been stimulated or that mucosal permeability was increased. Atropine inhibited the effects of pentagastrin, but guanethidine potentiated these effects; net secretion occurred at a dose of gastrin that only reduced absorption in the absence of guanethidine. Therefore, pentagastrin probably exerts much of its effects on intestinal absorption and blood flow through stimulation of the autonomic nervous system.

Histamine probably causes passive intestinal secretion through cardiovascular effects. Intraarterial histamine increases lymph flow (a characteristic of passive secretion) (16) and initially increases blood flow to both muscularis and mucosa-submucosa, but total blood flow gradually declines toward control primarily owing to decreases to the mucosa-submucosa (52). Lee and Silverberg (32) studied the effects of intraarterial histamine and found intestinal edema, protein in the secreted fluid, and entry of dye into the lumen from the blood. They also noted that arterial pressure had to be reduced below about 40 mm Hg before there was a reduction in secretion. These findings are consistent with filtration caused by decreases in the pre- to postcapillary resistance ratio or to increased capillary permeability.

Summary

Capillary plasma flow at the intestinal secretory site provides the substrate for both active and passive secretion. The rate of passive secretion is altered when Starling forces in the mucosal capillaries and interstitial space change. The conductances of the capillaries, interstitial space, and epithelium both affect and are affected by the rate of fluid movement between the blood and lumen. Active secretion is a transcellular process in which cellular mechanisms transport salts and water, originating in the plasma, from the interstitial space to the lumen. Active secretion can be inhibited or supported by concurrent changes in the same forces that affect passive secretion. Certain drugs and hormones have been shown to alter active or passive intestinal secretion, but the mechanism of other agents has not yet been defined.

REFERENCES

1. Beubler, E., and Juan, H., (1977): The function of prostaglandins in transmucosal water movement and blood flow in rat jejunum. *Naunyn Schmiedebergs Arch. Pharmacol.*, 299:89–94.
2. Bond, J. H., Levitt, D. G., and Levitt, M. D. (1977): Quantitation of countercurrent exchange during passive absorption from the dog small intestine. *J. Clin. Invest.*, 59:308–318.
3. Bowen, J., Pawlik, W., and Fang, W. (1975): Pharmacologic effects of gastrointestinal hormones on intestinal oxygen consumption and blood flow. *Surgery*, 78:515–519.
4. Brunsson, I., Eklund, S., Jodal, M., Lundgren, O., and Sjovall, H. (1979): The effect of vasodilation and sympathetic nerve activation on net water absorption in the cats small intestine. *Acta Physiol. Scand.*, 106:61–68.
5. Cassuto, J., Jodal, M., Tuttle, R., and Lundgren, O. (1981): On the role of intramural nerves in the pathogenesis of cholera toxin-induced intestinal secretion. *Scand. J. Gastroenterol.*, 16:377–384.
6. Chou, C. C., and Gallavan, R. H. (1982): Blood flow and intestinal motility. *Fed. Proc.*, 41:2090–2095.
7. Diana, J. W. (1982): Transcapillary water flux. *Physiologist*, 25:365–375.
8. Donowitz, M., and Madara, J. L. (1982): Effect of

extracellular calcium depletion on epithelial structure and function in rabbit ileum: A model for selective crypt or villous epithelial cell damage and suggestion of secretion by villous epithelial cells. *Gastroenterology*, 83:1231–1243.
9. Donowitz, M., Wicklein, D., Reynolds, D., Hynes, R., Charney, A., and Zinner, M. (1979): Effect of altered intestinal water transport on rabbit ileal blood flow. *Am. J. Physiol.*, 236:E482–E487.
10. Duffy, P. A., Granger, D. N., and Taylor, A. E. (1978): Intestinal secretion induced by volume expansion in the dog. *Gastroenterology*, 75:413–418.
11. Eklund, S., Jodal, M., Lundgren, W., and Sjoquist, A. (1979): Effects of vasoactive intestinal polypeptide on blood flow, motility and fluid transport in the gastrointestinal tract of the cat. *Acta Physiol. Scand.*, 105:461–68.
12. Farack, U., M., Kautz, U., and Loeschke, K. (1981): Loperamide reduces the intestinal secretion but not the mucosal CAMP accumulation induced by cholera toxin. *Naunyn Schmiedebergs Arch. Pharmacol.*, 317:178–179.
13. Fondacaro, J. D., Walus, K. M., Schwaiger, M., and Jacobson, E. D. (1981): Vasodilation of the normal and ischemic canine mesenteric circulation. *Gastroenterology*, 80:1542–1549.
14. Gore, R. W., and Bohlen, H. G. (1977): Microvascular pressures in rat intestinal muscle and mucosal villi. *Am. J. Physiol.*, 233:H685–H693.
15. Granger, D. N. (1981): Intestinal microcirculation and transmucosal fluid transport. *Am. J. Physiol.*, 240:G343–G349.
16. Granger, D. N., Cross, R., and Barrowman, J. A. (1982): Effects of various secretagogues and human carcinoid serum on lymph flow in the cat ileum. *Gastroenterology*, 83:896–901.
17. Granger, D. N., Kvietys, P. R., Mailman, D., and Richardson, P. D. I. (1980): Intrinsic regulation of functional blood flow and water absorption in canine colon. *J. Physiol.*, 307:443–451.
18. Granger, D., Kvietys, P., and Perry, M. (1982): Role of exchange vessels in the regulation of intestinal oxygenation. *Am. J. Physiol.*, 242:G570–G574.
19. Granger, D. N., Kvietys, P. R., Wilborn, W. H., Mortillaro, N. A., and Taylor, A. E. (1980): Mechanism of glucagon-induced intestinal secretion. *Am. J. Physiol.*, 239:G30–G38.
20. Granger, D. N., Mortillaro, N. A., Kvietys, P. R., Rutili, G., Parker, J. C., and Taylor, A. E. (1980): Role of the interstitial matrix during intestinal volume absorption. *Am. J. Physiol.*, 238:G183–G189.
21. Granger, D. N., Mortillaro, N. A., and Taylor, A. E. (1977): Interactions of intestinal lymph flow and secretion. *Am. J. Physiol.*, 232:E13–E18.
22. Granger, D. N., Sennett, M., McElearney, P., and Taylor, A. (1980): Effect of local arterial hypotension on cat intestinal capillary permeability. *Gastroenterology*, 79:474–480.
23. Granger, D. N., Shackelford, J. S., and Taylor, A. E. (1979): PGE_1-induced intestinal secretion: Mechanism of enhanced transmucosal protein efflux. *Am. J. Physiol.*, 236:E788–E796.
24. Granger, H. J., and Nyhof, R. A. (1982): Dynamics of intestinal oxygenation: Interactions between oxygen supply and uptake. *Am. J. Physiol.*, 243:G91–G96.
25. Holliger, C., Radzyner, M., Villiger, A., and Knoblauch, M. (1979): Effects of glucagon, vasoactive intestinal peptide (VIP) and lysine-vasopressine on villous microcirculation and superior mesenteric artery blood flow of the rat. *Bibl. Anat.*, 18:129–131.
26. Hubel, K. A. (1976): Intestinal ion transport: Effect of norepinephrine, pilocarpine and atropine. *Am. J. Physiol.*, 231:252–257.
27. Hubel, K. A., and Shirazi, S. (1982): Human ileal ion transport *in vitro*: Changes with electrical field stimulation and tetrodotoxin. *Gastroenterology*, 83:63–68.
28. Isaacs, P. E. T., and Turnberg, L. A. (1977): Failure of glucagon to influence ion transport across human jejunal and ileal mucosa in vitro. *Gut*, 18:1059–1061.
29. Johnson, P., and Hanson, K. (1966): Capillary filtration in the small intestine of the dog. *Circ. Res.*, 19:766–773.
30. Karlstrom, L., Cassuto, J., Jodal, M., and Lundgren, O. (1981): The effect of hexamethonium on the secretion induced by sodium deoxycholate in the rat jejunum. *Experentia*, 37:991–992.
31. Kvietys, P. R., Wilborn, W. H., and Granger, D. N. (1981): Effect of atropine on bile-oleic acid induced alterations in dog jejunal hemodynamics, oxygenation, and net transmucosal water movement. *Gastroenterology*, 80:31–38.
32. Lee, J. S., and Silverberg, J. W. (1976): Effect of histamine on intestinal fluid secretion in the dog. *Am. J. Physiol.*, 231:793–798.
33. MacFerran, S. N., and Mailman, D. (1977): Effects of glucagon on canine intestinal sodium and water fluxes and regional blood flow. *J. Physiol.*, 266:1–12.
34. Mailman, D. (1978): Effects of vasoactive intestinal polypeptide on intestinal absorption and blood flow. *J. Physiol.*, 279:121–132.
35. Mailman, D. (1980): Effects of pentagastrin on intestinal absorption and blood flow in the anaesthetized dog. *J. Physiol.*, 307:429–442.
36. Mailman, D. (1981): Fluid and electrolyte absorption. In: *Gastrointestinal Physiology*, edited by L. R. Johnson, 2nd ed. pp. 107–122. C. V. Mosby Co. St. Louis, Missouri.
37. Mailman, D. (1981): Tritiated water clearance as a measure of intestinal absorptive site and total blood flow. In: *Measurement of Blood Flow: Applications to the Splanchnic Circulation.*, edited by D. N. Granger, and G. B. Bulkley. Williams and Wilkins Co. Baltimore.
38. Mailman, D. (1982): Blood flow and intestinal absorption. *Fed. Proc.*, 41:2096–2100.
39. Mailman, D. (1982): Relationships between intestinal absorption and hemodynamics. *Annu. Rev. Physiol.*, 44:43–55.
40. Mailman, D. (1984): Pharmacological and hormonal influence on gastrointestinal regional blood flow. *Fed. Proc.*, 43:7–15.
41. Mailman, D., and Jordan, K. (1975): The effect of saline and hyperoncotic dextran infusion on canine ileal salt and water absorption and regional blood flow. *J. Physiol.*, 252:97–113.
42. Morris, A. I., and Turnberg, L. A. (1980): The influ-

ence of a parasympathetic agonist and antagonist on human intestinal transport in vivo. *Gastroenterology*, 79:861–866.
43. Morris, A. I., and Turnberg, L. A. (1981): Influence of isoproterenol and propranolol on human intestinal transport in vivo. *Gastroenterology*, 81:1076–1079.
44. Padula, R., Noble, P., and Camishion, R. (1968): Vascularity of the mucosa of the small intestine after vagotomy and splanchnicectomy. *Surg. Gynecol. Obstet.*, 122:41–48.
45. Pawlik, W. W., Fondacaro, J. D., and Jacobson, E. D. (1980): Metabolic hyperemia in canine gut. *Am. J. Physiol.*, 239:G12–G17.
46. Poitras, E., Modigliani, R., and Bernier, J. J. (1980): Effect of a combination of gastrin, secretin, cholecystokinin, glucagon, and gastric inhibitory polypeptide on jejunal absorption in man. *Gut*, 21:299–304.
47. Richardson, P. D. I. (1974): Drug induced changes in capillary filtration coefficient and blood flow in the innervated small intestine of the anaesthetized cat. *Br. J. Pharmacol.*, 52:481–498.
48. Richardson, P. D. I. (1975): The effects of glucagon and pentagastrin on capillary filtration coefficient in the innervated jejunum of the anaesthetized cat. *Br. J. Pharmacol.*, 54:225P.
49. Robinson, J. W. L., Winistorfer, B., and Mirkovich, V. (1980): Source of net water and electrolyte loss following intestinal ischaemia. *Res. Exp. Med.*, 176:263–275.
50. Shepherd, A. (1982): Role of capillary recruitment in the regulation of intestinal oxygenation. *Am. J. Physiol.*, 242:G435–G441.
51. Svanvik, J. (1973): Mucosal hemodynamics in the small intestine of the cat during regional sympathetic vasoconstrictor activation. *Acta Physiol. Scand.*, 89:19–29.
52. Walus, K. M., Fondacaro, J. D., and Jacobson, E. D. (1981): Mesenteric vascular reactivity to histamine receptor agonists and antagonists. *Dig. Dis. Sci.*, 26:438–443.
53. Walus, K. M., and Jacobson, E. D. (1981): Relation between small intestinal motility and circulation. *Am. J. Physiol.*, 241:G1–G15.
54. Wells, H. S., and Johnson, R. G. (1934): The intestinal villi and their circulation in relation to absorption and secretion of fluid. *Am. J. Physiol.*, 109:387–402.
55. Winne, D. (1970): Formal kinetics of water and solute absorption with regard to intestinal blood flow. *J. Theor. Biol.*, 27:1–18.
56. Winne, D. (1979): Influence of blood flow on intestinal absorption of drugs and nutrients. *J. Pharm. Thero.*, 6:333–393.
57. Yablonski, M. E., and Lifson, N. (1976): Mechanism of production of intestinal secretion by elevated venous pressure. *J. Clin. Invest.*, 57:904–915.

Permeability Characteristics of Intestinal Capillaries

*Michael A. Perry and **D. Neil Granger

*School of Physiology and Pharmacology, University of New South Wales, Kensington, NSW, 2033, Australia; and **Department of Physiology, College of Medicine, University of South Alabama, Mobile, Alabama 36688

The capillaries of the small intestine are predominantly fenestrated and ultrastructurally appear to be highly permeable. A very permeable vascular bed in the intestine is consistent with the primary function of this organ, which is the absorption of fluid and nutrients. However, the removal of absorbed fluid from the mucosal interstitium would be enhanced by a transcapillary oncotic pressure gradient that would draw fluid into the capillary lumen. The existence of such a gradient would require the intestinal capillaries to be relatively impermeable to plasma proteins. The capillaries of the small intestine appear to possess both these attributes, that is, they are very permeable to small solutes and at the same time restrict the movement of plasma proteins (16,35).

The permeability characteristics of the intestinal capillaries have been investigated by a number of different techniques. Small solute permeability has been studied with the osmotic transient and multiple indicator dilution techniques; macromolecule permeability has been investigated by steady state analysis of lymph and plasma samples as well as by the rate of washout of protein from the intestinal vasculature. In this chapter, we describe briefly each of the techniques used to assess vascular permeability in the intestine and review the information that each approach provides. The various applications of vascular permeability data to pore theory (including conditions that alter intestinal capillary permeability) are also described. Data obtained in the small intestine are compared with values obtained for other predominantly fenestrated capillary beds, such as the stomach, colon, and pancreas, as well as with the continuous capillary beds of the hindpaw or skeletal muscle.

PERMEABILITY OF INTESTINAL CAPILLARIES TO SMALL SOLUTES

Indicator Dilution Studies

Theory

The indicator dilution technique involves the injection of a mixture of tracers into the arterial supply of an organ and collection of venous samples at 0.5- to 2.0-sec intervals. The injected mixture contains a vascular tracer (i.e., one that during a single transit through the organ does not leave the vasculature) and one or more diffusible tracers that cross the capillary wall and distribute both in the intravascular volume and in part of the extravascular volume (Fig. 1, *left-hand panel*). The venous concentration curves obtained following the injection of a single bolus containing a vascular and a diffusible marker are represented in Fig. 1 (*upper right-hand panel*). Comparison of the relative concentration (relative to its concentration in the injected bolus) of the diffusible tracer (C_{diff}) to that of the vascular tracer (C_{ref}) gives the proportion of the diffusible molecule that left the circulation. This proportional loss is termed extraction (Fig. 1, *lower right-hand panel*) and is calculated as follows:

$$E = (C_{ref} - C_{diff})/C_{ref}. \quad (1)$$

The permeability-surface area product (PS) for the diffusible solute is calculated from the ex-

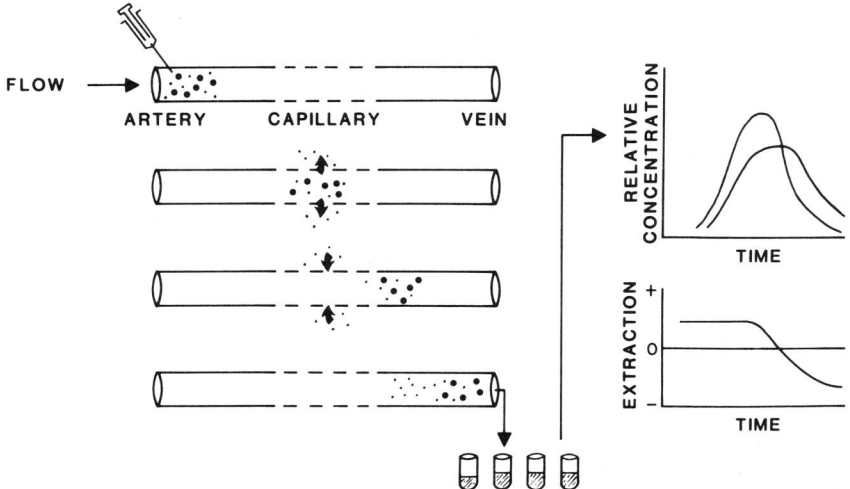

FIG. 1. Schematic representation of the extraction of a diffusible solute *(small dot)* relative to a vascular tracer *(large dot)* as the bolus of injected material passes through the vasculature. The relative concentrations of the two tracers in venous samples are shown in the *upper right-hand panel* and the pattern of extraction of the smaller tracer in the *lower right-hand panel* (From Granger and Perry, ref. 10, with permission.)

traction (E) and the plasma flow rate through the organ $(\dot{Q}_p)$ by an equation described originally by Renkin (38):

$$PS = \dot{Q}_p \ln(1 - E) \qquad (2)$$

Inclusion of two diffusible solutes in the injected bolus allows a comparison of the simultaneous estimates of PS for each diffusible solute. Under these conditions, the perfused capillary surface area (S) and plasma flow rate are the same for both solutes and $P_1/P_2 = \ln(1 - E_1)/\ln(1 - E_2)$. If both solutes diffuse freely from the circulation into a large extravascular volume without restriction at the capillary wall, then P_1/P_2 will be equal to the ratio of their respective free diffusion coefficients (D_1/D_2). However, if the larger of the two diffusible solutes (P_2) is restricted to some degree by the capillary wall, then P_1/P_2 will be greater than D_1/D_2. The degree of restricted diffusion $(P_1/P_2 \div D_1/D_2)$ can be used to calculate an "equivalent" or "effective" pore radius by the use of an equation that describes the effects of steric hindrance and frictional resistance on the diffusion of a solute through a cylindrical pore in the absence of hydraulic flow through the pore (37). If two diffusible solutes are injected simultaneously,

$$P_1/P_2 \div D_1/D_2 = \qquad (3)$$

$$\frac{(1-\alpha)^2[1 - 2.104\alpha + 2.09\alpha^3 - 0.95\alpha^5 \ldots]}{(1-\beta)^2[1 - 2.104\beta + 2.09\beta^3 - 0.95\beta^5 \ldots]},$$

where $\alpha = a_1/r$ and $\beta = a_2/r$ and a_1 and a_2 refer to the molecular radii of solutes 1 and 2, respectively, and r refers to the radius of the equivalent or effective pore in the capillary wall. The relationships between calculated effective or equivalent pore radii and their morphological counterparts in the capillary wall have not been established; however, they represent a convenient way of comparing the permeability characteristics of capillaries in different vascular beds. The equivalent pore dimensions calculated from indicator dilution data as well as those calculated from lymph studies (see below) appear to be sensitive indicators of changes in vascular permeability induced by various physiological and pathological stimuli.

Results

Small intestine

The multiple indicator dilution technique has been used to assess the permeability characteristics of capillaries in the isolated, perfused cat small intestine (35). The diffusible tracers used were raffinose (5.7 Å radius), inulin (15 Å radius), and β-lactoglobulin A (28 Å radius). The relative concentration curves for two of these diffusible tracers together with their extraction patterns are shown in Fig. 2. The extraction of the tracers remained relatively constant up to the peak of the vascular tracer curve, then declined. The initial plateau extraction value was used to calculate PS for each molecule. Plasma flow rate through the tissue was increased by local intraarterial infusions of isoproterenol (a selective mucosal vasodilator). Under resting conditions, approximately 80% of the blood flow is distributed to the mucosa-submucosa of the cat small intestine and 20% to the muscularis-serosa (13,24). Isoproterenol alters this distribution in favor of the mucosa-submucosa, therefore PS values obtained during isoproterenol infusion reflect predominantly the permeability characteristics of the fenestrated capillaries of the mucosal-submucosal region of the small intestine.

PS values for all three tracers increased with plasma flow rate. The relationship between PS and plasma flow through the intestine for inulin and β-lactoglobulin A is shown in Fig. 3. At the highest plasma flow rate studied (50 ml·min^{-1}·100 g^{-1}), the PS values for raffinose, inulin, and β-lactoglobulin A were 42, 23, and 3.5 ml·min^{-1}·100 g^{-1}, respectively. The increase in PS with increasing plasma flow resulted from recruitment of additional capillary surface area with increasing infusions of isoproterenol. Raffinose appeared to be flow-limited over the entire range of flow rates studied, that is, the PS value for raffinose was governed by plasma flow rate and not by the restrictive properties of the capillary wall. There was, however, restricted diffusion of β-lactoglobulin A compared with inulin, since the permeability ratio of inulin to lactoglobulin (7.6) was greater than the ratio of their respective free diffusion coefficients (1.73). These data are consistent with an equivalent pore radius of 59 Å for the fenestrated capillaries in the mucosa-submucosa of the small intestine. The PS values reported for the small intestine (Table 1) are 20 times larger than those observed in skeletal muscle for raffinose (44) and inulin (6,45). Even if the capillary surface area in the small intestine were as much as three- to fourfold greater than in skeletal muscle, this would mean that the fenestrated capillaries of the intestine are at least five to seven times more permeable to small solutes than the continuous capillaries of skeletal muscle.

The small intestine is composed of two ultrastructurally different capillary beds, the fenestrated capillaries of the mucosa-submucosa in parallel with the continuous capillaries of the muscularis. PS values recorded during isoproterenol infusion predominantly reflect the permeability characteristics of fenestrated capillaries, since isoproterenol redistributes blood flow in favor of the mucosa-submucosa. Adenosine, however, is known to selectively dilate the muscularis layer of the small intestine (17) and has recently been used in indicator dilution studies to investigate the permeability characteristics of capillaries in intestinal smooth muscle (35). The transit time of tracers through the muscularis vessels is less than through the tortuous vessels of the mucosa-submucosa. Therefore, during adenosine infusion, the initial samples on the indicator dilution curve predominantly represent blood from the muscularis region of the small bowel (47), whereas later samples mainly represent blood from the mucosal-submucosal region. The extraction patterns for raffinose and inulin observed in the cat small intestine during adenosine infusion are shown in Fig. 4. The initial samples of low extraction revealed restricted diffusion of inulin compared to raffinose; in subsequent samples there was unrestricted diffusion of the tracer pair, an observation consistent with the findings

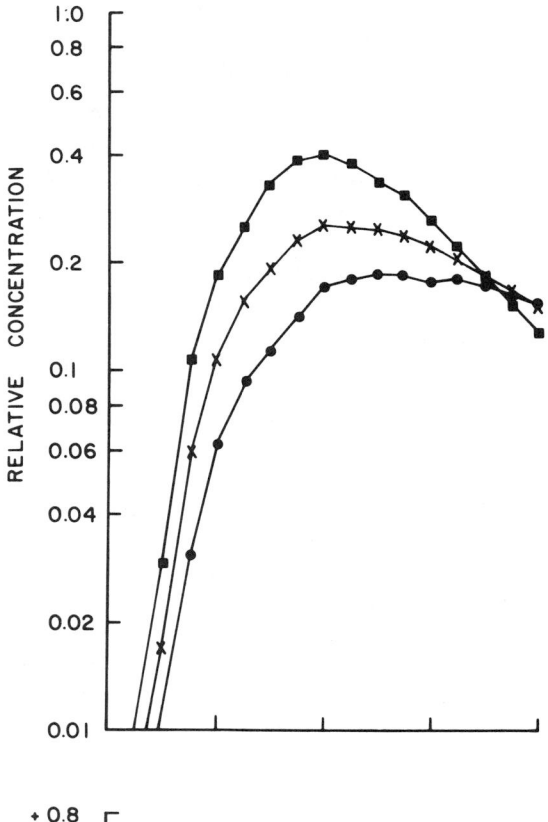
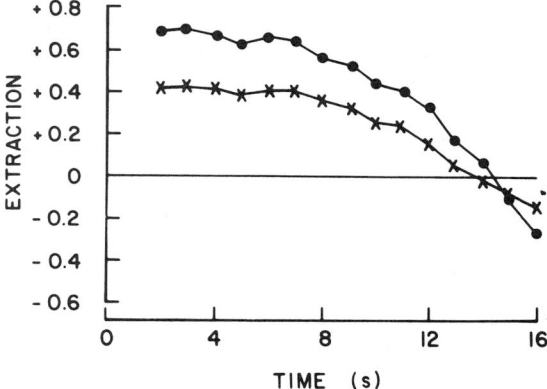

FIG. 2. Relative concentrations of vascular tracer (^{125}I-γ-globulin) *(squares)* and two diffusible tracers—^{3}H-raffinose *(circles)* and ^{14}C-inulin *(X's)*—in venous blood samples collected from small intestine. Extraction of diffusible tracers is shown in *lower panel*. (From Perry and Granger, ref. 35, with permission.)

during isoproterenol infusion. Although this approach does not allow complete separation of blood perfusing the muscularis from that perfusing the mucosal region of the small intestine, the results indicate that the equivalent pore dimensions of capillaries in the muscularis are close to the 40 to 45 Å radius observed in skeletal muscle capillaries and smaller than the 59 Å observed in mucosal capillaries.

Other splanchnic organs

Experiments similar to those described above for the small intestine have also been performed in the stomach and pancreas (Table 1). In the stomach, the PS values for raffinose, inulin, and β-lactogobulin A are three times larger than values reported for the intestine. However, the equivalent pore radius for gastric capillaries is 53 Å, a value similar to that observed in the

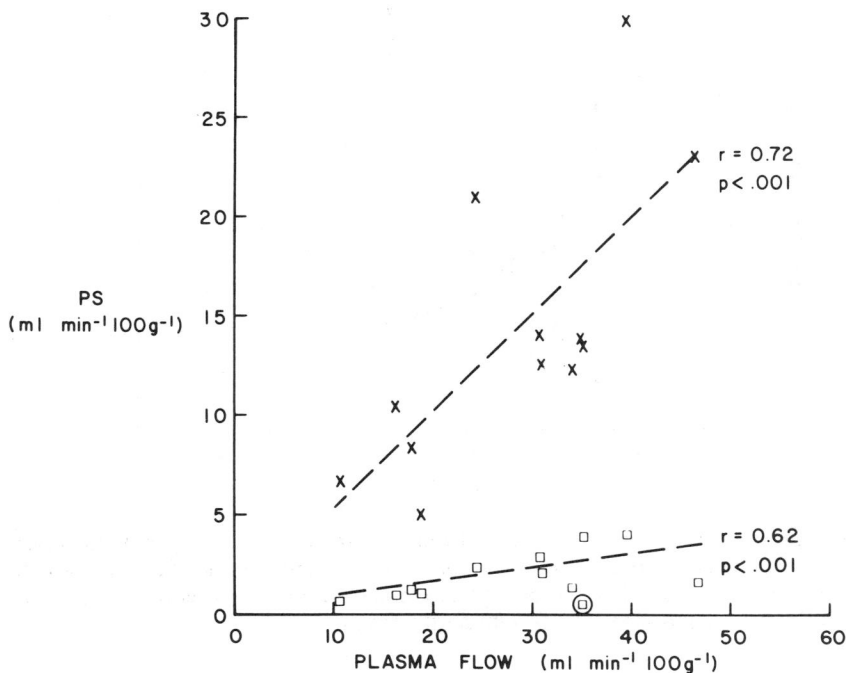

FIG. 3. Capillary permeability–surface area products (PS) for two simultaneously injected diffusible tracers—inulin *(X's)* and β-lactoglobulin A *(squares)*—plotted as a function of plasma flow through the cat small intestine. Circled value was omitted from all calculations. (From Perry and Granger, ref. 35, with permission.)

TABLE 1. *Capillary permeability–surface area products (ml · min^{-1} · 100 g^{-1}) and calculated equivalent pore radii (Å) for small intestine and other organs*

Tissue	PS$_{gluc}$	PS$_{raff}$	PS$_{inulin}$	PS$_{lactogl}$	Equiv pore radius	Ref.
Small intestine						
Cat		42.0	23.0	3.5	59	35
Rabbit		55.0[a]	26.0[a]			
Stomach						
Dog		140	70	8	53	33
Dog	23.2					47
Pancreas						
Dog			23.2	4.9	67	21
Pig	110[b]					19
Skeletal muscle						
Cat	17.6		0.7			6

PS, permeability–surface area product; gluc, glucose; raff, raffinose; lactogl, lactoglobulin.
[a]Data from M. A. Perry *(unpublished observations)*.
[b]Value for Cr-EDTA, a molecule of similar dimensions to sucrose. Data represent maximum PS values observed at the highest plasma flow rate studied.

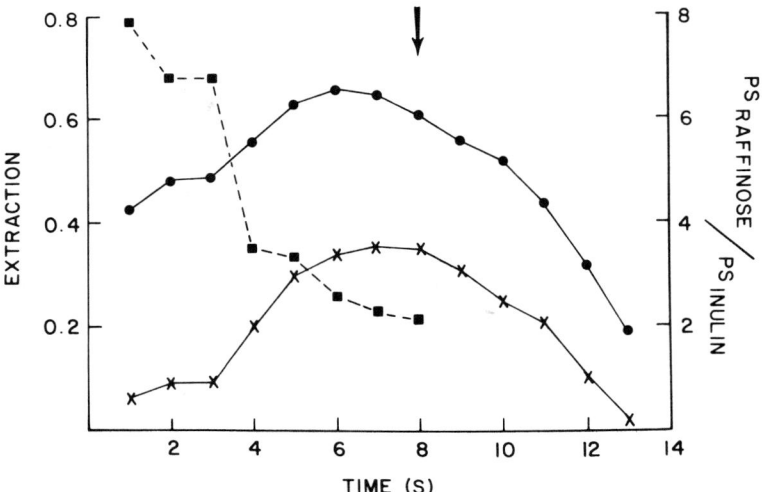

FIG. 4. Extraction pattern in the cat small intestine for raffinose *(circles)* and inulin *(X's)* obtained when tracers were injected during a constant infusion of adenosine. Ratio of permeability for raffinose to permeability for inulin (PS_{raff}/PS_{inulin}) *(broken line)* declined up until peak *(arrow)* of vascular tracer curve. (From Perry and Granger, ref. 35, with permission.)

small intestine. These results suggest that the restrictive properties of the gastric capillaries are similar to those of the small intestine but that the stomach possesses a greater capillary surface area for exchange. However, recent studies (32) have shown that increasing plasma flow rate through the type of stomach preparation used to study vascular permeability may cause recruitment of additional tissue along the border zones of the segment. This recruitment may explain the higher PS values obtained in the stomach compared with the small intestine. The permeability ratios from which the equivalent pore radius is calculated are independent of S and therefore unaffected by any recruitment of tissue.

PS values for the isolated perfused dog pancreas are similar to the values reported for the small intestine (Table 1). The data are consistent with an equivalent pore radius for pancreatic capillaries of 68 Å. Since one of the tracers in the pair (inulin) was flow-limited, this value represents a maximum pore size. The pancreas appears to differ markedly from other purely fenestrated vascular beds, for example, the salivary gland where the PS for inulin is approximately 176 ml·min^{-1}·100 g^{-1}, and the equivalent pore radius is 120 Å (26). Not only are the pancreatic capillaries less permeable but it also appears likely that there are either fewer capillaries or fewer fenestrae per capillary in the pancreas compared with the salivary gland. Unfortunately, there are not sufficient data on the ultrastructure of these two tissues to support this contention.

Factors Influencing Permeability

Certain conditions and agents are known to alter the permeability of intestinal capillaries to macromolecules (see below). The mechanism by which such changes occur is an increase in the dimensions of the large (200–250 Å) pores in the capillary wall. Indicator dilution estimates of equivalent pore radius reflect predominantly the dimensions of the far more numerous small pores (40–80 Å). There are no reports of circumstances under which the indicator dilution estimate of small pore radius is increased. Recent studies in our laboratory indicate that hypoxemia in the cat sufficient to reduce the arterial Po_2 from a control value of 118 mm Hg to 35 mm Hg for a period of 10 min caused a significant increase in the equivalent pore radius of intestinal capillaries from 59 to 67 Å (Fig. 5). This effect was sustained for at least 15 min after the intestinal preparation had been returned to normoxic conditions. Local intraarterial infusions of histamine (2 µg/min) also caused a significant increase in the effective pore radius from 58 to 76 Å. Lymph protein clearance increased sixfold during histamine infusion yet remained unchanged during hypoxemia, suggesting that hypoxemia affected only the small pore population whereas histamine increased the number or dimensions of the large pores as well as the small pores.

Osmotic Transient Studies

The osmotic transient technique has been used to investigate the permeability characteristics of capillaries in the small intestine (7). The technique is based on the assumption that the addition of an osmotically active solute to the plasma will cause removal of fluid from the tissue, depending on both the size of the solute molecule and the permeability of the capillary wall to the solute. An osmotically active solute that diffuses relatively freely across the capillary wall will exert little osmotic effect, whereas an impermeant solute (reflection coefficient = 1) will exert its full osmotic effect across the membrane. When urea, glucose, mannitol, and maltose were added to the blood supply of an isolated, perfused cat intestine preparation, the resulting weight changes and calculated reflection coefficients were extremely small. The low values were thought to result from the many difficulties associated with the osmotic transient technique, not the least of which is that the osmotic bolus was found to increase intestinal capillary permeability (7). Therefore, this technique does not appear to be a suitable means of investigating capillary permeability in the intestine.

PERMEABILITY OF INTESTINAL CAPILLARIES TO MACROMOLECULES

Lymph Studies

Theory

The use of lymph-to-plasma concentration ratios *(L/P)* for different size solute molecules as an indicator of vascular permeability was initially introduced by Grotte (18). This analysis assumes that steady state *L/P* values of an organ reflect the permeability characteristics of

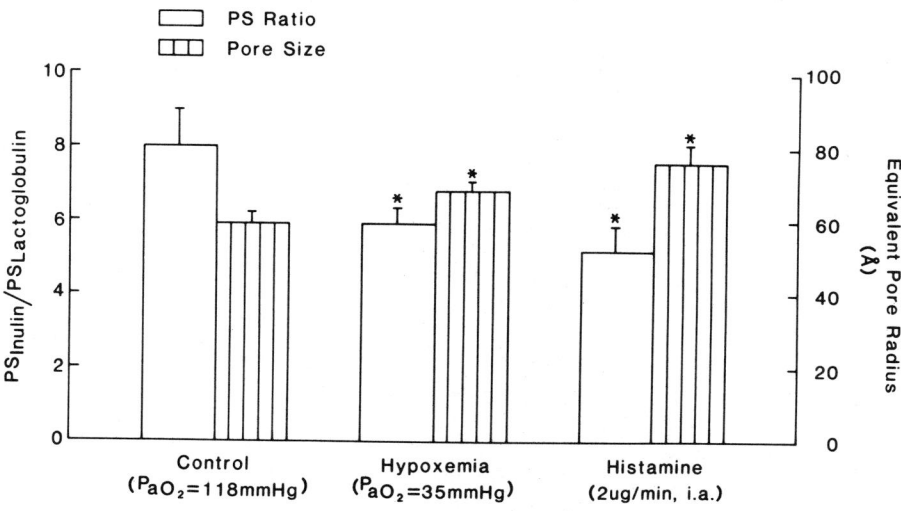

FIG. 5. Decline in the ratio of permeability for inulin to permeability for lactoglobulin and associated increase in calculated equivalent pore size following 10 min of arterial hypoxemia or histamine infusion *(unpublished observations).*

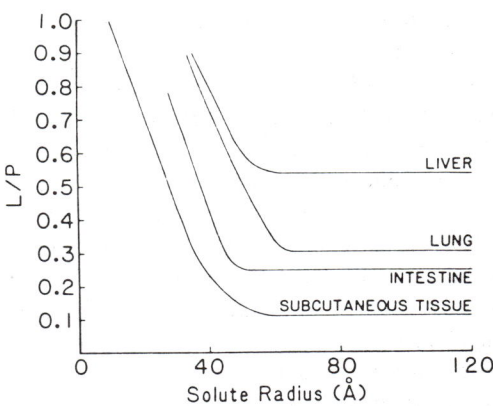

FIG. 6. Relationships between lymph-to-plasma ratio (L/P) and solute radius acquired at normal capillary filtration rates for subcutaneous tissue (42), small intestine (16), lung (29), and liver (9).

the capillary bed. Figure 6 illustrates the relationship between L/P and solute radius for several organs. The data presented in Fig. 6 indicate that the liver has the most permeable microvasculature; lung and intestine are of intermediate permeability; and the subcutaneous capillaries are the least permeable. Although this analysis provides a reasonable qualitative assessment of regional microvascular permeability, there are a number of serious limitations with the analysis. The steady state L/P values are influenced not only by the permeability of the capillary wall but also by the capillary filtration rate and the perfused capillary surface area. Therefore, interpretation of L/P data at normal filtration rates is difficult. For example, it is possible that the lung, which has a very high capillary surface area but relatively low lymph flow, may have L/P values that would exceed those of the small intestine even if the permeability to macromolecules were the same in both tissues.

Recently, the relationship between L/P and the filtration rate across the capillary wall or lymph flow rate was used as a means of assessing intestinal capillary permeability. When lymph flow is increased by graded increases in venous pressure, the L/P ratio for any given macromolecule decreases. This is called the filtration-rate-dependent portion of the relationship. At high lymph flows (above ten times control), the L/P ratio becomes constant despite further increases in lymph flow (filtration-rate-independent values). At a normal portal pressure, the exchange of macromolecules across the intestinal capillary wall occurs by both diffusion and convection. Elevation of venous pressure increases the convective movement of macromolecules across the capillary wall while at the same time the diffusive contribution to total exchange is reduced to a negligible level. Only when the L/P ratio is filtration-rate-independent can the true sieving characteristics of the capillary wall be assessed, at which time 1-L/P (filtration-rate-independent) is equal to the osmotic reflection coefficient (σ_d). Both theoretical and experimental evidence supports the contention that $\sigma_d = 1 - L/P$ at high capillary filtration rates (2,16).

The relationship obtained experimentally between total protein L/P ratio and lymph flow rate in the small intestine of cat and rat is shown in Fig. 7. The osmotic reflection coefficient for total protein (calculated from Fig. 7, assuming $\sigma_d = 1 - L/P$ when L/P is filtration-rate-independent) is 0.92. Analysis of the different molecular weight constituents of lymph and plasma has provided estimates of the osmotic reflection coefficients for a variety of different sized solute molecules (Table 2).

The osmotic reflection coefficients may be used to describe the permeability characteristics of the capillary bed in terms of equivalent pore theory (40). An example of such an analysis is shown in Fig. 8 where $1 - \sigma_d$ is plotted as a function of solute radius. The equation of Drake and Davis (4) was used to generate theoretical curves relating $1 - \sigma_d$ to solute radius for different sized equivalent pores. The plot shown in Fig. 8 can be described by fitting the data with two sets of equivalent pores. This is done by first fitting a theoretical "large pore line" to the points representing the large solutes. Then, by a curve-peeling process the resulting values of $1 - \sigma_d$ for smaller solutes are fitted with a smaller theoretical pore curve. The ordinate intercept predicts the percentage of total hy-

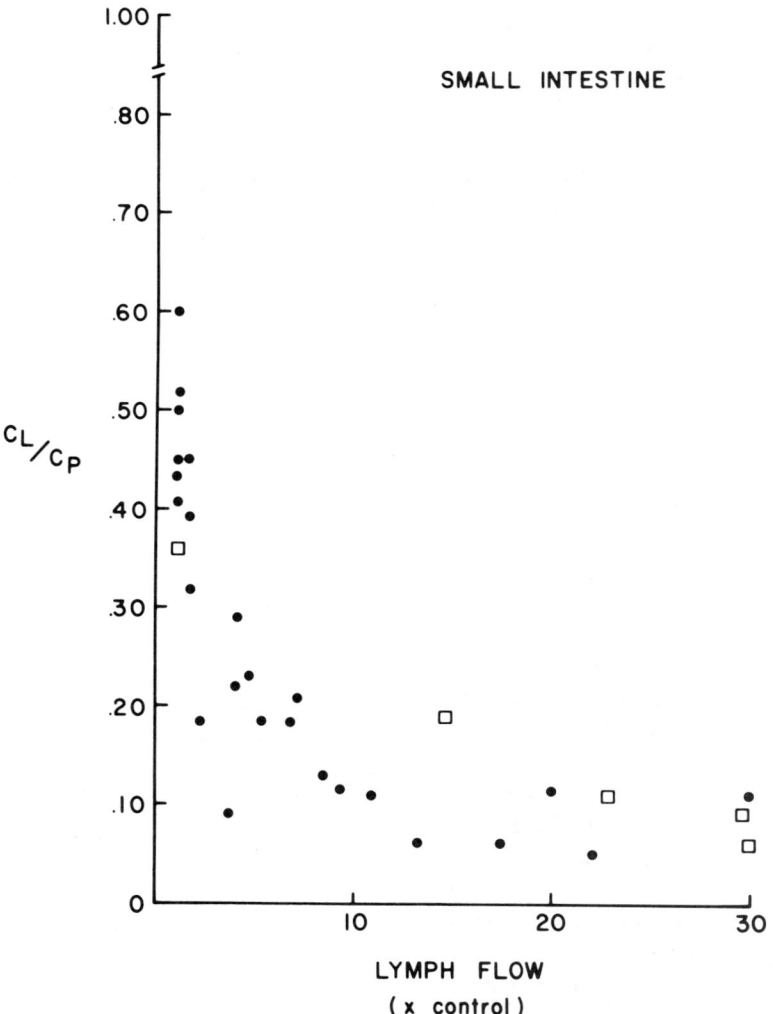

FIG. 7. Steady state relationship between C_L/C_P for total protein and lymph flow in the small intestine of the cat *(circles)* (16) and rat *(squares)* (23).

draulic conductance provided by each set of pores.

Results

Small intestine

The reflection coefficients of intestinal capillaries for various macromolecules are shown in Table 2. The value of σ_d for total protein in the small intestine indicates that 92% of the total colloid osmotic pressure of plasma acts across the capillary wall. There is a progressive increase in the reflection coefficient as the size of the solute increases from 37 Å (albumin) to 120 Å (β-lipoprotein). Clearly, this indicates that intestinal capillaries sieve macromolecules depending on molecular size. The permeability characteristics of intestinal capillaries are best described by two populations of equivalent pores with radii of 46 Å and 200 Å (Fig. 8). There are 6,400 small pores for every large pore, and 95% of the total hydraulic conductance across the capillary wall occurs through small pores but only 5% through large pores (Table 3). Comparison of the results presented in Tables 2 and 3 for the small intestine and the hind-paw

TABLE 2. *Reflection coefficients calculated using L/P data obtained at high capillary filtration rates in small intestine and other organs*

Solute radius (Å)	Small intestine (16)	Hindpaw (36)	Stomach (33)	Colon (41)	Pancreas[a] (a)
Total protein	0.92	0.90	0.78	0.85	0.85
37	0.90	0.87	0.73	0.75	
38	0.92		0.77		
39	0.94		0.78		
40		0.89		0.82	
42	0.96		0.79		
44		0.89		0.87	
48				0.88	
96	0.98		0.91		
100		0.96		0.95	
120	0.99	0.97	0.91	0.98	

[a]Data from P. R. Kvietys *(unpublished observations)*.

indicates that these two vascular beds have similar osmotic reflection coefficients for plasma proteins and similar equivalent pore radii. That is, the fenestrated capillaries of the small intestine are as impermeable to plasma proteins as the continuous capillaries of the hindpaw. Although the technique of lymphatic protein flux analysis provides information on the selectivity of a vascular bed and the ratio of small to large pore areas and numbers, it cannot, at present, be used to assess the absolute numbers of pores per unit surface area of endothelium. Therefore, the data presented in Tables 2 and 3 provide no indication of the far greater blood-lymph exchange of protein per unit mass of tissue that occurs in the intestine compared with the hindpaw. The large capacity for transcapillary exchange in the intestine is the result of a large "pore area" for exchange afforded by the fenestrae. In effect, the fenestrae increase the number of equivalent pores per unit surface area of endothelium; however, each pore remains as selective to plasma proteins as the equivalent pores observed in continuous capillaries. The high transcapillary exchange capacity of fenestrated vascular beds is readily apparent in the indicator dilution data presented in Table 1.

Other splanchnic organs

Filtration-rate-independent *L/P* ratios of endogenous macromolecules have been used to investigate the permeability characteristics of capillaries in other splanchnic organs (Table 2 and 3). The capillaries of the stomach, small intestine, and colon possess equivalent small pores of similar dimensions (46–53 Å radius). However, the microvasculature of the stomach appears to be more permeable to macromolecules than either the small intestine or colon. Gastric capillaries have equivalent large pores of 250 Å compared with 180 to 200 Å for the other two organs. Recently, Davenport and Wood (46) reported reflection coefficients for albumin and fibrinogen of 0.74 and 0.87. These values are the same as those reported by Perry et al. (33), and they support the contention that the stomach is more permeable to macromolecules than the small intestine or colon. The equivalent pore dimensions for the discontinuous vascular bed of the liver (Table 3) are much larger than the values for other splanchnic beds. The data for the liver were collected at a venous pressure of 0 to 2 mm Hg, since elevation of venous pressure causes a reduction in perm-selectivity in this organ (9).

Effect of Solute Charge

Until recently little was known about the charge-selective properties of the intestinal capillary wall. Studies of endogenous lactate de-

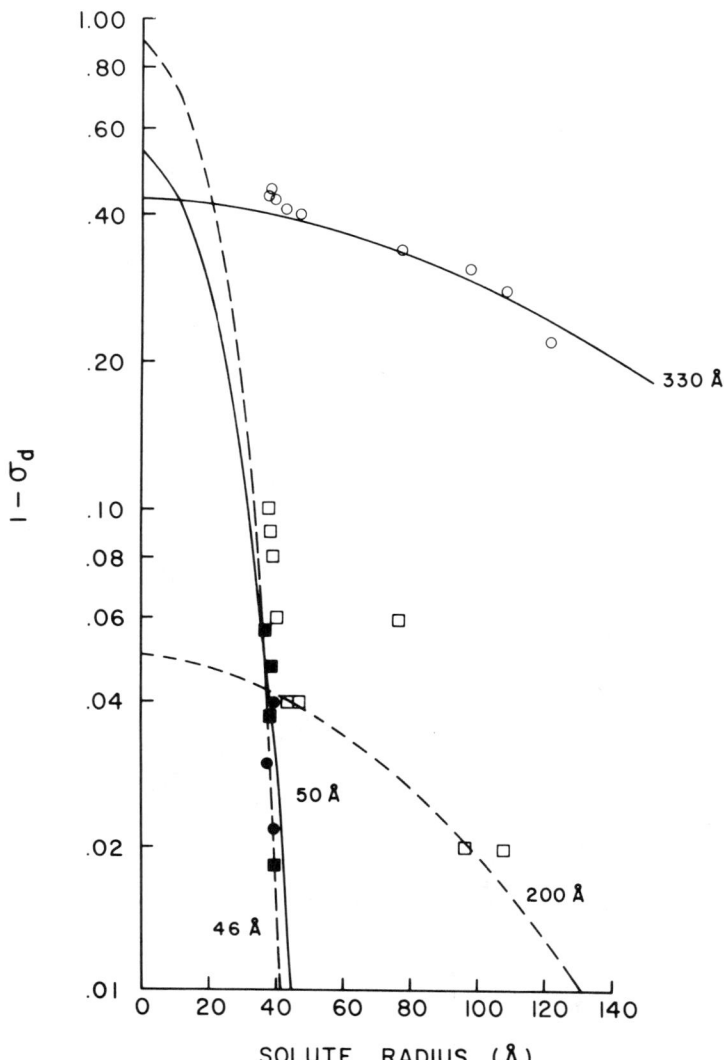

FIG. 8. Pore stripping analysis for lymphatic protein flux data from small intestine under control conditions *(squares)* and after 1 hr of ischemia *(circles)*. It was assumed that $\sigma_d = 1-C_L/C_P$ at the high capillary filtration rates studied. Note that the analysis predicts that ischemia selectively increases the size of the large pores.

hydrogenase (LDH) isoenzymes in plasma and intestinal lymph (25) indicate that the degree of restriction to blood-lymph exchange increases with increasing positive charge on the molecule (Fig. 9). Furthermore, the osmotic reflection coefficients for LDH isoenzymes decrease from 0.95 for the most-positive isoenzyme (pI = 8.3) to 0.71 for the most negative (pI = 5.2). That is, the blood-lymph barrier in the intestine behaves as if it were positively charged. Recent studies with charged dextran molecules (MW = 24,000) support this conclusion (31). The steady state L/P ratio of neutral dextran is twice that of positive dextran of the same molecular weight, indicating selective restriction of the positive compared to neutral dextran by the intestinal blood-lymph barrier (Fig. 10). Ultrastructural studies (43) indicate that plasmalemmal vesicles or transendothelial channels may represent the positively charged pathways

TABLE 3. Dimensions and relative frequencies of equivalent pores in capillaries of small intestine and other organs

Organ	Species	Small-pore radius[a] (Å)	Flow through small pores[b] (%)	Large-pore radius[a] (Å)	Flow through large pores[b] (%)	A_s/A_l,[c] (%)	N_s/N_l,[d]	Flow through other pathways[b]	Ref.
Small intestine	Cat	46	90	200	5	340/1	6,400/1	5	16,39
Hind-paw	Dog	47	82	195	13	114/1	2,064/1	5	36
Stomach	Cat	47	75	250	23	92/1	2,600/1	2	33
Colon	Dog	53	71	180	17	48/1	550/1	12	41
Liver	Cat	90[e]	20	330	80	3.4/1	46/1	0	9

[a] Equivalent pore radii were calculated by the graphic analysis (Fig. 4) of Renkin et al. (40).
[b] Percent of the total hydraulic flow across the capillary wall that analysis predicts will pass through small pores, large pores, or other hydraulically conductive pathways.
[c] Total area of small pores compared with total area of large pores (A_s/A_l).
[d] Relative number of small pores compared with large pores (N_s/N_l).
[e] Data for the liver did not provide a close fit to the predicted relationship for small pores and was compatible with small-pore radii in the range 70-110 Å.

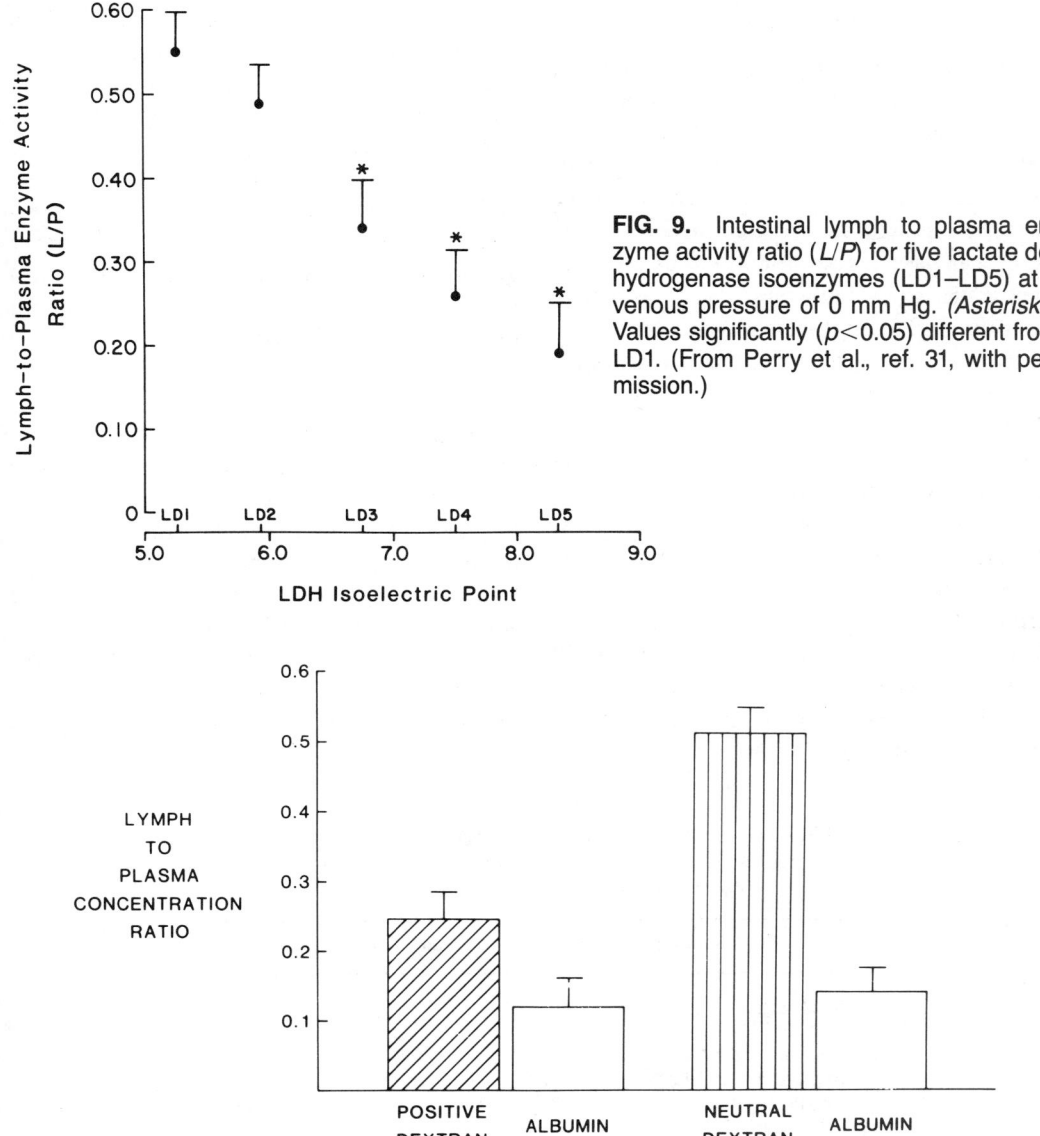

FIG. 9. Intestinal lymph to plasma enzyme activity ratio (L/P) for five lactate dehydrogenase isoenzymes (LD1–LD5) at a venous pressure of 0 mm Hg. *(Asterisks)* Values significantly ($p<0.05$) different from LD1. (From Perry et al., ref. 31, with permission.)

FIG. 10. Mean ($\pm$ SEM) lymph to plasma concentration ratios of positively charged dextran and simultaneously injected ^{125}I-albumin and neutral dextran with simultaneously-injected ^{125}I-albumin. The L/P for neutral dextran is significantly ($P=0.012$) greater than that for positive dextran. (From Perry et al., ref. 31, with permission.)

across intestinal capillaries, since cationic ferritin labeled all but these two structures in the endothelial cell wall. The findings in the intestine contrast with those in the kidney, where the existence of a negatively charged barrier is well established. The physiological significance of a positively charged barrier associated with intestinal capillaries may be to facilitate the movement of negatively charged proteins, for example, albumin, into the interstitium of the intestinal mucosa. This would be advantageous for certain absorbed nutrients, for instance, fatty acids, which leave the interstitium bound to proteins.

Factors Influencing Permeability

A variety of physiological, pharmacological, and pathological interventions are known to enhance capillary protein leakage in the intestine (Table 4). Whether the increased transcapillary protein flux is a result of an increase in the perfused capillary surface area or is due to an increase in vascular permeability is unknown in most instances. Many agents (e.g., histamine, bradykinin, glucagon) increase vascular permeability (reduce the reflection coefficient for total plasma protein); however, it is uncertain whether or not they also increase capillary surface area. Other substances such as isoproterenol and secretin increase capillary protein leakage without altering vascular permeability, suggesting that capillary recruitment occurs. Certain conditions that increase vascular permeability do so by preferentially increasing the dimensions of the large pores. During fat absorption (11) and following 1 hr of intestinal ischemia (Fig. 8), there is a reduction in the osmotic reflection coefficient values for endogenous proteins, a finding consistent with an increase in the size of the large pores from 200 Å to 300 to 330 Å. The mechanism by which these conditions selectively influence the large pore system is not readily apparent. *In vivo* microscopic studies in tissues such as mesentery indicate that various pharmacologic agents reversibly increase vascular leakage of tracers by forming large interendothelial gaps (large pores) in venous capillaries (1). The gaps are believed to be formed as a result of receptor-mediated contraction and subsequent separation of endothelial cells.

Electron microscopic studies of the fenestrated capillaries of the rat small intestine reveal a number of ultrastructural changes in response to physiological or pathological insults. Intraluminal placement of mustard oil causes the formation of large gaps between endothelial cells with little effect on the fenestrae (20). The gaps, like those observed in the mesentery, are reversible. However, perfusion of the vessels of the rat intestine with histamine causes partial removal of fenestral diaphragms, occasional de-

TABLE 4. *Effects of various physiologic and pharmacologic interventions on the osmotic reflection coefficient for total plasma protein in the intestinal circulation*

Experimental condition	Reflection coeff.	Ref.
Physiologic		
Control	0.92	16
Fat absorption	0.70	11
Drugs and hormones		
Isoproterenol	0.92	12
Bradykinin	0.65	12
Secretin	0.91	11
Cholecystokinin	0.89	11
Glucagon	0.81	8
Histamine	0.56	27
Cimetidine and histamine	0.90	27
Benadryl and histamine	0.56	27
Compound 48/80	0.76	5
Angiotensin II	0.93[a]	28
Pathologic		
Ischemia	0.59	15
Ischemia and superoxide dismutase	0.86	14
E. coli endotoxin	0.78	14
Goldblatt hypertension	0.55[a]	22
Arterial hyperglycemia (20 mM)	0.64	7

[a] Values derived from dog; all other values from cat.

tachment of the endothelium from the basement membrane, as well as focal separation of the junctions between endothelial cells (3). These changes presumably account for the reduction in σ_d for total proteins from 0.92 to 0.56 predicted from lymph protein studies in the intestine (27).

Vascular Washout Studies

Another technique that has been used to investigate the permeability to macromolecules of different vascular beds involves measuring the rate of movement of tracers between interstitium and blood (30,34). In these studies, the labeled macromolecule is allowed to circulate in the animal for 20 hr so the tracer can reach the interstitium. ^{51}Cr-labeled red cells are then injected into the animal, and the tissue under study is vascularly isolated and perfused with tracer-free artificial plasma. The rate of efflux of the labeled macromolecule from interstitium to blood is calculated from the tracer activity in venous effluent (after correction for vascular washout) and the residual activity in the organ. The efflux of gamma-globulin/cm^2 of capillary surface area in the intestine ($120 \times 10^{-6} \cdot \text{min}^{-1} \cdot \text{cm}^{-2}$) is similar to that observed in skeletal muscle ($113 \times 10^{-6} \cdot \text{min}^{-1} \cdot \text{cm}^{-2}$). These data confirm the findings of the lymphatic protein flux technique that the fenestrated capillaries of the intestine are as impermeable to macromolecules as the continuous capillaries of skeletal muscle (16).

ACKNOWLEDGMENTS

This work was supported by grants from the National Health and Medical Research Council of Australia, the National Heart Lung and Blood Institute (HL 26441), and the Alabama Affiliate, American Heart Association. D. N. G. is the recipient of a Research Career Development Award (HL00816) from the National Heart, Lung and Blood Institute.

REFERENCES

1. Arfors, K. E., Rutili, G., and Svensjo, E. (1979): Microvascular transport of macromolecules in normal and inflammatory conditions. *Acta. Physiol. Scand. (Suppl.)*, 463:93–103.
2. Bresler, E. H., and Groom, L. J. (1981): On equations for combined convective and diffusive transport of neutral solutes across porous membranes. *Am. J. Physiol.*, 241:F469–F476.
3. Clementi, F., and Palade, G. E. (1969): Intestinal capillaries. II. Structural effects of EDTA and histamine. *J. Cell. Biol.*, 42:706–714.
4. Drake, R., and Davis, E. (1978): A corrected equation for the calculation of reflection coefficients. *Microvasc. Res.*, 15:259.
5. Durbin, T. J., Mortillaro, N. A., and Wilborn, W. H. (1982): Effects of endogenous histamine on capillary permeability in the feline ileum. *Fed. Proc.*, 41:1742 (Abstract).
6. Garlick, D. G. (1970): Factors affecting the transport of extracellular molecules in skeletal muscle. In: *Capillary Permeability: Alfred Benzon Symposium II*, edited by C. Crone and N. A. Lassen, pp. 228–238. Munksgaard, Copenhagen.
7. Granger, D. N., Granger, J. P., Brace, R. A., Parker, R. E., and Taylor, A. E. (1979): Analysis of the permeability characteristics of intestinal capillaries. *Circ. Res.*, 44:335–344.
8. Granger, D. N., Kvietys, P. R., Wilborn, W. H., Mortillaro, N. A., and Taylor, A. E. (1980): Mechanism of glucagon-induced intestinal secretion. *Am. J. Physiol.*, 239:G30–G38.
9. Granger, D. N., Miller, T., Allen, R., Parker, R. E., Parker, J. C., and Taylor, A. E. (1979): Permselectivity of the liver blood-lymph barrier to endogenous macromolecules. *Gastroenterology*, 77:103–109.
10. Granger, D. N., and Perry, M. A. (1983): Permeability characteristics of the microcirculation. In: *The Physiology and Pharmacology of the Microcirculation*, edited by N. A. Mortillaro, pp. 157–208. Academic Press, New York.
11. Granger, D. N., Perry, M. A., Kvietys, P. R., and Taylor, A. E. (1982): Permeability of intestinal capillaries: Effects of fat absorption and gastrointestinal hormones. *Am. J. Physiol.*, 242:G194–G201.
12. Granger, D. N., Richardson, P. D. I., and Taylor, A. E. (1979): Effects of isoprenaline and bradykinin on capillary filtration in the cat ileum. *Br. J. Pharmacol.*, 67:361–366.
13. Granger, D. N., Richardson, P. D. I., and Taylor, A. E. (1979): Volumetric assessment of the capillary filtration coefficient in the cat small intestine. *Pfluegers Arch.*, 381:25–33.
14. Granger, D. N., Rutili, G., and McCord, J. M. (1981): Superoxide radicals in feline intestinal ischemia. *Gastroenterology*, 81:22–29.
15. Granger, D. N., Sennett, M., McElearney, P., and Taylor, A. E. (1980): Effect of local arterial hypotension on cat intestinal capillary permeability. *Gastroenterology*, 79:474–480.
16. Granger, D. N., and Taylor, A. E. (1980): Permeability of intestinal capillaries to endogenous macromolecules. *Am. J. Physiol.*, 238:H457–H464.

17. Granger, D. N., Valleau, J. D., Parker, R. E., Lane, R. S., and Taylor, A. E. (1978): Effects of adenosine on intestinal hemodynamics, oxygen delivery, and capillary fluid exchange. *Am. J. Physiol.*, 235:H707–H719.
18. Grotte, G. (1956): Passage of dextran molecules across the blood-lymph barrier. *Acta Chir. Scand. (Suppl)*, 211:1–84.
19. Haraldsson, B., Rippe, B., Moxham, B. J., and Folkow, B. (1982): Permeability of fenestrated capillaries in the isolated pig pancreas, with effects of bradykinin and histamine, as studied by simultaneous registration of filtration and diffusion capacities. *Acta Physiol. Scand.*, 114:67–74.
20. Hurley, J. V., and McQueen, A. (1971): The response of the fenestrated vessels of the small intestine of rats to aplication of mustard oil. *J. Pathol.*, 105:21–29.
21. Kvietys, P. R., Perry, M. A., and Granger, D. N. (1983): Permeability of pancreatic capillaries to small molecules. *Am. J. Physiol.*, 245:G519–524.
22. Laine, G. A., and Granger, H. J. (1981): Permeability of intestinal capillaries in chronic arterial hypertension. *Microvasc. Res.*, 21:248– (Abstract).
23. Lee, J. S. (1981): Lymph pressure in intestinal villi and lymph flow during fluid secretion. In: *Tissue Fluid Pressure and Composition*, edited by A. R. Hargens, pp. 165–172. Williams & Wilkins, Baltimore.
24. Lundgren, O. (1967): Studies on blood flow distribution and counter current exchange in the small intestine. *Acta Physiol. Scand. (Suppl.)*, 303:5–42.
25. McElearney, P. M., and Granger, D. N. (1979): Intestinal capillary wall as a charge selective filter. *Physiologist*, 22:85 (Abstract).
26. Mann, G. E., Smaje, L. H., and Yudilevich, D. L. (1979): Permeability of the fenestrated capillaries in the cat submandibular gland to lipid insoluble molecules. *J. Physiol.*, 279:335–354.
27. Mortillaro, N. A., Granger, D. N., Kvietys, P. R., Rutili, G., and Taylor, A. E. (1981): Effects of histamine and histamine antagonists on intestinal capillary permeability. *Am. J. Physiol.*, 240:G381–G386.
28. Nyhof, R. A., and Granger, H. J. (1982): The acute effects of angiotensin II (AII) on canine intestinal vascular permeability. *Physiologist*, 25:232– (Abstract).
29. Parker, J. C., Parker, R. E., Granger, D. N., and Taylor, A. E. (1981): Vascular permeability and transvascular fluid and protein transport in the dog lung. *Circ. Res.*, 48:549–561.
30. Perry, M. A. (1981): Transcapillary efflux of gamma globulin in skeletal muscle lung and small intestine of the rabbit. In: *Progress in Microcirculation Research*, edited by D. Garlick, pp. 249–260. Committee in Postgraduate Medical Education UNSW, Sydney.
31. Perry, M. A., Benoit, J. N., Kvietys, P. R., and Granger, D. N. (1983): Restricted transport of cationic macromolecules across intestinal capillaries. *Am. J. Physiol.*, G568–572.
32. Perry, M. A., Bulkley, G. B., Kvietys, P. R., and Granger, D. N. (1982): Regulation of oxygen uptake in resting and pentagastrin-stimulated canine stomach. *Am. J. Physiol.*, 242:G565–G569.
33. Perry, M. A., Crook, W. J., and Granger, D. N. (1981): Permeability of gastric capillaries to small and large molecules. *Am. J. Physiol.*, 241:G478–G486.
34. Perry, M. A., and Garlick, D. G. (1975): Transcapillary efflux of gamma globulin in rabbit skeletal muscle. *Microvasc. Res.*, 9:119–126.
35. Perry, M. A., and Granger, D. N. (1981): Permeability of intestinal capillaries to small molecules. *Am. J. Physiol.*, 241:G24–G30.
36. Perry, M. A., Navia, C. A., Granger, D. N., Parker, J. C., and Taylor, A. E. (1983): Calculation of effective pore radii in dog hind-paw capillaries using endogenous lymph and plasma proteins. *Microvasc. Res.*, 26:250–253.
37. Renkin, E. M. (1954): Filtration, diffusion and molecular sieving through porous cellulose membranes. *J. Gen. Physiol.*, 38:225–243.
38. Renkin, E. M. (1959): Transport of potassium-42 from blood to tissue in isolated mammalian skeletal muscles. *Am. J. Physiol.*, 197:1205–1210.
39. Renkin, E. M. (1980): Ambiguities and errors in evaluation of capillary pore sizes. *Am. J. Physiol.*, 240:H145–H146.
40. Renkin, E. M., Watson, P. D., Sloop, C. H., Joyner, W. L., and Curry, F. E., (1977): Transport pathways for fluid and large molecules in microvascular endothelium of the dog's paw. *Microvasc. Res.*, 14:205–214.
41. Richardson, P. D. I., Granger, D. N., Mailman, D., and Kvietys, P. R. (1980): Permeability characteristics of colonic capillaries. *Am. J. Physiol.*, 239:G300–G305.
42. Rutili, G., and Arfors, K-E. (1977): Protein concentration in interstitial and lymphatic fluids from the subcutaneous tissue. *Acta Physiol. Scand.*, 99:1–8.
43. Simionescu, N., Simionescu, M., and Palade, G. E. (1981): Differentiated microdomains on the luminal surface of the capillary endothelium. I. Preferential distribution of anionic sites. *J. Cell. Biol.*, 90:605–613.
44. Trap-Jensen, J., and Lassen, N. A. (1970): Capillary permeability for small hydrophilic tracers in exercising skeletal muscle in normal man and in patients with long-term diabetes mellitus. In: *Capillary Permeability: Alfred Benzon Symposium II*, edited by C. Crone and N. A. Lassen, pp. 135–152. Munksgaard, Copenhagen.
45. Trap-Jensen, J., and Lassen, N. A. (1971): Restricted diffusion in skeletal muscle capillaries in man. *Am. J. Physiol.*, 220:371–376.
46. Wood, J. G., and Davenport, H. W. (1982): Measurement of canine gastric vascular permeability to plasma proteins in the normal and protein-losing states. *Gastroenterology*, 82:725–733.
47. Yudilevich, D. L., Renkin, E. M., Alvarez, O. A., and Bravo, I. (1968): Fractional extraction and transcapillary exchange during continuous and instantaneous tracer administration. *Circ. Res.*, 23:325–336.

Microvascular Pressures in the Small Intestine

*H. Glenn Bohlen and **Robert W. Gore

*Department of Physiology, Indiana University School of Medicine, Indianapolis, Indiana 46223; and
**Department of Physiology University of Arizona College of Medicine, Tuscon, Arizona 85724

Measurements of microvascular pressures in the small intestine have added a vital dimension to our understanding of both transcapillary fluid exchange and regional vascular control. Various forms of the now classic isogravimetric-isovolumetric methods (8,9,26) have been used to determine the average intestinal capillary pressure as well as the pre- to postcapillary resistance ratio. More recently, direct measurements of pressure in individual microvessels with the Landis (20) and servo-null pressure measurement systems (15,28) have contributed to our knowledge of the distribution of pressures in the microvasculature. Information about the pressure distribution has also helped elucidate the possible differences in vascular regulation within the various parallel vasculatures of the intestinal wall (3,4,10). In this chapter, the available data on microvascular pressures will be examined to gain insight into the physiological regulation of the microvasculature in the small intestine.

PHYSICAL CONSIDERATIONS

What does the measurement of pressures in individual microvessels indicate about the vasculature in general? The pressure in a single vessel defines the fraction of the mean arterial pressure that exists at that point. Therefore, such measurements indicate on a relative basis the percentage of the total resistance that exists prior to the point of measurement, and they can be used to calculate the actual resistance to that point, if total blood flow is known. The resistance to any given point in the vasculature, to be called upstream resistance, is the pressure difference between the major arteries (Pa) and the point of measurement in the microcirculation (Px) divided by the total flow (F_T) in the circuit (Eq. 1):

$$R_{up} = \frac{Pa - Px}{F_T}. \quad (1)$$

The total resistance (R_T) of the vasculature is arterial pressure minus venous pressure (PV) divided by total flow (Eq. 2):

$$R_T = \frac{Pa - Pv}{F_T}. \quad (2)$$

If the upstream resistance is expressed as a ratio of the total resistance, then Eq. 3 results:

$$\frac{R_{up}}{R_T} = \frac{\dfrac{Pa - Px}{F_T}}{\dfrac{Pa - Pv}{F_T}}. \quad (3)$$

Total flow factors out of Eq. 3 to yield Eq. 4:

$$\frac{R_{up}}{R_T} = \frac{Pa - Px}{Pa - Pv}. \quad (4)$$

Equation 4 indicates one need only know arterial, venous, and microvascular pressures to calculate the fraction of the total resistance that occurs upstream from the point of measurement. However, the results of the equation do not provide information about the variables listed as assumptions. By repeatedly measuring pressure in each vessel type in the entire microvasculature, one can determine the percentage of total resistance contributed by each type of microvessel. This approach is rarely used, however, because it is much easier to plot the microvascular pressures versus the various types of microvessels and, from the shape of the curve, deduce qualitatively where the greatest pressure reductions and the major resistance sites are.

VASCULAR ANATOMY

The vast majority of microvascular pressure measurements in the small intestine have been made in rats, whereas most of the data available on intestinal vascular control have been obtained in cats and dogs. Although there is qualitative agreement regarding many physiological functions in rats and larger laboratory animals, such as cats and dogs, it is important to realize that differences exist. There is also the possibility that the vascular branching patterns in different species have effects on both microvascular pressures and vascular regulation.

The microvascular branching pattern in the rat, shown in Fig. 1, is characteristic of the majority of vertebrates in that the mesenteric vessels pierce the muscle layers to form a submucosal system of interconnected large and intermediate diameter arterioles (1,10). In larger animals (e.g., cats and dogs), the muscle layers have arterioles that branch from vessels analogous to the first- (1A) and second-order (2A) arterioles in the rat and that then supply the muscle layers. Large animals have a branching system of arterioles in the visceral muscle layer that rivals the complexity of vascular branching in skeletal muscle. In both large and small animals, the arteriolar supply of a villus begins as small side branches (15–30 μm) of arterioles (2A) that interconnect the largest radial arterioles. In rodents and similar small animals, the side branch vessels send one, or occasionally two, branches up to the muscle layers. Larger animals also have a similar vascular arrangement to perfuse the deepest sections of the muscle layers. The side branch arterioles (3A in rats) then descend through the submucosa and connect to deep submucosal vessels as well as to the main arteriole of one or more villi.

The branching pattern within a villus may be such that the bulk of capillary perfusion begins near the villus apex and cascades downward, as in rodents and cats (9,10,16,23,25), or capillaries may be formed along the main arteriole and run, in general, across and even up the villus as in rabbits and possibly man (9,16,25).

The venous system of the intestine usually begins within each villus as paired venules that coalesce to form a single venule (CV), which rises through the submucosa. Within the submucosa, venules from the submucosal and muscle layers join the collecting venules (CV) that arise from villi. An extensive interconnecting venous plexus formed in the superficial submucosa drains into large intramural venules that, in turn, drain into the mesenteric veins.

PRESSURE DISTRIBUTION

The distribution of pressures within the rat small intestine is presented in Fig. 2 (10). These pressure measurements were made in innervated preparations when the mean arterial pressure was in the range of 100 to 110 mm Hg. One of the most striking features of the pressure profile is that the pressure in the largest arterioles is about half the mean central arterial pressure. This observation has been confirmed in several studies (2,4). The large pressure drop prior to the intramural arterioles apparently occurs as mesenteric arteries form the arcade of small arteries and large arterioles along the mesenteric border of the bowel. Pressures measured in the mesenteric arteries prior to the arteriolar arcade are typically 80% to 90% of the mean arterial pressure.

Within the microvasculature, the pressure drop from first- (1A) to second-order arterioles (2A) is remarkably small, usually only 3 to 7 mm Hg (Fig. 2) (3,4,10). The second-order arterioles are collateral vessels between adjacent first-order arterioles; this may explain the minor drop in pressure from large to intermediate diameter vessels. Similar circumstances would be expected in larger animals because an extensive network of collateral arterioles with large diameters (70–120 μm) exists in cats, dogs, and rabbits (24).

The large pressure drop between the second- and third-order arterioles from 44.6 ± 2.9 to 32.4 ± 2.6 mm Hg occurs within 50 μm from

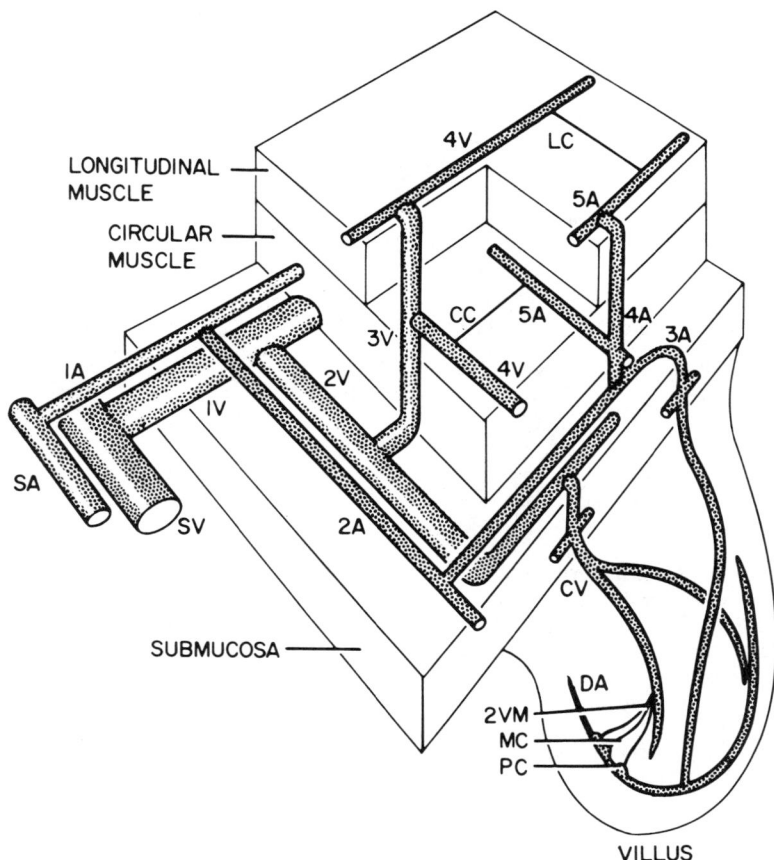

FIG. 1. Typical microvascular branching in the rat intestine. Large- and intermediate-diameter arterioles of the submucosa provide perfusion of small arterioles to the muscle, submucosal, and mucosal layers. In larger animals, a few large arterioles provide the bulk perfusion for a more complex muscle layer microvasculature. The mucosal vasculatures are simple branching systems in large and small species. SA, small artery of the mesentery; SV, small vein of the mesentery; 1A, first-order arteriole (submucosa); 2A, second-order arteriole (submucosa); 3A, third-order arteriole (submucosa); 4A, fourth-order arteriole (muscle); SA, fifth-order arteriole (muscle); LC and CC, longitudinal and circular muscle layer capillaries; MA, main arteriole of a villus; DA, distributing arteriole of a villus; PC, precapillary sphincter; 2VM, second-order venule by the mucosa; and CV, collecting venule of a villus. (From Gore and Bohlen, ref. 10, with permission.)

the origin of the third-order arteriole (10). This rapid dissipation of pressure across a branch point where the daughter vessel is substantially smaller than the parent vessel agrees with theoretical studies by Vawter et al. (27) of pressure dissipation at branch points. The pressure of 26.6 ± 2.0 mm Hg in fifth-order arterioles (5A) of the muscle layer decreases to 23.8 ± 1.5 mm Hg at the midpoint in capillaries of the longitudinal (LC) and circular muscle (CC) layers. From the pressure profile in Fig. 2, it is apparent that pressure dissipation occurs from the arteries to the capillaries in the muscle layers in two stages: outside the intestine in mesenteric arteries and at the transition from intermediate to small-diameter arterioles (2A and 3A). Although it may seem inefficient to position major determinants of capillary pressure at a great distance from the capillary, this arrangement spares the immediate precapillary arterioles from dissipating large hydrostatic pressures.

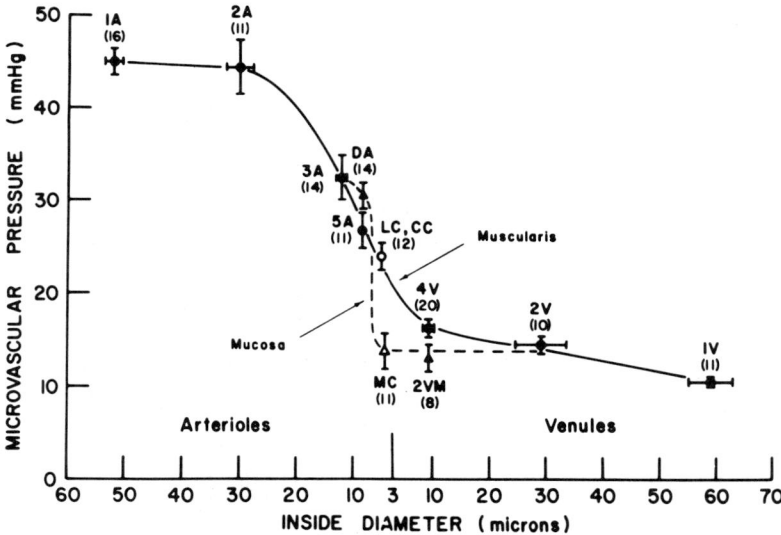

FIG. 2. Microvascular pressures (mean ± SEM) in the innervated small intestine of the rat at a mean arterial pressure of 104 ± 4 (SD) mm Hg. *(Circles)* Pressures in the intestinal muscle and submucosal vasculature; *(triangles)* mucosal microvascular pressures. For abbreviations, see legend to Fig. 1. *(Numbers in parentheses)* Number of observations in a total of 44 animals. (From Gore and Bohlen, ref. 10, with permission.)

Microvascular pressures within the villi, indicated by the dashed portion of the pressure profile in Fig. 2, show the substantial differences in pressure dissipation by the mucosal vasculature compared with the muscle vasculature. The pressure in the smallest mucosal arterioles is 30.6 ± 1.8 mm Hg compared with 32.4 ± 2.6 mm Hg in the third-order arterioles (3A) that are the origin of villus perfusion. The minimum distance over which the approximately 2 to 5 mm Hg pressure drop occurs is about 600 to 700 μm. Part of the reason for such a small arterial pressure drop is the very high resistance that the blood must encounter at the origin of mucosal capillaries. Note in Fig. 2 that mucosal capillary pressure is only 13.8 ± 2.2 mm Hg compared with 30.6 ± 1.8 mm Hg in the precapillary arterioles. The pressure drop of about 17 mm Hg occurs over a distance of only 20 to 50 μm from the origin of the capillary with a minor pressure drop from capillaries to mucosal venules (10). The entrance to many of the capillaries (>60%) is constricted by a structure analogous to a precapillary sphincter. The high resistance of the capillary origin is by no means fixed. Indeed, the constricted input segment can be made to dilate to the same diameter as the capillary (3.5–5 μm). The maintenance of low mucosal capillary pressures would minimize capillary filtration and, more probably, favor fluid absorption (10).

Dissipation of venous pressures within the intestinal microvasculature, at least in the rat, is very minor (3,4,10). A small drop in pressure occurs from the mucosal and muscle capillaries to the largest venules or IV (Fig. 2). The absence of a large resistance between the capillaries and venules leaves the capillaries vulnerable to elevated venous pressures. This facet of intestinal microvascular pressure is discussed below.

The data discussed thus far on microvascular pressures in the rat may be qualitatively, and perhaps quantitatively, relevant to other species. Königes and Ottó (19) in 1937 reported that average pressures in mucosal capillaries of the cat were 31.3 mm Hg and varied ± 15%. They mentioned that the tip diameters of micropipettes used to measure the pressures were 8 to

14 µm and that the vessels constricted when penetrated. It would be physically impossible to penetrate true capillaries with such large pipettes. Also, capillaries do not constrict when penetrated. Therefore, Königes and Ottó (19) probably measured pressures in the smallest arterioles of the villi. If this was the case, their pressure measurements of 31 to 32 mm Hg in cats compare remarkably well with the values of 30.6 ± 1.8 mm Hg in the smallest mucosal arterioles of rats (2,10).

A second line of evidence indicates qualitatively and perhaps quantitatively similar control of microvascular pressure occurs in the intestine of rats and cats. Capillary pressures measured with the isogravimetric method in cats and by direct micropuncture in the rat are similar. The isogravimetric method, which predicts an average capillary pressure in the intestine, includes contributions by the muscle, submucosal and mucosal capillaries and any other vessel that can exchange fluid. Average isogravimetric pressures of 13 to 15 mm Hg are reported typically with a range of pressures from 12 to 19 mm Hg (17,18,24). Gore and Bohlen (10) computed a weighted average of directly measured muscle and mucosal capillary pressures, based on the distribution of the total flow to both tissue regions, and obtained an average capillary pressure of 16.8 mm Hg. This weighted average was based on direct measurements when the intestine was filtering and, therefore, would be expected to be higher than isogravimetric conditions. However, the agreement of direct and isogravimetric estimates is sufficient to predict that large and small species not only have approximately equal capillary pressures but also similar pre- to postcapillary resistance ratios for the various parallel vascular beds.

CONTROL OF MICROVASCULAR PRESSURES

Three major facets of the interaction of intestinal vascular function and microvascular pressures will be considered: first, the effect of reflex activity by the sympathetic nervous system on microvascular pressures at normal and reduced arterial pressure; second, the influence of increased sympathetic activity on vascular behavior at normal arterial pressures; and, third, the effect of intestinal absorption on microvascular pressures.

The majority of studies of intestinal microvascular pressures with isogravimetric methods have used preparations that for technical reasons were denervated. Therefore, low-frequency direct sympathetic stimulation (2 Hz), which probably has the same effect on vascular resistance as normal resting sympathetic activity, is used to determine how background sympathetic activity affects the intestinal vasculature. Low-frequency stimulation reduces blood flow by 20% to 50% and decreases the capillary filtration coefficient (K_f) by nearly 30% (7,8). The reduction in K_f may be caused by reductions in capillary pressure as well as the number of capillaries available for flow. However, the effects of the vasodilation that results from the removal of sympathetic tone or the effects of resting sympathetic activity on microvascular pressures are controversial. For example, Granger et al. (13) have demonstrated that adenosine-induced vasodilation does not effect lymph production. This finding may indicate that mild vasodilation has a relatively minor effect on capillary pressure. In Fig. 3, the pressures in various intestinal vessels of the rat before and after acute denervation are compared (3). At normal arterial pressures of 100 to 110 mm Hg, acute denervation had no significant effect on arteriolar pressures and tended to lower pressure in capillaries and in some venules (4V and 2V), yet the vasculature dilated (3). Therefore, these studies (3,7,8,14) demonstrate that resting sympathetic activity does not disturb microvascular pressures in the intestine and that blood flow is maintained at a lower level than if the tissues were denervated.

The absence of a major effect of resting sympathetic activity on intestinal microvascular pressures is puzzling. The hemodynamic data seem to indicate that although mild sympathetic stimulation increases total resistance, it does not alter the ratio of pre- to postcapillary resistance. However, if the microvascular pressures before

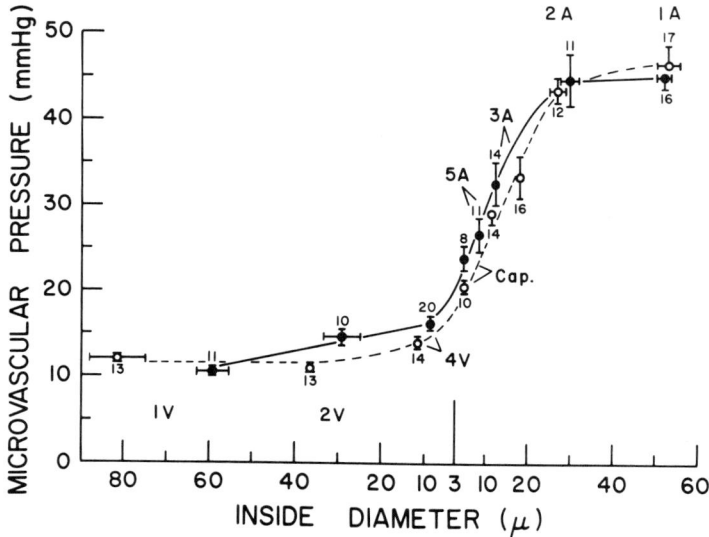

FIG. 3. Intestinal microvascular pressures (mean ± SEM) in innervated *(closed circles)* and acutely denervated *(open circles)* rat intestine at a mean arterial pressure of 105 ± 3 (SD) mm Hg. For abbreviations, see legend to Fig. 1. *(Numbers beside data points)* Number of observations in 28 innervated and 23 denervated preparations. (From Bohlen and Gore, ref. 3, with permission.)

and after denervation are not significantly different, some active mechanism may maintain a near-constant pressure profile regardless of resting sympathetic activity. There are various accounts in the literature of a weak mechanism to regulate capillary pressure, as measured by isogravimetric techniques, when the arterial or venous pressure changes (17,18,24). As shown in Figs. 4, 5, and 6, arteriolar, capillary, and venular pressures in the innervated and denervated rat intestine are simple, linear functions of arterial pressure (3). Although these observations (3) certainly do not discount the possibility of an active mechanism to control capillary and microvascular pressures in other species, they do indicate that the vasculature of the rat intestine lacks a control mechanism to precisely regulate capillary pressure as arterial pressure is lowered. Granger et al. (12) have reached a similar conclusion for the vasculature of the cat intestine in which capillary pressure is poorly regulated as arterial pressure is reduced. However, as discussed later, there are mechanisms in the intestinal vasculature that do prevent large vessel pressure changes from fully affecting capillary pressures.

The effect of strong sympathetic stimulation at a normal blood pressure is universally agreed to lower intestinal microvascular pressures. The basic question of interest is "Which vessels are responsible for the microvascular pressure changes?" In Fig. 7, the microvascular pressures in the rat intestinal microvasculature are presented for innervated and acutely denervated conditions as well as during direct sympathetic nerve stimulation at frequencies of 4, 8, and 16 Hz (4). As previously mentioned, acute denervation (Figs. 3–7) has essentially no effect on microvascular pressures, and stimulation at 4 Hz (Fig. 7) only slightly decreases microvascular pressures (2–4 mm Hg), although the majority of vessels constricted (4). However, at 8 Hz, there is a tendency for pressures to decrease throughout the vasculature. The predominate and statistically significant ($p<0.05$) pressure reduction is caused by the smallest arterioles (5A), and this effect extends to the remainder of the downstream vascular segments. In contrast, 16-Hz stimulation causes a dramatic decrease in all pressures, and the reduction is caused by constriction of the large and intermediate diameter arterioles (1A and 2A).

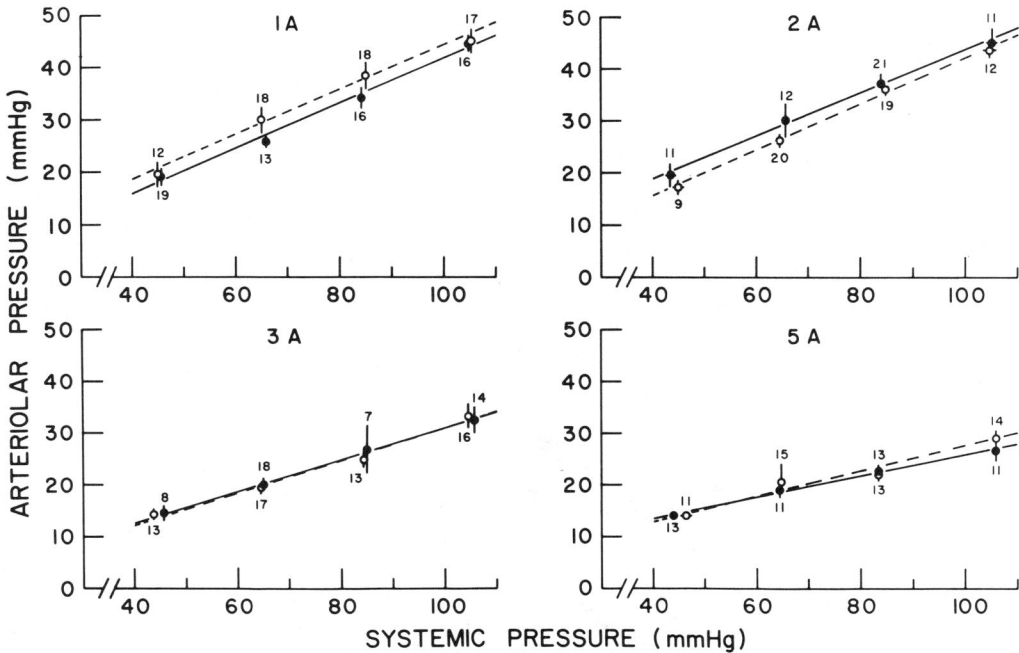

FIG. 4. Microvascular pressures (mean ± SEM) in rat intestinal arterioles from innervated *(closed circles)* and denervated *(open circles)* preparations as a function of the systemic arterial pressure. *(Numbers above and below data points)* Numbers of vessels studied. For abbreviations, see legend to Fig. 1. (From Bohlen and Gore, ref. 3, with permission.)

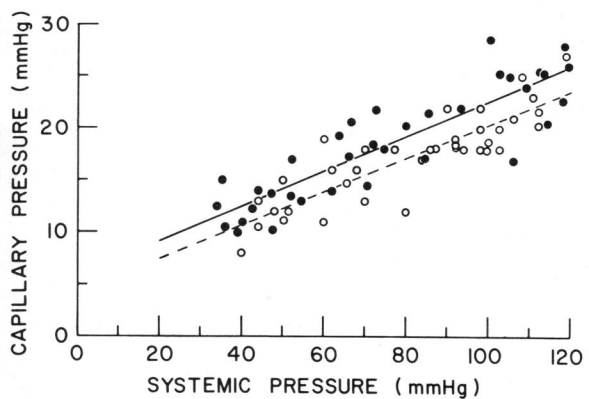

FIG. 5. Muscle layer capillary pressures in innervated *(closed circles, solid line)* and denervated *(open circles, dashed line)* rat intestine preparations at various systemic arterial pressures. (From Bohlen and Gore, ref. 3, with permission.)

Whether analogous behavior by small and large vessels at various rates of sympathetic stimulation occurs in other species is not known. In rats, low to moderate rates of sympathetic stimulation reduce capillary pressure by constricting the small arterioles, but larger arterioles become the predominate effector at high rates of sympathetic activity (4).

The influence of physiological vasodilation, such as during absorption of food, on microvascular pressures is of particular interest because capillary pressure affects transcapillary water exchange. At this time, no direct or indirect measurements of microvascular pressures have been made during absorptive activity as Granger has emphasized in his recent review (11). Therefore, the influence of vasodilation on microvascular pressures cannot be directly addressed, but several lines of evidence indicate that, at least in the mucosal capillaries, the pres-

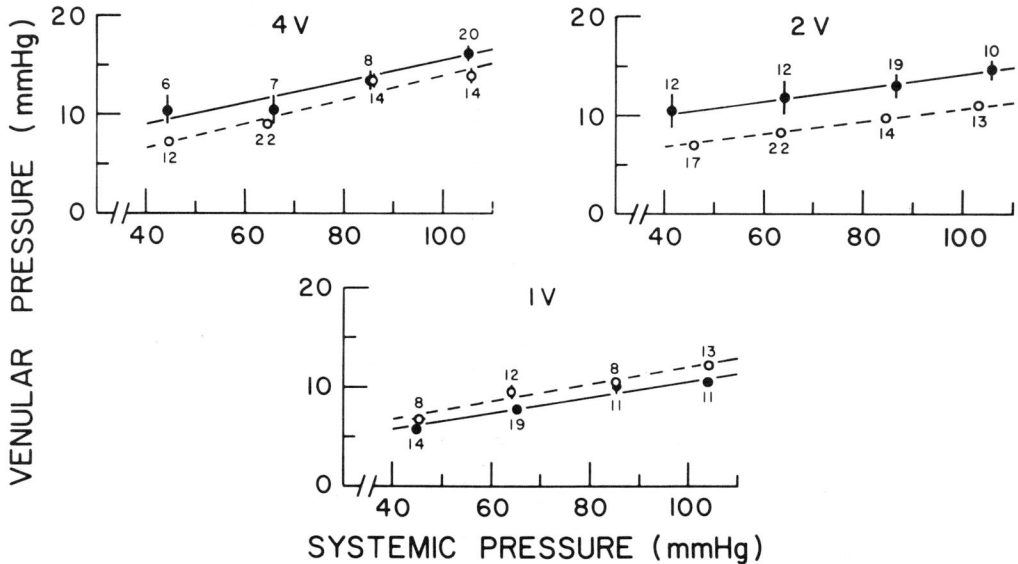

FIG. 6. Venular pressures in the innervated *(closed circles)* and denervated *(open circles)* rat intestine at various systemic arterial pressures. Note that denervation tends to lower pressure in small- and intermediate-diameter vessels (4V, 2V) and slightly increase pressure in large 1V venules. (From Bohlen and Gore, ref. 3, with permission.)

sure is probably not affected. Granger and coworkers (14) have reported that intraarterial infusion of adenosine in amounts that increased blood flow 60% to 70% had essentially no effect on capillary fluid exchange. Just how these data relate to vascular responses during natural absorption is not known. Adenosine caused mucosal flow to decrease rather than increase as typically occurs during absorption (14). However, the data (14) do demonstrate that vasodilation of at least part of the bowel wall does not necessarily influence capillary exchange. In a study by Brunsson et al. (5), the rate of lymph production during absorption was not influenced by blood flow up to five times the normal flow. If mucosal capillary pressure had been substantially elevated so that capillary absorption was converted to filtration, one would have expected lymph flow to increase, but it did not (5). The possible changes in capillary pressures, assuming that such changes occur, may be very difficult to detect without some form of direct or indirect method to measure capillary pressure during absorption. This point is raised because Granger and Taylor (13) have proposed the possibility that as fluid is absorbed from the lumen to the mucosal interstitium, the interstitial fluid pressure is increased and tissue oncotic pressure falls as interstitial proteins are diluted. Both of these events would tend to nullify capillary filtration due to an increase in mucosal capillary pressure. The increase in mucosal tissue pressure during absorption has been documented by Lee (21,22). Assuming this fluid is of lumenal origin, its presence, as noted by increased tissue pressure, would decrease the interstitial oncotic pressure. In effect, a safety system may exist to prevent capillary filtration during luminal absorption. Moreover, the hemodynamics of the mucosa may simply allow flow to change without inducing major changes in mucosal capillary pressure. A variety of studies by Lee (21,22) indicate that the lymphatic system of the intestinal mucosa is capable of transporting virtually all of the fluid absorbed from the lumen even if the blood flow is stopped. Therefore, the mucosal capillaries may be a "backup" system for absorption rather than the primary system responsible for introducing absorbed fluid during resting conditions into the vascular system (see Chapter 18).

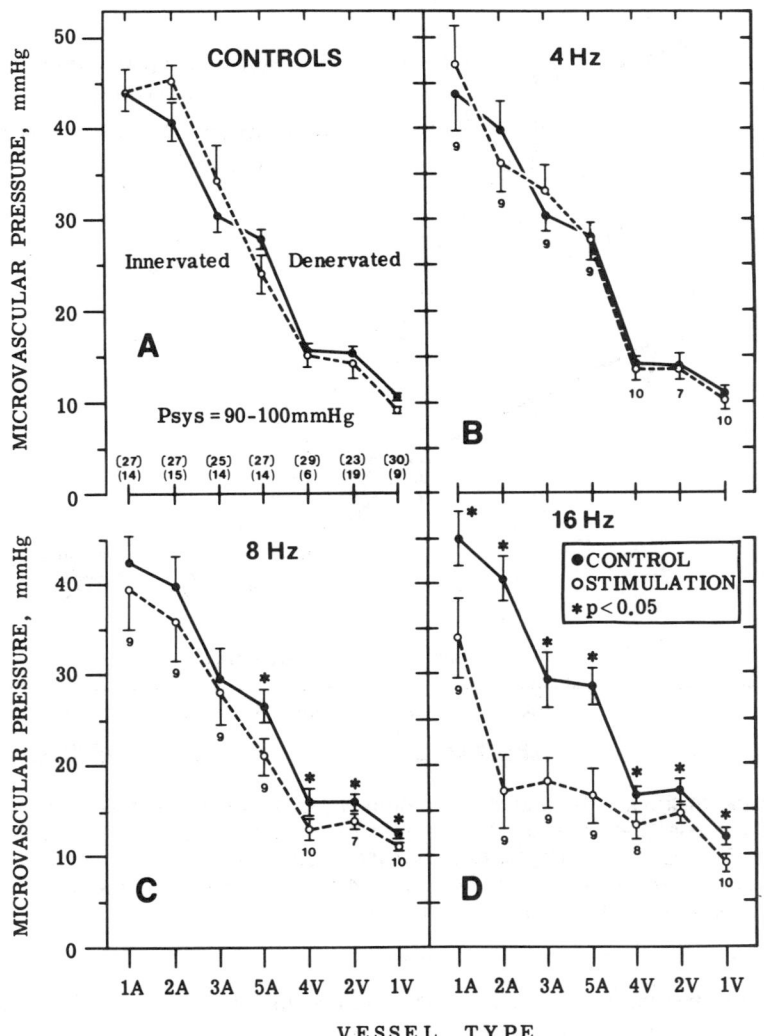

FIG. 7. Intestinal microvascular pressures during innervated and acutely denervated (**A:** *solid and dashed lines*) conditions at 4-**(B)**, 8-**(C)**, and 16-**(D)** Hz direct sympathetic stimulation *(dashed line)* of denervated preparations *(solid line)*. For abbreviations, see legend to Fig. 1. (From Bohlen and Gore, ref. 3, with permission.)

LOCAL REFLEX OR MYOGENIC MECHANISMS AND MICROVASCULAR PRESSURES

A myogenic mechanism that maintains constant microvascular pressures, blood flow, and vessel wall stress has been proposed for the small intestine (17,18). Studies by Johnson and Hanson (17), Johnson and Richardson (18), and Mortillaro and Taylor (24) imply that the intestinal vascular resistance changes attenuate the increase in capillary pressure caused by venous pressure elevation. The success of the capillary pressure defense is such that only 62% to 69% of a given change in venous pressure affects the overall intestinal capillary pressure (17,18,24). It should be emphasized that the protection afforded the capillary pressure is the result apparently of both pre- and postcapillary vascular responses (17,18,24). A recent study by Davis

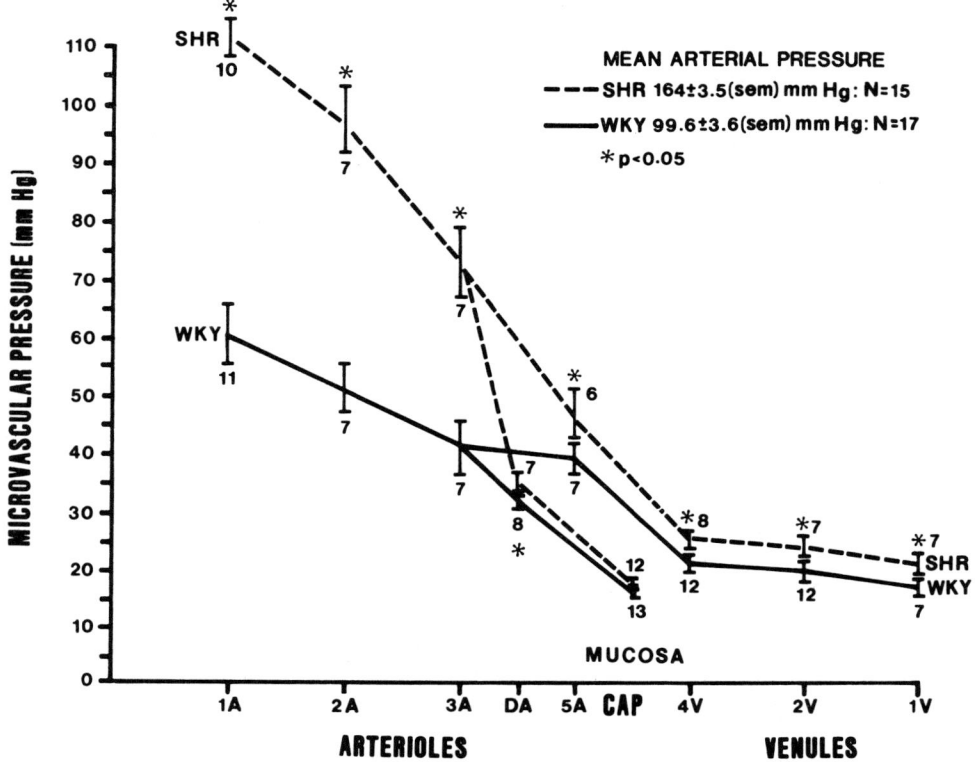

FIG. 8. Intestinal microvascular pressures in normal *(solid line)* and spontaneously hypertensive *(dashed line)* rat at age 18–21 weeks. Pressures in the majority of vessels in hypertensive animals are significantly ($P<0.05$) higher than normal. However, mucosal capillary pressure is normal ($P>0.05$), and muscle layer capillary pressure *(line from 5A to 4V)* is increased only about 15–20% for a 65% increase in mean arterial pressure. (From Bohlen, ref. 2, with permission.)

and Gore (6) indicates that in the rat intestine, the muscle layer capillary pressure increases by 72% and mucosal capillary pressure by 82% of the increase in venous pressure. What is of particular interest in the study by Davis and Gore (6) is that the large to intermediate diameter arterioles (15–35 μm) are the vessels primarily responsible for the increase in the arterial resistance. The small precapillary arterioles dilated as the venous pressure increased. The response of the large- to intermediate-diameter arterioles is of interest because it is these vessels that are in series with both the muscular and mucosal vasculatures. Therefore, these arterioles are ideally situated to influence both blood flow and arteriolar pressure at the inputs to the individual parallel circuits of the bowel wall.

HYPERTENSION AND INTESTINAL MICROVASCULAR PRESSURES

The effect of essential hypertension on the microvasculature has recently been one of the most intensively studied areas of vascular research. The spontaneously hypertensive rat (SHR), which has a form of hypertension with many of the characteristics of essential hypertension in man, has been used to assess the effects of systemic arterial hypertension on intestinal microvascular pressures.

The data presented in Fig. 8 were obtained in 18- to 21-week-old normal and SHR rats; the hypertensive syndrome is fully developed and stable at this age (2). The pressures in the 1A, 2A, and 3A arterioles of the SHR are substantially higher than in comparable vessels of normal animals. The pressures in the 5A of the muscle layer and smallest arterioles of the mucosa, DA, are higher than normal but only by a small amount. Therefore, capillary pressures, represented by the lines interconnecting the 5A and smallest venules, 4V, of the muscle layer and actual mucosal capillary pressure, are essentially normal because of the pressure drop across the arterioles. The measurement of vessel diameters in this study indicated that a generalized constriction of the arterioles in the SHR compared to normotensive rats was primarily responsible for the essentially normal capillary pressures in hypertensive animals. Whether these data indicate that the capillary pressure was maintained near normal during hypertension as a result of some active capillary pressure control mechanism or simply as a coincidence of vasoconstriction caused by the hypertensive process is unknown. However, it is of interest that of the vascular beds that can least tolerate elevated capillary pressures, with the possible exception of the brain, the intestine is essentially spared from a disruption of capillary pressure during hypertension.

SUMMARY

Measurements of microvascular pressures by both micropuncture and isogravimetric methods have been very useful in the analysis of intestinal vascular control and transcapillary fluid exchange. Although micropuncture methods have been almost exclusively limited to use in rats, the data obtained correlate qualitatively and, in many cases, quantitatively to measurements using indirect techniques in larger species. Therefore, our concepts of microvascular pressure control appear to be valid despite species differences in intestinal vascular physiology.

REFERENCES

1. Baez, S. (1959): Microcirculation in the intramural vessels of the small intestine in the rat. In: *The Microcirculation*, edited by S. Baez, pp. 114–125. Illinois Press.
2. Bohlen, H. G. (1983): Intestinal microvascular adaptation during maturation of spontaneously hypertensive rats. *Hypertension*, 5:739–745.
3. Bohlen, H. G., and Gore, R. W. (1977): Comparison of microvascular pressures and diameters in the innervated and denervated rat intestine. *Microvas. Res.*, 14:251–264.
4. Bohlen, H. G., and Gore, R. W. (1979): Microvascular pressures in rat intestinal muscle during direct nerve stimulation. *Microvas. Res.*, 17:27–37.
5. Brunsson, I., Eklund, S., Jodal, M., Lundgren, O., and Sjövall, H. (1979): The effect of vasodilation and sympathetic nerve activation on net water absorption in the cat's small intestine. *Acta Physiol. Scand.*, 106:61–68.
6. Davis, M. J., and Gore, R. W. (1983): Capillary pressures in rat intestinal muscle and mucosal villi during venous pressure elevation. *Am. J. Physiol. (In press)*.
7. Folkow, B., Lewis, D. H., Lundgren, O., Mellander, S., and Wallentin, I. (1964): The effect of graded vasoconstrictor fibre stimulation on the intestinal resistance and capacitance vessels. *Acta Physiol. Scand.*, 61:445–457.
8. Folkow, B., Lewis, D. H., Lundgren, O., Mellander, S., and Wallentin, I. (1964): The effect of the sympathetic vasoconstrictor fibres on the distribution of capillary blood flow in the intestine. *Acta Physiol. Scand.*, 61:458–466.
9. Gannon, B. J., Gore, R. W., and Rogers, P. A. W. (1981): Is there an anatomical basis for a vascular countercurrent mechanism in rabbit and human intestinal villi? *Biomed. Res. (Suppl.)*, 2:235–241.
10. Gore, R. W., and Bohlen, H. G. (1977): Microvascular pressures in rat intestinal muscle and mucosal villi. *Am. J. Physiol.*, 233:H685–H693.
11. Granger, D. N. (1981): Intestinal microcirculation and transmucosal fluid transport. *Am. J. Physiol.*, 240:G343–G349.
12. Granger, D. N., Mortillaro, N. A., Perry, M. A., and Kvietys, P. R. (1982): Autoregulation of intestinal capillary filtration rate. *Am. J. Physiol.*, 243:G475–G483.
13. Granger, D. N., and Taylor, A. (1978): Effects of solute-coupled transport on lymph flow and oncotic pressures in cat ileum. *Am. J. Physiol.*, 235:E429–E436.
14. Granger, D. N., Valleau, J. D., Parker, R. E., Lane, R. S., and Taylor, A. E. (1978): Effects of adenosine on intestinal hemodynamics, oxygen delivery, and capillary fluid exchange. *Am. J. Physiol.*, 235:H707–H719.
15. Intaglietta, M., Parvula, R. R., and Tompkins, W. R. (1970): Pressure measurement in the mammalian microvasculature. *Microvas. Res.*, 2:212–220.
16. Jacobson, L. F., and Noer, R. F. (1952): The vascular pattern of the intestinal villi in various laboratory animals and man. *Anat. Rec.*, 114:85–101.
17. Johnson, P. C., and Hanson, K. M. (1966): Capillary

filtration in the small intestine of the dog. *Circ. Res.*, 19:766–773.
18. Johnson, P. C., and Richardson, D. R. (1974): The influence of venous pressure on filtration forces in the intestine. *Microvas. Res.*, 7:296–306.
19. Königes, H. G., and Otto', M. (1937): Studies on the filtration mechanism of the intestinal lymph and on the action of acetylcholine on it and on the circulation of the intestinal villi. *Qu. J. Exp. Biol.*, 26:319–329.
20. Landis, E. M. (1927): The capillary pressure in frog mesentery as determined by microinjection methods. *Am. J. Physiol.*, 75:548–570.
21. Lee, J. S. (1973): Effects of pressures on water absorption and secretion in rat jejunum. *Am. J. Physiol.*, 224:1338–1344.
22. Lee, J. S. (1981): Lymph flow during fluid absorption from rat jejunum. *Am. J. Physiol.*, 240:G312–G316.
23. Mohiuddin, A. (1966): Blood and lymph vessels in the jejunal villi of the white rat. *Anat. Rec.*, 156:83–90.
24. Mortillaro, N. A., and Taylor, A. E. (1976): Interaction of capillary and tissue forces in the cat small intestine. *Circ. Res.*, 39:348–358.
25. Noer, R. J. (1943): The blood vessels of the jejunum and ileum: A comparative study of man and certain laboratory animals. *Am. J. Anat.*, 73:293–334.
26. Pappenheimer, J. R., and Soto-Rivera, A. (1948): Effective osmotic pressure of the plasma proteins and other quantities associated with the capillary circulation in the hindlimbs of cats and dogs. *Am. J. Physiol.*, 152:471–491.
27. Vawter, D., Fung, Y. C., and Zweifach, B. W. (1974): Distribution of blood flow and pressure from a microvessel into a branch. *Microvas. Res.*, 8:44–52.
28. Wiederhielm, C. A., Woodbury, J. W., Kirk, S., and Rushmer, R. F. (1964): Pulsatile pressures in the microcirculation of the frog's mesentery. *Am. J. Physiol.*, 207:173–176.

Microvascular Control of Intestinal Oxygenation

Harris J. Granger, Gerald A. Meininger, George E. Barnes, and Anthony H. Goodman

Microcirculation Research Institute and Department of Medical Physiology, College of Medicine, Texas A&M University, College Station, Texas 77843

The oxygenation of intestinal tissue is dependent on a well-organized hierarchy of transport processes and vasoregulatory mechanisms. From an engineering viewpoint, insight into the physiology of tissue oxygenation can be gained by applying the basic concepts of transport phenomena and control theory. The aim of this chapter is to analyze the dynamics of intestinal oxygenation. First, we describe a simple graphical approach to evaluating the steady state interactions between O_2 supply and utilization. Next, a mathematical model of local microvascular regulation of intestinal oxygenation is presented, and its behavior under different conditions is scrutinized. Finally, the limitations of current models are discussed, and potential new directions in mathematical simulation of intestinal O_2 transport and vasoregulatory processes are considered.

INTESTINAL OXYGENATION: BALANCE BETWEEN OXYGEN SUPPLY AND UPTAKE

The generation of an adequate supply of ATP in gastrointestinal tissues is required for maintenance of motility, secretion, and absorption. The formation of ATP in the parenchymal cells of the enteric tract is coupled to oxidative processes operating at the mitochondrial level. Thus, hypoxia of the bowel compromises the major functions of the digestive tract, and anoxia destroys the ability of these cells to perform chemical or mechanical work. To preserve digestive function over a wide range of physiological demands, the circulation of the intestine is controlled by the parenchymal cells in such a manner that tissue oxygenation does not limit ATP production. To gain insight into the nature of this coupling of tissue metabolism to the circulation, an understanding of the basic processes of oxygen supply and utilization is required.

Stages of Oxygen Transport

The translocation of oxygen from the main supply artery of the intestine to its final destination in the mitochondria of the parenchymal cells involves three separate and distinctive processes: (a) convection, (b) diffusion, and (c) chemical reaction (Fig. 1, *upper panel*). First, oxygen is carried from the major artery to the capillaries by convection in the stream of blood that courses through the microcirculation. Consequently, the rate of oxygen delivery ($J_{O_{2A}}$) to the capillary level is dependent on the flow (F_A) and the concentration ($[O_2]$) of the gas in arterial blood or

$$J_{O_{2A}} = F_A \cdot [O_2]_A. \quad (1)$$

Physiological control of oxygen convection is achieved by modulation of blood flow via appropriate alterations in vascular resistance. The potential range of flow in the small intestine is impressive; with total dilation, blood flow has been reported to increase eightfold from a control value of 30 to 50 ml·min^{-1}·100 g^{-1} in the nonabsorbing state (6). The homeostatic importance of flow control in the regulation of oxygen transport can best be appreciated by solving the Fick equation for venous oxygen concentration ($[O_2]_V$); the result is

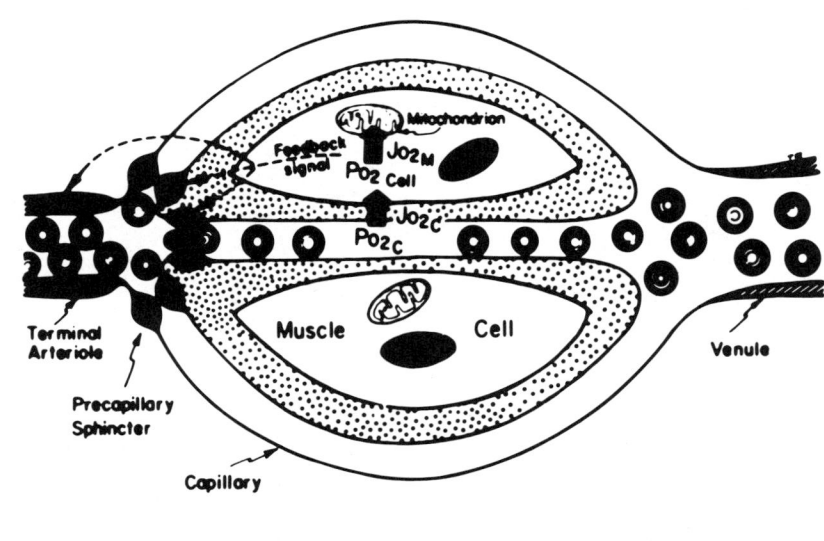
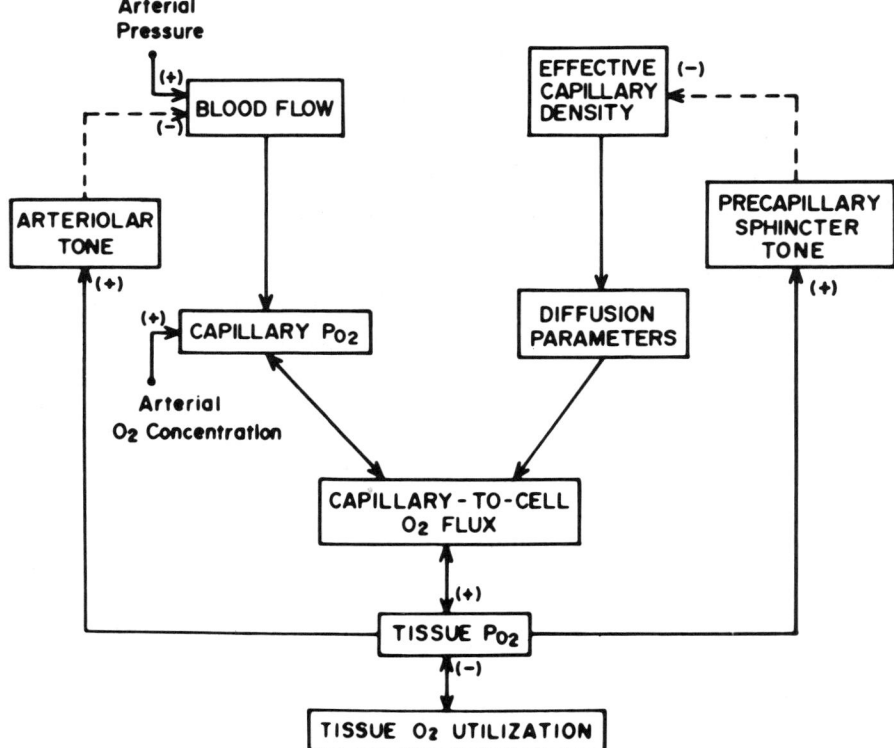

FIG. 1. Anatomical *(upper panel)* and physiological *(lower panel)* bases of mathematical model of intestinal oxygenation. From ref. 4.

$$[O_2]_V = [O_2]_A - (JO_{2D}/F_A), \quad (2)$$

where JO_{2D} is the transcapillary oxygen flux. Assume for the moment that venous oxygen levels reflect capillary oxygenation (i.e., capillary PO_2). Equation 2 states that, for a constant $[O_2]_A$, the oxygen uptake-to-blood-flow ratio is a primary determinant of capillary PO_2. In other words, by modulating convection in accordance with oxygen needs, the flow control system serves to stabilize the source Po_2, which drives oxygen out of the blood into the tissues.

The movement of oxygen from the capillaries into the cells is governed by the laws of diffusion. The major determinants of the diffusive oxygen flux (Jo_{2D}) are the capillary oxygen tension (Po_{2cap}), the oxygen tension in the cell (Po_{2cell}), and diffusion parameters including capillary surface area (A) and capillary-to-cell diffusion distance (ΔX). Thus,

$$Jo_{2D} = K_1 \cdot A \cdot (Po_{2cap} - Po_{2cell})/\Delta X, \quad (3)$$

where K_1 is a constant that includes the oxygen solubility and diffusion coefficients. In muscle tissue, the capillary distribution pattern with relationship to the parenchymal cells allows changes in both A and ΔX when the number of open capillaries (N) is altered (5). Thus, in muscle, A changes in proportion to capillarity (i.e., number of open capillaries) and ΔX in inverse proportion to the square root of N. As a consequence, the diffusive oxygen flux is proportional to $N^{3/2}$, and the rate of diffusion increases eightfold for a fourfold increment of functional capillary density. Therefore, for skeletal muscle and possibly intestinal smooth muscle, Eq. 3 reduces to

$$Jo_{2D} = K_2 \cdot N^{3/2} \cdot (Po_{2cap} - Po_{2cell}). \quad (4)$$

The vascular and parenchymal organization of gastrointestinal mucosa suggests that the arguments used to generate Eq. 4 from Eq. 3 are not appropriate for the luminal lining. The cells of the villus form a tissue cylinder surrounding an inner cylindrical meshwork of capillaries. The oxygen consumption of the tissue in the central core of the villus probably is minimal compared with the mucosal cells. Consequently, the exchange of oxygen between the capillary network and mucosal cells of the villus can best be approximated by viewing the system as a cylindrical sheet of blood surrounded by a larger cylindrical sheet of oxygen-consuming cells. Therefore, changes in the number of open capillaries in the layered vascular net should affect exchange surface area more than effective capillary-to-cell diffusion distance. With these considerations in mind, diffusive oxygen flux in mucosa may be better described by Eq. 5

$$Jo_{2D} = K_3 \cdot N \cdot (Po_{2cap} - Po_{2cell}). \quad (5)$$

Comparison of Eqs. 4 and 5 suggests that a given relative change in functional capillarity has a greater impact on oxygenation of muscularis than on mucosa. It should be emphasized that Eq. 5 is a gross approximation. This points out the need for a rigorous formulation of the diffusion problem in specialized structures such as villi. In intestine as a whole, filtration coefficient and permeability–surface area product measurements suggest that functional capillary density can increase two- to fourfold; thus, only 25% to 50% of the exchange vessels are perfused under normal conditions (1,5,6).

After oxygen diffuses into the cell, the gas acts as an electron acceptor and removes reducing equivalents from the terminal oxidase of the respiratory chain. Thus, the final stage of oxygen transport involves the process of chemical reaction. The rate of mitochondrial oxygen utilization (Jo_{2M}) is dependent on the concentration of electron acceptor (i.e., oxygen) and the concentration of reduced cytochrome $(a \cdot a_3)_R$, the electron donor. Hence,

$$Jo_{2M} = K \cdot [a \cdot a_3]_R \cdot Po_{2cell} \quad (6)$$

where K is a constant. Within the mitochondrion, cytochrome $a \cdot a_3$ exists in the interchangeable reduced and oxidized forms. At a resting metabolic rate, the fraction of $a \cdot a_3$ in the reduced form is small, for example, 0.1 or less. In such a state, reductions in cell Po_2 elicit a temporary decrease in conversion of reduced cytochrome oxidase to oxidized cytochrome oxidase. Consequently, $[a \cdot a_3]_R$ rises to compensate for the reduced cell Po_2, and mitochondrial oxygen uptake remains unchanged. With further reductions in cell Po_2, elevated $[a \cdot a_3]_R$ continues to stabilize Jo_{2M} until a cell Po_2 is reached at which all of the cytochrome $a \cdot a_3$ is reduced. Lowering cell Po_2 below this critical level results in a reduction of oxygen utilization, since further compensatory increases in $[a \cdot a_3]_R$ are not possible. As a consequence of Eq. 6, the kinetics of mitochondrial oxygen utilization can be described by

$$JO_{2M} = [PO_{2cell}/(K_M + PO_{2cell})] \cdot JO_{2max}, \quad (7)$$

where K_M is the cell PO_2 at which oxygen uptake is half the maximum rate (JO_{2max}) possible in the given metabolic state. In most tissues, K_M is less than 0.1 mm Hg. In intestinal mucosa, tissue PO_2 averages 12 to 15 mm Hg (1,3,6). Therefore, cell PO_2 in these tissues exceeds the K_M by two orders of magnitude, and JO_{2M} is independent of cell PO_2 until PO_2 in the tissue falls below 1 mm Hg.

Graphical Analysis of Oxygen Supply-Uptake Interactions

Although Eqs. 2, 3, and 7 provide a basis for examining the interactions of oxygen supply and demand, many physiologists are more comfortable with, and have a clearer understanding of, graphical analyses of functional relationships. In this section, we present a simple graphical representation of the basic concepts summarized above. The approach (3) consists of separating the diffusion and chemical reaction stages of oxygen transport at the level of the cell and utilizing cell PO_2 as the primary variable common to both processes. Figure 2 illustrates the method. The reader will recognize the chemical reaction curve as a restatement of the basic relation between mitochondrial oxygen uptake and cell PO_2. The diffusion curve simply states that, all other factors being constant, the rate of oxygen supply to the cell decreases in inverse linear fashion as PO_2 in the cell rises. In the steady state, supply and uptake are equal, as indicated by the intersection of the two curves. The x- and y-axis values of the intersection point represent the prevailing cell PO_2 *(point b)* and oxygen utilization rate, respectively. The intersection of the supply curve with the x-axis *(point c)* identifies the prevailing capillary PO_2. At this point, cell and capillary PO_2 are equal, and the diffusive oxygen flux is zero. Thus, the magnitude of the sector between points b and c provides a measure of the capillary-to-cell PO_2 difference. Finally, the length of the segment between points a (i.e., the critical PO_2) and b reflects the cell PO_2 reserve against development of tissue hypoxia.

Having established the basic relationships, let us consider the effects of different factors on the supply-uptake curves. As illustrated in Fig. 3, changes in blood flow and arterial PO_2 simply produce parallel shifts in the supply curve; increasing blood flow or arterial PO_2 shifts the curve to the right, whereas a shift to the left occurs with reduced arterial PO_2 or blood flow. Consider the graded effects of a reduction in blood flow. For both hypoperfusion states shown in Fig. 3, the capillary and cell PO_2 are reduced, the former reflecting augmented extraction of oxygen from the bloodstream. At moderate levels of reduction in flow, the capillary-to-cell PO_2 difference remains normal, and the cell PO_2 stabilizes above the critical value. Thus, oxygen uptake is maintained at the normal level owing to a passive increase in oxygen extraction made possible by the preexisting cell PO_2 reserve. Thus, the cell PO_2 reserve provides a "margin of safety" against development of tissue hypoxia; this safety factor is inherent to the cell and is available even in the absence of local vascular compensations. With more severe reductions in flow, the reserve is depleted, cell PO_2 falls below the critical level, and the capillary-to-cell PO_2 difference falls; consequently, oxygen uptake is compromised. Thus, in the second case, the increase in oxygen extraction is not sufficient to compensate for the flow reduction, and cell hypoxia results. By contrast, the hyperperfusion curve clearly illustrates that the oxygen uptake does not increase with augmented flow because the capillary-to-cell PO_2 difference remains constant in spite of dramatic increases in the prevailing tissue and capillary PO_2 values. From these examples, the value of an intrinsic flow control system is evident; stabilization of flow at an appropriate level helps to prevent development of tissue hypoxia and also eliminates the need for providing excessive resting flow as a means of effecting such protection.

As indicated earlier, functional capillary density is an important determinant of transmicro-

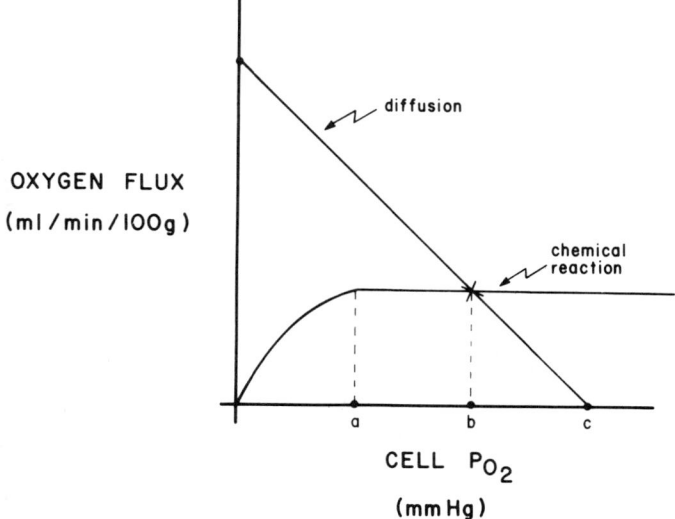

FIG. 2. Basic oxygen supply-uptake curves for graphic analysis of intestinal oxygenation. See text for explanation. From ref. 3.

a. critical cell P_{O_2}
b. normal cell P_{O_2}
c. capillary P_{O_2}
b-a. cell P_{O_2} reserve
c-b. capillary-to-cell P_{O_2} difference

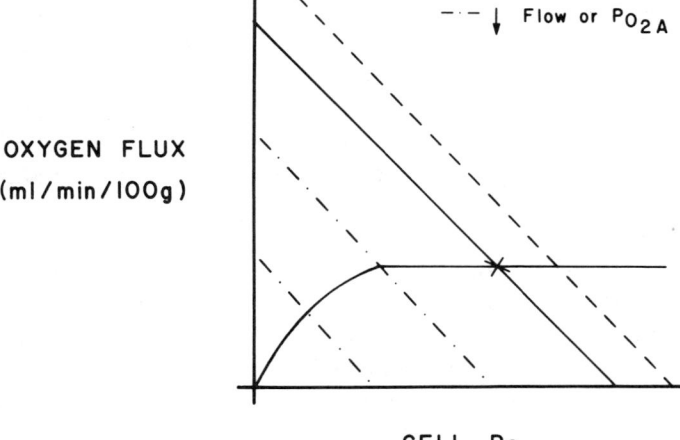

FIG. 3. Effect of changes in blood flow and arterial P_{O_2} on intestinal oxygen supply-uptake balance. From ref. 3.

vascular oxygen flux. Figure 4 shows how changing the number of perfused capillaries affects the supply curve. As indicated in the figure, changes in capillarity modify the slope of the supply relationship. Oxygen uptake is unchanged so long as the intersection of the supply-uptake relationships occurs in the plateau region of the uptake curve. For example, the curve labeled *increased capillarity* shows that augmentation of capillary density increases the

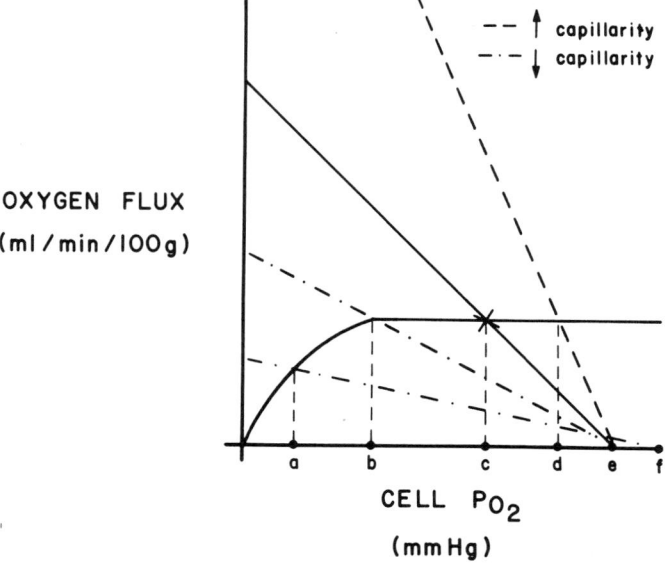

FIG. 4. Effect of changes in functional capillary density on intestinal oxygen supply-uptake relationships. From ref. 3.

slope of the supply curve and the magnitude of the prevailing cell P_{O_2} *(point d)*. Capillary P_{O_2} is unchanged *(point e)*, and the capillary-to-cell P_{O_2} difference is reduced *(e-d)*. However, owing to changes in the diffusion parameters, the P_{O_2} flux remains constant in the face of a reduced P_{O_2} difference. Hence, oxygen uptake is unaltered. Thus, with constant-flow perfusion, oxygen extraction is unchanged in the face of increased capillary density. Under these circumstances, changes in oxygen extraction do not provide a measure of altered capillarity. With small reductions of capillary density, the capillary-to-cell P_{O_2} difference is increased *(e-b)* in the face of a constant capillary P_{O_2}. Tissue P_{O_2} *(point b)* falls but not to the critical level. Thus, in this situation also, oxygen extraction and consumption remain normal. With further reductions in capillary density, the critical level is reached, and oxygen uptake is compromised *(intersection extending from point a)*. Under these conditions, not only is the slope reduced, but the supply curve is shifted to the right. The reason for the parallel shift can be appreciated by examination of Eqs. 2 and 3, the underlying bases for the supply curve. Note that the capillary P_{O_2} is dependent on the venous oxygen concentration described in Eq. 2, which, in turn, includes oxygen uptake as an independent variable. Thus, whenever the supply and uptake curves intersect at an oxygen uptake different from control, the supply curve shifts to the left if oxygen uptake is increased or to the right if oxygen uptake is decreased. Hence, in our example of a dramatic reduction in capillary density, capillary P_{O_2} is elevated above control *(point f)*, oxygen extraction is reduced, and oxygen uptake falls in spite of a large capillary-to-cell P_{O_2} difference *(f-a)*. In this case, the oxygen supply is diffusion-limited.

The impact of changes in oxygen demand is illustrated in Fig. 5. As expected, elevated oxygen demand results in an upward shift in the uptake curve. In addition, there is some evidence that the K_M is elevated; therefore, the critical P_{O_2} rises. As indicated above, the supply curve is shifted to the left when uptake increases above normal. The net effect is a decrease in tissue *(point a)* and capillary oxygen tensions *(point c)* with a greater reduction in the former than in the latter. Consequently, the capillary-to-cell P_{O_2} difference *(c-a)* and gradient are increased, and oxygen consumption is accelerated. With reductions of oxygen demand, the uptake curve is lowered, and the supply curve is shifted to the right. Thus, the oxygen tensions in the cells *(point e)* and capillaries *(point f)* are elevated, with the former

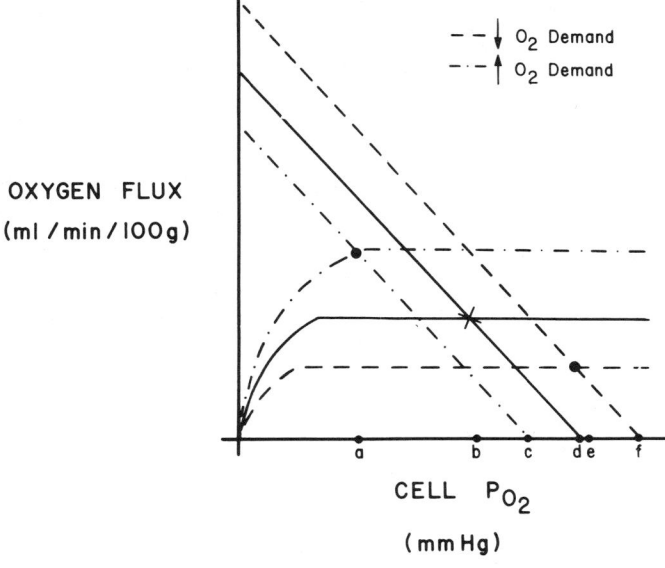

FIG. 5. Effect of altered oxygen demand on supply-uptake curves. From ref. 3.

rising more than the latter. Hence, the P_{O_2} difference is reduced *(f-e)*, and oxygen consumption is diminished.

A reexamination of Figs. 2 through 5 reveals an additional major feature of tissue oxygen dynamics. Under normal conditions, cell P_{O_2} is higher than the critical level, and oxygen flux is reaction-limited. In other words, increasing either tissue perfusion or exchange capacity does not alter oxygen uptake in the normal state. By contrast, tissue oxygen dynamics are transport-limited when oxygen uptake can be increased by elevating blood flow or opening more capillaries. Transport limitation is evident if the prevailing cell P_{O_2} is lower than the critical value. At such a low level of tissue oxygenation, improvement of the oxygen supply leads to accelerated mitochondrial uptake of oxygen.

LOCAL MICROVASCULAR CONTROL OF INTESTINAL OXYGENATION

General Considerations

The foregoing analyses clearly demonstrate that blood flow and functional capillary density are major determinants of intestinal oxygenation. These considerations led to the formulation of a conceptual and mathematical framework for analysis of vascular control of tissue oxygenation (1–6). The basic tenets of the model are simple. According to the metabolic theory of local vasoregulation, the tone of microvascular smooth muscle is modulated directly or indirectly by the prevailing level of tissue oxygenation (see Chapter 3). As a consequence of this metabolic linkage, tissue P_{O_2} is stabilized in the face of any stress tending to alter the balance between oxygen supply and demand (Fig. 1, *lower panel*). Active microvascular buffering of tissue oxygenation can be accomplished by local modulation of tissue blood flow or microvascular oxygen exchange capacity. In many tissues of the body, the major site of vascular resistance is in the small- to medium-size arterioles. Thus, local modulation of arteriolar tone at these loci allows intrinsic regulation of total blood flow through the microvascular network. In turn, the arteriolar flow-control system serves to buffer tissue oxygenation by stabilizing capillary P_{O_2}; this is achieved by matching blood flow to the oxygen demands of the tissue. Control of microvascular oxygen exchange capacity resides in the terminal ramifications of the precapillary network (i.e., terminal arterioles and precapillary sphincters). These microvascular effectors modulate the number of capillaries perfused at a given moment. The exchange control system stabilizes tissue oxygenation by modifying surface area and effective capillary-to-cell diffusion distance; this component of the local vasoregulatory system provides buffering capability even in the face of reduced capillary Po_2. By working in unison, the flow and exchange controllers provide a wide margin of safety against development of tissue hypoxia during stress.

The Mathematical Model

According to current concepts of functional differentiation of the microvasculature (Fig. 1, *upper panel*), the terminal vascular bed consists of three series-coupled and anatomically distinct segments: (a) the arteriolar or resistance section, (b) the capillary or exchange section, and (c) the venous or capacitance section. Blood flows through the rigid arterioles and capillaries into the venous capacitance vessels at a rate (F_A) determined by the arteriovenous pressure difference ($P_A - P_V$), arteriolar resistance (R_A), and capillary resistance (R_C); hence,

$$F_A = (P_A - P_V)/(R_A + R_C). \quad (8)$$

The outflow (F_V) from the venous compartment is a function of venous pressure (P_V), outflow pressure (P_O), and venous resistance (R_V):

$$F_V = (P_V - P_O)/R_V. \quad (9)$$

The volume (V_V) of blood in the veins at any time (t) is given by

$$V_v = V_{v_o} + \int (F_A - F_V) dt, \quad (10)$$

where V_{v_o} is the original venous volume. Venous pressure is a nonlinear function of venous blood volume. Assuming a parallel arrangement of capillaries, the capillary resistance is

$$R_c = (N_o/N)R_{c_o}, \quad (11)$$

where N is the instantaneous effective capillary density, N_o is the normal or initial effective capillary density, and R_{c_o} is the normal capillary resistance.

Assuming that each open capillary of radius r supplies oxygen to a circumscribed tissue cylinder of radius R, the diffusive flow of oxygen across a single capillary (jo_2) is a function of the capillary Po_2 (Po_{2c}), the cell Po_2 (Po_{2cell}), and the capillary-to-cell diffusion distance ($R - r$). Thus,

$$jo_{2c} = K_1(Po_{2cap} - Po_{2cell})/(R - r), \quad (12)$$

where K_1 is a constant. For any reference cross-sectional area (A) of tissue,

$$A = N\pi r^2, \quad (13)$$

or, expressing R in terms of effective capillary density (N),

$$R = K_2 N^{-1/2}, \quad (14)$$

where K_2 is a constant. Substituting Eq. 14 into Eq. 12 yields

$$jo_{2c} = K_1(Po_{2cap} - Po_{2cell})/(K_2 N^{-1/2} - r). \quad (15)$$

The total oxygen flux (Jo_{2c}) or oxygen delivery across all the open capillaries is thus

$$Jo_{2c} = N \cdot jo_{2c}, \quad (16)$$

Substituting Eq. 15 into Eq. 16 yields

$$Jo_{2c} = K_1 \cdot N(Po_{2cap} - Po_{2cell})/(K_2 N^{-1/2} - r). \quad (17)$$

The oxygen concentration of the capillary blood (Co_{2c}) is a function of arterial oxygen concentration (Co_{2A}) and transcapillary oxygen flux-to-arterial blood flow ratio. Assuming that venous oxygen concentration is a first approximation for Co_{2c},

$$Co_{2c} = Co_{2A} - (Jo_{2D}/F_A). \quad (18)$$

The capillary Po_2 is related to capillary oxygen concentration by the sigmoid hemoglobin dissociation curve; an adequate approximation of this relationship is given by the following:

$$Po_{2cap} = -20 \cdot \ln[1 - (Co_{2c}/Co_{2A})^{1/2}]. \quad (19)$$

After diffusing out of the capillaries, oxygen enters intestinal smooth muscle or mucosal cells, where it is consumed by the mitochondria. The relationship between cell Po_2 and mitochondrial oxygen utilization (Jo_{2M}) is nonlinear as defined above in Eq. 7.

The volume of oxygen in the cells (Vo_2) at a given time t is

$$V_{O_2} = V_{O_{2o}} + \int (J_{O_{2c}} - J_{O_{2M}})dt, \quad (20)$$

where $V_{O_{2o}}$ is the initial intracellular oxygen volume. The intracellular P_{O_2} is

$$P_{O_{2cell}} = K_3 \cdot V_{O_2}, \quad (21)$$

where K_3 is a constant that includes the intracellular fluid volume and the solubility coefficient of oxygen.

Several feedback mechanisms have been proposed to explain intrinsic metabolic regulation of the microcirculation. The proponents of the vasodilator theory maintain that vasoactive chemicals are released from parenchymal cells at a rate determined by the oxygen availability-to-demand ratio. These metabolites then diffuse to vascular smooth muscle cells and initiate appropriate hemodynamic responses, thus maintaining oxygen delivery in accordance with tissue demand. By contrast, other investigators state that intrinsic microvascular control is mediated through the direct effect of changes in interstitial P_{O_2} on vascular smooth muscle. At this time it is not possible to choose between these two mechanisms, nor is it necessary to do so, if we recognize that both mechanisms produce the same end result: Tissue oxygen delivery is maintained in accordance with metabolic demand. With this in mind we developed our feedback equations in terms of tissue oxygen delivery without specifying the exact mechanism.

The effects of altered O_2 supply/demand ratio on vascular resistance and microvascular exchange capacity in the intestine are compatible with the view that a local metabolic control system acts to maintain intracellular P_{O_2} in the parenchyma above the critical level by means of feedback regulation of arteriolar resistance and capillary density (Fig. 1, *lower panel*). Stated mathematically, the feedback relations are as follows:

$$\tau R \cdot dR_A/dt + R_A = K_{R1} \cdot P_{O_{2cell}} + K_{R2} \quad (22)$$

and

$$\tau R \cdot dN/dt + N = K_{N1} - K_{N2} \cdot P_{O_{2cell}}. \quad (23)$$

τR and τN are time constants describing the rate of change of resistance and capillary density following a perturbation of cell P_{O_2}. In the steady state, dR_A/dt and dN/dt are both zero, and the two feedback equations reduce to

$$R_A = K_{R1} \cdot P_{O_{2cell}} + K_{R2} \quad (24)$$

and

$$N = K_{N1} - K_{N2} \cdot P_{O_{2cell}}. \quad (25)$$

Thus, arteriolar resistance rises in direct proportion to cell P_{O_2}, the sensitivity factor being K_{R1}. When cell P_{O_2} is zero, a residual resistance remains and is equal to K_{R2}. On the other hand, capillary density falls in a linear fashion as tissue oxygenation increases, the sensitivity factor being K_{N2}. In anoxia, maximum capillary density is attained and is equal to K_{N1}.

A major feature of the model is the assumption that the P_{O_2} sensitivity of the microvascular elements controlling capillary density is greater than that of the arteriolar (resistance) segment. In our original model, this basic feature was a requirement for ensuring the predictive value of the analysis under a wide variety of experimental conditions.

Simulation of Flow Autoregulation

A sudden reduction of local perfusion pressure causes a rapid fall in intestinal blood flow, as illustrated in the left panel of Fig. 6. As a consequence of hypoperfusion, oxygen availability at the capillary level is diminished, and the rate of transmicrovascular O_2 flux falls. The temporary imbalance between O_2 delivery to the cells and intestinal O_2 consumption results in a decreased intracellular P_{O_2}, which elicits an automatic dilatation of intestinal arterioles and precapillary sphincters. In turn, the increments in vascular conductance and number of open capillaries augment O_2 transport to the intestinal cells via their effects on blood flow and O_2 diffusion parameters, respectively. Although intracellular P_{O_2} is not perfectly stabilized by the proportional control system, compensatory microvascular reactions are of sufficient magnitude to maintain tissue oxygenation above the critical P_{O_2}. Consequently, in

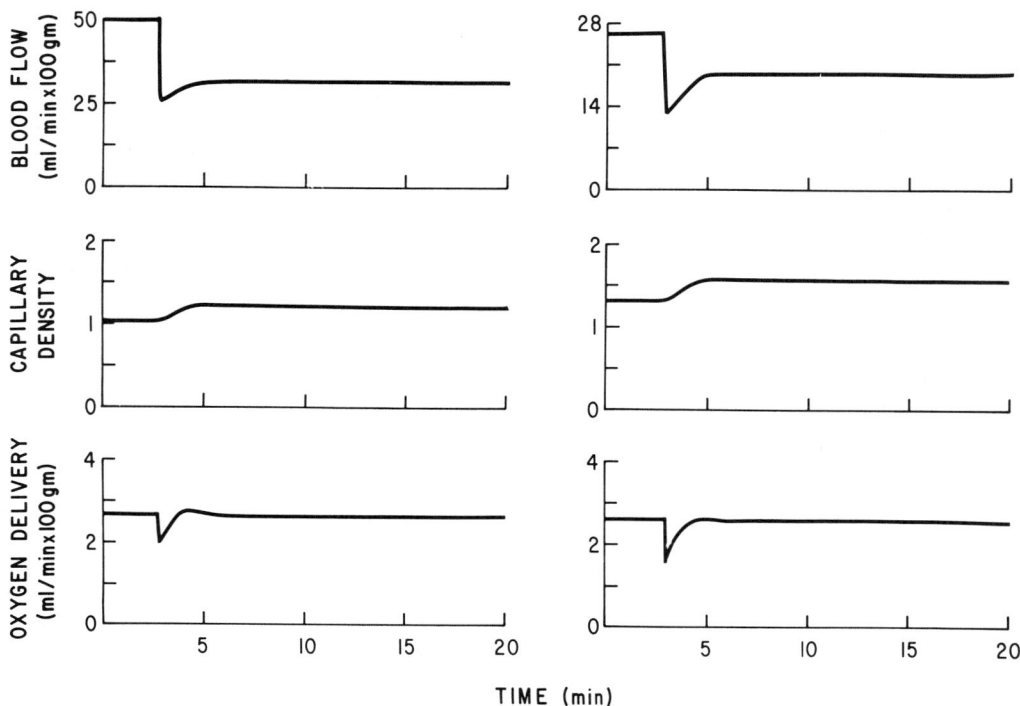

FIG. 6. Autoregulation of intestinal blood flow. Two transient responses of the model to a 50% step reduction in arterial perfusion pressure. *(Left)* Response of normal, nonabsorbing intestine. *(Right)* Response in intestine exhibiting higher than normal arteriolar tone and number of open capillaries. Note the higher degree of flow autoregulation in the right panel. From ref. 6.

the steady state, transcapillary O_2 flux and intestinal O_2 uptake return to normal despite a significant fall in cell Po_2.

The partial recovery of blood flow following a sudden step-change in arterial perfusion pressure is termed autoregulation of blood flow. According to the left panel of Fig. 6, the degree of flow autoregulation in the normal, nonabsorbing intestine is limited, representing only a 25% recovery of perfusion rate. Under these conditions, intestinal oxygenation is buffered mainly by passive encroachment on the intracellular Po_2 reserve and precapillary sphincter modulation of effective capillary density. The greater contribution of the precapillary sphincter mechanism in the resting intestine reflects the higher sensitivity of these microvascular elements to alterations in intracellular Po_2.

Intracellular oxygen tension and the capillary density reserve in the intestine are diminished in the postprandial state or any other condition characterized by a lowered O_2 availability/demand ratio. When such conditions exist, the magnitude of flow autoregulation is markedly increased, reflecting the greater participation of the flow-controlling arterioles in local regulation of intestinal oxygenation when stresses are severe (Fig. 6, *right panel*). Thus, although the relative contribution of the arteriolar and precapillary sphincter components of the control system varies with prevailing conditions, integration of the dual-component regulatory mechanism extends the range of effectiveness beyond that provided by the individual components operating alone (Fig. 7). Moreover, the strategy of integration ensures economy in terms of overall cardiovascular dynamics. That is, the first line of defense is based on improving O_2 extraction by redistributing the existing blood flow. Major alterations in intestinal blood flow, which affect

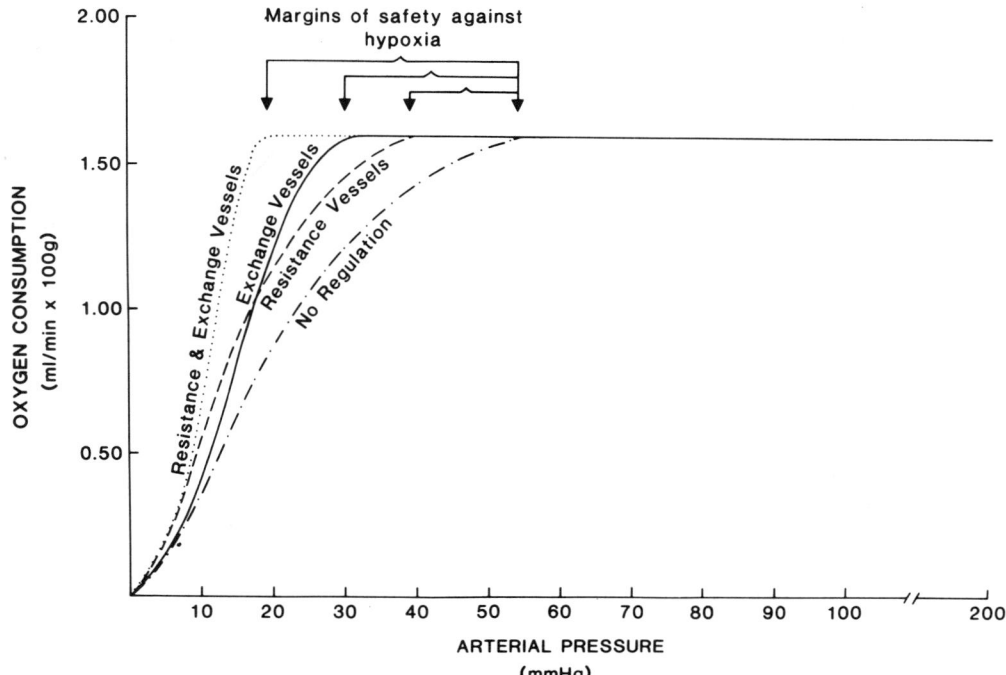

FIG. 7. Relative roles of passive factors, arteriolar feedback, and precapillary sphincter feedback in stabilization of intestinal O_2 uptake following graded changes in arterial pressure. Note that the margin of safety against development of hypoxia is greatest when all three components are operative. From ref. 1.

cardiac activity and overall cardiovascular behavior, are enlisted only after the redistribution mechanism approaches saturation.

Simulation of Postprandial Hyperemia

Oxygen uptake by intestinal cells increases after a meal, reflecting augmented solute absorption, motility, and active secretion. The acceleration of O_2 utilization produces a temporary imbalance between oxygen supply and demand, leading to a fall in intracellular Po_2. The relative tissue hypoxia triggers compensatory relaxation of arterioles and precapillary sphincters. Consequently, intestinal blood flow and arteriovenous O_2 difference increase, thereby augmenting O_2 supply to match intestinal demands.

Figure 8 illustrates responses of the model to graded increments of intestinal O_2 uptake above the normal level of 1.6 ml/min·100 g. In the absence of local microvascular control of intestinal flow and effective capillary density, transcapillary O_2 flux keeps stride with augmented O_2 demand by passive encroachment upon the 14-mm Hg margin of safety against hypoxia associated with a normal intracellular Po_2 of 15 mm Hg. Thus, although the capillary and cell oxygen tensions fall substantially, the capillary-to-cell Po_2 difference rises to provide the driving force for the accelerated O_2 flux. In intestine, the maximum increase in O_2 uptake observed in the postprandial state is less than 50%. Thus, it appears that the passive safety factor is just large enough to ensure adequate intestinal oxygenation in normal hypermetabolic states associated with feeding. However, hypoxia would result if an additional stress (i.e., reduced perfusion pressure, arterial hypoxemia) were applied to the system. In any event, the normal intestinal response to feeding *does* include increments in vascular conductance and number of open capillaries. As was the case for perfusion pressure reductions, the primary compensation during hypermetabolism is an in-

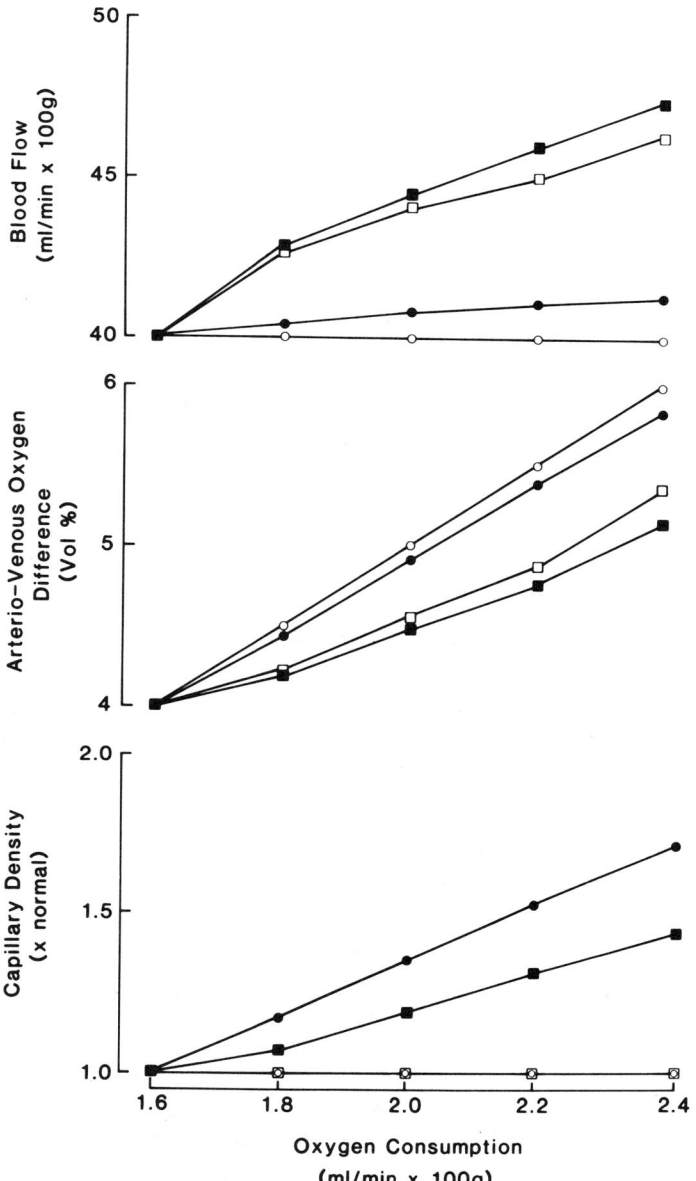

FIG. 8. Role of arteriolar feedback, precapillary sphincter feedback, and passive factors in augmenting transcapillary O_2 flux following graded elevations in intestinal O_2 demand. *(Open circles)* No regulation; *(closed circles)* exchange vessel regulation; *(open squares)* resistance vessel regulation; *(closed squares)* exchange and resistance vessel regulation. From ref. 1.

creased O_2 extraction dependent at least in part on locally mediated capillary recruitment. For example, O_2 extraction and intestinal blood flow increase 12.5% and 24%, respectively, following a 37.5% rise in parenchymal oxygen demand. Again, the lesser importance of postprandial hyperemia reflects the lower sensitivity of arterioles, in comparison to precapillary sphincters, to changes in intestinal oxygenation.

Other Local Control Phenomena

The model also simulates the dynamics of reactive hyperemia and hypoxemic vasodilation. With complete arterial occlusion, O_2 supply to the intestine falls to zero, and an intense feedback signal is perceived by the arterioles and sphincters, leading to relaxation of the microvascular elements governing resistance and exchange capacity. Upon release of the occlusion, blood flow overshoots above the normal value as a normal pressure head is reestablished across a dilated vascular bed. As cell Po_2 rises during the reactive hyperemia, a locally mediated vasoconstriction returns blood flow, exchange capacity, and intestinal oxygenation to normal. In hypoxemic vasodilation, the stimulus for local vasodilation is a fall in intracellular Po_2 secondary to a reduction of arterial oxygen content.

FUTURE DIRECTIONS

Although the graphical and systems analyses described above provide a useful framework for gross examination of the problem of intestinal oxygenation, several considerations suggest that substantial modifications of these models are required. First, the intestine is a heterogeneous organ consisting of mucosal, glandular, and smooth muscle cells, each served by individual microvasculatures connected in complex series or parallel arrangements. Moreover, an adequate mathematical description of O_2 transport in these specialized tissue units will require consideration of unit geometry and microvascular arrangement. At this time, enough anatomical and physiological information is available to begin consideration of a systems analysis of the intestine as a heterogeneous organ. Another limitation of existing models is the absence of the myogenic mechanism, which is known to play an important role in local regulation of the intestinal microcirculation. Finally, a detailed analysis of the nature of the feedback linkages between parenchymal metabolism and intestinal microvessels would enhance the predictive value of existing models. Unfortunately, this important step cannot be taken because knowledge in this area is virtually nonexistent. Consequently, development of a detailed model of circulation/metabolism coupling in the intestine is limited by the paucity of experimental data dealing with chemical mediation of the local microvascular reactions to altered tissue oxygenation.

REFERENCES

1. Granger, D. N., and Granger, H. J. (1983): Systems analysis of intestinal hemodynamics and oxygenation. *Am. J. Physiol.*, 245:G786–G796.
2. Granger, H. J. (1970): *Quantitative analysis of autoregulation and interstitial fluid dynamics*. PhD dissertation, University of Mississippi Medical Center, Jackson.
3. Granger, H. J., and Nyhof, R. A. (1982): Dynamics of intestinal oxygenation: Interactions between oxygen supply and uptake. *Am. J. Physiol.*, 243:G91–G96.
4. Granger, H. J., and Shepherd, A. P. (1973): Intrinsic microvascular control of tissue oxygen delivery. *Microvasc. Res.*, 5:49–72.
5. Granger, H. J., and Shepherd, A. P. (1979): Dynamics and control of the microcirculation. *Adv. Biomed. Eng.*, 7:1–63.
6. Shepherd, A. P., and Granger, H. J. (1973): Autoregulatory escape in the gut: A systems analysis. *Gastroenterology*, 65:77–91.

Mathematical Model of Intestinal Transcapillary Fluid and Protein Exchange

Joseph N. Benoit, Carlos A. Navia, Aubrey E. Taylor, and D. Neil Granger

Department of Physiology, College of Medicine, University of South Alabama, Mobile, Alabama 36688

Mathematical models have been developed for a wide variety of physiological systems. The circulatory system has proven to be particularly amenable to mathematical representation, since the physical principles describing hemodynamics are well defined. Blood flow, tissue oxygenation (9,19,22,28), and transcapillary exchange (8,24,26,29) have been the major focal points of mathematical models of the intestinal circulation. These systems analyses have improved our understanding of mechanisms involved in the regulation of intestinal hemodynamics and transcapillary exchange. Furthermore, the conceptual framework provided by these models has led to increased experimentation in the intestinal circulation.

The aspect of the intestinal circulation that has most frequently been simulated is transcapillary fluid and solute exchange (8,24,26,29). The major purpose of these models has been to describe the mechanisms involved in interstitial fluid volume regulation during periods of enhanced capillary filtration, absorption, and secretion. Although the simulations obtained from these models agree qualitatively with some of the experimental data in the literature, the quantitative predictive capability of these models has been limited by inadequate formulations and data regarding transcapillary protein exchange. The advent of new techniques for studying intestinal transcapillary exchange has eliminated the need for many of the assumptions inherent in earlier models. Data regarding the permeability characteristics of intestinal capillaries (e.g., the capillary osmotic reflection coefficient, capillary filtration coefficient, and capillary permeability-surface area product) are now available for the small intestine (15,17,27). This, coupled to recent revisions of thermodynamic formulations for transmembrane solute exchange, has prompted us to revise and expand our earlier model of intestinal transcapillary fluid and solute exchange (26). Unlike earlier models, the current model places greater emphasis on the role of transcapillary protein exchange in the regulation of interstitial fluid volume. In this chapter, we describe the model and compare the model's predictions with experimental results obtained from the cat small intestine during periods of enhanced capillary filtration (i.e., venous pressure elevation and plasma dilution), secretion, and absorption.

METHODS

General Considerations

The present computer model is based on a previous mathematical simulation of fluid and solute exchange in the cat small intestine (26). The model describes the intestine as three compartments: capillary, interstitium, and lumen. The capillary and mucosal membranes are considered freely permeable to water but relatively impermeable to plasma proteins. In addition, the interstitial compartment is connected to the lymphatic system via a membrane freely permeable to fluid and all solutes. The interstitial compartment behaves as an elastic chamber, the volume of which depends on the amount and direction of fluid movement across the membranes that surround it (Fig. 1).

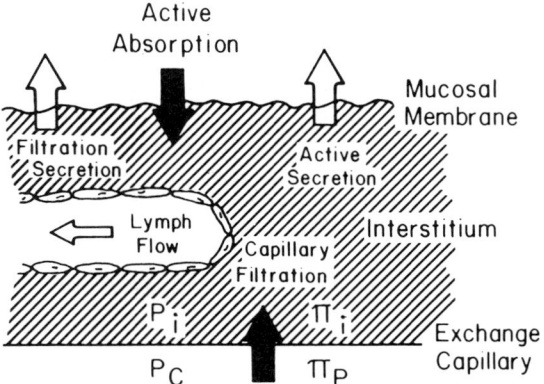

FIG. 1. Schematic representation of volume flows and forces governing the regulation of intestinal interstitial volume. (Modified from Granger et al., ref. 11, with permission.)

Several assumptions related to blood flow and capillary and mucosal membrane characteristics are incorporated into this model. Extrinsic regulatory mechanisms of intestinal blood flow (neural and humoral) are not considered. Intrinsic regulation is assumed to be consistent with the myogenic theory of local blood-flow regulation. The latter assumption is based on findings that in the isolated intestine perfused at constant pressure, precapillary resistance increases while the capillary filtration coefficient and permeability–surface area product for total plasma proteins decrease with venous pressure elevation (12). The osmotic and solvent drag reflection coefficients were assumed to be equal.

Tables 1 and 2 list the equations, variables, and parameters used to construct the model. Fig. 2 is a flow diagram of the model.

Fluid Flux

The Starling equilibrium (Eq. 1) was used to calculate transcapillary fluid flux ($J_{v,c}$). Capillary pressure (P_c) was calculated by Eq. 4 (12), where the postcapillary to precapillary resistance ratio (R_v/R_a) was assumed to be inversely related to venous pressure (P_v) (25). Tissue pressure (P_i) was derived from a previously reported interstitial compliance curve (25). The capillary osmotic reflection coefficient for total plasma proteins (σ_d) from the cat small intestine (17) was used and assumed to remain constant over the entire range of venous pressures. Plasma (π_P) and interstitial (π_i) oncotic pressures were calculated from equations relating cat plasma protein concentration to oncotic pressure (C. A. Navia, *unpublished observation*). Initial values for interstitial fluid volume (V_i) and quantity of interstitial protein (QP) were obtained from the literature (10). Lymph flow ($J_{v,L}$) was assumed to be related to interstitial hydrostatic pressure in a sigmoidal fashion (17,25).

Passive transmucosal fluid flux ($J_{v,mp}$) was also described by the Starling relationship (Eq. 8). The hydraulic conductivity (LP) of the mucosa was set at 0.0001 ml/min/mm Hg × 100 g for tissue pressures lower than 4.25 mm Hg and increased to 0.20 ml/min/mm Hg × 100 g for tissue pressures greater than 4.25 mm Hg (6,30).

The sum of the fluid fluxes on each iteration was integrated to calculate interstitial volumes (Eq. 9).

Protein Flux

Protein flux across the capillary membrane was calculated from the Patlak equation (Eq. 11) as rearranged by Bresler (2). This equation apparently can be divided into a convective,

$$J_{v,c}(1 - \sigma_d) C_P,$$

and a primarily diffusional component,

$$\frac{J_{v,c}(1 - \sigma_d)(C_p - C_i)}{e^x - 1},$$

where x is

$$(1 - \sigma_d) J_{v,c}/PS_c.$$

The capillary permeability–surface area product (PS_c) was assumed to be inversely related to venous pressure (17). Lymphatic solute flux ($J_{p,L}$) was calculated from Eq. 12. The Kedem-Katchalsky (19) equation (Eq. 13) was used to calculate transmucosal protein flux ($J_{p,m}$). The mucosal permeability–surface area product (PS_m) was set at 0.0001 and 0.05 ml/min × 100 g for tissue pressures of less than and greater than 4.25 mm Hg, respectively.

TABLE 1. *Variables used in simulation of transcapillary and transmucosal fluid and solute movement in the small intestine*

Symbol	Def. of variable	Initial numerical value	Units	Ref.
$J_{v,c}$	Capillary fluid flux	0.051	ml/min × 100 g	17
$K_{f,c}$	Capillary filtration coefficient	0.167	ml/min/mm Hg × 100 g	26
P_c	Capillary hydrostatic pressure	10.20	mm Hg	12
P_i	Interstitial hydrostatic pressure	−2.00	mm Hg	24
σ_d*	Capillary reflection coefficient	0.92	—	17
π_p	Plasma oncotic pressure	22.10	mm Hg	24
π_i	Interstitial oncotic pressure	9.24	mm Hg	24
P_a	Mesenteric arterial pressure	135.00	mm Hg	—
R_v	Postcapillary resistance	0.30	mm Hg/(ml/min) × 100 g	24
R_a	Precapillary resistance	3.70	mm Hg/(ml/min) × 100 g	24
P_v	Mesenteric venous pressure	0.00	mm Hg	—
C_p	Plasma protein concentration	7.10	g/100 ml	—
C_i	Interstitial protein concentration	3.60	g/100 ml	—
V_i	Interstitial volume	25.00	ml/100 g	10
$J_{v,L}$	Lymphatic fluid flux	0.051	ml/min × 100 g	17
$J_{v,mp}$	Passive mucosal fluid flux	0.00	ml/min × 100 g	—
$J_{v,aa}$	Active fluid absorption	0.00	ml/min × 100 g	—
$J_{v,sa}$	Active fluid secretion	0.00	ml/min × 100 g	—
$J_{p,c}$	Capillary solute flux	0.19	mg/min × 100 g	17
$J_{p,L}$	Lymphatic solute flux	0.19	mg/min × 100 g	17
$J_{p,m}$	Mucosal solute flux	0.00	mg/min × 100 g	—
PS_c	Capillary permeability–surface area product	0.05	ml/min × 100 g	17
PS_m	Mucosal permeability–surface area product	0.0001	ml/min × 100 g	17
LP	Mucosal hydraulic conductance	0.0001	ml/min/mm Hg × 100 g	—
σ_m*	Mucosal reflection coefficient	0.999	ml/min/mm Hg × 100 g	4
QP	Quantity of interstitial protein	90.00	g/100 ml	10
P_L	Luminal hydrostatic pressure	0.00	mm Hg	—

*For total plasma proteins.

Integration of protein fluxes as described in Eq. 14 was used to calculate new values of QP. Equation 15 was used to calculate interstitial protein concentration (C_i).

Computer Techniques

Equations describing the system were programmed in Applesoft BASIC on an Apple II⁺ microcomputer (Apple Computer, Inc., Cupertino, California). A function generator subroutine using a linear interpolation technique and described by the following equation was employed:

$$Z(x) = f(x_i) + \frac{x - x_i}{x_{i+1} - x_i} [f(x_{i+1}) - f(x_i)],$$

where $Z(x)$ is the interpolated value. The Euler rectangular method of integration was found to provide minimal execution time without significantly affecting the outcome of the model predictions. For all simulations, a time constant (dt) of 1.13 min was employed. This time constant was compared with lower and higher values and was not found to significantly affect the stability of the model.

A high-resolution video monitor provided an on-line graphic representation of capillary and lymphatic fluid fluxes, interstitial hydrostatic pressure, and interstitial volume. To expedite execution, the model was converted to machine language by the TASC Compiler (Microsoft, Inc., Bellevue, Washington). Copies of the model are available on request.

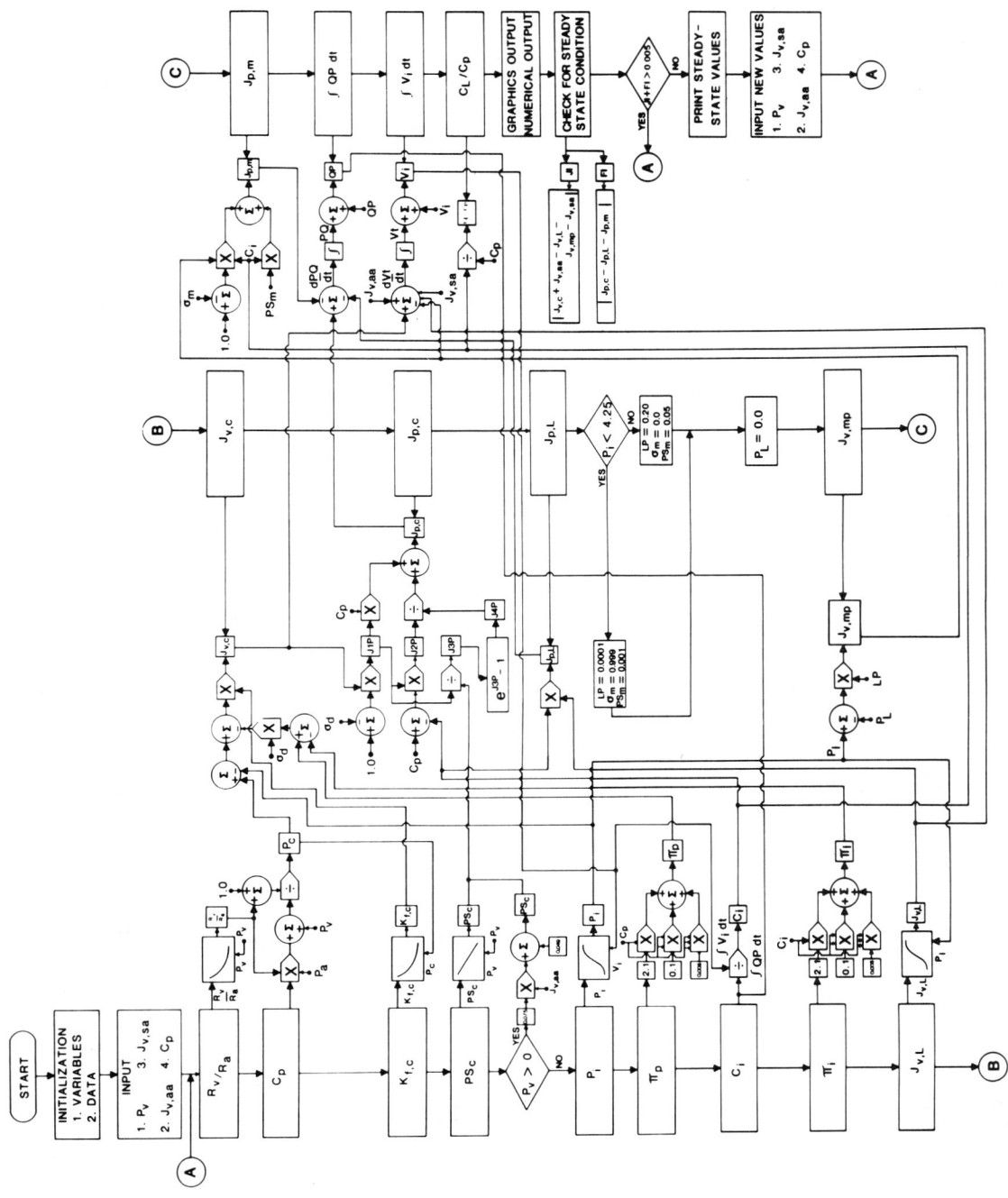

TABLE 2. *Systems equations describing transcapillary and transmucosal fluid and solute exchange in the small intestine*

Fluid exchange
1. $J_{v,c} = K_{f,c}[(P_c - P_i) - \sigma_d(\pi_c - \pi_i)]$
2. $K_{f,c} = f(P_c)$
3. $R_v/R_a = f(P_v)$
4. $P_c = \dfrac{P_a(R_v/R_a) + P_v}{R_v/R_a + 1}$
5. $P_i = f(V_i)$
6. $\pi_c = 2.1\, C_p + 0.1\, C_p^2 + 0.006\, C_p^3$
7. $\pi_i = 2.1\, C_i + 0.1\, C_i^2 + 0.006\, C_i^3$
8. $J_{v,mp} = LP(P_i - P_L)$
    if $P_i < 4.25$ mm Hg, $LP = 0.0001$
    $P_i > 4.25$, $LP \times 0.20$
9. $V_i = V_{io} + \int(J_{v,c} + J_{v,aa} - J_{v,L} - J_{v,mp} - J_{v,sa})dt$
10. $J_{v,L} = f(P_i)$

Protein exchange
11. $J_{p,c} = J_{v,c}(1-\sigma_d)C_p + \dfrac{J_{v,c}(1-\sigma_d)(C_p - C_i)}{e^x - 1}$,
    where $x = (1-\sigma_d)J_{v,c}/PS_c$
12. $J_{p,L} = J_{v,L}(C_i)$
13. $J_{p,m} = J_{v,mp}(1-\sigma_m)C_i + PS_m(C_i)$
14. $PS_c = f(P_v)$
15. $QP = QP_0 + \int(J_{p,c} - J_{p,L} - J_{p,m})dt$
16. $C_i = QP/V_i$

SIMULATIONS AND DISCUSSION

Venous Pressure Elevation and Plasma Dilution

Figure 3 depicts simulations of either elevating venous pressure or decreasing plasma oncotic pressure on interstitial volume and interstitial hydrostatic pressure (**A**), capillary (lymphatic) and mucosal fluid and solute fluxes (**B, C**), capillary filtration coefficient, and interstitial oncotic pressure (**D**). Elevations in venous pressure increase capillary hydrostatic pressure and precapillary resistance, but plasma dilution lowers plasma oncotic pressure without altering capillary pressure or vascular resistance. Both perturbations disrupt the normal Starling equilibrium to cause net capillary fluid filtration and fluid accumulation in the interstitium (Fig. 3 **A,B**). Larger perturbations of the system produce higher capillary filtration rates, interstitial volumes, interstitial hydrostatic pressures, and lymph flows. Figure 3 (**C**) also demonstrates that capillary protein flux increases when capillary filtration rate is enhanced by venous pressure elevation but not by plasma dilution. The increased capillary protein flux observed with venous pressure elevation reflects an enhanced convective flux of proteins. The fact that plasma dilution does not alter capillary protein flux can be explained by the lower plasma protein concentration that limits the amount of protein traversing the capillary. In either case, accumulation of fluid in the interstitium lowers the transcapillary hydrostatic pressure gradient and increases the oncotic pressure gradient, thereby opposing further fluid filtration from the capillary. An additional buffering capacity against interstitial edema is provided by the reduction in the capillary filtration coefficient associated with venous pressure elevation (25,27). This response is believed to be a myogenic regulatory mechanism that helps maintain fluid homeostasis across the capillary, but it does not occur with plasma dilution.

As previously mentioned, higher capillary filtration rates elevate interstitial volume and hydrostatic pressure. Higher tissue hydrostatic pressures enhance the rate of lymph formation, thereby removing fluid and protein from the interstitium. In most instances (i.e., venous pressures lower than 39 mm Hg or plasma oncotic pressures greater than 7.65 mm Hg), an equilibrium is reached between capillary and lymphatic fluid and protein fluxes (Fig. 3 **B,C**). When the capillary filtration rate exceeds maximal lymph flow, fluid accumulates in the interstitium at a greater rate. Tissue hydrostatic pressure is, in turn, driven towards a critical value. When this value (4.25 mm Hg) is reached, the mucosal membrane ruptures, causing the hydraulic conductivity of the membrane to increase (from 0.0001 to 0.20 ml/min/mm Hg × 100 g) (3,29,30). Figure 3 shows that upon reaching

FIG. 2. Flow chart of mathematical model. See Table 2 for definitions of symbols.

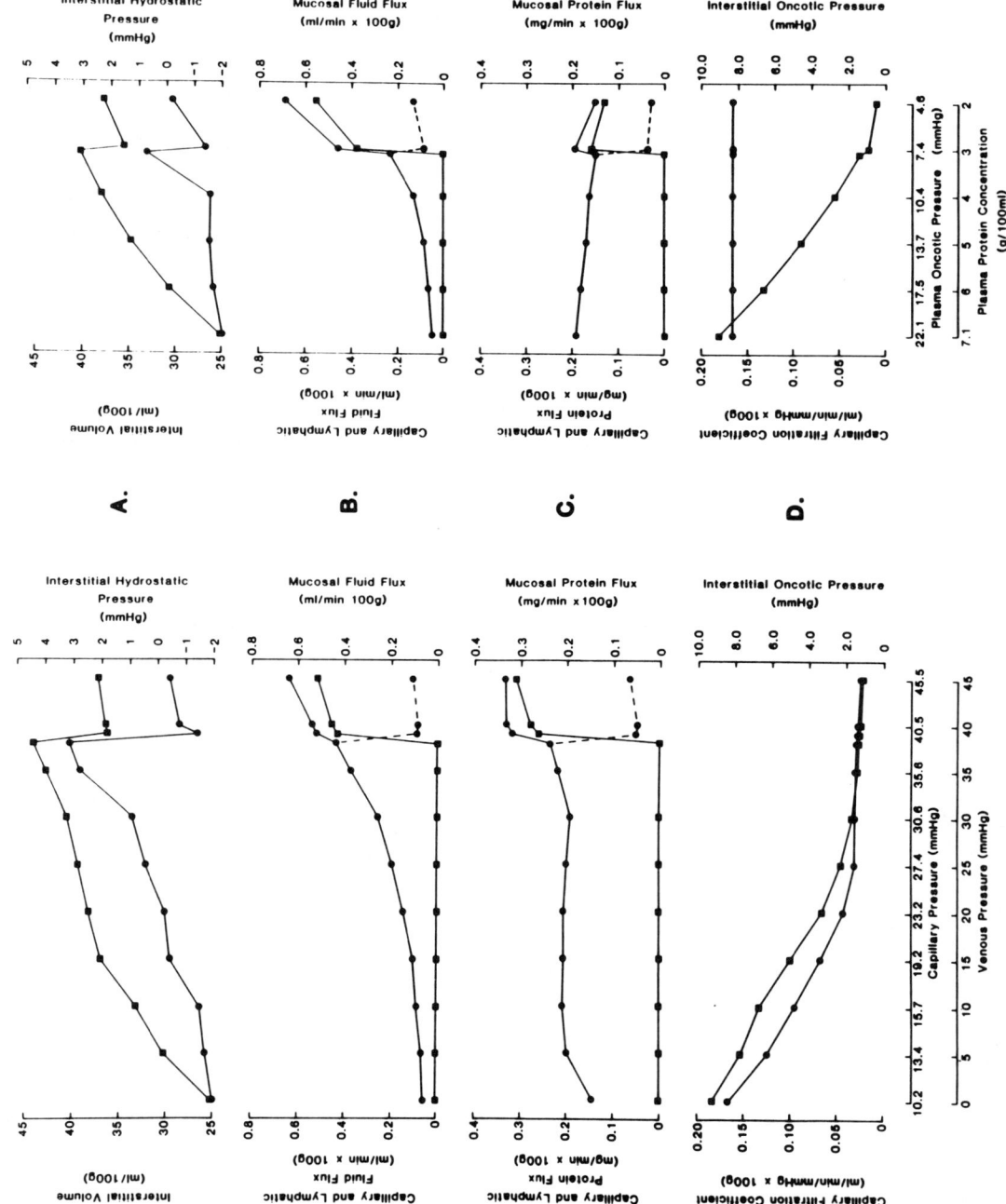

the critical value, transmucosal fluid and protein fluxes (filtration secretion) rapidly increase, interstitial volume and hydrostatic pressure decrease, and lymphatic fluid and protein fluxes fall. The drop in lymphatic fluxes associated with the onset of filtration secretion have been explained by a decreased lymphatic filling pressure (i.e., tissue hydrostatic pressure) caused by the greater fluid flux across the mucosa (13).

The changes in P_c and π_p required to produce the critical tissue pressure for filtration secretion were 28 and 14.5 mm Hg, respectively. For an osmotic reflection coefficient of 0.92, a 31-mm Hg oncotic pressure gradient should be required to produce the critical tissue hydrostatic pressure for filtration secretion. However, since an oncotic pressure gradient of 31 mm Hg is not possible (plasma oncotic pressure is 22.1 mm Hg), the discrepancy between the hydrostatic and oncotic pressure gradients necessary to produce filtration secretion can only be explained by the capillary derecruitment associated with venous pressure elevation. The lymphatic safety factor associated with venous pressure elevation (18.8 mm Hg) is higher than the lymphatic safety factor associated with plasma dilution (2.50 mm Hg) because capillary derecruitment is associated with the former condition but not the latter.

In summary, elevations in capillary pressure (produced by venous pressure elevation) or decreases in plasma oncotic pressure (produced by plasma dilution) increase capillary fluid flux, interstitial volume, interstitial hydrostatic pressure, and lymph flow. At higher filtration rates, interstitial volume increases, forcing interstitial hydrostatic pressure towards a critical value. Once the critical value is reached, the mucosal membrane ruptures and filtration secretion begins. In all instances, a greater imbalance in Starling forces is required to approach the critical value by elevating venous pressure than by diluting plasma colloids. This observation is explained by the decrease in the capillary filtration coefficient and permeability surface area product associated with venous pressure elevation but not with plasma dilution. Therefore, the ability of the lymphatic system to buffer changes in capillary pressure (caused by venous pressure elevation) is greater than the ability of this system to buffer changes in plasma oncotic pressure (caused by plasma dilution).

Relationship Between Lymph-to-Plasma Protein Concentration Ratio and Capillary Filtration Rate

Recently, a technique has been developed for determining the osmotic reflection coefficient of intestinal capillaries from the steady state relationship between lymph-to-plasma protein concentration ratio (C_L/C_P) and capillary filtration rate (or lymph flow) (17). As illustrated in Fig. 4A, when capillary filtration rate is increased from its normal value (by elevating venous pressure or decreasing plasma colloids), C_L/C_P decreases (filtration-rate-dependent) until sufficiently high lymph flows are obtained at which C_L/C_P is no longer influenced by further increases in lymph flow (filtration-rate-independent). When C_L/C_P becomes filtration-rate-independent, it can be assumed that convective exchange accounts for all solute movement across the capillaries because diffusive exchange is essentially zero, and the lymph-to-plasma protein concentration ratio represents the true separative capacity of the capillary membrane. Therefore, when C_L/C_P is filtration-independent,

$$\sigma_d = 1 - C_L/C_P.$$

Our model predicts that C_L/C_P becomes filtration-independent at values of 0.083 and 0.10 when capillary filtration is increased by venous pressure elevation and plasma dilution, respectively (Fig. 4B). The relationship between C_L/C_P and the capillary filtration rate, as well as

FIG. 3. Model predictions of effects of venous pressure elevation *(left panels)* or plasma dilution *(right panels)* on intestinal transcapillary fluid and solute exchange. *(Circles and squares)* Scales on the left and right ordinates, respectively. *(Broken lines)* The deviation of capillary and lymphatic flux that accompany the onset of filtration secretion.

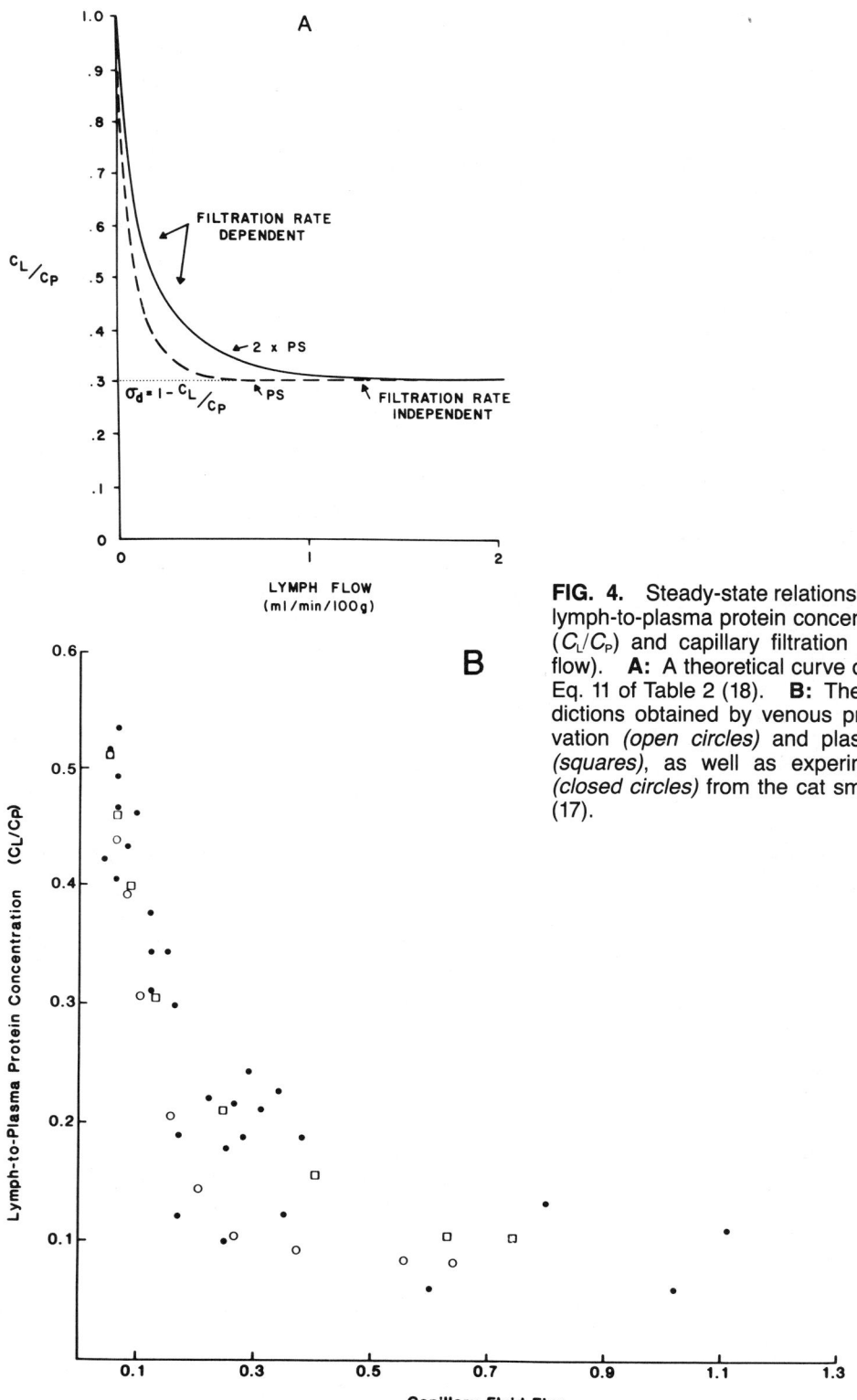

FIG. 4. Steady-state relationship between lymph-to-plasma protein concentration ratio (C_L/C_P) and capillary filtration rate (lymph flow). **A:** A theoretical curve derived from Eq. 11 of Table 2 (18). **B:** The model predictions obtained by venous pressure elevation *(open circles)* and plasma dilution *(squares)*, as well as experimental data *(closed circles)* from the cat small intestine (17).

the osmotic reflection coefficient predicted by the model (Fig. 4B), are in excellent agreement with experimental data from the cat small intestine (17). Of interest, is the model prediction that plasma dilution requires a higher capillary filtration rate for C_L/C_P to reach filtration-independence. This may be explained by the fact that capillary derecruitment does not occur with plasma dilution. The reduced exchange area associated with capillary derecruitment allows diffusive exchange to approach zero at lower capillary filtration rates.

Active Secretion

Considerable experimental evidence indicates that stimulation of active solute-coupled fluid movement into the intestinal lumen (secretion) significantly alters the factors that regulate intestinal interstitial fluid volume (7,13,21). For example, the Starling forces are altered in a manner consistent with enhanced capillary fluid filtration and interstitial dehydration during cholera toxin-induced secretion. Villus lymph (lacteal) pressure and total intestinal lymph flow decrease after exposure of the mucosa to cholera toxin (13,21) and other active secretagogues (7). These observations suggest that interstitial fluid pressure is reduced because of interstitial dehydration. Therefore, in the actively secreting small intestine, steady states are achieved when the rates of capillary filtration and active secretion are equal.

The model was used to evaluate the current hypothesis regarding the influence of active fluid secretion on capillary and interstitial forces. Figure 5 shows the effects of active fluid secretion on interstitial volume, interstitial hydrostatic pressure, transcapillary and lymphatic fluid and protein fluxes, and interstitial oncotic pressure for venous pressures of 0.0 and 20.0 mm Hg. For each set of simulations, venous pressure was held constant and secretory rate raised from 0.0 to 2.0 ml/min × 100 g. In both instances (venous pressures of 0 and 20 mm Hg), the simulations are inconsistent with the data in the literature. An explanation for this discrepancy may lie in the model's prediction that blood-to-interstitium protein movement increases with secretion rate. The resulting accumulation of protein in the interstitium leads to a rise in capillary filtration, interstitial volume, tissue hydrostatic pressure, and lymph flow. The effects of secretion rate on transcapillary protein exchange and interstitial volume were essentially reversed at a venous pressure of 20 mm Hg. The reason for this reversal appeared to be the reduced capillary surface area for fluid and protein exchange caused by venous pressure elevation. To more fully assess this possibility, we ran additional simulations at a venous pressure of 0 mm Hg while maintaining the capillary filtration coefficient at a reduced value (0.01 ml/min/mm Hg × 100 g). Under these conditions, interstitial fluid volume and lymph flow decreased significantly at all secretion rates studied. These findings are consistent with the literature. Whether or not there is a physiologic equivalent to the latter simulation remains to be determined. Further experimentation is required to resolve this discrepancy between the model predictions and available data.

Active Absorption

Considerable evidence indicates that the forces governing the rate of fluid exchange across intestinal capillaries are altered during periods of net transmucosal water absorption (1,5,6,14,16,23). The available data support the hypothesis that, in the absorbing small bowel, the balance of forces across the capillary wall is altered to favor the movement of absorbed water from interstitium to blood. This imbalance of forces across the capillaries is generally considered to be caused by a rise in interstitial hydrostatic pressure and a decline in interstitial oncotic pressure, both resulting from expansion of the interstitial spaces by absorbed fluid. The increased interstitial hydrostatic pressure also enhances lymph production, thereby providing another route for the removal of absorbed fluid from the interstitium.

The final series of simulations were designed to test the predictive capability of the model during active fluid absorption. Figure 6 illus-

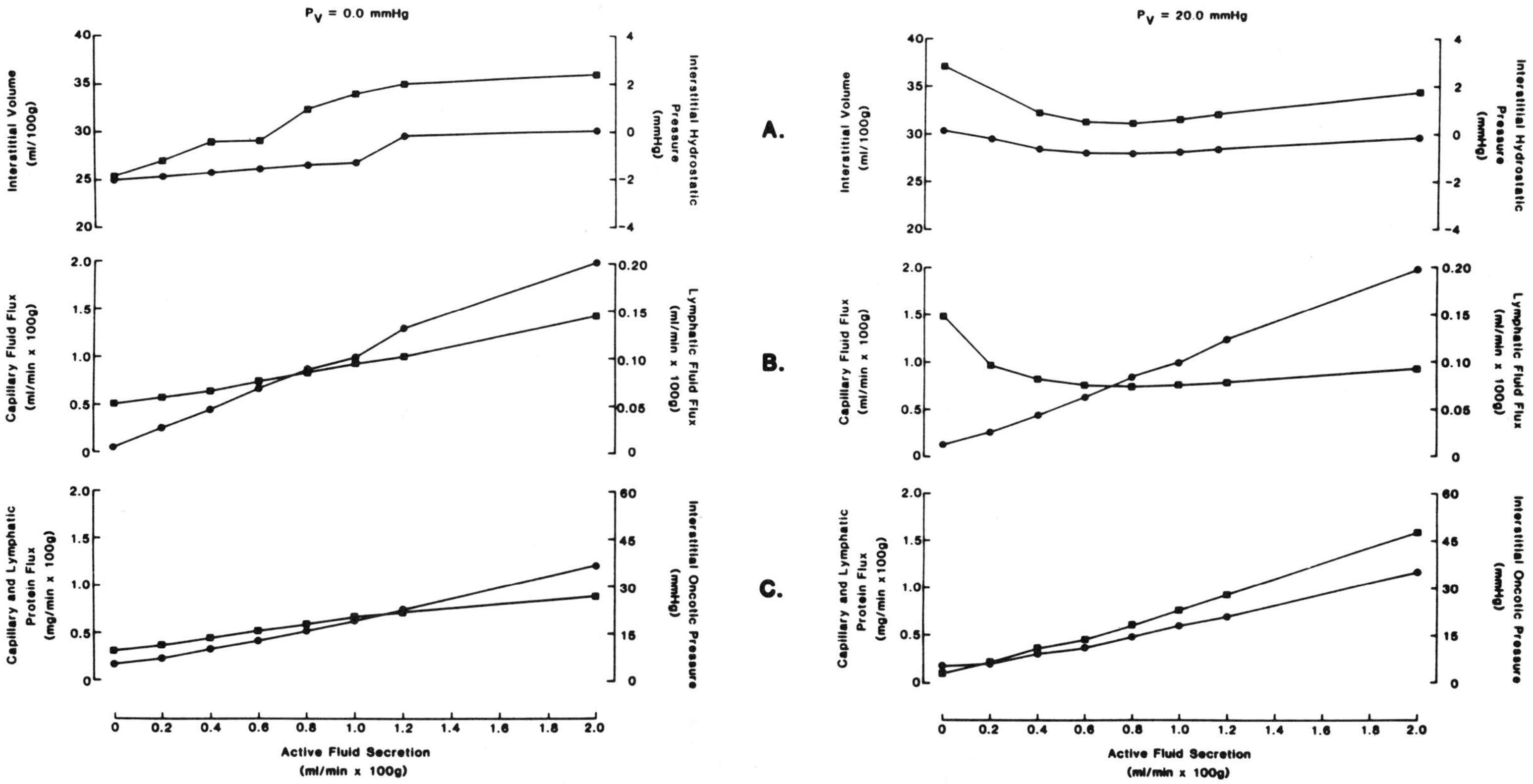

FIG. 5. Model predictions of effects of active fluid secretion on intestinal transcapillary fluid and solute exchange at venous pressures of 0.0 and 20.0 mm Hg. (*Circles and squares*) The left and right ordinates, respectively.

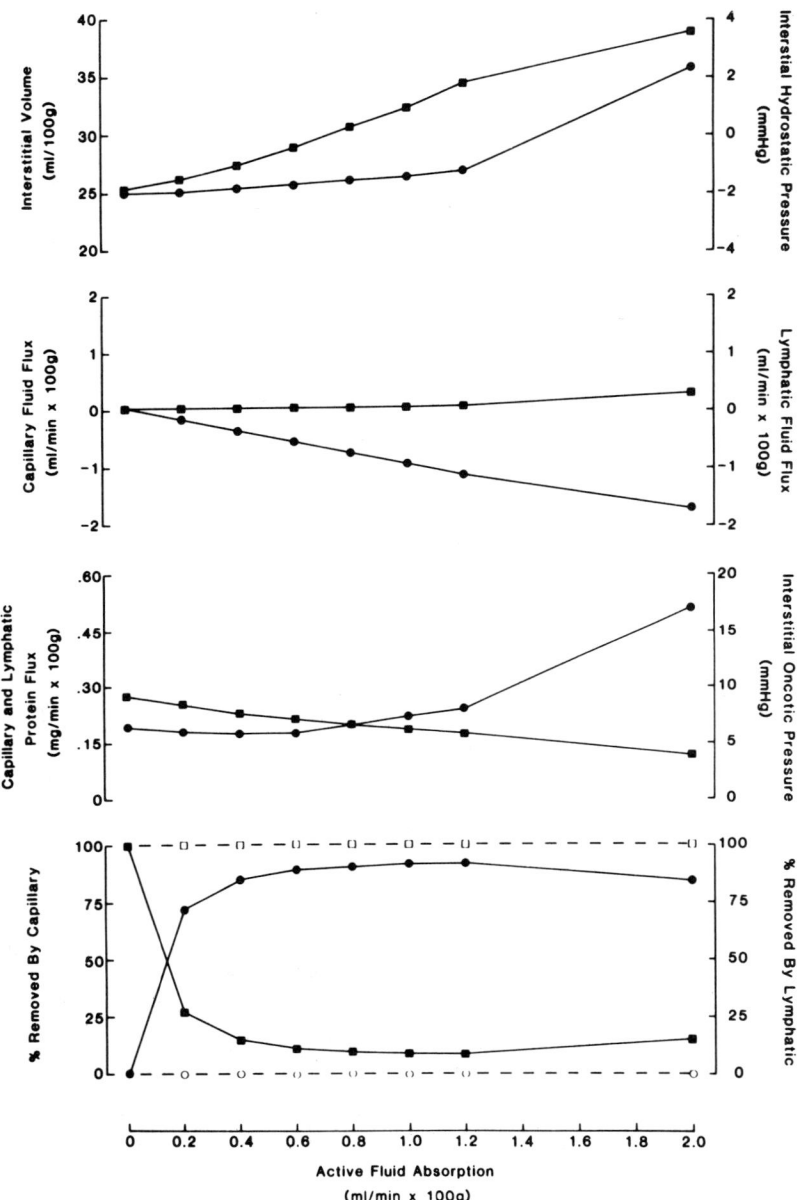

FIG. 6. Model predictions of the effects of active fluid absorption intestinal transcapillary fluid *(closed circles and closed squares)* and solute exchange *(open circles and open squares)*. *(Circles and squares)* The left and right ordinates, respectively.

trates the steady state values obtained for interstitial volume, interstitial hydrostatic pressure, and the fluxes of fluid and protein across the capillaries and lymphatics for absorption rates ranging from 0.0 to 2.0 ml/min × 100 g.

The model predicts that active absorption is accompanied by an increase in interstitial volume, which reduces interstitial oncotic pressure and raises tissue hydrostatic pressure (6). These alterations in the interstitial forces oppose capillary filtration and convert filtering capillaries to absorbing ones. Furthermore, the rise in tissue fluid pressure increases the rate of lymphatic filling and lymph flow. Therefore, during absorption both the capillaries and lymphatics serve to remove fluid and solute from the interstitium. The model predicted that during fluid absorption, the capillaries carry approximately 90% of the absorbed fluid whereas the remaining 10% is removed by the lymphatics. In the absorptive state, proteins can be removed from the interstitium either by the capillaries (via the interstitium-to-blood convective flux) or by the lymphatics. We observed a continuous reduction in the quantity of interstitial protein (QP) during absorption when the capillary permeability–surface area product (PS_c) remained at its control value (0.005 ml/min × 100 g). However, when the PS product was allowed to increase as a function of absorption rate, as reported in the literature (15), QP remained relatively constant. This observation supports the contention that either capillary permeability or surface area must increase during active fluid absorption.

SUMMARY AND CONCLUSIONS

We have presented a mathematical model of intestinal transcapillary fluid and protein exchange based on current concepts of microvascular transport. The predictive capabilities of this model exceed those of previous model (8,24,26,29) because of the revised formulations for transmembrane solute exchange and the new data on which the model is based. The predictions of the model are generally consistent with experimental data reported in the literature. Therefore, the model is conceptually sound. The fact that the simulations of active fluid secretion are inconsistent with experimental observations is not surprising in light of the limited information available on this topic. Nonetheless, this discrepancy (and others) between the model and experimental observations emphasizes the need for systematic quantitative analyses of the effects of various physiologic and pathologic conditions on intestinal transcapillary fluid and solute exchange.

Although the model presented in this chapter has been useful for comparing and integrating experimental findings with current concepts of transcapillary fluid and protein exchange, like other models, it is limited by the assumptions and data on which it is based. Additional experimentation is required to test the validity of these assumptions and to extend the analysis to incorporate the influences of intestinal microvascular and tissue heterogeneity. Now that techniques are available for measuring capillary pressure, the capillary filtration coefficient, and the osmotic reflection coefficient of single capillaries, data that permit treatment of the intestinal circulation as a heterogenous vascular bed may soon be available.

ACKNOWLEDGMENTS

The authors are grateful to Penny Cook, Sharon Miller, and Sandy Worley for their clerical assistance. This work was supported by a grant from the National Heart, Lung and Blood Institute (HL 26441).

REFERENCES

1. Barrowman, J. A. (1978): *Physiology of the Gastrointestinal Lymphatic System.* Cambridge University Press, Cambridge.
2. Bresler, E. H., Mason, E. A., and Wendt, R. P. (1976): Appraisal of equations for neutral solute flux across porous sieving membranes. *Biophys. Chem.*, 4:229–236.
3. Duffy, P. A., Granger, D. N., and Taylor, A. E. (1978): Intestinal secretion induced by volume expansion in the dog. *Gastroenterology*, 75:413–418.
4. Fordtran, J. S., Rector, F. C., and Ewton, M. F. (1965): Permeability characteristics of the human small intestine. *J. Clin. Invest.*, 44:1935–1944.
5. Granger, D. N. (1981): Intestinal microcirculation and transmucosal fluid transport. *Am. J. Physiol.*, 240:G343–G349.
6. Granger, D. N., and Barrowman, J. A. (1983): Microcirculation of the alimentary tract. I. Physiology of transcapillary fluid and solute exchange. *Gastroenterology*, 84:846–868.
7. Granger, D. N., Cross, R., and Barrowman, J. A. (1982): Effects of various secretagogues and human carcinoid serum on lymph flow in the cat ileum. *Gastroenterology*, 83:896–901.
8. Granger, D. N., Gabel, J. C., Drake, R. E., and Taylor, A. E. (1977): A mathematical model describing interstitial volume and protein regulation. In: *Proceedings of the Summer Computer Simulations Con-*

ference, pp. 572–576. Simulations Councils, Inc., La Jolla.
9. Granger, D. N., and Granger, H. J. (1983): Systems analysis of intestinal hemodynamics and oxygenation. *Am. J. Physiol.*, 245:G786–789.
10. Granger, D. N., Mortillaro, N. A., Kvietys, P. R., Rutili, G., Parker, J. C., and Taylor, A. E. (1980): Role of the interstitial matrix during intestinal volume absorption. *Am. J. Physiol.*, 238:G183–G189.
11. Granger, D. N., Mortillaro, N. A., Kvietys, P. R., and Taylor, A. E. (1980): Regulation of interstitial fluid volume in the small bowel. In: *Tissue Fluid Pressure*, edited by A. Hargens, pp. 173–183. Williams and Wilkins, Baltimore.
12. Granger, D. N., Mortillaro, N. A., Perry, M. A., and Kvietys, P. R. (1982): Autoregulation of intestinal capillary filtration rate. *Am. J. Physiol.*, 243:G475–G483.
13. Granger, D. N., Mortillaro, N. A., and Taylor, A. E. (1977): Interactions of intestinal lymph flow and secretion. *Am. J. Physiol.*, 232(1):E13–E18.
14. Granger, D. N., Perry, M. A., and Kvietys, P. R. (1983): The intestinal microcirculation and fluid transport in digestive organs. *Fed. Proc.*, 42:1667–1672.
15. Granger, D. N., Perry, M. A., Kvietys, P. R., and Taylor, A. E. (1981): Interstitium-to-blood movement of macromolecules in the absorbing small intestine. *Am. J. Physiol.*, 241(4):G31–G36.
16. Granger, D. N., and Taylor, A. E. (1978): Effects of solute-coupled transport on lymph flow and oncotic pressures in cat ileum. *Am. J. Physiol.*, 235(4):E429–E436.
17. Granger, D. N., and Taylor, A. E. (1980): Permeability of intestinal capillaries to endogenous macromolecules. *Am. J. Physiol.*, 238:H457–H464.
18. Granger, D. N., and Taylor, A. E. (1980): Permselectivity of intestinal capillaries. *Physiologist*, 23(1):47–52.
19. Granger, H. J., and Shepherd, A. P. (1979): Dynamics and control of the microcirculation. *Adv. Biomed. Eng.*, 7:1–63.
20. Kedem, O., and Katchalsky, A. (1961): A physical interpretation of the phenomenological coefficients of membrane permeability. *J. Gen. Physiol.*, 45:143–179.
21. Lee, J. S., and Silverberg, J. W. (1973): Effect of cholera toxin on fluid absorption and villus lymph pressure in dog jejunal mucosa. *Gastroenterology*, 62:993–1000.
22. Levitt, D. C., Bond, J. H., and Levitt, M. D. (1980): Use of a model of small bowel mucosa to predict passive desorption. *Am. J. Physiol.*, 239:G23–G29.
23. Mailman, D. (1982): Blood flow and intestinal absorption. *Fed. Proc.*, 41:2096–2100.
24. Mortillaro, N. A., and Granger, H. J. (1977): Myogenic control of intestinal circulation and its relation to capillary fluid exchange. In: *Proceedings of the Summer Computer Simulations Conference*, pp. 557–565. Simulations Councils, Inc., La Jolla.
25. Mortillaro, N. A., and Taylor, A. E. (1976): Interactions of capillary and tissue forces in the cat small intestine. *Circ. Res.*, 39(3):348–358.
26. Quillen, E. W., Granger, J. P., Granger, D. N., and Taylor, A. E. (1977): A mathematical simulation of interstitial volume and protein regulation in the small intestine. In: *Proceedings of the Summer Computer Simulations Conference*, pp. 566–571. Simulations Councils, Inc., La Jolla.
27. Richardson, P. D. I., and Granger, D. N. (1981): Capillary filtration coefficient as a measure of perfused capillary density. In: *Measurement of Blood Flow: Applications to the Splanchnic Circulation*, edited by D. N. Granger and G. B. Bulkley, pp. 321–335. Williams and Wilkins, New York.
28. Shepherd, A. P., and Granger, H. J. (1973): Autoregulatory escape in the gut: A systems analysis. *Gastroenterology*, 65:77–91.
29. Taylor, A. E., and Mortillaro, N. A. (1974): Re-evaluation of the filtration hypothesis in intestine. In: *Proceedings of the Summer Computer Simulations Conference*, pp. 673–677. Simulations Councils, Inc., La Jolla.
30. Yablonski, M. E., and Lifson, N. (1976): Mechanisms of production of intestinal secretion by elevated venous pressure. *J. Clin. Invest.*, 57:904–915.

Models of the Relationship Between Drug Absorption and Intestinal Blood Flow

Dietrich Winne

Division of Molecular Pharmacology, Department of Pharmacology, University of Tübingen, D-7400 Tübingen 1, Federal Republic of Germany

This chapter presents a series of mathematical models that have been proposed to describe quantitatively the relationship between intestinal absorption and blood flow. In these models, which have been reviewed previously (28), the real situation in the gut is simplified. Therefore, the models do not adequately simulate all physiological and experimental conditions. Furthermore, each model stresses different aspects of intestinal absorption and perfusion. Thus, experimental data can be consistent with one model, but not with another. Some models are special cases of a more general model; others are combinations of simpler models. The advantages of models are that the investigator is forced to define exactly the factors involved and that complicated interrelationships can be subdivided into easier partial problems. The mathematical treatment leads finally to a comprehensive description of the whole problem.

The models described in this chapter consider only the washout effect of blood flow on intestinal absorption because only this influence has been included in the mathematical treatments up to now. To facilitate comparison of the models, only the absorption of a passively transported, nonmetabolized nonelectrolyte in the absence of a net water flux is discussed, and the lymph drainage is neglected. For the same reason a uniform notation is used. Therefore, the symbols do not correspond to the symbols in the original articles. The derived equations are valid for a small section of the intestine assuming a constant luminal solute concentration. The absorption rate and the relevant areas are related to wet tissue weight (an example of normalization used in absorption experiments). Only the basic and final equations with few intermediate steps are given. For more general equations covering a broader range of experimental conditions and for the detailed derivations of the equations, the reader is referred to the original articles. To prevent confusion the numbering of the models coincides with the numbering used in the previous review (28).

MODELS WITH ONE ABSORPTIVE SITE AND WITHOUT COUNTERCURRENT EXCHANGE

Description of the Models and Derivation of the Equations

The first models of the relationship between intestinal absorption and blood flow assume one absorptive site, the subepithelial capillaries. Thus, absorptive site blood flow represents the fraction of the total blood flow that reaches these capillaries. The substance leaving the intestinal lumen is removed completely by the subepithelial blood. Thus, the "disappearance rate from the intestinal lumen" is equal to the "appearance rate in the intestinal venous blood."

Model 1

In model 1 proposed by Winne and Ochsenfahrt (22,31), two barriers are distinguished between the bulk phase of the intestinal lumen and the blood in the subepithelial capillaries (Fig. 1). The first barrier reaches from the luminal

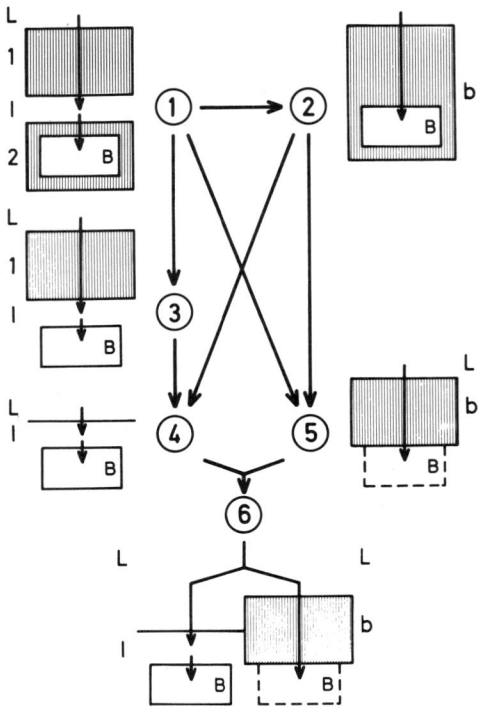

FIG. 1. Six models of intestinal blood flow and absorption. Interrelationships among models 1–6 are shown. *(Hatched areas)* Barriers with effective transport resistance; *(solid lines)* barriers without effective transport resistance; *(broken lines)* a capillary when the influence of blood flow is not effective. 1, first barrier (mucosal unstirred layer and epithelium); 2, second barrier (capillary wall); b, fused first and second barrier; B, blood in subepithelial capillaries; I, interstitial space between epithelium and subepithelial capillaries; L, luminal bulk phase; *(circled figures)* number of model.

bulk phase to the subepithelial interstitial space and includes the mucosal unstirred layer (the aqueous and mucous part) and the epithelium (cell membranes, cell content, basal membrane). The second barrier is the wall of the absorptive site capillaries. The permeation rate of a passively transported substance through the first barrier is proportional to the concentration difference. Hence,

$$\Phi_L = k_1 A_1 (C_L - C_I), \quad (1)$$

where Φ_L is the permeation rate through the first barrier related to wet tissue weight (mole min^{-1} g^{-1}), and k_1 is the permeability coefficient of the first barrier (cm min^{-1}). A_1 is the weight-normalized area of the first barrier (cm^2 g^{-1}). More precisely it is the cross-sectional area normal to the permeation direction inside the first barrier. Finally, C_L and C_I are the concentrations (mole ml^{-1}) in the luminal bulk phase and in the interstitial space near the capillary wall, respectively.

Assuming that all the subepithelial capillaries have the same dimensions, we can extrapolate the result from one capillary easily to the whole population. The permeation through the capillary wall is also proportional to the concentration difference. Thus,

$$d\Phi_B = k_2(C_I - C_W)dA_2 = \alpha a_1 \dot{V}_B dC_W, \quad (2)$$

where Φ_B is the permeation rate through the second barrier related to wet tissue weight (mole min^{-1} g^{-1}), k_2 is the capillary permeability coefficient (cm min^{-1}), A_2 is the capillary surface area (cm^2 g^{-1}), α is the fraction of total blood flow rate at absorptive site, a_1 is the blood-to-plasma water concentration ratio (considering protein binding and the distribution in red cells), $\dot{V}_B$ is the weight-normalized total blood flow of the intestinal segment under study (ml min^{-1} g^{-1}), and C_W is the concentration in plasma water (mole ml^{-1}). While C_I is assumed to be constant, C_W increases from the arterial to the venous ends of the capillaries. The differential form used in Eq. 2 indicates that the equation is valid for a small section with area dA_2. Integration yields finally

$$\Phi_B = \alpha a_1 \dot{V}_B E_1 (C_I - C_A) \quad (3)$$

with

$$E_1 = 1 - e^{-k_2 A_2 / \alpha a_1 \dot{V}_B} \quad (4)$$

where C_A is the concentration in the arterial plasma water (mole ml^{-1}). A more detailed derivation is given elsewhere (28,31).

At steady state the permeation rate through the first barrier is equal to the rate through the capillary walls: $\Phi_L = \Phi_B$. The unknown concentration C_I in the interstitial space is derived from Eqs. 1 and 3. The result introduced into Eq. 1 or 3 yields the relationship between blood flow and the permeation or absorption rate from the luminal bulk phase to blood. Thus,

$$\Phi_L = \Phi_B = \frac{C_L - C_A}{1/k_1A_1 + 1/\alpha a_1 \dot{V}_B E_1} \quad (5)$$

$$= \alpha a_1 \dot{V}_B (C_V - C_A), \quad (5)$$

where C_V is the concentration in venous plasma water (mole ml^{-1}) at the venous ends of the absorbing capillaries. The right-hand part of Eq. 5 describes the fact that under the conditions of model 1 the absorption rate is the arteriovenous concentration difference at the absorptive site times the absorptive site blood flow. The denominator of the middle part of Eq. 5 can be considered the total resistance to transport in analogy with Ohm's Law. The two terms in the denominator represent the partial resistances of the first barrier (bulk phase to interstitial space) and of the washout system (capillary wall and washout capacity). The first partial resistance can be further subdivided into partial resistances (e.g., unstirred layer and epithelium). From Eq. 3 and the right-hand part of Eq. 5, it follows that

$$E_1 = (C_V - C_A)/(C_I - C_A). \quad (6)$$

The quantity E_1 approaches unity when equilibrium is reached between the concentrations in the interstitial space and in plasma at the venous end of the capillaries ($C_V = C_I$). Thus, E_1 characterizes the approach to equilibrium.

The model of Druckrey and Küpfmüller (10) corresponds to model 1 with the difference that the substance tranverses the capillary wall only by solvent drag and not by diffusion.

Model 2

In model 2 discussed by Berggren and Goldberg (2), Coburn (6), Dobson et al. (9), and Forster (11), the first barrier and the capillary wall are considered to be fused so that one barrier is assumed between the luminal bulk phase and capillary blood (Fig. 1). The absorption rate can be derived analogously to Eqs. 2 through 5 starting with

$$d\Phi_B = k_b(C_L - C_W)dA_b = \alpha a_1 \dot{V}_B dC_W, \quad (7)$$

where k_b is the permeability coefficient (cm min^{-1}) of the total barrier between luminal bulk phase and blood, and A_b is the corresponding area related to wet tissue weight (cm^2g^{-1}). Integration of Eq. 7 yields

$$\Phi_L = \Phi_B = \alpha a_1 \dot{V}_B E_2 (C_L - C_A) \quad (8)$$

$$= \alpha a_1 \dot{V}_B (C_V - C_A),$$

where

$$E_2 = 1 - e^{-k_b A_b / \alpha a_1 \dot{V}_B} \quad (9)$$

Model 2 can also be derived from model 1 by expanding the second barrier up to the luminal bulk phase, and the first barrier is reduced until it is vanishingly small. Mathematically Eq. 5 of model 1 changes into Eq. 8, when $1/k_1$ approaches 0 and k_2A_2 approaches k_bA_b ($E_1 \rightarrow E_2$). In Fig. 2 the interrelationships of the equations are summarized. The intermediate and right-hand parts of Eq. 8 yield

$$E_2 = (C_V - C_A)/(C_L - C_A). \quad (10)$$

The quantity E_2 represents the approach to the equilibrium between luminal bulk phase and plasma water at the venous ends of the absorptive site capillaries.

Models 1 and 2 differ in the following ways. In model 2, the concentration gradient across the barrier reaches from the luminal bulk phase to the capillary blood (28). This gradient is steeper at the arterial end of the capillaries than at the venous end. In model 1, we have two concentration gradients and between them the uniform concentration in the subepithelial interstitial space. That means a rapid mixing is assumed in this space. The concentration gradient through the first barrier is uniform while the gradient through the capillary wall decreases from the arterial to the venous end.

The model of Barr and Riegelman (1) corresponds formally to model 2 with the difference that the luminal fluid and a part of the neighboring tissue are combined into one compartment.

By means of model 2, Winne (30) investigated the influence of absorptive site blood flow on unidirectional fluxes measured *in vivo*. If

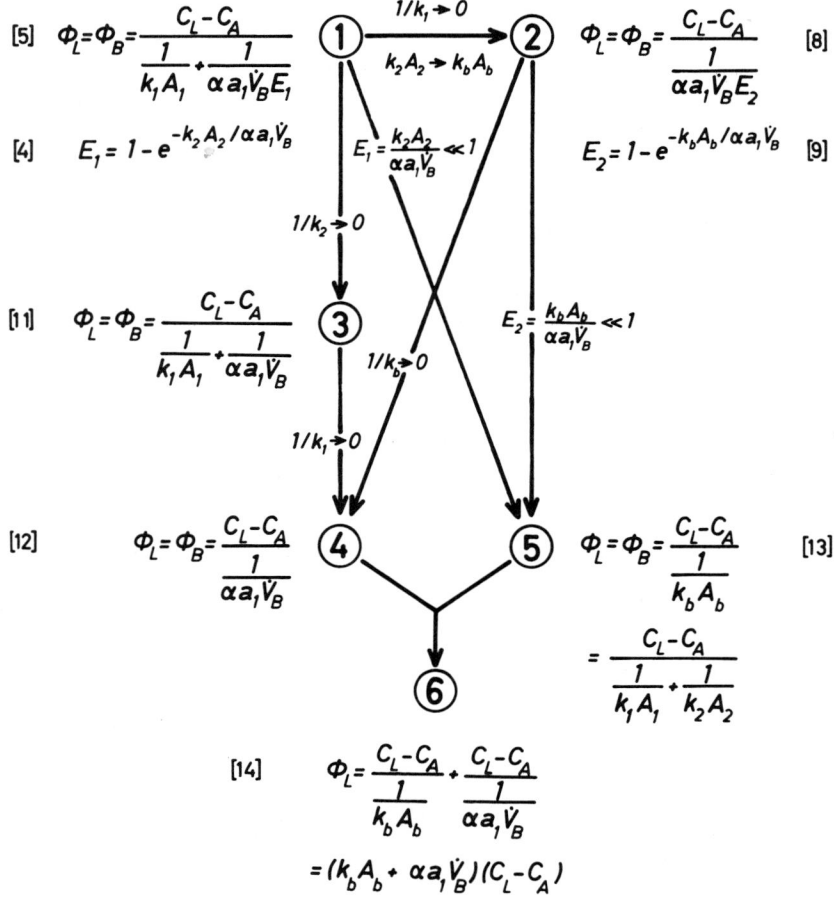

FIG. 2. Interrelationships among the equations describing the dependence of intestinal absorption on blood flow. Equations shown are from models 1–6.

changes in unidirectional fluxes are observed, they can be attributed to variations in blood flow or to changes in the permeation characteristics of the barrier between the bulk phase and the blood of the absorbing capillaries. However, the flux ratio is independent of blood flow provided the blood-to-lumen flux of a substance is proportional to, and the lumen-to-blood flux independent of, the concentration in the capillaries. In that case, changes of the flux ratio point to effects on the permeation characteristics of the barrier.

Model 3

Model 3 derived by Winne and Ochsenfahrt (31) can be interpreted as special case of model 1 (Figs. 1 and 2) when the resistance of the second barrier, the capillary wall, is very small $(1/k_2 \rightarrow 0)$. The equilibrium between the interstitial space and plasma water at the venous end of the capillaries is nearly reached, so that the quantity E_1 approaches unity. Thus, we obtain from Eq. 5

$$\Phi_L = \Phi_B = \frac{C_L - C_A}{1/k_1 A_1 + 1/\alpha a_1 \dot{V}_B} \qquad (11)$$

Since the walls of the capillaries in the intestinal villi are highly permeable (19), the conditions of model 3 may often be fulfilled.

Model 4

Model 4 mentioned or tested by Forster (11), Hamilton et al. (12), and Levitt and Levitt (14) represents a limiting case of models 1, 2, and 3 (Figs. 1 and 2). When the resistance of the barriers between the luminal bulk phase and the blood becomes negligible ($1/k_1 \to 0$, $1/k_2 \to 0$, $1/k_b \to 0$), the absorption rate is proportional to the absorptive site blood flow (effective mucosal blood flow). Hence,

$$\Phi_L = \Phi_B = \alpha a_1 \dot{V}_B (C_L - C_A). \quad (12)$$

This situation is also called "blood-flow-limited absorption." The venous plasma water at the absorptive site is equilibrated with the luminal bulk phase ($C_V = C_L$). On the other hand, the absorptive site blood flow can be determined by measuring the absorption or secretion rate of a suitable substance (6,7,9,11,12,16) if the conditions of model 4 are fulfilled.

Model 5

When the permeability of the layers between luminal bulk phase and blood decreases (more strictly $k_2 A_2 / \alpha a_1 \dot{V}_B \ll 1$, $k_b A_b / \alpha a_1 \dot{V}_B \ll 1$), the influence of the washout system on absorption also decreases. In the limiting case, models 1 and 2 change into model 5, which has been used by Levitt and Levitt (14). The absorption rate becomes independent of blood flow (Figs. 1 and 2).

$$\Phi_L = \Phi_B = \frac{C_L - C_A}{1/k_1 A_1 + 1/k_2 A_2} \quad (13)$$

$$= k_b A_b (C_L - C_A).$$

Since the diffusion through the first and second barrier represents the rate-limiting step, the situation of model 5 is called "diffusion-limited absorption."

Predictions of the Models

In general, the equations of models 1 to 3 describing the dependence of intestinal absorption on blood flow represent nonlinear curves that start at the origin, ascend, and level off into a horizontal section. The left panel of Fig. 3 demonstrates curves predicted by model 3. The permeability term $k_1 A_1$ of the first barrier was varied whereas the fraction α of the absorptive site blood flow was held constant. We have to bear in mind that under experimental conditions the absorptive site blood flow does not always vary in parallel with total blood

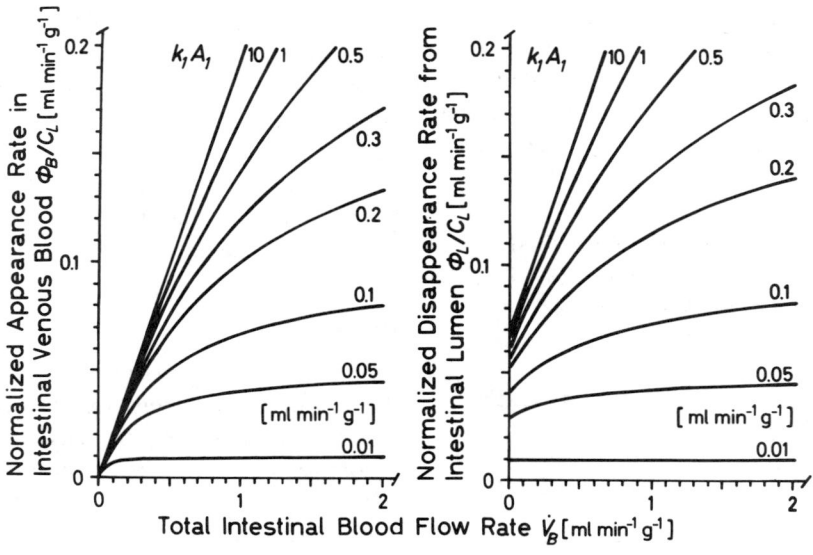

FIG. 3. Left: Dependence of appearance rate in intestinal venous blood on blood flow. Curves predicted by model 3 were calculated from Eq. 11 with $C_A = 0$, $a_1 = 1$, $\alpha = 0.2$, as value of $k_1 A_1$ was changed. **Right:** Dependence of disappearance rate from intestinal lumen on blood flow. Curves predicted by model 9 were calculated from Eq. 16 with $C_A = 0$, $a_1 = 1$, $\alpha = 0.2$, $k_3 A_3 = 0.07$ ml min^{-1} g^{-1}, as $k_1 A_1$ was altered. With increasing permeability of a substance, the blood-flow-independent or diffusion-limited absorption changes to the blood-flow-limited absorption.

flow. This fact renders the interpretation of experimental data more difficult. The absorption rate is normalized by the luminal concentration assuming zero arterial concentration, Φ/C_L. Models 1, 2, and 3 yield similar curves (28). Discriminating between these models is practically impossible. The shape of the curves depends on the permeability term k_1A_1 or k_bA_b and of blood flow, absorption is independent of blood flow ("blood-flow-independent absorption" or "diffusion-limited absorption"). The first term in the denominator of Eq. 11 is large compared with the second one; thus, blood flow loses its influence on the absorption rate. In the limiting mines the absorption rate. In the limiting case of model 4, we have a straight line and the absorption is blood-flow-limited. In the case of a substance with a low permeability coefficient, the horizontal section of the curve starts near the origin. Throughout almost the whole range of blood flow, absorption is independent of blood flow ("blood-flow-independent absorption" or "diffusion-limited absorption"). The first term in the denominator of Eq. 11 is large compared with the second one; thus, blood flow loses its influence on the absorption rate. In the limiting case, we have model 5.

The appearance rate of several substances in the intestinal venous blood of rat jejunum depends on total blood flow in the jejunal segment as predicted by models 1 to 5 (18,25,32,33) (see Fig. 4).

MODELS WITH MORE THAN ONE ABSORPTIVE SITE OR PATHWAY AND WITHOUT COUNTERCURRENT EXCHANGE

Description of the Models and Derivation of the Equations

Model 6

Levitt and Levitt (14) applied several models to the intestinal absorption of inert gases. The best fit was obtained with model 6, which combines models 4 and 5 (Fig. 1). According to this model, one fraction of a gas is absorbed in proportion to absorptive site blood flow, since

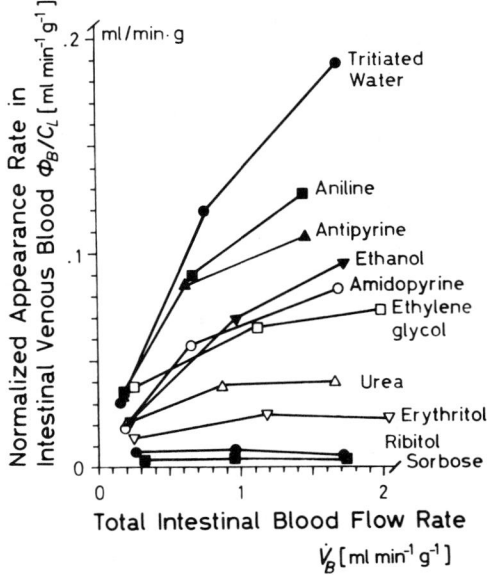

FIG. 4. Dependence of appearance rate in rat jejunal blood on total intestinal blood flow. (From Winne, ref. 28, with permission.)

the venous blood equilibrates fully with the gas in the intestinal lumen. Additionally, a second fraction is absorbed independently of blood flow, presumably in deeper layers of the mucosa. Thus, two pathways and absorptive sites are distinguished in model 6. The combination of Eqs. 12 and 13 yields (Fig. 2)

$$\Phi_L = (k_bA_b + \alpha a_1 \dot{V}_B)(C_L - C_A). \quad (14)$$

In recent investigations the authors have refined and extended the model (see model 12).

Model 9

Intestinal absorption experiments in rats have shown that under certain experimental conditions (e.g., intestinal segment placed outside the abdominal cavity) the appearance rate in the intestinal venous blood is smaller than the disappearance rate from the intestinal lumen (17,32,33). The luminally administered substance penetrates partially through the intestinal wall into the moistened tissue covering the segment or into a serosal bath. To take into account this experimental finding, Winne (23,24) extended model 1 to model 9 (see Fig. 5). After penetrating the epithelium, one fraction of the substance is removed by the blood in the absorptive site capillaries; the other fraction migrates through the subepithelial layers to the serosal side. The removal pathway thus is split into two branches. In this model, the vessels in the deeper layers of the intestinal wall and their washout capacity are ignored (see model 8).

The permeation through the first barrier is described by Eq. 1. The "appearance rate in the serosal fluid" Φ_S related to wet tissue weight (mole min^{-1} g^{-1}) is assumed to be proportional to the concentration difference between serosal fluid (C_S) and interstitial space (C_I).

$$\Phi_S = k_3 A_3 (C_I - C_S), \quad (15)$$

where k_3 is the permeability coefficient (cm min^{-1}) and A_3 is the corresponding area related to wet tissue weight (cm^2 g^{-1}). Since at steady state, $\Phi_L = \Phi_B + \Phi_S$, the unknown concentration C_I can be derived from Eqs. 1, 3, and 15. The result introduced into Eq. 1 yields tne "disappearance rate from the intestinal lumen."

$$\Phi_L = \frac{C_L - (\alpha a_1 \dot{V}_B E_1 C_A + k_3 A_3 C_S)/(\alpha a_1 \dot{V}_B E_1 + k_3 A_3)}{1/k_1 A_1 + 1/(\alpha a_1 \dot{V}_B E_1 + k_3 A_3)}. \quad (16)$$

From Eq. 3 it follows that the "appearance rate in the intestinal venous blood" is

$$\Phi_B = \frac{C_L + C_S k_3 A_3/k_1 A_1 - (1 + k_3 A_3/k_1 A_1) C_A}{1/k_1 A_1 + (1 + k_3 A_3/k_1 A_1)/\alpha a_1 \dot{V}_B E_1}. \quad (17)$$

From Eq. 15 the "appearance rate in the serosal fluid" is derived. Hence,

$$\Phi_S = \frac{C_L + C_A \alpha a_1 \dot{V}_B E_1/k_1 A_1 - (1 + \alpha a_1 \dot{V}_B E_1/k_1 A_1) C_S}{1/k_1 A_1 + (1 + \alpha a_1 \dot{V}_B E_1/k_1 A_1)/k_3 A_3}. \quad (18)$$

The three rates are all normalized to wet tissue weight.

Eq. 5 of model 1 can be derived from Eqs. 16 and 17 by setting $k_3 = 0$. That means the permeation into the serosal fluid is insignificant. In Fig. 6, the interrelationships of the equations are demonstrated using the restriction $C_S = C_A$ for convenience. When blood flow is stopped, we have the typical *in vitro* situation, and the only pathway is the penetration into the serosal bath. In the case of zero blood flow ($\dot{V}_B = 0$), Eqs. 16 and 18 change to

$$\Phi_L = \Phi_S = \frac{C_L - C_S}{1/k_1 A_1 + 1/k_3 A_3}. \quad (19)$$

The disappearance rate from the intestinal lumen equals the appearance rate in the serosal bath. It should be pointed out that in all models accumulation and metabolism in the intestinal wall are excluded. The denominator of Eq. 19 represents the resistance of the total intestinal wall. The two terms are the partial resistances of the first barrier and of the layers betweer. subepithelial interstitial space and serosal bath.

A modified version of model 9 has been derived and applied to experiments in which tritiated water moved simultaneously from the blood to the intestinal lumen and into moistened tissue on the serosal side (26).

Model 8

The disadvantage of model 9 is overcome in model 8 derived by Winne (24). The washout by blood is not restricted to the subepithelial region as in model 9 but reaches up to the serosa (Fig. 5). After traversing the first barrier, the molecules diffuse through the subepithelial tissue towards the serosa. They are removed by a spatial network of capillaries. The derivation of the absorption equations is more complicated and is described in detail elsewhere (24,28). The permeation through the first barrier is given by Eq. 1, where C_{I0} is substituted for $C_I \cdot C_{I0}$ is the concentration just below the epithelium. The rate of washout by blood in the tissue volume $A_3 dx$ with average density ρ (g ml^{-1}) follows from Eq. 3:

$$\Phi_B \rho A_3 dx = \alpha_2 a_1 \dot{V}_B \rho E_1 (C_I - C_A) A_3 dx, \quad (20)$$

where x is the perpendicular distance (cm) from the first barrier assuming a uniform thickness of the subepithelial tissue. α_2 is substituted for α, since the washout is not restricted to the subepithelial region but reaches to the serosa. α_2 represents the fraction of blood flow passing exchange vessels; the flow through shunts is not included in α_2. The density ρ is introduced because the absorption rate is related to wet tissue weight, and Eq. 20 was derived for a volume. The temporal change of an amount of substance in the volume $A_3 dx$ is given by

$$\frac{\partial C_I}{\partial t} A_3 dx = D \frac{\partial^2 C_I}{\partial x^2} A_3 dx \quad (21)$$
$$- \alpha_2 a_1 \dot{V}_B \rho E_1 (C_I - C_A) A_3 dx,$$

where the first term on the right-hand side of the equation represents the diffusion in the interstitial space with the diffusion constant D (cm^2 s^{-1}) and the second term is the removal by blood. t is the time (min). At steady state, Eq. 21 is equal to zero and the differential equation can be solved for the boundary conditions: $x = 0$, $C_I = C_{I0}$; $x = d$, $C_I = C_S$. d is the thickness (cm) of the subepithelial tissue and C_S is the concentration in the serosal fluid or bath. The solution of the differential equation describes the concentration in the subepithelial tissue as function of the distance from the first barrier. C_{I0} is unknown and can be calculated from Eq. 22:

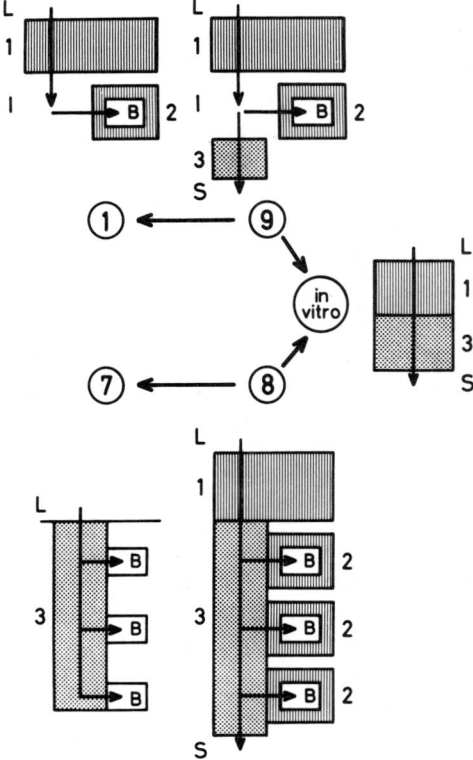

FIG. 5. Interrelationships among models 1, 7–9 for the dependence of intestinal absorption on blood flow. *(Dotted areas)* Subepithelial barrier with effective transport resistance. 3, subepithelial layers up to serosa; S, serosal fluid or bath. For further details, see legend to Fig. 1.

$$\Phi_L = k_1 A_1 (C_L - C_{I0}) = \quad (22)$$
$$- DA_3 \left[\frac{dC_I}{dx} \right]_{x=0}.$$

This equation shows that the flux through the first barrier is equal to the diffusional flux in the subepithelial tissue at $x = 0$. The result for C_{I0} is introduced into the middle part of Eq. 22 and yields the "disappearance rate from the intestinal lumen:"

$$\Phi_L = \frac{C_L - C_S/\cosh \psi - (1 - 1/\cosh \psi) C_A}{\dfrac{1}{k_1 A_1} + \dfrac{d \tanh \psi}{D A_3 \psi}}, \quad (23)$$

where

$$\psi = (\alpha_2 a_1 \dot{V}_B E_1 d/DA_3)^{1/2}. \tag{24}$$

Integration of Eq. 20 from $x = 0$ to $x = d$ delivers the "appearance rate in the intestinal venous blood."

$$\Phi_B = \frac{C_L + \left[1 + \dfrac{\psi DA_3}{k_1 A_1 d}\left(\dfrac{1 + \cosh\psi}{\sinh\psi}\right)\right]C_S - \left[2 + \dfrac{\psi DA_3}{k_1 A_1 d}\left(\dfrac{1 + \cosh\psi}{\sinh\psi}\right)\right]C_A}{\dfrac{\cosh\psi}{\cosh\psi - 1}\left[\dfrac{1}{k_1 A_1} + \dfrac{d\tanh\psi}{DA_3 \psi}\right]}. \tag{25}$$

The "appearance rate in the serosal fluid" is the difference between Φ_L and Φ_B:

$$\Phi_S = \frac{C_L - (\cosh\psi + \dfrac{\psi DA_3}{k_1 A_1 d}\sinh\psi)C_S + (\cosh\psi + \dfrac{\psi DA_3}{k_1 A_1 d}\sinh\psi - 1)C_A}{\cosh\psi \left[\dfrac{1}{k_1 A_1} + \dfrac{d\tanh\psi}{DA_3 \psi}\right]}. \tag{26}$$

In Eqs. 23, 25, and 26 the partial resistances of the first barrier and the subepithelial tissue can be recognized easily.

When blood flow $\dot{V}_B$ approaches zero, Eqs. 23 and 26 change to

$$\Phi_L = \Phi_S = \frac{C_L - C_S}{1/k_1 A_1 + d/DA_3}, \tag{27}$$

since $\tanh\psi/(\psi/d) \rightarrow d$, $\cosh 0 = 1$, $\sinh 0 = 0$ (see also Fig. 6). Comparison of Eqs. 19 and 27 show that D/d is equivalent to k_3, the permeability coefficient of the subepithelial tissue from model 9.

Model 7

Levitt and Levitt (14) attempted to fit the model of Van Liew (21) to their data, but the fit was worse than that of model 6. Model 7 has been proposed for the absorption of gases from subcutaneous pockets. It can be derived from model 8, when the resistances of the first barrier and the capillary wall are neglected, and the substance is removed completely by blood (Fig. 5). With $1/k_1 \rightarrow 0$, $1/k_2 \rightarrow 0$, $d \rightarrow \infty$, and $C_S = C_A$, it follows from Eq. 23 or 25 that

$$\Phi_L = \Phi_B = (\alpha_2 a_1 \dot{V}_B \rho D)^{1/2} A_3 (C_L - C_A), \tag{28}$$

since $1/\cosh\psi \rightarrow 0$, $\tanh\psi \rightarrow 1$, $E_1 \rightarrow 1$, $\psi/d = (\alpha_2 a_1 \dot{V}_B \rho/D)^{1/2}$ with $\rho = 1/A_3 d$ (see also Fig. 6).

Predictions of the Models

Since model 6 combines models 4 (blood-flow-limited absorption) and 5 (blood-flow-independent absorption), Eq. 14 represents an increasingly straight line starting from a point above the origin according to the blood-flow-independent component (28).

Models 8 and 9 have been derived to cover the discrepancy between the appearance rate in the intestinal blood and the disappearance rate from the intestinal lumen. The right panel of Fig. 3 shows the disappearance rates predicted by model 9. In contrast to the left panel, the curves do not converge on the origin but intersect the ordinate at positive values representing the mucosal-serosal flux at zero blood flow rate. The disappearance rates measured in rat jejunum do not deviate substantially from the

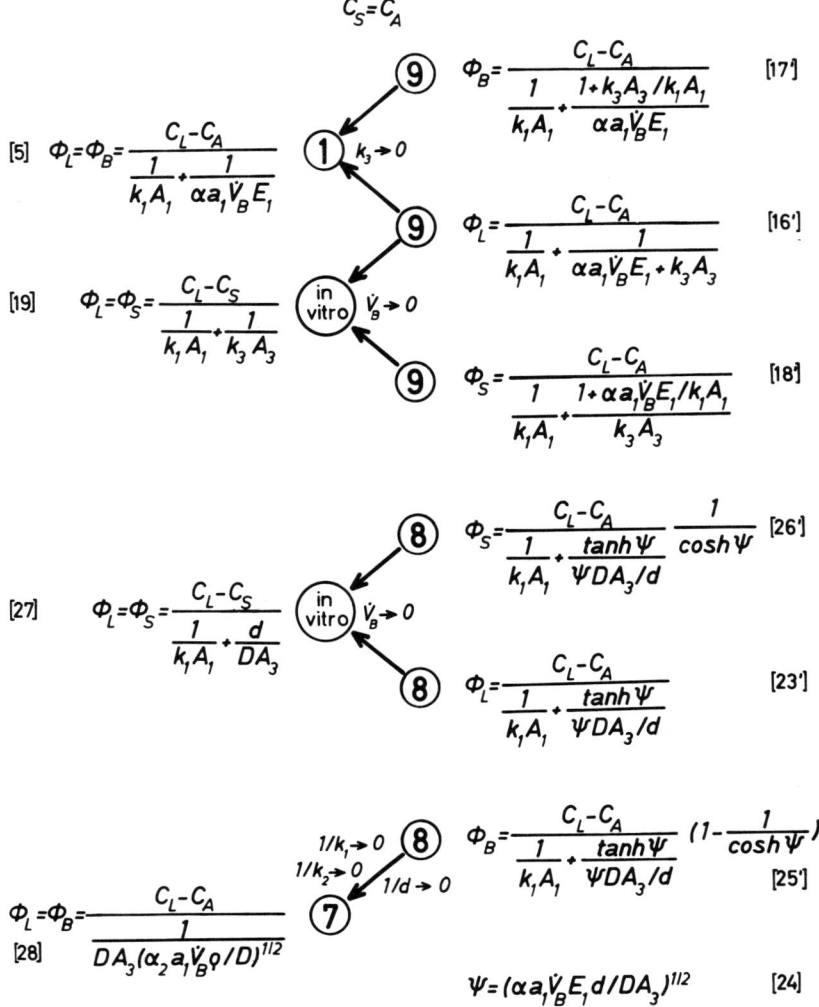

FIG. 6. Interrelationships among the equations describing the dependence of intestinal absorption on blood flow in models 1 and 7–9.

predictions of model 9, indicating that this model describes sufficiently the experimental situation (32,33).

The curves derived from model 8 are similar to the curves in the right panel of Fig. 3 (28). Model 7 predicts nonlinear curves starting from the origin similar to the intermediate curves in the left panel of Fig. 3 (28).

MODELS WITH COUNTERCURRENT EXCHANGE

The detection of an extravascular shunt between the arterial and venous limbs of the villous vessels in the small intestine (15) requires an extension of the models in order to consider the countercurrent exchange.

Description of the Models and Derivation of the Equations

Countercurrent Exchange

In the presence of countercurrent exchange in the intestinal villi, a substance that has entered the villous capillaries is not carried away but diffuses from the venous to the arterial limbs of the villous vessels (Fig. 7, models 10–12) where it is carried back to the absorptive site capillaries. Consequently, its absorption is

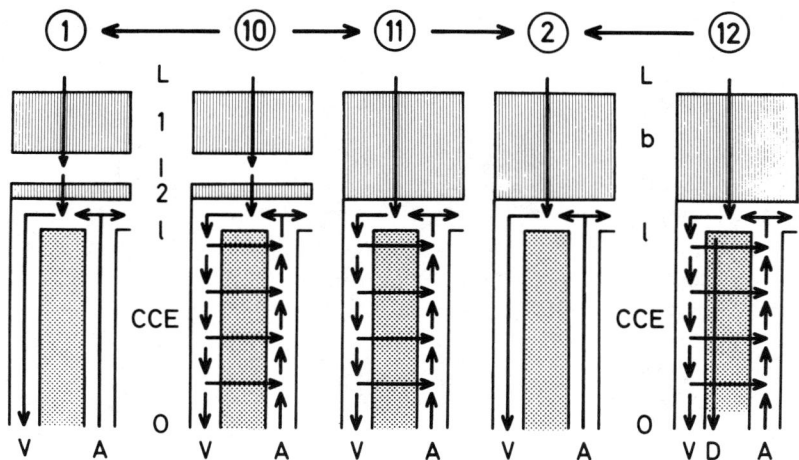

FIG. 7. Comparison of countercurrent models 1, 2, 10–12. A and V, arterial and venous limb of villous vessels; CCE, countercurrent exchange region; 0, proximal ending of CCE (base of villus); 1, distal ending of CCE. For further details see legend of Fig. 1.

retarded in nonsteady state conditions and reduced at steady state.

The mathematical treatment of the villous contercurrent exchange by Winne (27) starts with the following equation:

$$-\alpha a_1(-\dot{V}_B)dC_V = k_E(C_V - C_A)dA_E \\ = \alpha a_1 \dot{V}_B dC_A. \quad (29)$$

The amount of substance leaving a small section of the venous limbs (left-hand part of Eq. 29) traverses the tissue and reaches the arterial vessel (right-hand part of Eq. 29). The minus sign assigned to $\dot{V}_B$ in the left-hand part considers the fact that the direction of the venous blood flow is opposite to arterial flow, which is defined as positive. The extravascular shunt is proportional to the arteriovenous concentration difference in plasma water, the permeability coefficient k_E (cm min^{-1}), and the corresponding area dA_E related to wet tissue weight (cm^2 g^{-1}) (see intermediate part of Eq. 29). It is assumed that the exchange flux occurs only in the cross-section perpendicular to the villous axis. Any flux in the longitudinal direction is neglected. Eq. 29 represents two differential equations. With the boundary conditions $C_A = C_{A0}$ and $C_V = C_{V0}$ at the villous base and $C_A = C_{Al}$ and $C_V = C_{Vl}$ at the tip before entering the absorptive site, the solutions of the differential equations are

$$C_{Al} - C_{A0} = (C_{V0} - C_{A0})k_E A_E/\alpha a_1 \dot{V}_B \quad (30)$$

and

$$C_{Vl} - C_{A0} \\ = (C_{V0} - C_{A0})(1 + k_E A_E/\alpha a_1 \dot{V}_B). \quad (31)$$

The exchange flux Φ_E (mole min^{-1} g^{-1}) follows from the increase of the concentration in the arterial blood passing the exchange region:

$$\Phi_E = \alpha a_1 \dot{V}_B (C_{Al} - C_{A0}) \\ = k_E A_E (C_{V0} - C_{A0}). \quad (32)$$

The right-hand part of Eq. 32 is obtained by substitution from Eq. 30 for $C_{Al} - C_{A0}$. At the villous base the final net rate transported by blood Φ_B (mole min^{-1} g^{-1}) is

$$\Phi_B = \alpha a_1 \dot{V}_B (C_{V0} - C_{A0}). \quad (33)$$

From Eqs. 32 and 33 it follows that

$$\Phi_E/\Phi_B = k_E A_E/\alpha a_1 \dot{V}_B. \quad (34)$$

The ratio of the exchange flux to final net flux is equal to the ratio of the exchange permeability to the plasma water flux.

In the case of cylindrical villi, the exchange permeability term can be specified in more detail (4), since the tissue between the arterial and venous blood can be approximated by a hollow cylinder. Thus,

$$k_E A_E = nD2\pi l/\ln(r_V/r_A), \quad (35)$$

where n is the number of villi per unit wet tissue weight (g^{-1}), D is the diffusion constant of the substance in the exchange region ($cm^2 \, sec^{-1}$), l is the length of the exchange region (cm), r_A is the inner radius of the arterial vessel (cm), and r_V is the distance of the inner surface of the venous vessels from the villous axis (cm).

Model 10

When the permeation of a substance into the absorptive site capillaries is described according to model 1 (see Fig. 7), we have to substitute C_{Al} for C_A in Eq. 5. From Eqs. 5, 30, and 33 it follows after several rearrangements that

$$\Phi_L = \Phi_B = \frac{C_L - C_{A0}}{1/k_1 A_1 + 1/\alpha a_1 \dot{V}_B E_1 + k_E A_E/(\alpha a_1 \dot{V}_B)^2}. \quad (36)$$

$$\text{①} \quad \Phi_L = \Phi_B = \frac{C_L - C_{A0}}{\dfrac{1}{k_1 A_1} + \dfrac{1}{\alpha a_1 \dot{V}_B E_1}} \quad [5]$$

$$\text{⑩} \quad \Phi_L = \Phi_B = \frac{C_L - C_{A0}}{\dfrac{1}{k_1 A_1} + \dfrac{1}{\alpha a_1 \dot{V}_B E_1} + \dfrac{k_E A_E}{(\alpha a_1 \dot{V}_B)^2}} \quad [36]$$

$$\text{⑪} \quad \Phi_L = \Phi_B = \frac{C_L - C_{A0}}{\dfrac{1}{\alpha a_1 \dot{V}_B E_2} + \dfrac{k_E A_E}{(\alpha a_1 \dot{V}_B)^2}} \quad [37]$$

$$\text{②} \quad \Phi_L = \Phi_B = \frac{C_L - C_{A0}}{\dfrac{1}{\alpha a_1 \dot{V}_B E_2}} \quad [8]$$

$$\text{⑫} \quad \Phi_L = \Phi_B + \Phi_D = \frac{(C_L - C_{A0})\left(1 + k_D A_D \dfrac{k_E A_E}{(\alpha a_1 \dot{V}_B)^2}\right)}{\dfrac{1}{\alpha a_1 \dot{V}_B E_2} + \dfrac{k_E A_E}{(\alpha a_1 \dot{V}_B)^2}} \quad [39]$$

$$E_1 = 1 - e^{-k_2 A_2/\alpha a_1 \dot{V}_B} \quad [4] \qquad E_2 = 1 - e^{-k_b A_b/\alpha a_1 \dot{V}_B} \quad [9]$$

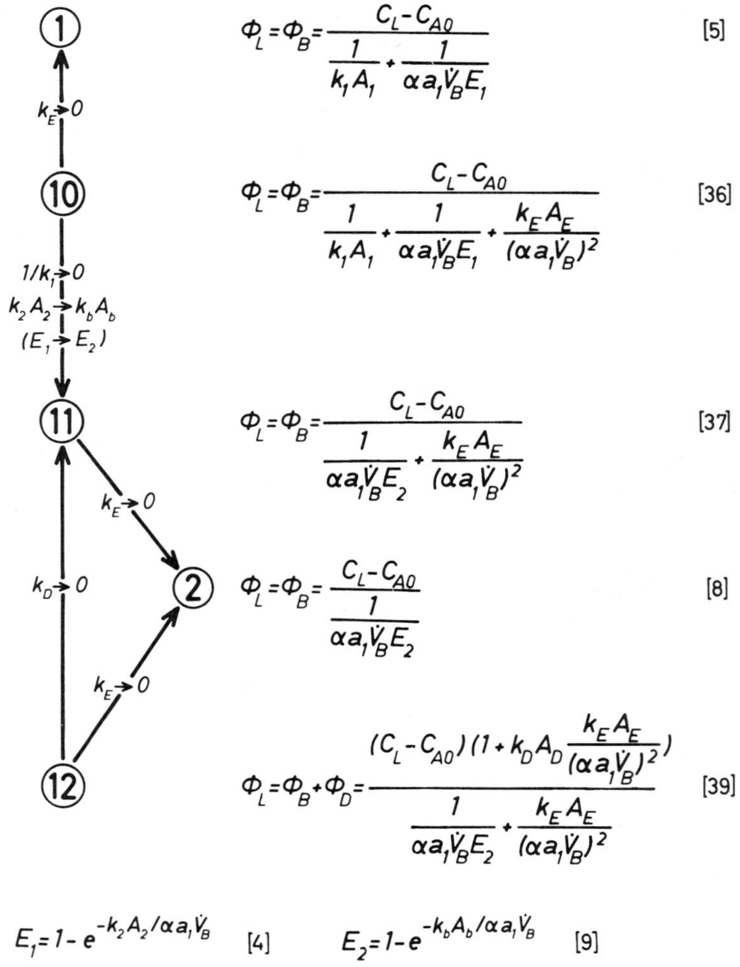

FIG. 8. Interrelationships among the equations that comprise models 1, 2, and 10–12.

Comparing Eq. 36 and Eq. 5 reveals that in the case of effective countercurrent exchange the denominator includes a third term, the "resistance" due to countercurrent exchange. For $k_E \to 0$, model 10 changes to model 1 (Figs. 7 and 8). Model 10 with and without net water flux has been discussed in more detail by Winne (27).

Model 11

When the permeation of a substance into the absorptive site capillaries is described according to model 2 (see Fig. 7), we obtain with $1/k_1 = 0$ and $k_2A_2 \to k_bA_b$ ($E_1 \to E_2$) from Eq. 36:

$$\Phi_L = \Phi_B = \frac{C_L - C_{A0}}{1/\alpha a_1 \dot{V}_B E_2 + k_E A_E/(\alpha a_1 \dot{V}_B)^2} \quad (37)$$

The second term of the denominator represents the resistance to transport attributable to countercurrent exchange. When the extravascular shunt vanishes ($k_E \to 0$), model 11 reverts to model 2 (Figs. 7 and 8).

Model 12

Bond et al. (4) extended model 11 by adding a diffusional component in the longitudinal direction of the villi (Fig. 7). This flux is taken up by subvillous blood flow. Assuming a linear longitudinal concentration gradient, the authors (13) approximated the diffusional flux Φ_D (mole min^{-1} g^{-1}) as follows:

$$\Phi_D = k_D A_D (C_{V1} - C_{V0}), \quad (38)$$

where k_D is the permeability coefficient for the diffusion in the villi in the longitudinal direction (cm min^{-1}), and A_D is the corresponding area related to wet tissue weight (cm^2 g^{-1}). Using Eqs. 31, 37, and 38 we obtain finally for the sum of the two fluxes

model 12 changes to model 11. When the countercurrent exchange vanishes ($k_E = 0$), model 2 is obtained (Figs. 7 and 8). Whereas in models 10 and 11 a longitudinal diffusional flux in the villi is excluded, this flux is added in model 12. It should be pointed out that Eq. 37 is used in model 12 for the flux component transported by blood. However, this equation has been derived under the assumption of *no* longitudinal flux. Therefore, Eq. 39 represents only an approximation of radial and longitudinal diffusion in the tissue of the villi.

Predictions of the Models

The influence of villous countercurrent exchange on intestinal absorption shall be discussed by means of model 10 (see also Chapter 7). According to Eq. 36, countercurrent exchange represents an additional resistance reducing the absorption rate. The broken lines in the left panel of Fig. 9 demonstrate the relationship between absorption and blood flow in the absence of countercurrent exchange according to model 3. The permeability of the first barrier ($k_1 A_1$) is varied from 0.01 to 10 ml min^{-1} g^{-1}. Although at $k_1 A_1 = 0.01$ ml min^{-1} g^{-1} an effect of the countercurrent exchange is not detected, the absorption rate is reduced with higher permeability ($k_1 A_1 = 0.1$ or 0.5 ml min^{-1} g^{-1}), as indicated by the deviation from the solid lines. Especially at low blood flow the reduction in the absorption rate is more pronounced. The shape of the curves near the origin changes from concave to convex. A highly permeable substance ($k_1 A_1 = 10$ ml min^{-1} g^{-1})

$$\Phi_L = \Phi_B + \Phi_D = \frac{(C_L - C_{A0})[1 + k_D A_D k_E A_E/(\alpha a_1 \dot{V}_B)^2]}{1/\alpha a_1 \dot{V}_B E_2 + k_E A_E/(\alpha a_1 \dot{V}_B)^2} \quad (39)$$

$k_D A_D$ can be specified more strictly (4) by

$$k_D A_D = n D \, 2 R^2 \pi/l, \quad (40)$$

where R is the radius of the villi (cm).

When the diffusional flux is neglected ($k_D = 0$),

is absorbed less efficiently than a substance with smaller permeability. This is the consequence of the diffusive countercurrent shunting that "traps" the highly permeable substance in the villus.

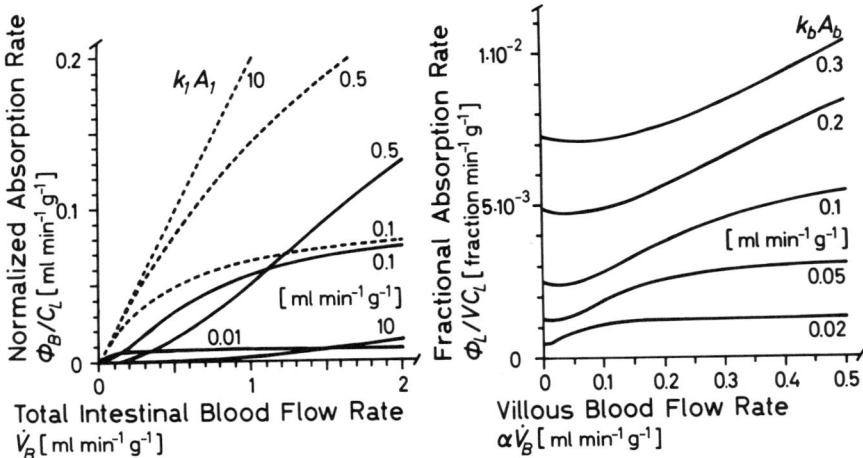

FIG. 9. Predicted effects of countercurrent exchange on intestinal absorption. **Left:** Dependence of intestinal absorption rate on blood flow in the absence *(broken lines)* and presence *(solid lines)* of countercurrent exchange according to model 10. Curves were generated from Eq. 36 with $C_{A0} = 0$, $a_1 = 1$, $\alpha = 0.2$, $E_1 = 1$, $k_E A_E / k_1 A_1 = 0$ and 1, respectively. A countercurrent exchange reduces the absorption rate especially at low blood flow and for highly permeable substances. **Right:** Dependence of intestinal absorption on villous blood flow according to model 12. Curves were calculated from Eq. 39. Φ_L / VC_L was plotted with $C_{A0} = 0$, $a_1 = 1$, $V = 15$ ml, $k_E A_E / k_b A_b = 5.5$, $k_D A_D / k_b A_b = 0.36$. In the presence of a countercurrent exchange, the curves change their shape from concave to convex when the permeability ($k_b A_b$) increases.

The right panel of Fig. 9 shows the relationship between absorption rate and villous blood flow predicted by model 12. The permeability of the first barrier and of the exchange region (radial and longitudinal direction) are varied in parallel. The curves start above the origin because of the longitudinal diffusional flux, and their shape changes from concave to convex when the permeability increases.

A convex curve nas been observed for the relationship between krypton absorption in cat jejunum and villous blood flow, a finding that indicates a significant influence of a countercurrent exchange (3). Dobson (8) compared the predictions of models 2, 3, and 10 to the observed dependence of tritiated water absorption on subepithelial blood flow in the rumen of sheep. The best fit of experimental data was obtained with the countercurrent exchange model 10. Levitt et al. (13) measured the disappearance rates of the gases He, H_2, CH_4, and Xe from the canine jejunum in normal and hypotensive states. There was reasonably good agreement between the experimental data and the predictions from model 12 using morphological and physical data.

CONCLUDING REMARKS

An essential condition for a washout effect of the blood flow on intestinal absorption is that the unidirectional flux from blood to lumen increases and decreases with increasing and decreasing concentration of the permeating substance in the blood; proportionality, however, is not necessary. That means a reduction of the washout capacity by diminishing the blood flow rate increases the concentration on the contraluminal side of the first barrier and, in consequence, augments the blood-to-lumen flux. We can also say that the concentration gradient through the first barrier is flattened, consequently reducing the net flux. If a permeation from blood to lumen were not possible, the absorption rate would be determined only by the lumen-to-blood transport and the washout effect of blood flow would be absent.

It should be mentioned that the models discussed consider only the washout effect of blood flow. An impairment of an active transport component by an insufficient oxygen supply in ischemia would additionally diminish the permeability terms.

The models discussed in this chapter describe the influence of the blood flow rate on intestinal absorption. But the inverse influence exists also, as shown by the increase of intestinal blood flow, when nutrients are absorbed: the postprandial hyperemia. However, this relationship is rather complicated (5,20), so that a mathematical treatment cannot be considered at present.

A comprehensive review on the influence of blood flow on the intestinal absorption of drugs and nutrients has been published previously (29).

REFERENCES

1. Barr, W. H., and Riegelman, S. (1970): Intestinal drug absorption and metabolism. I. Comparison of methods and models to study physiological factors of in vitro and in vivo intestinal absorption. *J. Pharm. Sc.*, 59:154–163.
2. Berggren, S. M., and Goldberg, L. (1940): The absorption of ethyl alcohol from the gastro-intestinal tract as a diffusion process. *Acta Physiol. Scand.*, 1:246–270.
3. Biber, B., Lundgren, O., and Svanvik, J. (1973): The influence of blood flow on the rate of absorption of ^{85}Kr from the small intestine of the cat. *Acta Physiol. Scand.*, 89:227–238.
4. Bond, J. H., Levitt, D. G., and Levitt, M. D. (1977): Quantitation of countercurrent exchange during passive absorption from dog small intestine. Evidence for marked species differences in the efficiency of exchange. *J. Clin. Invest.*, 59:308–318.
5. Chou, C. C., and Kvietys, P. R. (1981): Physiological and pharmacological alterations in gastrointestinal blood flow. In: *Measurement of Blood Flow, Applications to the Splanchnic Circulation*, edited by D. N. Granger and G. B. Bulkley, pp. 475–509. Williams and Wilkins, Baltimore.
6. Coburn, R. F. (1968): Carbon monoxide uptake in the gut. *Ann. NY Acad. Sci.*, 150:13–21.
7. Csáky, T. Z., and Varga, F. (1975): Subepithelial capillary blood flow estimated from blood-to-lumen flux of barbital in ileum of rats. *Am. J. Physiol.*, 229:549–552.
8. Dobson, A. (1979): The choice of models relating tritiated water absorption to subepithelial blood flow in the rumen of sheep. *J. Physiol. (Lond.)*, 297:111–121.
9. Dobson, A., Sellers, A. F., and Thorlacius, S. O. (1971): Limitation of diffusion by blood flow through bovine ruminal epithelium. *Am. J. Physiol.*, 220:1337–1343.
10. Druckrey, H., and Küpfmüller, K. (1949): *Dosis und Wirkung*, pp. 528–533. Editio Cantor, Berlin.
11. Forster, R. E. (1967): Measurement of gastrointestinal blood flow by means of gas absorption. *Gastroenterology*, 52:381–386.
12. Hamilton, J., Dawson, A. M., and Webb, J. P. W. (1967): Limitations in the use of inert gases in the measurement of small gut mucosal blood flow. *Gut*, 8:509–521.
13. Levitt, D. G., Bond, J. H., and Levitt, M. D. (1980): Use of a model of small bowel mucosa to predict passive absorption. *Am. J. Physiol.*, 239:G23–G29.
14. Levitt, M. D., and Levitt, D. G. (1973): Use of inert gases to study the interaction of blood flow and diffusion during passive absorption from the gastrointestinal tract of the rat. *J. Clin. Invest.*, 52:1852–1862.
15. Lundgren, O. (1967): Studies on blood flow distribution and countercurrent exchange in the small intestine. *Acta Physiol. Scand. Suppl.*, 303:1–42.
16. Mailman, D. (1981): Tritiated water clearance as a measure of intestinal absorptive site and total blood flow. In: *Measurement of Blood Flow, Applications to the Splanchnic Circulation*, edited by D. N. Granger and G. B. Bulkley, pp. 339–361. Williams and Wilkins, Baltimore.
17. Ochsenfahrt, H. (1979): The relevance of blood flow for the absorption of drugs in the vascularly perfused, isolated intestine of the rat. *Naunyn Schmiedebergs Arch. Pharmacol.*, 306:105–112.
18. Ochsenfahrt, H., and Winne, D. (1969): Der Einfluss der Durchblutung auf die Resorption von Arzneimitteln aus dem Jejunum der Ratte. *Naunyn Schmiedebergs Arch. Pharmacol.*, 264:55–75.
19. Renkin, E. M. (1977): Brief reviews: Multiple pathways of capillary permeability. *Circ. Res.*, 41:735–743.
20. Shepherd, A. P. (1982): Local control of intestinal oxygenation and blood flow. *Annu. Rev. Physiol.*, 44:13–27.
21. Van Liew, H. D. (1968): Coupling of diffusion and perfusion in gas exit from subcutaneous pocket in rats. *Am. J. Physiol.*, 214:1176–1185.
22. Winne, D. (1966): Der Einfluss einiger Pharmaka auf die Darmdurchblutung und die Resorption tritiummarkierten Wassers aus dem Dünndarm der Ratte. *Naunyn Schmiedebergs Arch. Pharmacol.*, 254:199–224.
23. Winne, D. (1970): Formal kinetics of water and solute absorption with regard to intestinal blood flow. *J. Theor. Biol.*, 27:1–18.
24. Winne, D. (1971): Die Pharmakokinetik der Resorption bei Perfusion einer Darmschlinge mit variabler Durchblutung. *Naunyn Schmiedebergs Arch. Pharmacol.*, 268:417–433.
25. Winne, D. (1972): The influence of blood flow and water net flux on the absorption of tritiated water from the jejunum of the rat. *Naunyn Schmiedebergs Arch. Pharmacol.*, 272:417–436.
26. Winne, D. (1972): The influence of blood flow and water net flux on the blood-to-lumen flux of tritiated water in the jejunum of the rat. *Naunyn Schmiedebergs Arch. Pharmacol.*, 274:357–374.
27. Winne, D. (1975): The influence of villous counter current exchange on intestinal absorption. *J. Theor. Biol.*, 53:145–176.

28. Winne, D. (1978): Blood flow in intestinal absorption models. *J. Pharmacokin. Biopharm.*, 6:55–78.
29. Winne, D. (1979): Influence of blood flow on intestinal absorption of drugs and nutrients. *Pharmacol. Ther.*, 6:333–393.
30. Winne, D. (1981): Unidirectional fluxes and blood flow. *J. Theor. Biol.*, 93:987–996.
31. Winne, D., and Ochsenfahrt, H. (1967): Die formale Kinetik der Resorption unter Berücksichtigung der Darmdurchblutung. *J. Theor. Biol.*, 14:293–315.
32. Winne, D., and Remischovsky, J. (1971): Der Einfluss der Durchblutung auf die Resorption von Harnstoff, Methanol und Äthanol aus dem Jejunum der Ratte. *Naunyn Schmiedebergs Arch. Pharmacol.*, 268:392–416.
33. Winne, D., and Remischovsky, J. (1971): Der Einfluss der Durchblutung auf die Resorption von Polyalkoholen aus dem Jejunum der Ratte. *Naunyn Schmiedebergs Arch. Pharmacol.*, 270:22–40.

The Small Bowel in Arterial Hypotension and Shock

*Ulf Haglund, **Mats Jodal, and **Ove Lundgren

*Department of Surgery, University of Lund, Malmö General Hospital, S-214 01 Malmö, Sweden; and
**Department of Physiology, University of Göteborg, S-400 33 Göteborg, Sweden

This chapter reviews the hemodynamic changes in the small intestine during ischemia and shock. The most striking event in the intestine is the development of mucosal ulcerations 1 or 2 hr after the onset of severe hypotension. These lesions indicate an extreme vulnerability of the mucosa to hypoxia. Therefore, we discuss the pathophysiology of the mucosal lesions as well as their functional implications.

For obvious reasons, most of our knowledge concerning the intestinal circulation in shock and ischemia is based on animal experiments. Unfortunately, there are, at least quantitatively, important species-differences in the small intestinal reactions to hypotension (29,44,81). The dog is the animal in which intestinal ischemia has been most extensively studied. In our opinion, the dog has certain marked disadvantages as a model of ischemic pathophysiology in the small intestinal circulation. The canine small intestine reacts to hypotension in several important ways that differ from the responses of cat, monkey, and most likely man. The cat is probably a more useful experimental animal for studies of the intestinal circulation because the vascular reactions of the cat and human small intestine are very similar physiologically (42,43). This review, therefore, is based mainly on experimental data obtained in cats. However, functionally important species-differences are pointed out and discussed.

INTESTINAL HEMODYNAMICS IN ISCHEMIA AND SHOCK

As pointed out by Folkow (21), the small intestinal vascular bed consists of several circuits coupled in parallel. Each of these circuits can be divided into different sections that are coupled in series, that is, the different layers of the small intestinal wall (the villi, the crypts, the submucosa, and the muscularis layers) constitute separate vascular circuits composed of functionally specialized series-coupled sections. These sections include the *resistance vessels*, which regulate local blood flow, the *precapillary sphincters*, which determine the number of capillaries open for flow at a given time, and the *exchange vessels* or the true capillaries, in which the exchange between tissue and blood takes place. The *postcapillary resistance vessels* contribute relatively little to the total resistance to blood flow. The resistance in this section is, nevertheless, very important because it affects the pre- to postcapillary resistance ratio and, hence, the mean capillary hydrostatic pressure. The reactions of the *capacitance vessels* determine the local blood volume.

The Series-coupled Vascular Sections

Resistance Vessels

Following hemorrhage, intestinal vascular resistance increases, although not nearly as much as in skeletal muscle. For example, bleeding an anesthetized cat to reduce its estimated blood volume 35% increases intestinal resistance 20% to 30% as arterial pressure falls from 140 to 70 mm Hg (30). The comparatively small vascular response in the intestine is due to several mechanisms. First, the smooth muscle of the small intestinal resistance vessels can greatly adjust its tone depending on the intravascular pressure and thus maintain blood flow despite reductions in perfusion pressure. This autoregulation is most pronounced in denervated segments (34,48–50,62). Second, the sympathetic vasoconstriction in the intestine evoked by stimulating the splanchnic nerves increases resistance 100% at most, even at maximal firing rate and normal perfusion pressure (22). This vasoconstriction is trivial compared to the five- to tenfold increase in skeletal muscle (67). Third, the difference between the vascular reactions in skeletal muscle and intestine may also be due to disparate rates of firing in the regional sympathetic vasoconstrictor fibers during hypotension. However, experimental observations do not substantiate this view (52). During the course of hemorrhagic hypotension, intestinal vascular resistance decreases steadily, reaching control values within 2 hr, a reaction that is partly explained by fading of the sympathetic vasoconstrictor response (36). This phenomenon is usually explained as an accumulation of "local metabolites," but it could also possibly reflect a depletion of neurotransmitter in the vasoconstrictor fibers. After retransfusion, blood flow usually increases to a value above the "resting" level (36).

A sympathetic influence on the resistance vessels during hemorrhage was clearly established in the cat experiments summarized above, since the vasoconstriction could not be demonstrated in animals in which the splanchnic nerves had been cut (30,36). This sympathetic influence can, in principle, be exerted via a direct nervous action on the vascular smooth muscles or via a release of circulating vasoconstrictor agents (adrenaline, noradrenaline, angiotensin via a release of renin). We have earlier proposed that the vasoconstrictor fibers are the main controllers of the resistance vessels (29,30,35). However, recent observations (S. Redfors and H. Sjövall, *in preparation*) suggest that the sympathetic control of the intestinal resistance vessels during a pronounced hemorrhagic hypotension is mainly exerted via circulating vasoconstrictor agents. Here it should also be pointed out that there are researchers who believe that the intestinal innervation and adrenal medullary secretions play no significant part in the control of the resistance vessels during hemorrhage (66). (See Chapter 5.)

Precapillary Sphincters

The number of perfused intestinal capillaries seems to increase or remain within the preshock control range when the small intestine is subjected to local ischemia or to generalized hemorrhagic or septic shock. The alterations in capillary density have been recorded by changes in capillary filtration coefficient, K_f (17,30,34–36). The increased K_f, however, may be explained in part by an augmented capillary hydraulic conductivity (27; see below). These observations indicate that the number of patent intestinal capillaries is not reduced in arterial hypotension.

Exchange Vessels

Activation of the sympathetic nerves to a skeletal muscle vascular bed induces a rapid reduction of the local blood volume followed by a slow, continuous reduction of tissue volume (67). This second slow reduction is due to an increase in the pre- to postcapillary resistance ratio. The resulting fall in mean hydrostatic capillary pressure, in turn, leads to absorption of fluid from the interstitium into the blood (67). Thus, activation of the sympathetic nerves in skeletal muscle leads to an "autotransfusion," at least during the 1st hr of hypotension (55, 60,68). This autotransfusion amounts to about 0.5 liters in an adult human. Later during the course of the shock, the absorption of fluid into the vascular compartment is reduced and is eventually changed to an outward filtration during a decompensated phase of shock (55,60, 68). A similar chain of events in the intestinal vascular bed would induce large changes in total blood volume (57) because the intestine has a much larger capillary surface area (24). Furthermore, the capillary hydraulic conductivity expressed per unit capillary surface area also seems to be higher in the intestine than in skeletal muscle (3). However, activation of the sympathetic nerves does not change the pre- to postcapillary resistance ratio in the small intestine at normal arterial pressure or during arterial hypotension (23,35,36). Thus, mean hydrostatic capillary pressure remains largely unchanged to judge from recordings of tissue volume. There seems to be no significant net fluid filtration across the capillary wall of the small intestine in local or hemorrhagic hypotension regardless of whether the local sympathetic nerves are activated or not (30,34–36). This also holds true in septic shock (17). However, the sympathetic nervous system increases net fluid transport from the intestinal lumen (80), thereby compensating for the fluid loss in hemorrhage (73).

The above description is based mainly on experiments performed on the feline small bowel. Again, the response seems to be different in the dog. Observations in the dog suggest that mean capillary hydrostatic pressure increases in shock (57). Furthermore, in the rat, direct pressure measurements in the different parts of the intestinal vascular tree have been made by Bohlen et al. (5). Measurements in the muscle layer at various arterial pressures demonstrate that capillary pressure is linearly correlated with arterial pressure. These findings may be reconciled with the observations described above, if one assumes that "autoregulation of mean capillary pressure" occurs mainly in the extensive capillary network in the mucosa.

Järhult (45) demonstrated that hemorrhage led to an increase in the blood glucose concentration, which, in turn, "mobilized" fluid from the extravascular space by an osmotic effect. However, this mechanism is also mainly confined to the skeletal muscle vascular bed and is negligible in the intestine.

After the hypotensive period, a slow, continuous increase in total intestinal volume is found (30,35,36,45). To a large extent, this volume increase is probably explained by an increased fluid volume in the lumen associated with a villous damage (29,36). However, assuming it to be entirely due to an increase of mean capillary pressure, an augmentation of capillary pressure of 1 to 4 mm Hg would suffice to explain the increased volume. Furthermore, recent data obtained by measuring intestinal lymph flow and the ratio of lymph to plasma protein concentrations indicate that intestinal capillary permeability is increased after 1 hr of hypotension (26,27). This would provide an additional possible explanation of the increased intestinal tissue volume, since the effective colloid osmotic pressure is decreased as a result of the decreased osmotic reflection coefficient for plasma proteins. This increased capillary leakiness probably occurs in the venous end of the capillary and is induced by superoxide free radicals (see below).

Capacitance Vessels

Reducing arterial pressure per se causes only small changes in the regional blood volume of the denervated small intestine (34). Stimulation of the splanchnic nerves induces a rapid 30% to 40% reduction in the intestinal blood volume (22). During the course of local or hemorrhagic hypotension, this response gradually diminishes (35,36), and after about 2 hr of hypotension the sympathetic capacitance response is only about 30% of that seen in resting, normotensive states. In the innervated small intestine, severe bleeding, that is, a 35% reduction of the total blood volume, causes an initial rapid fall (40–50%) in the regional blood volume (30). The changes in regional blood volume in the initial phase of acute bacteriemia are less pronounced (17). Late in shock, when the capacitance response to sympathetic stimulation is reduced (36), the intestinal blood volume gradually increases (30), probably because of the fading sympathetic effect on capacitance vessels.

In the dog, "pooling" of blood in the intestinal capacitance vessels occurs late in hemorrhagic or septic shock (57,83,84). To some extent this might be due to an increase in portal venous pressure, which seems to be specific for this species (17,40,53). After a portal-caval shunt operation, which neutralizes the effects of constriction of the sphincter muscles in the canine hepatic veins, significant intestinal congestion seems to be absent (25).

Extensive investigations in the cat intestine do not in any way suggest that fluid and blood stagnation occur in hemorrhage in sufficient magnitude to explain the "irreversibility of shock" (29,30,34–36). Moreover, such stagnation does not occur in man or in any other experimental animals (44,81), except possibly the dog.

Parallel-coupled Vascular Sections

The distribution of blood flow among the different vascular circuits of the intestinal wall has not been studied as extensively as, for example, the reactions of the resistance vessels. The distribution of injected radioactivity labeled microspheres has been used to fractionate the intramural blood flow distribution (2,6), but dynamic changes in the vascular beds are difficult to assess with microspheres, since one can only measure flows at predetermined times and only two to five times during an experiment. Furthermore, this method has lately been criticized on technical grounds (78).

We recently analyzed the intramural blood flows during hypotension with two different methods. One is based on the indicator dilution principle and involves the intraarterial injection of a radioactively labeled plasma tracer (^{198}Au-labeled colloids). The tracer's transit through the villi is recorded by a semiconductor detector in the intestinal lumen. Plasma flow, plasma volume, and plasma mean transit time in the villi can be determined as described in detail by Biber et al. (3). In the other technique, absorbtive site ("villous") blood flow is measured by estimating the uptake of carbon monoxide (CO) from the intestinal lumen as described by Micflikier et al. (65). Blood flow in the muscularis externa is determined from the elimination of ^{85}Kr detected by a Geiger-Müller tube at the antimesenteric border (51). Total blood flow is recorded simultaneously with a venous drop counter.

The plasma tracer method and the CO clearance technique have given similar results when studying the blood flow distribution at "rest" and during sympathetic vasoconstriction. During nervous vasoconstriction villous plasma and red blood cell flows are unaltered even at maximal physiological rates of nerve activation (80,82). The most striking observation made during hypotension is that even when total intestinal blood flow is reduced, villous plasma and red blood cell flows are barely depressed. Thus, when perfusion pressure to the small intestine is lowered to 40 mm Hg by partially occluding the superior mesenteric artery, villous plasma flow is maintained at the control level (61). Furthermore, lowering mesenteric arterial pressure to 25 to 30 mm Hg while stimulating the regional sympathetic fibers at 6 Hz decreased "absorptive site" blood flow, but red blood cell flow in the superficial parts of the mucosa was reduced only to about 80% of the control value (73; see Table 1) because plasma skimming in the intestine is abolished at low blood flows (46). In the same study, there was no difference with regard to "absorptive" red blood cell flow between animals that developed mucosal ulcerations ("damaged" group; see be-

TABLE 1. *Red blood cell flow estimated from rate of CO absorption before, during, and after a 2-hr period of simulated intestinal shock[a]*

	Control	Intestinal hypotension		Posthypotensive control
		1 hr	2 hr	
Undamaged mucosa $n = 6$	1.7 ± 0.3	1.3 ± 0.2	1.5 ± 0.3	2.6 ± 0.4
Mucosal damage $n = 9$	1.8 ± 0.3	1.5 ± 0.4	1.5 ± 0.3	2.3 ± 0.5

[a] Arterial pressure = ~30 mm Hg; electrical stimulation of regional vasoconstriction fibers at 6 Hz. Flow is expressed in ml × min^{-1} × 100 g^{-1} intestine.
Mean ± SE.
From Redfors et al. (73), with permission.

low) and those that did not ("undamaged" group in Table 1). These observations suggest that factors other than flow per se are important for the development of the mucosal ulcerations seen in the intestines in arterial hypotension (see below). The measurement of muscle layer blood flow demonstrated that arterial hypotension is accompanied by a decrease in muscle blood flow (13).

The above description of villous hemodynamics represents, in some respects, an oversimplification, since both methods simultaneously record blood flow to a large number of villi. However, in the "resting" feline intestine, blood flow in the villi is not homogeneous; some villi are well perfused and others are hypoperfused (3). Lowering perfusion pressure relaxes the "precapillary" sphincters and most of the villi are then perfused. The latter hemodynamic adjustment is reflected as an increase of both villous plasma volume and villous transit time (61). This can be easily demonstrated by injecting Evans blue intraarterially and observing a homogeneous coloring of the intestinal mucosa *(unpublished observation)*. Hence, blood flow in a single villus oscillates at rest, but is constant with a low linear velocity during hypotension. Over a longer period of time, *mean* villous blood flow is similar in the two situations. This description of villous hemodynamics is based on studies in the feline intestine in which the precapillary sphincters are located upstream from the villus. It may not entirely be applicable to those species with precapillary sphincters in the villi, for instance, the rat (5). However, our knowledge of rat villous hemodynamics in hypotension is less detailed than for the cat.

The details of the villous circulation are of particular interest because of the countercurrent exchanger in the villus. This mechanism is discussed in detail in Chapter 7; here only major points are discussed. The countercurrent exchanger depends on the anatomical arrangement of the villous vasculature with a central unbranched supply vessel surrounded by an extensive subepithelial capillary network (Fig. 1). When more villi are being perfused at low arterial pressure, the exchange area is increased.

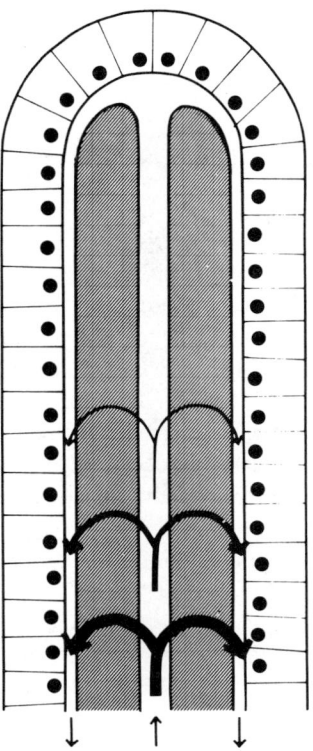

FIG. 1. Schematic illustration of the villous vascular anatomy and the shortcircuiting of oxygen in the villous countercurrent exchanger. For details, see text.

Furthermore, the time spent in the central vessel is greatly prolonged; the transit time for plasma in the whole villus increases from 5 to 15 to 20 sec. Hence, area and time for exchange are both increased (47).

The most important result of the increased effectiveness of the villous exchanger during arterial hypotension is that more oxygen is exchanged in the way illustrated in Fig. 1. The driving force of this extravascular "shunting" of oxygen is the Po_2 difference between the central vessel and the capillary network. The Po_2 difference is created by arterial inflow and by the epithelial consumption of oxygen, taking place along the full length of the villus. The low oxygen tension at the villus tip is present at normal resting perfusion pressure (4; see Chapter 7) and is lower still during hypotension. An increased countercurrent exchange of oxygen may, therefore, explain the mucosal ulcerations that develop at the villus tips even though villous blood flow appears normal.

INTESTINAL MUCOSAL DAMAGE

In all species, including man, intestinal ischemia induces characteristic damage to the small intestinal mucosa within a rather short period of time. The lesions are localized to the villi but may also be detected macroscopically as mucosal bleeding. This is often the case in the dog, in which bloody diarrhea is a common sequel to shock. Intestinal ischemia also affects epithelial transport processes (for review, see 63,75), but here only the intestinal lesions are discussed.

The development of intestinal lesions in hypotension has been described in detail by Chiu and co-workers (14), who devised a six-level grading system. The first sign of ischemic mucosal damage (grade 1) is the development of a subepithelial space at the very tip of the villus, the so-called Grühagen's space (14; see Fig. 2). An extension of the subepithelial space with moderate lifting of the epithelial layer from the lamina propria then becomes apparent (grade 2). As ischemia is prolonged, massive epithelial lifting occurs along the sides of the villi (grade 3), and a large number of the villi becomes denuded (grade 4). Full scale ischemic mucosal damage is characterized by loss of the entire villous layer (grade 5). It is typical that even in pronounced phases of mucosal damage, the deeper layers of the intestinal wall are histologically normal.

There is general agreement that these lesions are common in all forms of experimental shock (9,39,63). Most investigators believe that similar mucosal damage also occurs in man (9,33, 63), but both their incidence and their functional importance are unknown. However, in experimental animals, the mucosal damage causes decreased intestinal net fluid and electrolyte absorption (73). The pathogenesis of these lesions is controversial. Three major pathophysiological factors have been implicated: tissue hypoxia, superoxide radicals, and pancreatic proteases.

Tissue Hypoxia

Hypoxia at the tips of the villi is generally agreed to be important for the development of the mucosal damage in hypotensive states. This conclusion is supported by the observation that intraluminal administration of oxygen prevents the mucosal lesions in standardized shock models (1,31,74,79), whereas luminal perfusion itself does not prevent the damage (31). The cause of tissue hypoxia is a matter of discussion. Originally, a constriction of the mesenteric vascular bed was thought to be the mechanism underlying the small intestinal mucosal lesions in shock (57,72). A correlation between the degree of mucosal damage and total intestinal blood flow has been demonstrated (14,31). However, if villous blood flow is maintained, a direct flow-induced hypoxia appears less likely. Local denervation of the small intestine of dogs and rabbits seems to prevent mucosal lesions in hemorrhagic shock (54,70), but we have not been able to demonstrate any role of sympathetic vasoconstriction in mucosal ulceration (38). Extravascular short-circuiting of oxygen in the villous countercurrent exchanger offers another explanation to the hypoxia present in the tips as discussed in detail above (see also Chapter 7).

Portal hypertension is another factor suggested as a possible cause of mucosal damage (15). However, mucosal damage is found in experimental situations in which portal hypertension can certainly be excluded (19,31,40,57).

Superoxide Radicals

Growing evidence indicates that intestinal mucosal lesions can be aggravated not only during a hypotensive period but also in the immediate posthypotensive period. In regional intestinal ischemia, significant hyperemia is evident during the first minutes following restored pressure (34,35). In this situation, provided the local hypotension has not been severe enough to create fully developed microscopic damage (28), the villous damage is aggravated during the hyperemic period (Fig. 3; 76,77). This worsening of the intestinal damage can be prevented by pretreatment with superoxide dis-

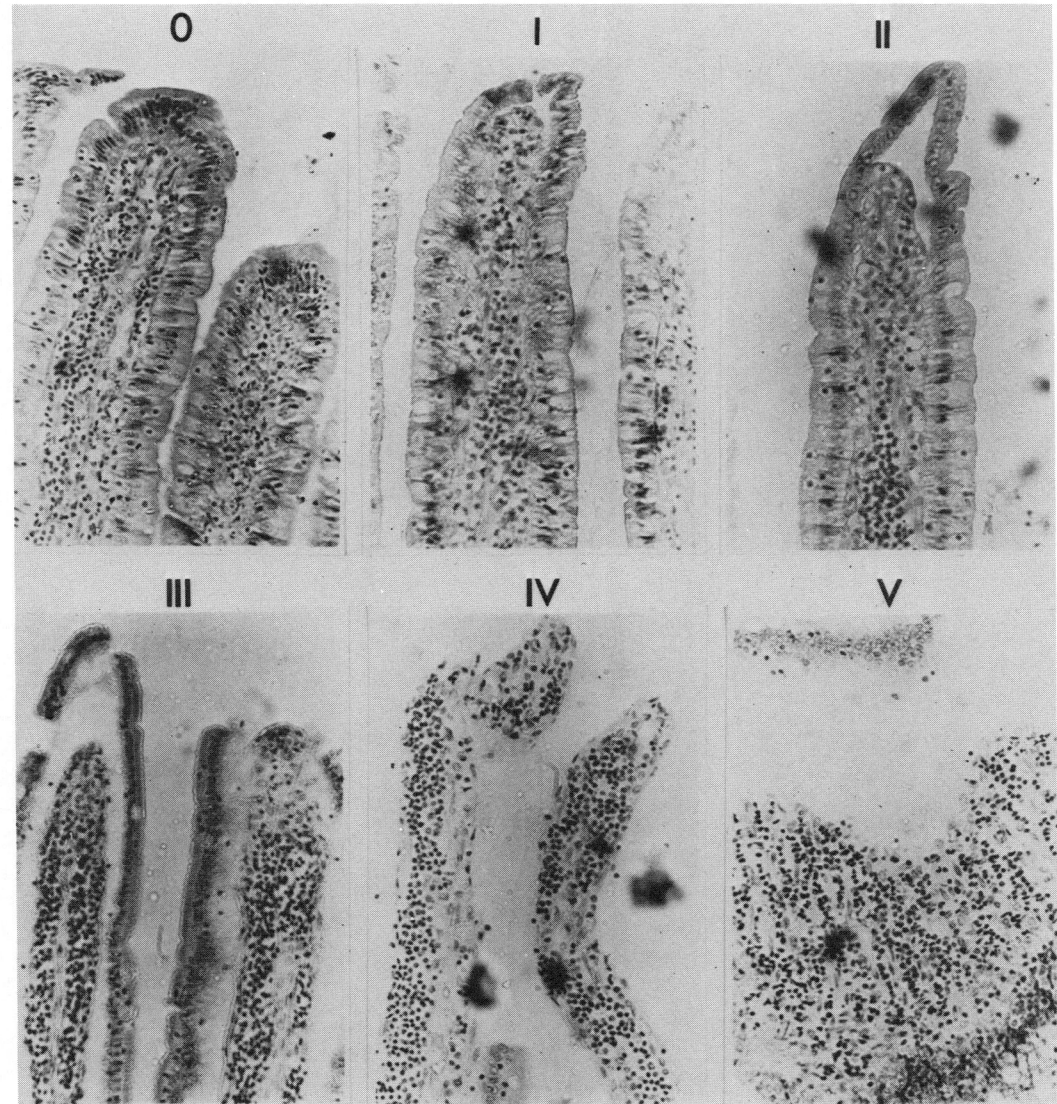

FIG. 2. Representative photomicrographs of the small intestinal mucosa illustrating the grading system used for the mucosal damage in hypotensive states. (From Falk et al., ref. 19, with permission.)

mutase (SOD), a superoxide radical scavenging enzyme (Fig. 4). Parks et al. (71) reported that the histological damage seen 1 hr after a 3-hr period of intestinal hypotension was ameliorated by SOD treatment. The oxygen free radicals, superoxide anion, hydroxyl radical, singlet oxygen, and hydrogen peroxide, are capable of causing extensive tissue and endothelial damage (64). Cytotoxic effects of superoxide radicals presumably result from peroxidation of lipid components of cellular and mitochondrial membranes. Superoxide radicals are also produced normally, but the defense mechanisms dismutate them immediately. This dismutation can proceed spontaneously, or it can be catalyzed by SOD, which may explain the findings described above. The enzyme xanthine oxidase may be a key enzyme in the production of superoxide radicals in the ischemic small intestine (see Fig. 4; 71). The substrate for this

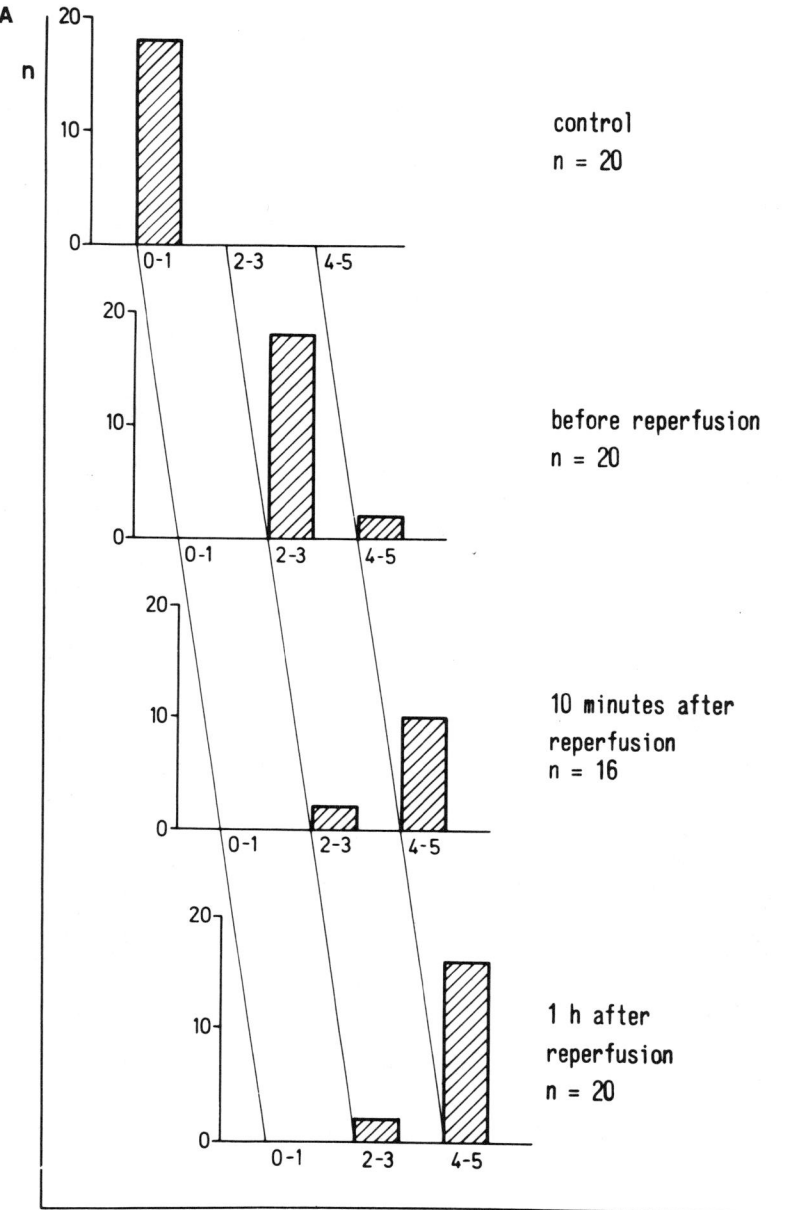

FIG. 3A. The degree of small intestinal mucosal damage found before, during, and after regional hypotension (30 mm Hg) with stimulation of the regional sympathetic nerves at 6 Hz for 2 hr in cats.

enzyme, hypoxanthine, accumulates as a result of ATP catabolism in ischemic tissues (16), including the ischemic small intestine (76,85). In favor of this hypothesis is the finding that the mucosal damage after local intestinal hypotension is ameliorated by allopurinol, a competitive xanthine oxidase inhibitor (71).

The reports summarized above favor the view that oxygen free radicals are involved in the pathogenesis of the intestinal mucosal lesions.

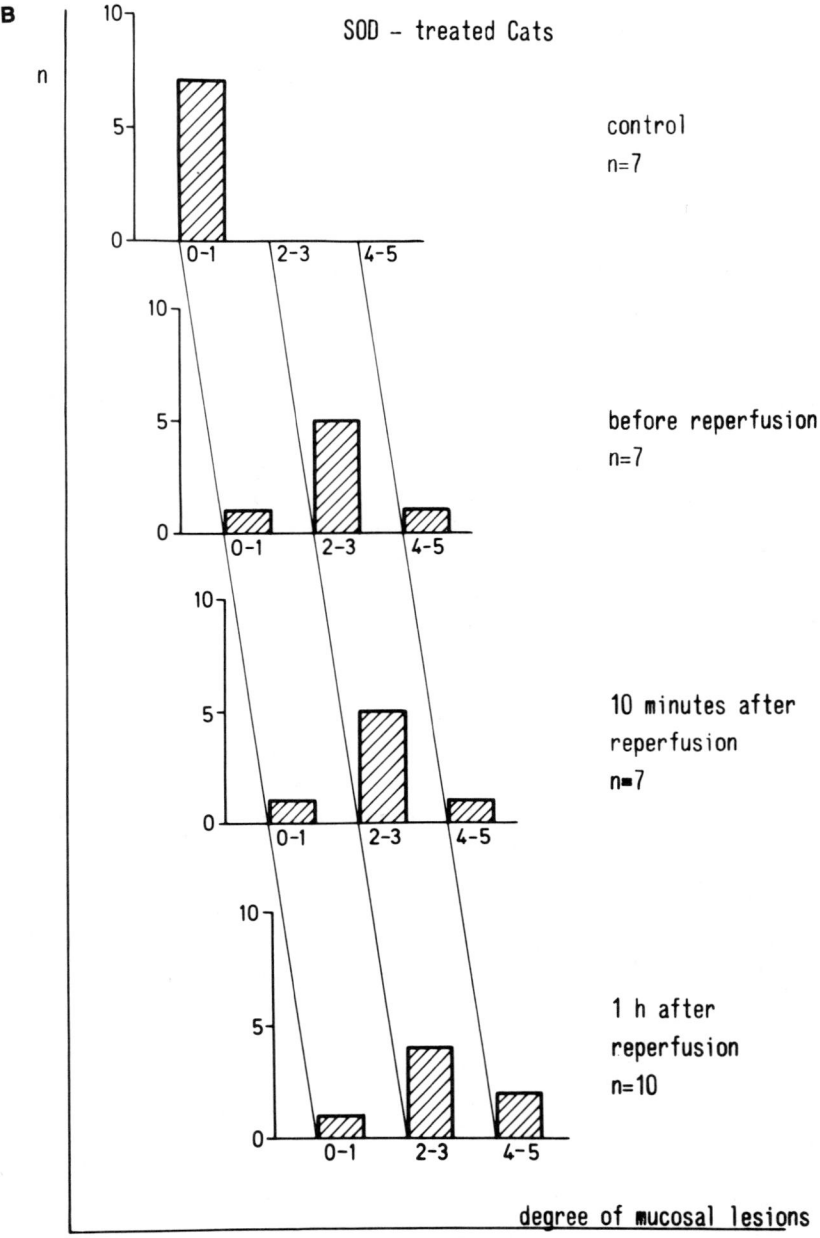

FIG. 3B. Data were obtained from cats that were given yeast superoxide dismutase (SOD) i.v. (15,000 U/kg body weight) after 60 min hypotension. (From M. H. Schoenberg and U. Haglund, *unpublished*, with permisson.)

This may be particularly true in regional ischemia of short duration and possibly following embolectomy of the superior mesenteric artery. If, however, the local hypotension is severe enough, the entire villous layer might already be destroyed before the reperfusion period (see 28). Mucosal damage is also reported following septic shock without reperfusion (19) and dur-

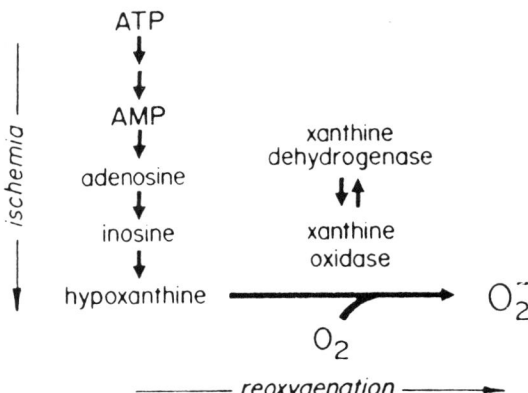

FIG. 4. Proposed mechanism for superoxide production in the ischemic bowel. (From Granger et al., ref. 26, with permission.)

ing the period of intestinal hypotension (Fig. 3; see 73). These observations indicate that the generation of superoxide free radicals is not necessary for the development of mucosal damage in ischemia and shock.

Pancreatic Proteases

Bounous and co-workers have proposed that the presence of intraluminal pancreatic proteases is important for the development of mucosal lesions in ischemia and shock (7–9). The ischemic small intestine ceases to produce mucus. Thus, the epithelial lining becomes vulnerable to the intraluminal enzymes, particularly trypsin and chymotrypsin. Intraluminal application of a proteases inhibitor, aprotinin (Trasylol), has been reported to prevent mucosal damage (7,11,69) or to minimize it (31). Intraluminal injections of trypsin, on the other hand, aggravate the mucosal lesions (11). The damaging action is attributed to enzymes already present along the intestinal wall before shock, since acute pancreatectomy has no effect on the mucosal lesions (9,10). However, pancreatectomy or pancreatic duct ligation 1 week before hemorrhagic shock prevents the mucosal lesions (9,10).

From the discussion above, it can be concluded that several mechanisms exist through which microscopic mucosal damage can be induced in hypotensive states. Hypoxia, the destructive actions of intraluminal proteases, and the posthypotensive generation of oxygen free radicals are all important factors in the pathogenesis. The relative importance of each single factor probably varies from one hypotensive shock situation to another, but it seems likely that hypoxia is the single most important factor in the pathophysiology of the small intestinal mucosal lesions.

GENERAL CARDIOVASCULAR EFFECTS OF INTESTINAL ISCHEMIA

The reactions of the small intestine during ischemia and shock have been of particular interest throughout the years because these reactions may be important for survival in shock (84). Lillehei (56) demonstrated that crossperfusing the small intestine of a dog during a period of hemorrhagic hypotension with blood from a healthy donor dog prevented the development of the bleeding lesions of the mucosa and reduced mortality from 80% to 10%. The "intestinal factor of irreversible hemorrhagic shock" was considered by Lillehei to be stagnation and pooling of blood and fluid in the small intestinal vascular bed and in the intestinal tissues (57). An intestinal loss of fluid of significant magnitude to cause hypovolemia may be important in the dog, but it is unlikely in most other species, including man (see 29,39).

Another suggested explanation for the "intestinal factor in irreversible shock" is that the damage to the mucosal epithelium eliminates the barrier that prevents bacteria and endotoxins from invading the intestinal vessels and the organism (20). According to this hypothesis, intestinal ischemia and shock would ultimately be converted to endotoxin shock, which, if not properly counteracted, could become irreversible. It was later demonstrated, however, that germ-free animals are as susceptible as normal ones to a standardized hemorrhagic insult (12). Consequently, the endotoxin theory is no longer considered a valid general mechanism in shock and intestinal ischemia.

More recently it has been demonstrated that the arterial pressure fall and circulatory de-

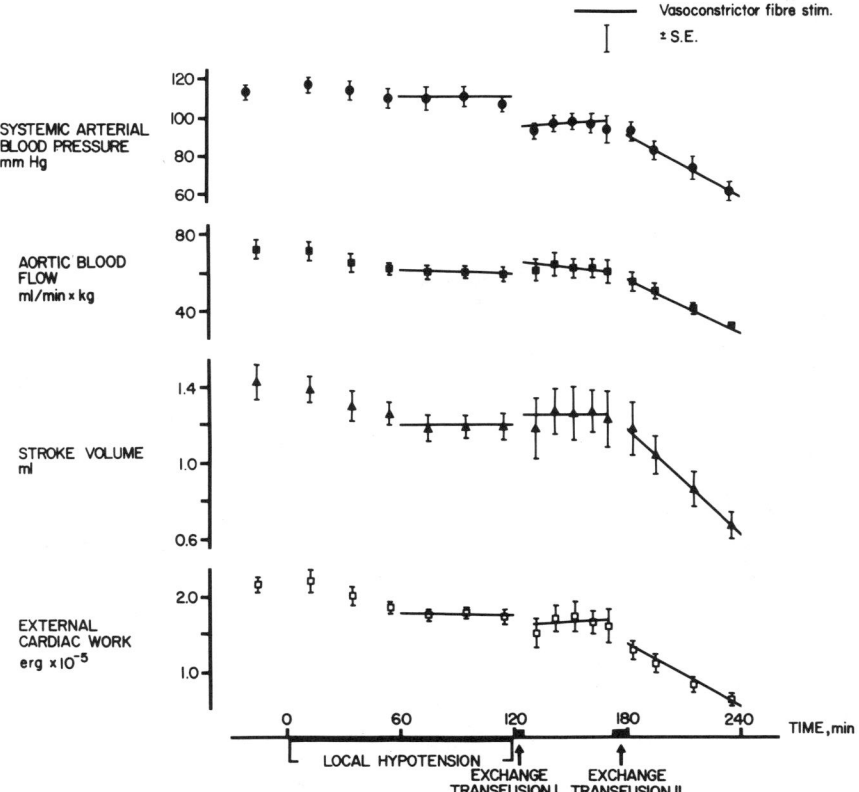

FIG. 5. Cardiac performance in cats subjected to regional intestinal hypotension for 120 min. During the first 5 min following restoration of regional arterial blood pressure, the intestinal venous outflow was collected and replaced. It was returned 45 min later in a second exchange transfusion. (From Haglund and Lundgren, ref. 37, with permission.)

terioration that regularly follow a period of regional intestinal ischemia can be prevented if the mucosal damage is avoided by perfusing the intestinal lumen with oxygenated saline (32). A good correlation is found between the degree of mucosal damage and the drop in arterial pressure 1 hr after regional intestinal ischemia (32). Furthermore, if the intestinal venous blood is collected during the first 5 min following a 2-hr period of regional intestinal ischemia and replaced with blood from a healthy donor cat, the general circulatory consequences of intestinal ischemia are also prevented (37), as illustrated in Fig. 5. Upon returning the collected intestinal venous blood (exchange transfusion II in Fig. 5), a general cardiovascular derangement develops.

The studies summarized above strongly suggest that the ischemic intestine releases into blood material "toxic" to the circulatory system, probably from the ulcerated villi. *In vitro* experiments show that the intestinal venous blood collected immediately after a period of regional hypotension contains substances that exert a negative inotropic effect on the heart (28,58,59). Following local intestinal hypotension as well as septic shock, cardiotoxic activity in the intestinal venous blood has also been detected in the *in situ* cat heart bioassay (18,41).

Figure 6 summarizes the mechanism we proposed to explain the role of the small intestine in so-called irreversible shock. Mucosal ulcerations develop during arterial hypotension secondary to, among other things, increased oxygen "shunting" in the countercurrent exchanger. This,

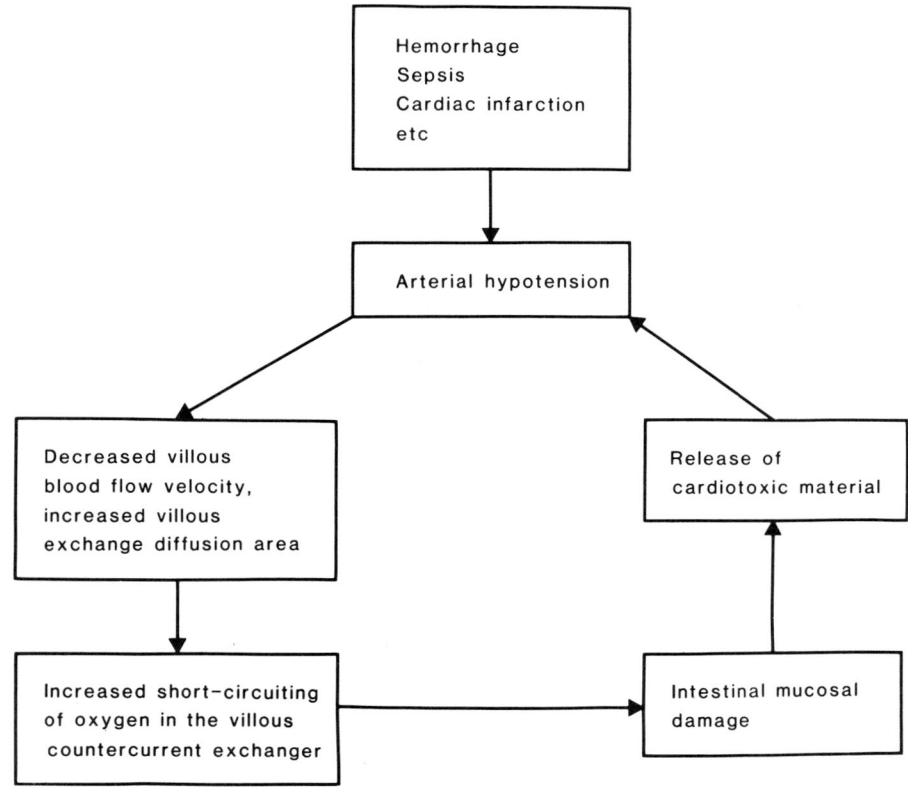

FIG. 6. Proposed chain of events explaining the role of the small intestine in the development of so-called irreversible shock.

in turn, leads to the release of cardiotoxic material, which further aggravates the arterial hypotension and the mucosal ulcerations. The cardiotoxic material released from the ischemic intestine has been tentatively characterized (58); it has a molecular weight of 500 to 1,000 daltons and is water-soluble. Further biochemical characterization has revealed that it is not a single myocardic depressant but several such substances *(unpublished observations)* as originally suggested by Haglund and Lundgren (37).

REFERENCES

1. Åhrén, C., and Haglund, U. (1973): Mucosal lesions in the small intestine of the cat during low flow. *Acta Physiol. Scand.*, 88:541–550.
2. Arvidsson, S., Lindblad, B., Esquivel, C., Fält, K., Lindström, C., Bergqvist, D., and Haglund, U. (1983): The effects of dihydroergotamine on the feline cardiovascular response to i.v. infusion of live E. coli bacteria. *Eur. Surg. Res. (in press)*.
3. Biber, B., Lundgren, O., Stage, L., and Svanvik, J. (1973): An indicator-dilution method for studying intestinal hemodynamics in the cat. *Acta Physiol. Scand.*, 87:433–447.
4. Bohlen, H. G. (1980): Intestinal tissue PO_2 and microvascular responses during glucose exposure. *Am. J. Physiol.*, 238:H164–H171.
5. Bohlen, H. G., Hutchins, P. M., Rapela, C. E., and Green, H. D. (1975): Microvascular control in intestinal mucosa of normal and hemorrhaged rats. *Am. J. Physiol.*, 229:1159–1164.
6. Bond, J. H., Levitt, D. G., and Levitt, M. D. (1977): Quantitation of countercurrent exchange during passive absorption from the dog small intestine. Evidence for marked species differences in the efficiency of exchange. *J. Clin. Invest.*, 59:308–318.
7. Bounous, G. (1967): Role of the intestinal contents in the pathophysiology of acute intestinal ischemia. *Am. J. Surg.*, 114:368–375.
8. Bounous, G. (1969): "Tryptic enteritis": Its role in the pathogenesis of stress ulcer and shock. *Can. J. Surg.*, 12:397–409.
9. Bounous, G. (1982): Acute necrosis of the intestinal mucosa. *Gastroenterology*, 82:1457–1467.

10. Bounous, G., Brown, R. A., Mulder, D. S., Hampson, L. G., and Gurd, F. N. (1965): Abolition of "tryptic enteritis" in the shocked dog. *Arch. Surg.*, 91:371–375.
11. Bounous, G., Hampson, L. G., and Gurd, F. N. (1964): Cellular nucleotides in hemorrhagic shock: Relationship of intestinal metabolic changes to hemorrhagic enteritis and the barrier function of intestinal mucosa. *Ann. Surg.*, 160:650–668.
12. Carter, D., and Einheber, A. (1966): Intestinal ischemic shock in germ-free animals. *Surgery*, 122:66–76.
13. Cassuto, J., Cedgård, S., Haglund, U., Redfors, S., and Lundgren, O. (1979): Intramural blood flows and flow distribution in the feline small bowel during arterial hypotension. *Acta Physiol. Scand.*, 106:335–342.
14. Chiu, C. J., McArdle, A. H., Brown, R., Scott, H. J., and Gurd, F. N. (1970): Intestinal mucosal lesion in low-flow states. *Arch. Surg.*, 101:478–483.
15. Crowell, J. W., and Nelson, K. M., Jr. (1975): Mechanism of bloody diarrhea in shock. *Circ. Shock*, 2:21–28.
16. DeWall, R. A., Vasko, K. A., Stanley, E. L., and Kezdi, P. (1971): Responses of the ischemic myocardium to allopurinol. *Am. Heart J.*, 82:362–370.
17. Falk, A., Kaijser, B., Myrvold, H., and Haglund, U. (1980): Intestinal vascular and central hemodynamic responses following i.v. infusion of live E. coli bacteria. *Circ. Shock*, 7:239–250.
18. Falk, A., Myrvold, H. E., and Haglund, U. (1982): Cardiopulmonary function as related to intestinal mucosal lesions in experimental septic shock. *Circ. Shock*, 9:419–432.
19. Falk, A., Myrvold, H. E., Lundgren, O., and Haglund, U. (1982): Mucosal lesions in the feline small intestine in septic shock. *Circ. Shock*, 9:27–35.
20. Fine, J. (1967): The intestinal circulation in shock. *Gastroenterology*, 52:454–458.
21. Folkow, B. (1967): Regional adjustments of intestinal blood flow. *Gastroenterology*, 52:423–432.
22. Folkow, B., Lewis, D. H., Lundgren, O., Mellander, S., and Wallentin, I. (1964): The effect of graded vasoconstrictor fibre stimulation on the intestinal resistance and capacitance vessels. *Acta Physiol. Scand.*, 61:445–457.
23. Folkow, B., Lewis, D. H., Lundgren, O., Mellander, S., and Wallentin, I. (1964): The effect of sympathetic vasoconstrictor fibres on the distribution of capillary blood flow in the intestine. *Acta Physiol. Scand.*, 61:458–466.
24. Folkow, B., Lundgren, O., and Wallentin, I. (1963): Studies on the relationship between flow resistance, capillary filtration coefficient and regional blood volume in the intestine of the cat. *Acta Physiol. Scand.*, 57:270–283.
25. Frank, H. A., Glotzer, P., Jacob, S. W., and Fine, J. (1951): Traumatic shock. XIX. Hemorrhagic shock in eck-fistula dogs. *Am. J. Physiol.*, 167:508–513.
26. Granger, D. N., Rutili, G., and McCord, J. (1981): Superoxide radicals in feline intestinal ischemia. *Gastroenterology*, 81:22–29.
27. Granger, D. N., Sennett, M., McElearney, P., and Taylor, A. E. (1980): Effect of local arterial hypotension on cat intestinal capillary permeability. *Gastroenterology*, 79:474–480.
28. Haglind, E., Haglund, U., Lundgren, O., and Scherstén, T. (1981): Graded intestinal vascular obstruction. IV. Analysis of the pathophysiology in the development of refractory shock. *Circ. Shock*, 8:635–646.
29. Haglund, U. (1973): The small intestine in hypotension and hemorrhage. An experimental cardiovascular study in the cat. *Acta Physiol. Scand. (Suppl.)*, 387:1–37.
30. Haglund, U. (1973): Vascular reactions in the small intestine of the cat during hemorrhage. *Acta Physiol. Scand.*, 89:129–141.
31. Haglund, U., Abe, T., Åhrén, C., Braide, I., and Lundgren, O. (1976): The intestinal mucosal lesions in shock: I. Studies on the pathogenesis. *Eur. Surg. Res.*, 8:435–447.
32. Haglund, U., Abe, T., Braide, I., Åhrén, C., and Lundgren, O. (1976): The intestinal mucosal lesions in shock: II. The relationship between the mucosal lesions and the cardiovascular derangement following regional shock. *Eur. Surg. Res.*, 8:448–460.
33. Haglund, U., Hultén, L., Lundgren, O., and Åhrén, C. (1975): Mucosal lesions in the human small intestine in shock. *Gut*, 16:979–984.
34. Haglund, U., and Lundgren, O. (1972): Reactions within consecutive vascular sections of the small intestine of the cat during prolonged hypotension. *Acta Physiol. Scand.*, 84:151–163.
35. Haglund, U., and Lundgren, O. (1972): The effects of vasoconstrictor fibre stimulation on the consecutive, vascular sections of the small intestine of the cat during prolonged local hypotension. *Acta Physiol. Scand.*, 85:547–558.
36. Haglund, U., and Lundgren, O. (1973): The effects of vasoconstrictor fibre stimulation on consecutive vascular sections of cat small intestine during hemorrhagic hypotension. *Acta Physiol. Scand.*, 88:95–108.
37. Haglund, U., and Lundgren, O. (1973): Cardiovascular effects of blood borne material released from the cat small intestine during simulated shock conditions. *Acta Physiol. Scand.*, 89:558–570.
38. Haglund, U., and Lundgren, O. (1977): The significance of sympathetic nervous activity for the development of the intestinal mucosal lesions in shock. *Acta Chir. Scand.*, 143:139–143.
39. Haglund, U., and Lundgren, O. (1978): Intestinal ischemia and shock factors. *Fed. Proc.*, 37:2729–2733.
40. Haglund, U., and Lundgren, O. (1979): On the protective role of the liver in the hypotensive state following intestinal ischemia. *Circ. Shock*, 6:89–97.
41. Haglund, U., Myrvold, H., and Lundgren, O. (1978): Cardiac and pulmonary function in regional intestinal shock. *Arch. Surg.*, 113:963–969.
42. Hultén, L., Jodal, M., Lindhagen, J., and Lundgren, O. (1976): Blood flow in the small intestine of cat and man as analyzed by an inert gas washout technique. *Gastroenterology*, 70:45–51.
43. Hultén, L., Lindhagen, J., and Lundgren, O. (1977): The sympathetic nervous control of intramural blood flow in the feline and human intestines. *Gastroenterology*, 72:41–48.
44. Jacobsson, E. D. (1972): Are adrenergic overactivity

and splanchnic vasoconstriction the prime pathophysiological events in shock? In: *The Fundamental Mechanisms of Shock*, edited by L. B. Hinshaw, and B. G. Cox, pp. 109–112. Plenum Publishing, New York.
45. Järhult, J., (1975): Osmolar control of the circulation in hemorrhagic hypotension. An experimental study in the cat. *Acta Physiol. Scand. (Suppl.)*, 423:1–84.
46. Jodal, M., and Lundgren, O. (1970): Plasma skimming in the intestinal tract. *Acta Physiol. Scand.*, 80:50–60.
47. Jodal, M., Lundgren, O., Sjöqvist, A., and Haglund, U. (1978): Countercurrent controversy. *Gastroenterology*, 75:767–769.
48. Johnson, P. C. (1960): Autoregulation of intestinal blood flow. *Am. J. Physiol.*, 199:311–318.
49. Johnson, P. C. (1964): Origin, localization and homeostatic significance of autoregulation in the intestine. *Circ. Res. (Suppl.)*, 15(1):225–232.
50. Johnson, P. C. (1968): Autoregulatory responses of cat mesenteric arterioles measured in vivo. *Circ. Res.*, 22:199–212.
51. Kampp, M., Lundgren, O., and Nilsson, N. J. (1968): Extravascular shunting of oxygen in the small intestine of the cat. *Acta Physiol. Scand.*, 72:396–403.
52. Kendrick, E., Öberg, B., and Wennergren, G. (1972): Vasoconstrictor fibre discharge to skeletal muscle, kidney, intestine and skin at varying levels of arterial baroreceptor activity in the cat. *Acta Physiol. Scand.*, 85:464–476.
53. Kuida, H., Gilbert, R. P., Hinshaw, L. B., Brunson, J. G., and Visscher, M. B. (1961): Species differences in effect of gram-negative endotoxin on circulation. *Am. J. Physiol.*, 200:1197–1202.
54. Kwan, A., Chiu, C. J., Mersereau, W., and Hinchey, E. J. (1974): The roles of intraluminal chyme and vasomotor response in the pathogenesis of non-occlusive intestinal infarcts. *Ann. Surg.*, 179:877–882.
55. Lewis, D. H., and Mellander, S. (1962): Competitive effects of sympathetic control and tissue metabolites on resistance and capacitance vessels and capillary filtration in skeletal muscle. *Acta Physiol. Scand.*, 56:162–188.
56. Lillehei, R. C. (1957): The intestinal factor in irreversible hemorrhagic shock. *Surgery*, 42:1043–1054.
57. Lillehei, R. C., Longerbeam, J. K., Bloch, J. H., and Manax, W. G. (1964): The nature of irreversible shock: Experimental and clinical observations. *Ann. Surg.*, 160:682–708.
58. Lundgren, O., and Haglund, U. (1978): On the chemical nature of the blood borne cardiotoxic material released from the feline small bowel in regional shock. *Acta Physiol. Scand.*, 103:59–70.
59. Lundgren, O., Haglund, U., Isaksson, O., and Abe, T. (1976): Effects on myocardial contractility of blood borne material released from the feline small intestine in simulated shock. *Circ. Res.*, 38:307–315.
60. Lundgren, O., Lundwall, J., and Mellander, S. (1964): Range of sympathetic discharge and reflex vascular adjustments in skeletal muscle during hemorrhagic hypotension. *Acta Physiol. Scand.*, 62:380–390.
61. Lundgren, O., and Svanvik, J. (1973): Mucosal hemodynamics in the small intestine of the cat during reduced perfusion pressure. *Acta Physiol. Scand.*, 88:551–563.
62. Lutz, J., and Henrich, H. (1970): Gefässreaktionen in situ bei druck- und stromkonstanter Perfusion der intestinalen Strombahn und ihre Abhängigkeit vom Ausgangsdruck. *Pflüegers Arch.*, 319:68–81.
63. Marston, A. (1977): *Intestinal Ischaemia*. Edward Arnold Ltd., London.
64. McCord, J. M., and Fridovich, I. (1978): The biology and pathology of oxygen radicals. *Ann. Intern. Med.*, 89:122–127.
65. Micflikier, A. B., Bond, J. H., Sircar, B., and Levitt, M. D. (1976): Intestinal villus blood flow measured with carbon monoxide and microspheres. *Am. J. Physiol.*, 230:916–919.
66. McNeill, J. R., Stark, R. D., and Greenway, C. V. (1970): Intestinal vasoconstriction after hemorrhage; roles of vasopressin and angiotensin. *Am. J. Physiol.*, 219:1342–1347.
67. Mellander, S. (1960): Comparative studies on the adrenergic neuro-hormonal control of resistance and capacitance blood vessels in the cat. *Acta Physiol. Scand. (Suppl.)*, 50(176):1–86.
68. Mellander, S., and Lewis, D. H. (1963): Effect of hemorrhagic shock on the reactivity of resistance and capacitance vessels and on capillary filtration transfer in cat skeletal muscle. *Circ. Res.*, 13:105–118.
69. Messmer, K., Klövekorn, W. P., Sunder-Plassman, L., and Brendel, W. (1971): Studies concerning the effect of trasylol in a standardized model of hemorrhagic shock in dogs. In: *New Aspects of Trasylol Therapy. Protease inhibition in Shock Therapy*, edited by W. Brendel and G. L. Haberland, pp. 25–32. F. K. Schattauer Verlag, Stuttgart.
70. Palmerio, C., Zetterström, B., Shammash, J., Euchbaum, E., Frank, E., and Fine, J. (1963): Denervation of the abdominal viscera for the treatment of traumatic shock. *N. Engl. J. Med.*, 269:709–716.
71. Parks, D. A., Bulkley, G. B., Granger, D. N., Hamilton, S. R., and McCord, J. (1982): Ischemic injury in the cat small intestine: Role of superoxide radicals. *Gastroenterology*, 82:9–15.
72. Penner, A., and Bernheim, A. I. (1939): Acute postoperative enterocolitis. A study on the pathologic nature of shock. *Arch. Pathol.*, 27:966–983.
73. Redfors, S., Hallbäck, D-A., Haglund, U., Jodal, M., and Lundgren, O. (1984): Blood flow distribution, villous tissue osmolality and fluid and electrolyte transport in the cat small intestine during regional hypotension. *Acta Physiol. Scand. (in press).*
74. Robinson, J. W. L., and Mirkovitch, V. (1977): The roles of intraluminal oxygen and glucose in the protection of the rat intestinal mucosa from the effects of ischaemia. *Biomedicine*, 27:60–62.
75. Robinson, J. W. L., Mirkovitch, V., Winistörfer, B., and Saegesser, F. (1981): Response of the intestinal mucosa to ischaemia. *Gut*, 22:512–527.
76. Schoenberg, M., Younes, M., Muhl, E., Haglund, U., Sellin, D., and Schildberg, F. W. (1983): Free radical involvement in ischemic damage of the small intestine. In: *Oxyradicals and Their Scavenger Systems. Vol II. Cellular and Medical Aspects*, edited by R. A. Greenwald and G. Cohen, pp. 154–158. Elsevier Science Publishing Co. Inc. New York.
77. Schoenberg, M. H., Muhl, E., Sellin, D., Younes, M., Schildberg, F. W., and Haglund, U. (1984): Post-

hypotensive generation of superoxide free radicals—Possible role in the pathogenesis of the intestinal mucosal damage. *Acta Chir. Scand. (in press).*
78. Shepherd, A. P., Maxwell, L. C., and Jacobson, E. D. (1981): Limitations of the microsphere technique to fractionate intestinal blood flow. In: *Measurements of Blood Flow*, edited by D. N. Granger and G. B. Bulkley, pp. 195–200. Williams & Wilkins, Baltimore.
79. Shute, K. (1976): Effect of intraluminal oxygen on experimental ischaemia of the intestine. *Gut*, 17:1001–1006.
80. Sjövall, H., Redfors, S., Jodal, M., and Lundgren, O. (1983): The effect of splanchnic nerve stimulation on blood flow distribution, villous tissue osmolality and fluid and electrolyte transport in the small intestine of the cat. *Acta Physiol. Scand.*, 117:359–365.
81. Swan, K. G., Barton, R. W., and Reynolds, D. G. (1972): Splanchnic blood flow in experimental shock. In: *The Fundamental Mechanisms of Shock*, edited by L. B. Hinshaw and B. G. Cox, pp. 87–103. Plenum Publishing, New York.
82. Svanvik, J. (1973): Mucosal hemodynamics in the small intestine of the cat during regional sympathetic vasoconstrictor activation. *Acta Physiol. Scand.*, 89:19–29.
83. Weil, M. H., MacLean, L. D., Visscher, M. B., and Spink, W. W. (1956): Studies on the circulatory changes in the dog produced by endotoxin from gram-negative microorganisms. *J. Clin. Invest.*, 35:1191–1198.
84. Wiggers, C. J. (1950): *The Physiology of Shock*. Commonwealth Fund, New York.
85. Younes, M., Schoenberg, M. H., Jung, H., Fredholm, B., Haglund, U. and Schildberg, F. W. (1984): Oxidative tissue damage following regional intestinal ischemia and reperfusion in the cat. *Res. Exp. Med. (in press).*

The Effects of Luminal Distension and Obstruction on the Intestinal Circulation

Ulf Öhman

Department of Surgery, Karolinska Hospital,
S-104 01 Stockholm, Sweden

Bowel obstruction impairs the blood circulation in the gut wall by several different mechanisms. Strangulation denotes, by definition, an interruption of the intestinal blood supply. Closed-loop obstructions and certain simple large-bowel obstructions involve impressive levels of intraluminal pressure that compromise the mucosal circulation. Bands and adhesions may cause localized pressure necroses in the gut wall. Other mechanisms causing local circulatory impairment in bowel obstruction are hypothetical and less well understood. Although simple mechanical obstruction is defined as blockage of the lumen of the bowel without compromise of its blood supply, it is generally assumed and conceptually attractive that progressive distension should impair the intramural circulation of the bowel (106); however, it is difficult to find experimental evidence in support of this concept (23).

Several routes of animal experimentation have been pursued to explore this topic. Essentially, the intestinal blood circulation has been studied in response to artificial distension, bowel obstruction, and a combination of these assaults. Both *in vivo* and *in vitro* systems have been used. Current knowledge of these issues is reviewed in this chapter.

EFFECTS OF ARTIFICIAL DISTENSION

Artificial distension of the small bowel impedes the regional blood flow, as demonstrated in early studies involving microscopic observations (6,77,78,89,131) and blood-flow measurements (22,33,34,65). More recent investigations have quantitated these influences. Distension of the dog small bowel to 30 cm water reduced blood flow in the superior mesenteric artery by 30% (43). Stepwise distension of isolated canine small bowel segments reduced regional blood flow in a stepwise fashion (7,116,124); however, 20% to 35% of resting flow remained even at an intraluminal pressure of 100 to 200 mm Hg. Distension of canine jejunal loops at constant blood flow produced, for each incremental step of distension, a linear increase in inflow pressure (59). The linearity of the response and the absence of readjustment suggested simple mechanical compression of the blood vessels.

Microvessels of the villi progressively deteriorate when luminal pressure is raised and become virtually extinguished at 100 mm Hg (116). Findings suggestive of arteriovenous shunting at the villus base have been demonstrated in the dog at a luminal pressure of 40 mm Hg (116).

Changes in lymph pressure and flow reflect capillary filtration in the small bowel. Over a physiological range of distension pressures (0–20 mm Hg), lymph pressure and flow increased with a concomitant decrease in blood flow, whereas higher lumen pressures resulted in a progressive reduction in lymph flow (36).

We have studied denervated and homologously perfused feline small bowel. Stepwise distension of the gut reduced blood flow in a stepwise fashion (81) as in previous studies. We also attempted, however, to evaluate quantitatively the regional microcirculation. Capillary filtration was determined with a volumetric method (30,71) adapted from the original gravimetric method (92). Two-thirds of a venous pressure elevation is transmitted backwards to the capillary level (53,76). A sudden and rather small (38) elevation of venous pressure produces a known elevation of the capillary pressure and a biphasic volume increase of the specimen. Whereas the rapid phase represents filling of capacitance vessels, the slow component is solely the result of transcapillary fluid movement (21,31,38,55–58,76). Thus, the capillary filtration coefficient (CFC) can be calculated as an index of the capillary area open to perfusion. CFC calculated by this method corresponds well with hard observational data (14).

Capillary perfusion, as opposed to total blood flow, was not reduced by distension to 20 mm Hg, whereas higher levels of intraluminal pressure reduced flow rate and CFC in parallel (81). At 100 mm Hg distension, 30% of basal flow remained (Fig. 1), but only 15% of the capillaries were open to flow (Fig. 2). Regional oxygen uptake parallelled the blood-flow rate; 30% of basal uptake remained at 100 mm Hg distension (Fig. 3). Rapid deflation of the bowel from 100 mm Hg to atmospheric pressure revealed a discrepancy between blood flow and capillary perfusion: total flow did not regain predistension levels, whereas transcapillary exchange and oxygen uptake returned within 5 min to basal levels.

The discrepancy between total blood flow and capillary perfusion and the nonresumption of flow after deflation prompted a study with prolonged distension to 20 mm Hg (83), a value that corresponds approximately to mean capillary pressure in the intestine (30,55–58). Both flow and CFC were reduced by about 50%; specimens with a low basal flow exhibited an early and pronounced reduction of transcapillary exchange, whereas those with a high basal flow showed insignificant reductions of CFC (83).

The model was complicated by reflex contractile phenomena. Distension stimulated intestinal motility, which atropine abolished in denervated but not in innervated specimens (83). Stress relaxation or "delayed compliance" was also observed, that is, the addition of each volume increment caused a steep rise in gut pressure, whereupon the bowel relaxed to accommodate the increased volume, thus reducing the intraluminal pressure. Relaxation was followed by immediate resumption of blood flow and CFC (81,83). Similarly, maintenance of a

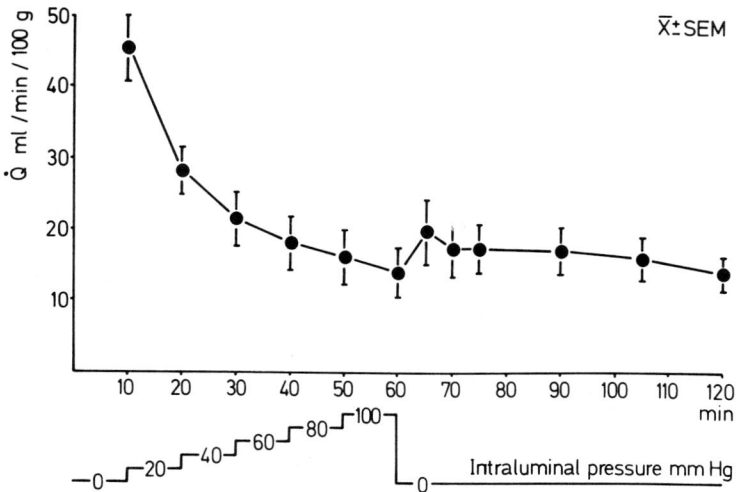

FIG. 1. Regional blood flow (ml/min × 100 g) during *in vitro* homologous perfusion of denervated feline small bowel upon artificial distension to 100 mm Hg. Mean and SEM from 11 experiments. (From Öhman, ref. 81, with permission.)

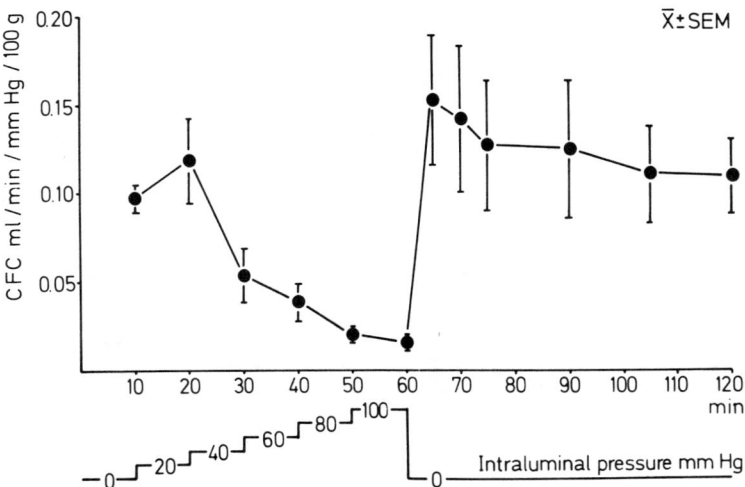

FIG. 2. Capillary filtration coefficient (ml/min × mm Hg × 100 g) during *in vitro* homologous perfusion of denervated feline small bowel upon artificial distension to 100 mm Hg. Mean and SEM from 11 experiments. (From Öhman, ref. 81, with permission.)

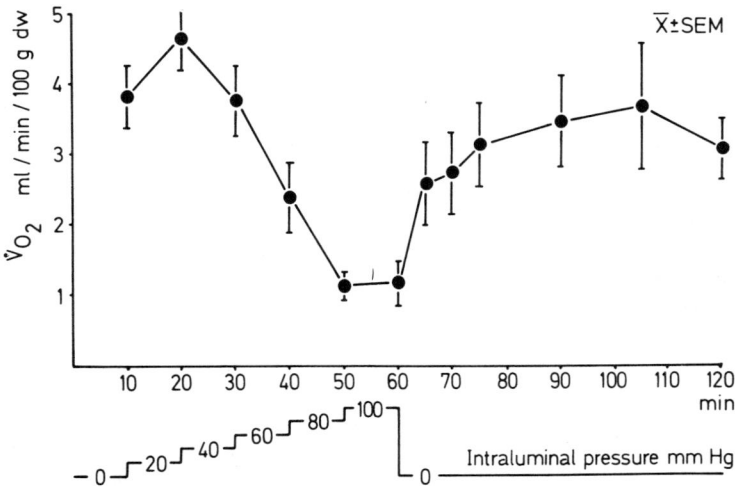

FIG. 3. Oxygen consumption (ml/min × 100 g dry weight) during *in vitro* homologous perfusion of denervated feline small bowel upon artificial distension to 100 mm Hg. Mean and SEM from 11 experiments. (From Öhman, ref. 81, with permission.)

fixed level of intraluminal pressure required repeated increments of distension until a steady level was reached. At this plateau stable reductions in the hemodynamic variables were noted (81,83). In autoperfused segments of canine small intestine, the major factor responsible for recovery of flow and resistance following distension was the decrease in extravascular pressure that occurred as a result of delayed gut wall compliance (15,44).

The contractions elicited by distension make it difficult to isolate blood-flow changes caused by distension from those caused by motility. Spontaneous rhythmic bowel contractions are reported to have little effect on blood flow and resistance (11,44,51,59,60,130). This is essentially true, but a reservation must be added: each single contraction exerts a subtle flow-reducing effect (Fig. 4). Thus, rhythmic contractions do have an effect on regional blood

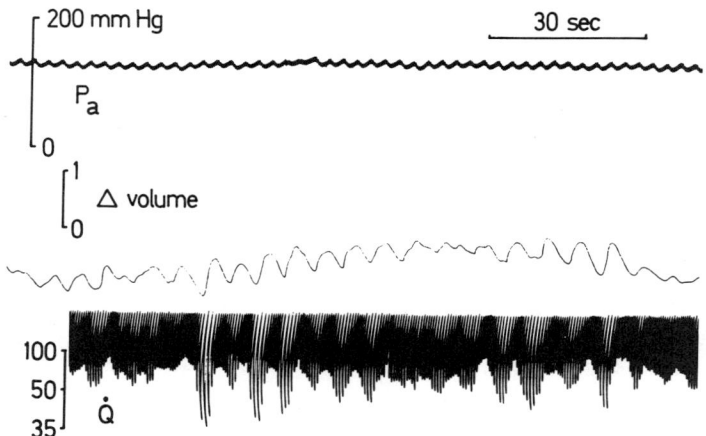

FIG. 4. Relations between contractile bowel activity and regional blood flow. Contractions elicited by distension to 20 mm Hg of *in vitro* homologously perfused feline small bowel. Each bowel contraction is recorded as a reduction in volume and a concomitant decrease in flow rate, whereas bowel relaxations present as augmentations of volume and flow. Markings from top: arterial perfusion pressure (mm Hg), volume change of specimen (ml/100 g), and regional blood flow rate (ml/min × 100 g). (From Öhman, ref. 83, with permission.)

flow, but the integrated net effect on mean blood flow is *nil* (15,83,87).

Experiments with acetylcholine have clarified the motility issue (60,96,110); a low dose augments blood flow, whereas a high dose reduces flow through tonic bowel contractions. Rhythmic contractions increase flow in the muscular layer, suggesting an "exercise" hyperemia of the contracting muscle, whereas physostigmine-induced tonic contractions and increased gut wall tension divert the blood flow away from the mucosal and submucosal layers (17).

The relations between motility and blood flow can thus be summarized (15,83,87): an active increase in gut pressure, such as that seen in rhythmic gut contractions, does not affect regional vascular resistance unless the contractions are vigorous enough to impede blood flow mechanically. On the other hand, a passive elevation of gut pressure, that is, an artificial distension of the intestine, augments regional vascular resistance through extravascular compression and thereby reduces blood flow.

Relations between luminal pressure and blood flow have also been studied in the large bowel. The results agree with those from small bowel studies. Distension reduces blood flow and abolishes autoregulation (19,45,46). Distension of the canine colon to 60 mm Hg produced ischemic mucosal injury, as did a difference of more than 30 mm Hg between systemic and distending pressures (8). Moderate systemic hypotension alone and moderate colonic distension alone produced no such injuries.

Bowel distension within the closed abdomen might reproduce physiologic conditions better than distension of the bowel at laparotomy (24). Studies on piglets with the abdomen closed demonstrated pressure-related decreases in blood flow to the small intestine (105). At 60 mm Hg luminal pressure, blood flow was reduced to 25% of the basal value. At 15 mm Hg luminal pressure, mucosal blood flow was reduced to less than half, whereas blood flow to the muscular layer was greatly increased. At high luminal pressures, only 18% of mucosal blood flow remained (105), a finding in agreement with the reduction to 15% of CFC in grossly distended feline small bowel (81).

Ileal mucosal blood flow in rabbits with closed abdomens was not significantly changed by a distending pressure of 30 cm water, whereas distension to 60 cm water reduced it to a nondetectable value (121). In rats with closed abdomens, distension to 20 mm Hg did not decrease small bowel blood flow, whereas 40 mm Hg reduced it to 22% of preinflation level (24).

A significant difference between *in vivo* and *in vitro* systems is noted with respect to the responses following deflation of the bowel. A slight hyperemic response was noted in piglets with closed abdomens (105), whereas preinflation flow values were not restored in the isolated feline preparations (81,83). This has been ascribed to bowel wall edema that results from perfusion as well as distension (81,83). Another conceivable explanation is the difference between intact and denervated intestine, the latter having possibly lost its autoregulatory capabilities (105).

Oxygen uptake by the intestine is independent of blood flow within rather wide limits in the "resting" condition (39,41,62,64,86,111). Oxygen uptake by the feline small bowel was not affected by distension to 20 mm Hg (83), nor was it changed by the same distension to which isolated canine jejunal loops were subjected (59,116). At this moderate distension, however, oxygen uptake became a function of blood flow (Fig. 5) (86) as it also does at low flow rates (62). Marked distension reduces the oxygen uptake significantly (64,81,83,99,116). An autoregulation of oxygen uptake (39–41,112) aims to satisfy the oxygen need of the bowel irrespective of the current blood flow rate. The ability to autoregulate blood flow (37,52,54) deteriorates upon distension of the bowel (44–46). Evidently, autoregulation of oxygen uptake is also diminished by distension (86).

In summary, the intestinal circulation deteriorates when intraluminal pressure is artificially raised above physiological levels. This deterioration predominantly affects mucosal blood flow and transcapillary exchange. Because of the unique properties of the bowel wall, however, it is highly uncertain whether these responses are pertinent to the course of events in clinical and experimental bowel obstruction.

EFFECTS OF INTESTINAL OBSTRUCTION

From the hemodynamic point of view, distension of the bowel would seem to be the salient feature of intestinal obstruction. Thus, artificial distension seems the appropriate procedure to evaluate hemodynamic changes produced by obstruction. This view, unfortunately, is too simple. The small bowel has a pronounced ability to distend and thus prevent intraluminal pressure from reaching inappropriate levels. Distension, however, creates an appreciable tension within the gut wall (23). Compliance is probably a better index of gut wall tension than luminal pressure (16).

Sustained basal pressure in the small intestine is 2 to 4 mm Hg in man (23), cat (79), and dog (116,122,125). Simple small bowel obstruction in the dog created sustained luminal pressures of 8 to 12 cm water (125). Luminal pressure in clinical cases was around 10 cm water in small bowel obstruction and somewhat higher, 10 to 25 cm water, in colonic obstruction (125).

Despite the demonstration, more than 50 years ago, that gut pressures necessary to arrest blood flow are in excess of those observed in obstructed bowel (13), it has been an almost universal misconception that obstruction creates a harmful increase in sustained gut pressure (73,85). The truth is that sustained pressure is rather low despite considerable distension. Experiments on rats (61), cats (79,84), rabbits (128), dogs (4,66,73,91,118), and piglets (104) show that *sustained* gut pressure in simple small bowel obstruction ranges from 5 to 10 mm Hg, commonly around the former level and virtually never exceeding the latter. Luminal pressure in the presence of constant peristalsis is about 15 mm Hg (116), and pharmacologically induced peristalsis causes a major rise in luminal pressure even in obstruction (79,116).

Feline bowel specimens were investigated in an organ perfusion chamber 30 min after release of a 72-hr obstruction. Blood flow, vascular resistance, capillary filtration, and oxygen consumption were determined. No differences were observed between obstructed and nonob-

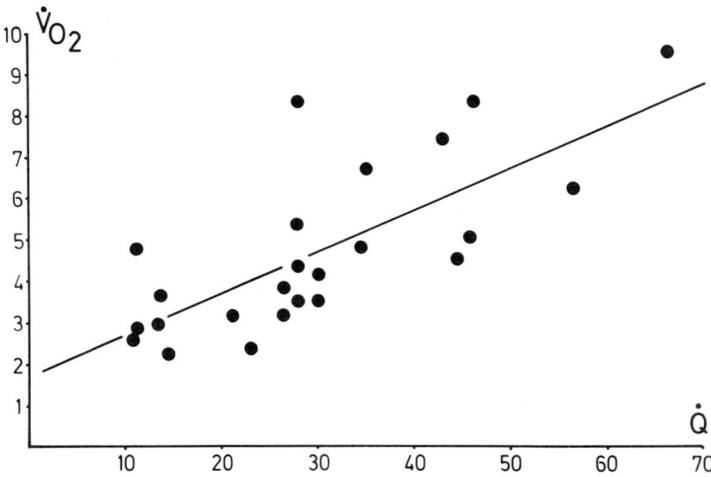

FIG. 5. Regional blood flow (ml/min × 100 g wet weight) vs oxygen consumption (ml/min × 100 g dry weight) in denervated and *in vitro* homologously perfused feline small bowel upon distension to 20 mm Hg. (From Öhman, ref. 86, with permission.)

structed specimens (80). Even when studied in the presence of continuing distension after 72 hr of obstruction, hemodynamic and microcirculatory variables were within normal ranges (84). Determinations of blood flow with the microsphere method in piglets (104) and rats (24) with closed abdomens demonstrated a doubling of intestinal blood flow in the presence of a 48-hr simple obstruction.

The effects of experimental bowel obstruction on intestinal hemodynamic variables can be summarized as follows: perfusion experiments *in vitro* after bowel obstruction *in vivo* show that neither blood flow nor capillary perfusion deteriorate (82,84). Blood flow determinations *in vivo* even suggest that blood flow in the bowel wall is increased during obstructive conditions (24,104).

Unimpaired intestinal blood flow in mechanical obstruction (24,73,80,82,84,104) and adynamic ileus (1,95) are compatible with the histological findings: apart from a progressive reduction of the villus capillary bed (20,128) without increased capillary permeability (47,126), the histological picture of the bowel wall is virtually normal (13,32,72–74,114).

The insignificance of the hemodynamic changes in obstruction are somewhat surprising with respect to the results of distension procedures. Evidently, artificial distension of the bowel does not duplicate an *in vivo* obstruction. It is probable that the rate of stretch plays an important role in this discrepancy (27,84). Whereas a rapid artificial distension augments vascular resistance in the intestine, the slowly increasing distension of obstruction does not. Recent results (24,104) even suggest vascular resistance falls in the obstructed bowel. This concept receives support from the fact that bowel obstruction leads to enhanced distensibility of the gut wall, that is, a certain level of luminal pressure produces a greater distension, and hence a greater gut wall tension, in the obstructed than in the nonobstructed gut (23,82,84). The intraintestinal volume needed to produce a stable luminal pressure of 20 mm Hg in obstructed feline gut was twice the volume required in control specimens (84); this can be regarded as an expression of delayed compliance.

It is tempting to attribute the hyperemia of obstructed bowel (24,104) to the increased secretion observed in response to elevated gut pressure proximal to the obstruction (12,35,63, 73,75,84,114,119,120,129). This secretion may be a local rather than a systemic effect (120) that consists of a passive filtration-secretion augmented by increased tissue permeability and increased effective capillary surface area (121). Whether secretion induces the hyperemia or vice versa is not clear. Both may be caused by a common, possibly humoral, factor (24). Indomethacin prevents the secretion induced by distension of rat small bowel (70) and the secretion produced in closed-loop obstruction in the rat *(unpublished observation)*. These findings suggest that prostaglandins may be mediators of such secretion, which possibly is an exaggeration of the general "entero-pooling" produced by prostaglandins (100).

In summary, simple obstruction involves distension of the bowel but only a modest increase of gut pressure. Neither total blood flow nor capillary perfusion deteriorates with obstruction. On the contrary, vascular resistance may be significantly reduced in the occluded bowel.

COMBINED EFFECTS OF OBSTRUCTION AND DISTENSION

Stepwise distension of the feline small bowel after 72 hr of *in vivo* obstruction produced hemodynamic responses similar to those of nonobstructed specimens (82). However, two subtle differences were noted. The first increment of distension (20 mm Hg) reduced the CFC in obstructed bowel but not in controls, and obstructed specimens consumed less oxygen during distension than did control specimens (Fig. 6).

To evaluate these findings further, obstructed specimens were subjected to prolonged 20 mm Hg distension (84). Two protocols were followed: distension added to the continuing distension of obstruction and distension after an intervening decompression (Fig. 7). The additional and uninterrupted distension to 20 mm Hg caused a profound (80–90%) reduction of the CFC, a response that, for several reasons (69,85), indicates the perfused capillary surface area was reduced to virtually zero. In speci-

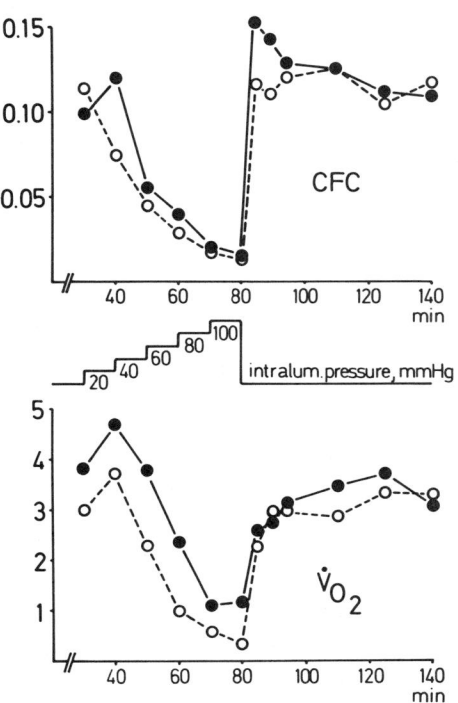

FIG. 6. Effects of distension to 100 mm Hg on capillary filtration coefficient (ml/min × mm Hg × 100 g) and oxygen consumption (ml/min × 100 g dry weight) in denervated feline small bowel, homologously perfused *in vitro*. *(Solid symbols)* Nonobstructed specimens, mean of 11 experiments. *(Open symbols)* After 72 hr of *in vivo* obstruction, mean of 11 experiments. (From Öhman, ref. 85, with permission.)

mens given the opportunity to "recover" during an intervening decompression, the same level of distension produced smaller (40–50%) and rather variable reductions in CFC (84). Oxygen consumption by the bowel was virtually unaffected by the experimental procedure, that is, the specimens utilized oxygen despite a pronounced reduction in the surface area of perfused capillaries.

The procedure has been repeated in rats with closed abdomens (24). Intestinal blood flow was determined after 48 hr of obstruction. The results from the feline model were confirmed: distension of the obstructed gut to 10 mm Hg did not reduce blood flow, whereas distension to 20 and 40 mm Hg reduced flow by 50% and 95%, respectively.

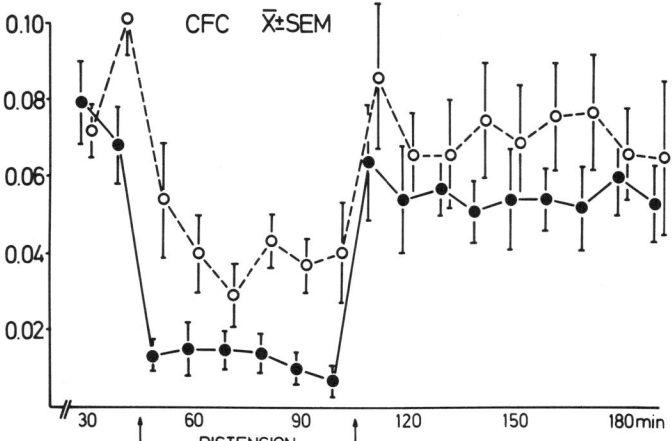

FIG. 7. Capillary filtration coefficient (ml/min × mm Hg × 100 g) during *in vitro* homologous perfusion of feline small bowel after 72 hr of *in vivo* obstruction. Specimens artificially distended to 20 mm Hg. *(Solid symbols)* Continuous distension, mean and SEM of 12 experiments *(Open symbols)* After intraoperative decompression, mean and SEM of 12 experiments. (From Öhman, ref. 84, with permission.)

The effects of bowel obstruction on the gut wall are strikingly similar to those produced by the administration of papaverine. Distensibility of the canine small bowel was significantly increased following papaverine, and blood flow in papaverine-treated gut declined more rapidly in response to increasing gut pressure than did flow in control specimens (44).

It can be concluded from these studies that simple obstruction per se, although not a threat to bowel microcirculation or viability, renders the gut wall vulnerable to further distension or ischemia. The effects of papaverine on the gut wall responses to distension are strikingly similar to those observed in simple obstruction.

EFFECTS OF DECOMPRESSION OF OBSTRUCTED BOWEL

Two experimental studies have addressed the decompression question. The protocol mentioned in the preceding paragraph compared continuously distended with intermittently decompressed bowel after 72 hr of obstruction *in vivo* (84). Intraoperative decompression opened a significant number of capillaries and increased the capacity of the capillary bed to withstand renewed moderate distension. Two further effects of decompression were noted. Oxygen uptake in decompressed intestine was twice the uptake in distended specimens (86), and blood flow in the postdistension phase tended to be lower in decompressed specimens (84). Furthermore, the autoregulatory capacity lost as a result of obstruction and distension was reestablished following decompression of the gut (86).

In a study on piglets after 48 hr obstruction, mean sustained gut pressure was less than 10 mm Hg and did not differ significantly from normal (104). Blood flow in the obstructed gut doubled from the preobstruction level, and decompression of the distended bowel reduced flow to one-third of this enhanced level. Mucosal and muscular perfusion were equally affected by the reduction in total flow (104).

Thus, decompression of the obstructed bowel seems to cause edema and to augment vascular resistance but concomitantly opens a significant number of capillaries, thereby restoring the capacities for autoregulation and oxygen uptake.

DISCUSSION AND CLINICAL IMPLICATIONS

Clinical inference from animal research is fraught with danger and should be exercised with caution. The investigations reviewed in this chapter seem to be physiologically relevant; no critical evidence has appeared to devalue their relevance to man (123). Furthermore, the present author contends that the close qualitative and quantitative similarities between man and the cat with respect to gut morphology (26) and the mesenteric circulation (48–50,67) permit some guarded inferences from the feline experiments to the clinical condition of intestinal obstruction.

Since luminal pressure is kept within a rather "physiological" range during the course of simple obstruction, the condition does not per se produce any harmful effects in the intestinal circulation. This lack of a blood-flow response must be considered a very appropriate protective mechanism, since the bowel mucosa, despite its tremendous regenerative potential, demonstrates a most unusual and extreme sensitivity to acute ischemia (101–103).

Whereas obstruction may thus involve bowel distension without affecting bowel microcirculation or viability, it also involves an increased distensibility of the bowel wall, that is, a certain level of luminal pressure produces a greater distension, and hence a greater gut wall tension, in obstructed than in nonobstructed bowel. The anticipation that this might lead to an increased susceptibility of the intramural circulation to any further increase in luminal pressure was substantiated by the experimental findings. An additional and rather modest increment of luminal pressure in the already obstructed gut caused a profound reduction in the surface area of perfused capillaries. This CFC reduction was readily reversible upon deflation of the bowel, and its functional significance is not known. However, it is tempting to speculate that a prolonged capillary closure of this magnitude might threaten bowel viability. The clinical correlate to the experimental situation is a mechanical obstruction complicated postoperatively by a functional obstruction, such as that seen when the return of bowel motility is delayed after the relief of an obstruction (66,97).

The experimental findings indicate a solution to this hypothetical problem: an intraoperative decompression of the obstructed bowel may occasion some degree of gut wall edema and a slight augmentation of vascular resistance but may also enhance the capacity of the capillary bed to withstand, with retained function, a renewed distension of the gut. Two points should be noted from a clinical point of view. The first is that an intraoperative decompression does not necessarily mean an open decompression with its conceivable contamination of the abdominal cavity (18). Closed aseptic decompression with a long intestinal tube serves the same purpose (107). The second point is that decompression of the obstructed gut involves some unwanted effects, such as gut wall edema (35,115), augmentation of regional vascular resistance (84, 104), and, possibly, a slower return of postoperative gut motility (127). Although decompression of obstructed bowel is generally recommended (107,116), it is not clear whether the possible benefits to the microcirculation should take precedence over these potentially harmful effects.

Vast clinical experience suggests that, in the ordinary case of simple obstruction, the relieved small bowel is perfectly capable of handling its luminal pressure and contents. Thus, the two lines of action are equally applicable. The decision to decompress the intestine is preferably left to the discretion of the operating surgeon and is dictated more by technical circumstances than by subtle physiological considerations, even if one study suggests a more rapid return to a "physiological state" following decompression (117). The simple truth may be that "the benefits of decompression are solely those of access and easy closure of the abdominal wall" (115).

Adverse effects of increased luminal pressure per se have been postulated. For example, pressure waves of high amplitude and long duration might cause, by impairing the mucosal circulation, the bowel lesions of ulcerative colitis (25). It has also been speculated that the exaggerated flow of lymph from obstructed and distended large bowel may promote tumor dissemination and thus contribute to the poor outcome in patients with obstructing malignancy (2). Indeed, the enhanced incidence of lymph node involvement in obstructing versus nonobstructing colorectal carcinomas (88) supports this hypothesis.

Some concluding speculations will be issued. Moderate distension of the feline small intestine produced early, profound reductions of transcapillary exchange in specimens with a low basal flow, whereas the reductions were transient and insignificant in those with a brisk flow (83).

Therefore, a low flow may predispose the bowel to microcirculatory derangement following distension and precipitate the clinical syndrome of "nonocclusive mesenteric ischemia" (3,9,10,28,42,90,98).

The capacity of the obstructed and subsequently distended feline small intestine to consume oxygen at a normal rate despite a pronounced reduction of the CFC (84) also deserves comment. Evidently, reduced capillary perfusion can be associated with different levels of oxygen utilization; although adequate during obstruction (84,86) and "autoregulatory escape" (5,29,68,108,113), oxygenation may be deficient after the administration of cardiac glycosides (93,94). This discrepancy might explain the frequent restitution in bowel obstruction and the poor outcome in cases of "nonocclusive mesenteric ischemia," a condition often involving an element of digitalis intoxication (10,28,42,109).

SUMMARY

Effects of luminal distension and obstruction on intestinal blood flow and oxygen uptake have been studied in animal experiments.

Distending pressures of 20 mm Hg or less impair regional blood flow and augment the oxygen uptake but do not reduce the capillary area open to perfusion, whereas pressures in excess of this level cause concomitant decreases in blood flow, oxygen uptake, and capillary perfusion. At 100 mm Hg distension, only 30% of basal flow and 15% of capillary perfusion remain.

However, the distension of obstruction, as opposed to artificial distension, only modestly increases intraluminal pressure and reduces, rather than augments, vascular resistance. This discrepancy invalidates artificial distension as a model for studying the hemodynamic effects of intestinal obstruction. The difference in the hemodynamic effects may be caused by different rates of stretch; a rapid artificial distension augments vascular resistance, whereas the slow distension of obstruction does not, since the distensibility of the gut wall is greatly enhanced.

Although simple obstruction per se does not threaten the bowel's microcirculation or its viability, obstruction renders the gut wall vulnerable to further distension. Thus, a moderate additional distension virtually abolishes the perfused capillary surface area. An intervening decompression seems to restore the capacity of the capillary bed to withstand renewed distension.

Some cautious clinical inferences are drawn from these animal experiments: an intraoperative decompression of obstructed intestine, although causing some degree of gut wall edema and a slight augmentation of vascular resistance, might enable the microcirculation to withstand renewed distension of the intestine. Finally, some of these findings may increase our understanding of "nonocclusive mesenteric ischemia."

ACKNOWLEDGMENTS

The work presented was carried out in the experimental research laboratory of the Department of Surgery, Karolinska Hospital, and supported by grants from the Swedish Medical Research Council (B75-17X-2022-09).

REFERENCES

1. Abe, H., Appert, H. E., and Howard, J. M. (1974): Hemodynamic observations of adynamic ileus in the conscious dog. *Ann. Surg.*, 179:332–338.
2. Ackerman, N. B. (1974): The influences of mechanical factors on intestinal lymph flow and their relationship to operations for carcinoma of the intestine. *Surg. Gynecol. Obstet.*, 138:677–682.
3. Aldrete, J. S., Han, S. Y., Laws, H. L., and Kirklin, J. W. (1977): Intestinal infarction complicating low cardiac output states. *Surg. Gynecol. Obstet.*, 144:371–375.
4. Antoncic, R. F., and Lawson, H. (1941): The muscular activity of the small intestine, in the dog, during acute obstruction. *Ann. Surg.*, 114:415–423.
5. Baker, R., and Mendel, D. (1967): Some observations on 'autoregulatory escape' in cat intestine. *J. Physiol (Lond.)*, 190:229–240.
6. van Beuren, F. T., Jr. (1926): The mechanism of intestinal perforation due to distention. *Ann. Surg.*, 83:69–78.
7. Boley, S. J., Agrawal, G. P., Warren, A. R., Veith, F. J., Levowitz, B. S., Treiber, W., Dougherty, J., Schwartz, S. S., and Gliedman, M. L. (1969): Pathophysiologic effects of bowel distention on intestinal blood flow. *Am. J. Surg.*, 117:228–234.
8. Bookstein, J. J. (1978): Non-occlusive ischemic co-

8. litis: angiographic aspects in a canine model. *Invest. Radiol.*, 13:506–513.
9. Bounous, G. (1982): Acute necrosis of the intestinal mucosa. *Gastroenterology*, 82:1457–1467.
10. Britt, L. G., and Cheek, R. C. (1969): Nonocclusive mesenteric vascular disease: Clinical and experimental observations. *Ann. Surg.*, 169:704–711.
11. Brobmann, G. F., Jacobson, E. D., and Brecher, G. A. (1970): Intestinal vascular responses to gut pressure and acetylcholine in vitro. *Angiologica*, 7:129–139.
12. Caren, J. F., Meyer, J. H., and Grossman, M. I. (1974): Canine intestinal secretion during and after rapid distention of the small bowel. *Am. J. Physiol.*, 227:183–188.
13. Carlson, H. A., and Wagensteen, O. H. (1932): Histologic study of the intestine in simple obstruction. *Proc. Soc. Exp. Biol. Med.*, 29:421–424.
14. Casley-Smith, J. R., O'Donoghue, P. J., and Crocker, K. W. J. (1975): The quantitative relationships between fenestrae in jejunal capillaries and connective tissue channels: proof of "tunnel-capillaries". *Microvasc. Res.*, 9:78–100.
15. Chou, C. C. (1982): Relationship between intestinal blood flow and motility. *Annu. Rev. Physiol.*, 44:29–42.
16. Chou, C. C., and Dabney, J. M. (1967): Interrelation of ileal wall compliance and vascular resistance. *Am. J. Dig. Dis.*, 12:1198–1208.
17. Chou, C. C., and Grassmick, B. (1978): Motility and blood flow distribution within the wall of the gastrointestinal tract. *Am. J. Physiol.*, 235:H34–H39.
18. Davis, S. E., and Sperling, L. (1969): Obstruction of the small intestine. *Arch. Surg.*, 99:424–426.
19. Dencker, H., Lingårdh, G., Muth, T., and Olin, T. (1969): Massive gangrene of the colon secondary to carcinoma of the rectum. *Acta Chir. Scand.*, 135:357–361.
20. Derblom, H., Johansson, H., and Nylander, G. (1963): Vascular pattern of intestinal villi in the obstructed small bowel of the rat. *Surgery*, 54:780–783.
21. Diana, J. N., and Shadur, C. A. (1973): Effect of arterial and venous pressure on capillary pressure and vascular volume. *Am. J. Physiol.*, 225:637–650.
22. Dragstedt, C. A., Lang, V. F., and Millet, R. F. (1929): The relative effects of distention on different portions of the intestine. *Arch. Surg.*, 18:2257–2263.
23. Duthie, H. L. (1972): Intestine. In: *Scientific Basis of Surgery*, 2nd ed., edited by W. T. Irvine, pp. 69–100. Churchill Livingstone, Edinburgh, London.
24. Enochsson, L., Nylander, G., and Öhman, U. (1982): Effects of intraluminal pressure on regional blood flow in obstructed and unobstructed small intestines in the rat. *Am. J. Surg.*, 144:558–561.
25. Fairburn, R. A. (1973): On the aetiology of ulcerative colitis (a vascular hypothesis). *Lancet*, 1:697–699.
26. Fischer, H., and Seesemann, E. (1961): Die Strukturprinzipien der Wand des Katzendünndarms im Vergleich mit dem Darm des Menschen. *Morph. Jb.*, 102:257–280.
27. Fleisher, D. R. (1970): On the measurement of intestinal tonus. *Gastroenterology*, 58:685–691.
28. Fogarty, T. J., and Fletcher, W. S. (1966): Genesis of nonocclusive mesenteric ischemia. *Am. J. Surg.*, 111:130–137.
29. Folkow, B., Lewis, D. H., Lundgren, O., Mellander, S., and Wallentin, I. (1964): The effect of the sympathetic vasoconstrictor fibres on the distribution of capillary blood flow in the intestine. *Acta Physiol. Scand.*, 61:458–466.
30. Folkow, B., Lundgren, O., and Wallentin, I. (1963): Studies on the relationship between flow resistance, capillary filtration coefficient and regional blood volume in the intestine of the cat. *Acta Physiol. Scand.*, 57:270–283.
31. Friedman, J. J. (1976): Transcapillary protein leakage and fluid movement; effect of venous pressure. *Microvasc. Res.*, 12:275–290.
32. Gage, M., and Hosoi, K. (1935): Histological changes observed in the intestinal wall following simple mechanical obstruction in rabbits. *Proc. Soc. Exp. Biol. Med.*, 32:1651–1653.
33. Gatch, W. D., and Culbertson, C. G. (1935): Circulatory disturbances caused by intestinal obstruction. *Ann. Surg.*, 102:619–635.
34. Gatch, W. D., Trusler, H. M., and Ayers, K. D. (1927): Effects of gaseous distention on obstructed bowel. *Arch. Surg.*, 14:1215–1221.
35. Grace, R. H. (1971): The handling of water and electrolytes by the small bowel following the relief of intestinal obstruction. *Br. J. Surg.*, 58:760–764.
36. Granger, D. N., Kvietys, P. R., Mortillaro, N. A., and Taylor, A. E. (1980): Effect of luminal distension on intestinal transcapillary fluid exchange. *Am. J. Physiol.*, 239:G516–G523.
37. Granger, D. N., Richardson, P. D. I., Kvietys, P. R., and Mortillaro, N. A. (1980): Intestinal blood flow. *Gastroenterology*, 78:837–863.
38. Granger, D. N., Richardson, P. D. I., and Taylor, A. E. (1979): Volumetric assessment of the capillary filtration coefficient in the cat small intestine. *Pflügers Arch.*, 381:25–33.
39. Granger, H. J., Goodman, A. H., and Cook, B. H. (1975): Metabolic models of microcirculatory regulation. *Fed. Proc.*, 34:2025–2030.
40. Granger, H. J., and Nyhof, R. A. (1982): Dynamics of intestinal oxygenation: Interactions between oxygen supply and uptake. *Am. J. Physiol.*, 243:G91–G96.
41. Granger, H. J., and Shepherd, A. P., Jr. (1973): Intrinsic microvascular control of tissue oxygen delivery. *Microvasc. Res.*, 5:49–72.
42. Haglund, U., and Lundgren, O. (1979): Non-occlusive acute intestinal vascular failure. *Br. J. Surg.*, 66:155–158.
43. Hahnloser, P. B., Burns, G. P., Tibblin, St., and Schenk, W. G., Jr. (1970): Kreislaufdynamik bei experimenteller Überdehnung des Magens, des Dünndarms und der Abdominalhöhle. *Helv. Chir. Acta*, 37:259–265.
44. Hanson, K. M. (1973): Hemodynamic effects of distension of the dog small intestine. *Am. J. Physiol.*, 225:456–460.
45. Hanson, K. M., and Moore, F. T. (1969): Effects of intraluminal pressure in the colon on its vascular pressure-flow relationships. *Proc. Soc. Exp. Biol. Med.*, 131:373–376.
46. Hanson, K. M., and Moore, F. T. (1969): Pressure-volume relationships and blood flow in the distended colon. *Am. J. Physiol.*, 217:35–39.

47. Herczeg, B. (1973): Extravascular circulation of albumin in experimental intestinal obstruction. *Z. Exp. Chir.*, 6:337–345.
48. Hultén, L., Jodal, M., Lindhagen, J., and Lundgren, O. (1976): Colonic blood flow in cat and man as analyzed by an inert gas washout technique. *Gastroenterology*, 70:36–44.
49. Hultén, L., Jodal, M., Lindhagen, J., and Lundgren, O. (1976): Blood flow in the small intestine of cat and man as analyzed by an inert gas washout technique. *Gastroenterology*, 70:45–51.
50. Hultén, L., Lindhagen, J., and Lundgren, O. (1977): Sympathetic nervous control of intramural blood flow in the feline and human intestines. *Gastroenterology*, 72:41–48.
51. Jacobson, E. D., Brobmann, G. F., and Brecher, G. A. (1970): Intestinal motor activity and blood flow. *Gastroenterology*, 58:575–579.
52. Johnson, P. C. (1960): Autoregulation of intestinal blood flow. *Am. J. Physiol.*, 199:311–318.
53. Johnson, P. C. (1965): Effect of venous pressure on mean capillary pressure and vascular resistance in the intestine. *Circ. Res.*, 16:294–300.
54. Johnson, P. C. (1967): Autoregulation of blood flow in the intestine. *Gastroenterology*, 52:435–443.
55. Johnson, P. C., and Hanson, K. M. (1962): Effect of arterial pressure on arterial and venous resistance of intestine. *J. Appl. Physiol.*, 17:503–508.
56. Johnson, P. C., and Hanson, K. M. (1963): Relation between venous pressure and blood volume in the intestine. *Am. J. Physiol.*, 204:31–34.
57. Johnson, P. C., and Hanson, K. M. (1966): Capillary filtration in the small intestine of the dog. *Circ. Res.*, 19:766–773.
58. Johnson, P. C., and Richardson, D. R. (1974): The influences of venous pressure on filtration forces in the intestine. *Microvasc. Res.*, 7:296–306.
59. Kachelhoffer, J., Pousse, A., Marescaux, J., Hurizaga, M., and Grenier, J. F. (1978): Effects of motility and luminal distension on dog small intestine hemodynamics. *Eur. Surg. Res.*, 10:184–193.
60. Kewenter, J. (1971): Effects of graded acetylcholine infusions on intestinal motility, volume, and blood flow. *Scand. J. Gastroenterol.*, 6:434–440.
61. Kubrová, J., Robinson, J. W. L., and Mirkovitch, V. (1973): La fonction de la muqueuse après une occlusion aiguë de l'intestin grêle du rat. *Res. Exp. Med.*, 160:321–325.
62. Kvietys, P. R., and Granger, D. N. (1982): Relation between intestinal blood flow and oxygen uptake. *Am. J. Physiol.*, 242:G202–G208.
63. Larsson, M., Nylander, G., and Öhman, U. (1981): Effects of intestinal obstruction on plasma water and extracellular fluid volumes in the rat. *Surg. Gynecol. Obstet.*, 152:331–334.
64. Lawson, H., and Ambrose, A. M. (1942): The utilization of blood oxygen by the distended intestine. *Am. J. Physiol.*, 135:650–659.
65. Lawson, H., and Chumley, J. (1940): The effect of distention on blood flow through the intestine. *Am. J. Physiol.*, 131:368–377.
66. de Lorimier, A. A., Norman, D. A., Gooding, C. A., and Preger, L. (1973): A model for the cinefluoroscopic and manometric study of chronic intestinal obstruction. *J. Pediatr. Surg.*, 8:785–791.
67. Lundgren, O. (1974): The circulation of the small bowel mucosa. *Gut*, 15:1005–1013.
68. Lundgren, O., and Jodal, M. (1975): Regional blood flow. *Annu. Rev. Physiol.*, 37:395–414.
69. Lundgren, O., and Wallentin, I. (1964): Local chemical and nervous control of consecutive vascular sections in the mesenteric lymph nodes of the cat. *Angiologica*, 1:284–296.
70. MacGregor, I. L., and Lavigne, M. E. (1979): Inhibition by indomethacin of intestinal distension induced secretion in the rat. *J. Surg. Res.*, 26:167–170.
71. Mellander, S. (1960): Comparative studies on the adrenergic neuro-hormonal control of resistance and capacitance blood vessels in the cat. *Acta Physiol. Scand. (Suppl.)*, 176:1–86.
72. Merkle, P., Bindewald, H., and Betzler, M. (1975): Tierexperimentelle Untersuchungen zur Absorption und Durchblutung beim mechanischen Dünndarmileus. *Langenbecks Arch. Chir. (Suppl. Chir. Forum 1975)*, 279–282.
73. Mirkovitch, V., Cobo, F., Robinson, J. W. L., Menge, H., and Gomba, Sz. (1976): Morphology and function of the dog ileum after mechanical occlusion. *Clin. Sci. Molec. Med.*, 50:123–130.
74. Mirkovitch, V., Robinson, J. W. L., Menge, H., and Cobo, F. (1976): The consequences of ischaemia after mechanical obstruction of the dog ileum. *Res. Exp. Med.*, 168:45–55.
75. Mishra, N. K., Appert, H. E., and Howard, J. M. (1974): The effects of distention and obstruction on the accumulation of fluid in the lumen of small bowel of dogs. *Ann. Surg.*, 180:791–795.
76. Mortillaro, N. A., and Taylor, A. E. (1976): Interaction of capillary and tissue forces in the cat small intestine. *Circ. Res.*, 39:348–358.
77. Noer, R. J., and Derr, J. W. (1949): Effect of distention on intestinal revascularization. *Arch. Surg.*, 59:542–549.
78. Noer, R. J., Robb, H. J., and Jacobson, L. F. (1951): Circulatory disturbances produced by acute intestinal distention in the living animal. *Arch. Surg.*, 63:520–528.
79. Öhman, U. (1975): Studies on small intestine obstruction. I. Intraluminal pressure in experimental low small bowel obstruction in the cat. *Acta Chir. Scand.*, 141:413–416.
80. Öhman, U. (1975): Studies on small intestinal obstruction. II. Blood flow, vascular resistance, capillary filtration, and oxygen consumption in denervated small bowel after obstruction. *Acta Chir. Scand.*, 141:417–423.
81. Öhman, U. (1975): Studies on small intestinal obstruction. III. Circulatory effects of artificial small bowel distension. *Acta Chir. Scand.*, 141:536–544.
82. Öhman, U. (1975): Studies on small intestinal obstruction. IV. Circulatory effects of artificial small bowel distension after obstruction. *Acta Chir. Scand.*, 141:545–549.
83. Öhman, U. (1975): Studies on small intestinal obstruction. V. Blood circulation in moderately distended small bowel. *Acta Chir. Scand.*, 141:763–770.
84. Öhman, U. (1975): Studies on small intestinal ob-

struction. VI. Blood circulation in moderately distended small bowel after obstruction. *Acta Chir. Scand.*, 141:771–779.
85. Öhman, U. (1975): Studies on small intestinal obstruction. Blood circulation in obstructed and artificially distended small intestine in the cat. *Acta Chir. Scand. (Suppl.)*, 452:1–41.
86. Öhman, U. (1976): Blood flow and oxygen consumption in the feline small intestine; responses to artificial distension and intestinal obstruction. *Acta Chir. Scand.*, 142:329–333.
87. Öhman, U. (1979): Intestinal motility and regional blood flow. *Opusc. Med.*, 24:72–73.
88. Öhman, U. (1982): Prognosis in patients with obstructing colorectal carcinoma. *Am. J. Surg.*, 143:742–747.
89. Oppenheimer, M. J., and Mann, F. C. (1943): Intestinal capillary circulation during distension. *Surgery*, 13:548–554.
90. Ottinger, L. W. (1974): Nonocclusive mesenteric infarction. *Surg. Clin. N. Am.*, 54:689–698.
91. Owings, J. C., McIntosh, C. A., Stone, H. B., and Weinberg, J. A. (1928): Intra-intestinal pressure in obstruction. *Arch. Surg.*, 17:507–520.
92. Pappenheimer, J. R., and Soto-Rivera, A. (1948): Effective osmotic pressure of the plasma proteins and other quantities associated with the capillary circulation in the hindlimbs of cats and dogs. *Am. J. Physiol.*, 152:471–491.
93. Pawlik, W., and Jacobson, E. D. (1974): Effects of digoxin on the mesenteric circulation. *Cardiovasc. Res. Center Bull.*, 12:80–84.
94. Pawlik, W., Shepherd, A. P., Mailman, D., and Jacobson, E. D. (1974): Effects of ouabain on intestinal oxygen consumption. *Gastroenterology*, 67:100–106.
95. Póka, L., Földi, E., Czirbusz, G., Farkas, I., Bartek, I., and Lukács, L. (1969): Changes of mesenteric microcirculation in malabsorption during gastrointestinal paralysis. *Acta Chir. Acad. Sci. Hung.*, 10:311–319.
96. Price, W. E., Shehadeh, Z., Thompson, G. H., Underwood, L. D., and Jacobson, E. D. (1969): Effects of acetylcholine on intestinal blood flow and motility. *Am. J. Physiol.*, 216:343–347.
97. Rennie, J. A., Christofides, N. D., Mitchenere, P., Fletcher, D., Stockley-Leathard, H. L., Bloom, S. R., Johnson, A. G., and Harding Rains, A. J. (1980): Neural and humoral factors in postoperative ileus. *Br. J. Surg.*, 67:694–698.
98. Renton, C. J. C. (1972): Non-occlusive intestinal infarction. *Clin. Gastroenterol.*, 1:655–673.
99. Richter, H., Jostarndt, L., Tichai, I., and Thermann, M. (1976): Die Beeinflussung der Sauerstoffversorgung des Dünndarmes im Ileusmodell. *Chirurg*, 47:328–330.
100. Robert, A. (1981): Prostaglandins and the gastrointestinal tract. In: *Physiology of the Gastrointestinal Tract*, edited by L. R. Johnson, pp. 1407–1434. Raven Press, New York.
101. Robinson, J. W. L., Haroud, M., Winistörfer, B., and Mirkovitch, V. (1974): Recovery of function and structure of dog ileum and colon following two hours' acute ischaemia. *Eur. J. Clin. Invest.*, 4:443–452.
102. Robinson, J. W. L., and Mirkovitch, V. (1972): The recovery of function and microcirculation in small intestinal loops following ischaemia. *Gut*, 13:784–789.
103. Robinson, J. W. L., Mirkovitch, V., Winistörfer, B., and Saegesser, F. (1981): Response of the intestinal mucosa to ischaemia. *Gut*, 22:512–527.
104. Ruf, W., Suehiro, G., Suehiro, A., and McNamara, J. J. (1980): Small intestine blood flow after 48 hours ileus, prostigmin and manual decompression. *Z. Exp.Chir.*, 13:267–273.
105. Ruf, W., Suehiro, G. T., Suehiro, A., Pressler, V., and McNamara, J. J. (1980): Intestinal blood flow at various intraluminal pressures in the piglet with closed abdomen. *Ann. Surg.*, 191:157–163.
106. Schrock, T. R. (1981): Small intestine. In: *Current Surgical Diagnosis and Treatment*, 5th ed., edited by J. E. Dunphy and L. W. Way, pp. 547–571. Lange Medical Publications, Los Altos.
107. Schwartz, S. I., and Storer, E. H. (1979): Manifestations of gastrointestinal disease. In: *Principles of Surgery*, 3rd ed., edited by S. I. Schwartz, G. T. Shires, F. C. Spencer, and E. H. Storer, pp. 1039–1079. McGraw-Hill Book Co., New York.
108. Shanbour, L. L., and Jacobson, E. D. (1971): Autoregulatory escape in the gut. *Gastroenterology*, 60:145–148.
109. Shanbour, L. L., and Jacobson, E. D. (1972): Digitalis and the mesenteric circulation. *Am. J. Dig. Dis.*, 17:826–828.
110. Shehadeh, Z., Price, W. E., and Jacobson, E. D. (1969): Effects of vasoactive agents on intestinal blood flow and motility in the dog. *Am. J. Physiol.*, 216:386–392.
111. Shepherd, A. P. (1978): Intestinal O_2 consumption and ^{86}Rb extraction during arterial hypoxia. *Am. J. Physiol.*, 234:E248–E251.
112. Shepherd, A. P. (1982): Local control of intestinal oxygenation and blood flow. *Annu. Rev. Physiol.*, 44:13–27.
113. Shepherd, A. P., and Granger, H. J. (1973): Autoregulatory escape in the gut: A systems analysis. *Gastroenterology*, 65:77–91.
114. Shields, R. (1965): The absorption and secretion of fluid and electrolytes by the obstructed bowel. *Br. J. Surg.*, 52:774–779.
115. Shields, M. A., and Dudley, H. A. F. (1971): Effects of open and closed decompression on the water content and motility of experimentally obstructed small bowel in the rabbit. *Br. J. Surg.*, 58:337–339.
116. Shikata, J., Shida, T., Amino, K., and Ishioka, K. (1983): Experimental studies on the hemodynamics of the small intestine following increased intraluminal pressure. *Surg. Gynecol. Obstet.*, 156:155–160.
117. Singleton, A. O., Jr., and Montalbo, P. (1968): Effects of decompression during removal of intestinal obstruction. *Ann. Surg.*, 167:909–911.
118. Sperling, L., Paine, J. R., and Wangensteen, O. H. (1935): Intra-enteric pressure in experimental and clinical intestinal obstruction. *Proc. Soc. Exp. Biol. Med.*, 32:1504–1506.
119. Sung, D. T. W., and Williams, L. F., Jr. (1971): Intestinal secretion after intravenous fluid infusion in small bowel obstruction. *Am. J. Surg.*, 121:91–95.
120. Swabb, E. A., Hynes, R. A., and Donowitz, M. (1982):

Elevated intraluminal pressure alters rabbit small intestinal transport in vivo. *Am. J. Physiol.*, 242:G58–G64.
121. Swabb, E. A., Hynes, R. A., Marnane, W. G., McNeil, J. S., Decker, R. A., Tai, Y.-H., and Donowitz, M. (1982): Intestinal filtration-secretion due to increased intraluminal pressure in rabbits. *Am. J. Physiol.*, 242:G65–G75.
122. Tasaka, K., and Farrar, J. T. (1976): Intraluminal pressure of the small intestine of the unanesthetized dog. *Pflügers Arch.*, 364:35–44.
123. Tepperman, B. L., and Jacobson, E. D. (1981): Mesenteric circulation. In: *Physiology of the Gastrointestinal Tract*, edited by L. R. Johnson, pp. 1317–1336. Raven Press, New York.
124. Tunick, P. A., Treiber, W. F., Jr., Frank, M., Veith, F. J., Gliedman, M. L., and Boley, S. J. (1970): Pathophysiological effects of bowel distention on intestinal blood flow (II). *Curr. Top. Surg. Res.*, 2:59–69.
125. Wangensteen, O. H. (1955): *Intestinal Obstructions*, 3rd ed. Charles C Thomas, Springfield.
126. Wetterfors, J. (1965): Some aspects of the behaviour of serum albumin in intestinal obstruction. *Acta Chir. Scand.*, 130:521–536.
127. Wickstrom, P., Haglin, J. J., and Hitchcock, C. R. (1973): Intraoperative decompression of the obstructed small bowel. *Surgery*, 73:212–219.
128. Wójtowicz, J., Wirga, Z., and Wirga, E. (1975): Angiographic patterns in experimental obstruction of the small bowel. *Invest. Radiol.*, 10:583–594.
129. Wright, H. K., O'Brien, J. J., and Tilson, M. D. (1971): Water absorption in experimental closed segment obstruction of the ileum in man. *Am. J. Surg.*, 121:96–99.
130. Zeigler, M. G., Barton, R. W., and Swan, K. G. (1973): Mesenteric blood flow and small intestinal motility in the dog. *Surgery*, 73:649–656.
131. van Zwalenburg, C. (1907): Strangulation resulting from distention of hollow viscera. *Ann. Surg.*, 46:780–786.

Portal Hypertension

Charles L. Witte and Marlys H. Witte

Department of Surgery, University of Arizona College of Medicine, Tucson, Arizona 85724

One of the most serious and vexing disorders of the splanchnic circulation is hepatic portal venous hypertension. What makes it serious are potentially life-threatening complications of gastrointestinal hemorrhage and intraabdominal fluid accumulation. What makes it vexing is the complexity of portal system hemodynamics and the relative inaccessibility of the visceral circulation to direct measurement.

Strategically situated between the digestive tract and liver, the portal system is both an outlet for intestinal, pancreatic, and splenic venous blood and the dominant blood supply to the liver. Some investigators (7) propose that portal "artery" is a better term for this anomalous arrangement, perhaps in an analogy to the pulmonary artery, which transports blood from systemic veins while perfusing the lungs. But with a low intraluminal pressure (≈ 10 mm Hg), a relatively thin vascular wall, and marked pressure sensitivity to comparatively small resistance shifts downstream, the designation portal "vein" seems appropriate.

In this chapter, we examine varix hemorrhage and ascites, the two major clinical sequelae of portal hypertension, and we explore their underlying pathomechanisms and current approaches to treatment.

VARIX HEMORRHAGE

Gastrointestinal hemorrhage from rupture of large varicose veins at the lower end of the esophagus and upper stomach is prima facie evidence of portal hypertension. Most commonly an outward manifestation of hepatic cirrhosis, varix hemorrhage also develops in conjunction with isolated portal vein thrombosis, nonfibrosing liver disease (e.g., nodular transformation or hyperplasia), and a wide spectrum of hematologic and congenital disorders with prominent splenomegaly and hyperdynamic splenic blood flow. Whereas bleeding varices are generally viewed as a direct consequence of portal hypertension and the latter, in turn, of obstructed portal blood flow, the precise hemodynamic derangements responsible for elevated portal pressure and the specific factors initiating esophagogastric hemorrhage are unclear. For example, progressive occlusion of the portal vein in animals rarely raises portal pressure chronically to the high level (>25 mm Hg) typically encountered in patients with cirrhosis or long-standing extrahepatic portal block. Furthermore, rupture of varices has not been reproduced experimentally despite diverse circulatory maneuvers designed to simulate the dynamics of portal hypertension (16). Moreover, there is no direct correlation in patients with cirrhosis between bleeding from varices and the level of portal pressure or severity of hepatic fibrosis. To some extent these apparent inconsistencies are rooted in long-held but overly simplified concepts of the pathogenesis of portal hypertension and its complications.

Portal venous pressure depends on intrahepatic resistance and the magnitude of splanchnic blood flow. Because of the unique anatomical configuration of the visceral circulation, however, the pressure at any given moment reflects a fluctuating but interrelated set of blood flows and vascular resistances in the hepatic, intestinal, splenic, and systemic circuits. Nonetheless, extensive anatomic and physiologic studies indicate that a constant component of clinical portal hypertension is heightened resistance to portal blood flow, and despite proliferation of an enormous collateral network linking the portal and systemic circulations, portal pressure gradually rises. Although the portal system is commonly said to be "stagnant" or "passively congested," these designations are misleading. In contrast to congestive heart failure or sudden experimental narrowing of the portal vein, where blood flow slows and venous oxygen saturation falls, splanchnic venous blood is well oxygenated in patients with long-standing portal hypertension, and intestinal and splenic blood flow are rapid (15). Indeed, high cardiac output at rest, lowered systemic vascular resistance, and "spider" angiomata, signs of a hyperdynamic circulation, are common in hepatic cirrhosis. Hyperdynamic splanchnic blood flow is also a major component of portal hypertension associated with large splenic, hepatic, or intestinal arterioportal fistulae as well as myeloproliferative disorders with massive splenomegaly (16). In these conditions, fistula closure or splenectomy not only controls the hyperdynamic circuit but often alleviates varix hemorrhage and ascites. On the basis of these examples and the relation between congestive splenomegaly (another complication of portal hypertension) and hyperdynamic splenic blood flow, it has been suggested that the dominant hemodynamic abnormality in portal hypertension is rapid splanchnic blood flow rather than a restriction to portal flow (6).

Although obstruction to portal venous flow alone (backward theory) is probably an oversimplified explanation for portal hypertension, so, too, is hyperdynamic visceral arterial flow (forward theory). Experimentally, doubling or even tripling splanchnic blood flow induces only mildly elevated portal pressure, whereas clinically infusion of vasoactive drugs restricting splanchnic inflow or ligation of gastrosplenic arteries rarely if ever eliminates portal hypertension (16). Although hepatic arterial flow may be disproportionately elevated in patients with cirrhosis and although high volume flow after portacaval shunt has a favorable prognosis (3), adjustments in hepatic arterial flow probably derive from autoregulatory responses to diminishing transhepatic portal flow or alternatively from neovascularization to regenerating nodules and Glisson's capsule in the cirrhotic liver (16). Because the absolute level of portal pressure depends on both splanchnic blood flow and portal venous resistance, coexistent derangements in both visceral vascular compartments probably contribute to portal hypertension (15) (Fig. 1). In the portal stenotic rat, for example, splanchnic arteriolar dilation accompanies elevated portal pressure and high-grade portasystemic shunting (2,12). Moreover, portal hypertension in patients derives from a wide spectrum of hemodynamic patterns ranging from near-complete obstruction of portal venous flow (e.g., far advanced cirrhosis or portal vein occlusion), to mild restriction of portal flow but with markedly hyperdynamic splanchnic blood flow (e.g., Gaucher's Disease), to moderate elevation in both splanchnic blood flow and portal venous resistance (e.g., myeloproliferative disorders; see Table 1).

Whereas increased resistance to portal flow is probably a prerequisite for severe portal hypertension, the magnitude of splanchnic arterial flow ultimately controls the height of portal pressure (i.e., "active congestion"). In other words, as resistance to transhepatic portal flow rises, splanchnic venous flow is rerouted through small caliber high-resistance venous collaterals under greater pressure rather than through the low-pressure hepatic sinusoids. In this setting, a small increment in splanchnic blood flow (e.g., alcohol ingestion or food consumption), ordinarily having little effect on venous pressure because of substantial reserve compliance of large visceral veins, sharply raises portal pressure. In accordance with hydraulic principles, when intraluminal pressure raises wall tension beyond the bursting potential of thin-wall collateral veins, bleeding of esophageal varices ensues. Lack of direct correlation between portal pressure and varix bleeding does not refute this "explosive theory" because bursting also depends on muscular thickness of the vein and surrounding esophageal wall. Thus, the venous channel with the greatest wall tension is the wide-lumen portal vein, which with acquired

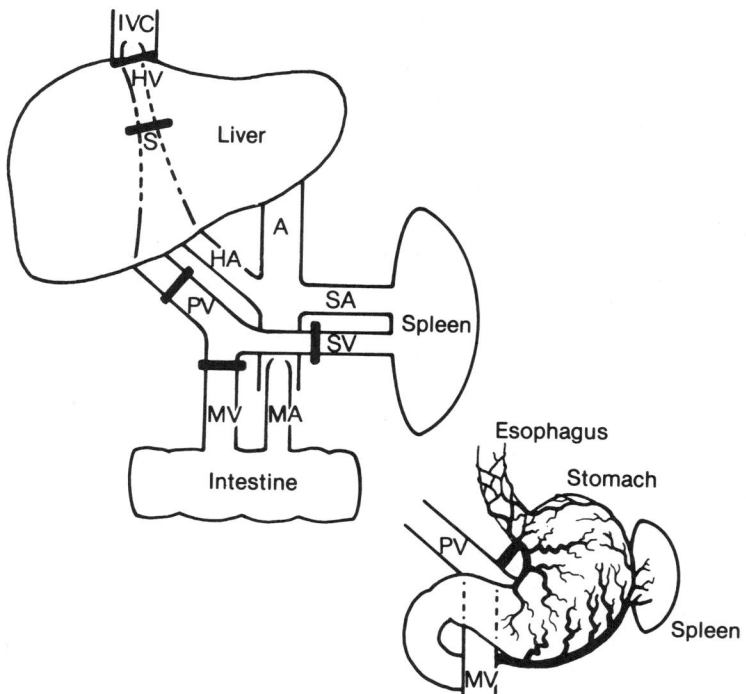

FIG. 1. Schematic diagram of visceral circulation in portal hypertension, including collateral venous tributaries from the portal (PV), mesenteric (MV), and splenic (SV) veins to the distal esophagus and stomach (esophagogastric varices). Although elevated resistance to portal territorial flow occurs at various sites *(bars)*, increased splenic (SA), mesenteric (MA), or hepatic (HA) arterial inflow may also contribute to elevated portal pressure. A, aorta; HV, hepatic vein; S, hepatic sinusoid; IVC, inferior vena cava. (See Table 1 for clinical manifestations and text for discussion of "active" vs "passive" congestion in this syndrome.)

phlebosclerosis and thicker muscle, however, never spontaneously disrupts. On the other hand, thinner collateral varices of lesser lumen size and muscle content may burst with lower tensile strength at the same intraluminal pressure. Also, contrary to common teaching, when varix bleeding is massive, blood is often seen to move en masse from submucosa to gastric lumen, appearing as a diffuse ooze from a reddened stomach rather than emanating from a discrete bleeding vein. When these examples of so-called diffuse gastritis, nonspecific gastric erosions, and no single bleeding site are grouped with clearly identified variceal rupture, more than 85% of gastrointestinal bleeding in patients with known esophagogastric varices is ultimately traceable to elevated portal pressure (10). Furthermore, venous decompression by portacaval shunt promptly arrests digestive tract hemorrhage in these individuals, corroborating that portal hypertension is the predominant cause of the bleeding (10).

NONOPERATIVE THERAPY

The treatment of bleeding varices particularly from liver disease is notoriously difficult. Hepatocellular function is marginal at the outset, and hypovolemia, tranfusion of blood and blood products, and a gastrointestinal tract filled with blood further aggravate metabolic derangements. Jaundice, blood-clotting deficiencies, confusion and coma ("ammonia intoxication") result. A major operation under these conditions is clearly hazardous. Sometimes bleeding spontaneously ceases presumably from sudden reduction in splanchnic blood flow during oligemia. Continued bleeding, however, requires prompt

TABLE 1. *Portal hemodynamics and major clinical manifestations*

Primary circulatory derangement	Clinical example	Varix hemorrhage	Ascites	Splenomegaly
I. Portal system block				
a. Hepatic veins	Budd-Chiari Syndrome	+ +	+ + + +	Moderate
b. Hepatic sinusoid	Hepatic cirrhosis	+ + + +	+ + + +	Marked
c. Portal vein	Venous thrombosis	+ + + +	+	Marked
d. Splenic vein	Venous thrombosis	+ + +	Absent	Variable
e. Superior mesenteric vein	Venous thrombosis	Absent	+ +[a]	Absent
II. Hyperdynamic visceral flow				
a. Spleen				
1. No PSB	Hereditary spherocytosis	Absent	Absent	Marked
2. With PSB (Ia,b,c, or d)	Myeloid metaplasia	+ + +	+ +	Massive
b. Intestine				
1. No PSB	Traumatic A-V fistula	?	?	Absent
2. With PSB (Ia,b,c, or d)	A-V fistula with liver fibrosis	+ + +	+ +	Marked
c. Liver				
1. No PSB	Hepatic A-P fistula	Absent	+	Absent
2. With PSB (Ia or b)	Cirrhosis; hepatic A-P fistula with liver fibrosis	+ + + +	+ + + +	Marked

A-V, arteriovenous; PSB, portal system blockade; A-P, arterioportal; + + + +, very common; + + +, common; + +, variable incidence; +, rare; ?, questionable occurrence.
[a]Usually bloody with bowel infarction.

pharmacologic or mechanical manipulation to restrict gastric blood flow or alternatively to compress and thereby disconnect high-pressure collateral channels linking the portal vein to azygos system at the lower end of the esophagus (Table 2). Intravenous infusion of vasopressin, a potent splanchnic vasoconstrictor, is usually initially effective (see Chapter 31). This hormone has only mild, transient adverse effects on hepatic arterial flow, but unfortunately it is a powerful coronary artery vasoconstrictor with undesirable effects on cardiac rhythm and performance. Simultaneous with parenteral vasopressin, gastric lavage with iced saline further decreases distal esophageal blood flow. Perhaps best known but potentially dangerous is the intragastric balloon tube. This device positioned in the upper stomach with the gastric balloon inflated with a large volume of air effectively compresses gastric venous collaterals. Varix hemorrhage usually stops immediately not only providing stop-gap control for up to 48 hr but also confirming the source and site of bleeding.

Although not strictly noninvasive, other approaches directly attack varices without formal thoracotomy or laparotomy. Analogous to percutaneous transhepatic cholangiography for anatomic delineation of bile ducts, percutaneous transhepatic (or alternatively transumbilical) portography has undergone extensive testing both as a method to unravel portal hemodynamics as well as to treat bleeding varices. Under fluoroscopy, a catheter is threaded over a flexible wire through the liver substance into the portal system. In addition to portal pressure measurement, visualization of variant natural shunt pathways and directional determinations of flow, the superselective catheter placement into collateral veins traversing the esophagogastric juncture allows intravariceal instillation of thrombogenic agents. With combinations of concentrated dextrose, thrombin, gelatin sponge, or rapid-congealing cyanoacrylates, occlusion of large varices and arrest of hemorrhage are possible, albeit transitory because of venous recanalization or neocollateralization. Moreover, the procedure is not without risk, including immediate or delayed portal vein thrombosis (1). A similar approach undergoing strong resurgence is transendoscopic sclerosis of esoph-

TABLE 2. *Treatment modalities in portal hypertension*

Approach	Non-operative	Operative
Varix hemorrhage		
Decrease visceral arterial inflow	Vasopressin, propranolol, iced gastric lavage	Splenectomy, ligation GSA, balloon occlusion SMA
Obliterate varices	Balloon tube tamponade	Sclerosis (endoscopic, transhepatic), P-A disconnection (staple-gun)
Decrease portal venous resistance		
Total PSS	—	P-C, M-C, proximal S-R
Segmental PSS	—	Coronary V-C, distal S-R
Ascites		
Decrease lymph formation Increase lymph absorption	Salt-water restricted diet, diuretic drugs	P-C shunt Peritoneovenous shunts, abdominal paracentesis, TD-S reconstruction

GSA, gastrosplenic arteries; SMA, superior mesenteric artery; P-A, portal-azygos; PSS, portasystemic shunt; P-C, portacaval; M-C, mesocaval; S-R, splenorenal; V-C, venacaval; TD-S, thoracic duct-subclavian venous.

ageal varices. Here, as with varicosities of the legs, irritating drugs are instilled through a rigid or flexible endoscope into the lower esophageal veins repeatedly over months or even years to stimulate thrombosis and obliteration.

Recently, long-term oral administration of a β-blocker (e.g., propranolol) has been advocated to control varix hemorrhage (8) by reducing cardiac output and, secondarily, splanchnic blood flow. This "new" approach thereby reemphasizes curtailment of inflow rather than lowering elevated venous resistance for portal decompression.

OPERATIVE THERAPY

Conventional operations for varix bleeding can be divided into two major categories: "shunt" and "nonshunt." The objective of various portasystemic shunt operations is to decrease varix pressure indirectly by lowering outflow resistance to portal, mesenteric, or splenic venous flow. Nonshunt procedures, like nonoperative approaches, are directed at restricting arterial inflow or obliterating the bleeding site (Table 2). Portasystemic shunts can be further subdivided into "total" and "selective." Because the portal system is valveless, decompression of the entire venous network including varices is feasible provided the shunt is large enough to accommodate the considerable flow of blood. After construction of a side-to-side anastomosis, the portal vein functions as an outflow tract, and both gut and liver are decompressed. An end-to-side portacaval shunt, however, fully decompresses only the extrahepatic splanchnic bed, and though this procedure has been criticized particularly when ascites coexists, the clinical outcome of different total shunts are comparable.

Despite the undisputed success of portasystemic shunts in alleviating varix hemorrhage, long-term survival has been discouraging particularly in cirrhosis. A persistent lifestyle of drunkenness and poor diet subjects these individuals to fatal auto accidents, barroom brawls, infections, malnutrition, and progressive hepatocellular dysfunction. In others, both alcoholic and nonalcoholic, abstract thinking and mental acuity may be severely impaired, reflecting either marginal hepatic function or high blood levels of nitrogenous substances bypassing the liver.

Because total portal diversion carries a high morbidity and mortality, and because varix hemorrhage typically occurs at the esophagogastric juncture, attention has turned to selective decompression of lesser splanchnic veins (i.e., gastrosplenic) with maintenance of greater splanchnic (mesenteric) portal hypertension and transhepatic portal flow. Although manipulation of venous flow at one site might be expected to exert a similar response throughout a valveless system, a strategically located but small venous shunt can nonetheless decompress esophagogastric varices directly without concomitantly diverting a substantial fraction of portal blood flow. However, variability in size and accessibility of accessory coronary veins and difficulty with long-term patency sharply limit gastrocaval shunting.

Perhaps a sounder operation along these lines is the distal splenorenal shunt (13). Recognizing that segmental obstruction of the splenic vein may precipitate esophagogastric hemorrhage despite patency of the mesenteric-portal system (hence the designation sinistral or left-sided portal hypertension), Warren et al. (13) propose selective decompression of esophageal varices by division of the splenic vein and anastomosis of the *distal* segment into the renal vein. Along with ligation of major bridging veins between greater and lesser splanchnic systems (e.g., gastroepiploic, coronary, umbilical veins), esophagogastric varices are decompressed with preservation of mesenteroportal flow into the liver. Although technically difficult, distal splenorenal shunts thus far show a lower incidence of severe postshunt encephalopathy compared with total shunts (13). Survival of alcoholic patients, however, has not been improved, raising the specter once again that alcoholism is crucial in mortality regardless of treatment. Moreover, unless coexistent ascites is readily manageable with diuretic drugs and salt restriction beforehand, segmental shunting is probably unwise. Portal hypertension persists in the greater splanchnic system and after transection of congested lymphatic trunks at the root of the mesentery and over the pancreas, intractable ascites and renal failure may ensue (see Ascites).

Although a distal splenorenal shunt seemingly has little advantage over a total shunt in management of pure extrahepatic portal block, some transhepatic portal flow is usually reestablished around the site of obstruction. Because a total shunt removes this quantum (albeit small) of portal perfusion, a distal splenorenal shunt has also been advocated for extrahepatic portal block and even far-advanced cirrhosis with marginal portal flow to the liver (13).

Because shunt operations are technically demanding with substantial immediate and delayed morbidity and mortality, a variety of nonshunt operations have been recommended to control bleeding while preserving liver function. In massive hemorrhage, the most direct approach is to oversew the bleeding site, that is, varicosities in the lower esophagus. Unfortunately, direct transthoracic ligation has an unacceptably high early rebleeding rate, and transabdominal varix ligation combined with high gastric bisection (Tanner's operation), even when done using rapid-fire stapling guns, has a prohibitive mortality. From an extensive experience in Japan, Sigiura and Futagawa (11) advocate thoracoabdominal exploration with meticulous ligation of all visible portal-azygos collateral veins, esophageal transection, and reanastomosis, vagotomy, pyloroplasty, and splenectomy. The operation is formidable, the hazards great, and as yet, no other major center describes comparable results.

Because flow dynamics in patients with portal hypertension vary, the pathophysiology and optimal treatment of varix hemorrhage remain controversial. For example, some surgeons, impressed with the hyperdynamic or "forward" features of splanchnic blood flow in liver disease, manage varix hemorrhage by interruption of major arteries to the upper stomach (ascending left gastric, short gastrics, gastroepiploics, and splenic) and splenectomy (6). However, as in earlier attempts to stem variceal bleeding by ligating gastrosplenic arteries, this approach disregards the torrent of blood passing into the portal system via mesenteric arteries and independently reaching esophagogastric varices. Others (5) advocate transthoracic transposition of the engorged spleen (another feature of portal hypertension) to stimulate collateralization between perisplenic veins and superior vena caval tributaries. Still others suggest occlusion of splenic arterial inflow, sometimes combined with splenic transposition into the lateral abdominal wall, to facilitate retrograde diversion of mesenteric flow from esophageal varices into the splenic vein and newly acquired collaterals (16). Although sporadically successful, these procedures as a group have a higher incidence of rebleeding but not necessarily lower patient survival compared with shunt operations.

ASCITES

Palpable fluid within the peritoneal cavity is the other major complication of portal hypertension. Whereas ascites rarely accompanies portal hypertension from extrahepatic portal block, it is common in hepatic cirrhosis. Starling's Law of the capillary makes it clear that accumulation of extracellular fluid in tissues (edema) or body cavities (effusion) represents an imbalance between net capillary filtration and its return as lymph to the bloodstream. Suffusion associated with absent or obstructed lymphatics traditionally is termed lymphedema or low output failure of lymph flow. However, accumulation of extracellular fluid from excessive capillary filtration with accelerated but insufficient lymph return is another type of imbalance—high output failure of lymph flow, of which ascites in hepatic cirrhosis is a prototype (17). Fluid retention is largely restricted to the peritoneal cavity, and elevation in portal venous but not central venous pressure with markedly increased thoracic duct lymph flow indicates that increased leakage of fluid from visceral capillaries is the primary abnormality. At the same time, progressive weight gain with accumulation of excess body fluid reflects abnormal renal retention of ingested salt and water. Not surprisingly, therefore, the typical patient with "cirrhotic" ascites shows limited ability to excrete salt and water in the urine along with high serum renin activity and aldosterone level. Salt and water homeostasis is complex, but the end result of this renal dysfunction is to expand extracellular fluid, aggravate the imbalance in capillary dynamics from portal hypertension, and further increase lymph formation, thereby leading to greater sequestration of peritoneal fluid (Fig. 2). From this unifying hypothesis of ascites formation, it follows that treatment designed to restore balance in lymph dynamics, either by diminishing lymph formation or enhancing lymph return, is likely to ameliorate ascites.

DIURETIC DRUGS

The simplest approach to reduce the burden of lymph is to reverse renal salt and water retention by promoting a diuresis and natriuresis. By periodic contraction of the plasma compartment with indirect reduction in visceral capillary pressure and total surface area for transcapillary exchange, diuresis lowers the "driving" force for fluid movement, retards lymph formation, and potentiates resorption of trapped abdominal fluid into the bloodstream. Intermittent administration of these agents (furosemide, ethacrynic acid, spironolactone, or triamterene), especially when combined with dietary salt restriction, brings lymph dynamics into balance and improves ascites despite persistent hepatocellular dysfunction (17).

PORTASYSTEMIC SHUNT

In contrast to diuretic drugs and salt restriction, a portasystemic shunt decreases lymph formation directly by eliminating the predominant force (elevated hydrostatic pressure) favoring fluid transudation. Although this procedure is no longer justified solely for ascites from liver disease, past experience bears directly on pathomechanisms. Moreover, the physiologic effects of various venous shunt operations are of utmost importance in deciding a course of action when ascites accompanies life-threatening varix bleeding or results from hepatic vein occlusion (Budd-Chiari syndrome), a disorder of intense liver congestion.

Because experimental portal vein obstruction is rarely complicated by ascites whereas prolonged constriction of the hepatic veins or inferior vena cava above but not below the diaphragm promotes "weeping" of lymph from the hepatic surface into the peritoneal cavity, the liver has been considered the most likely source of ascites in patients with hepatic disease. Paucity of hepatic vein radicles in cast corrosions of

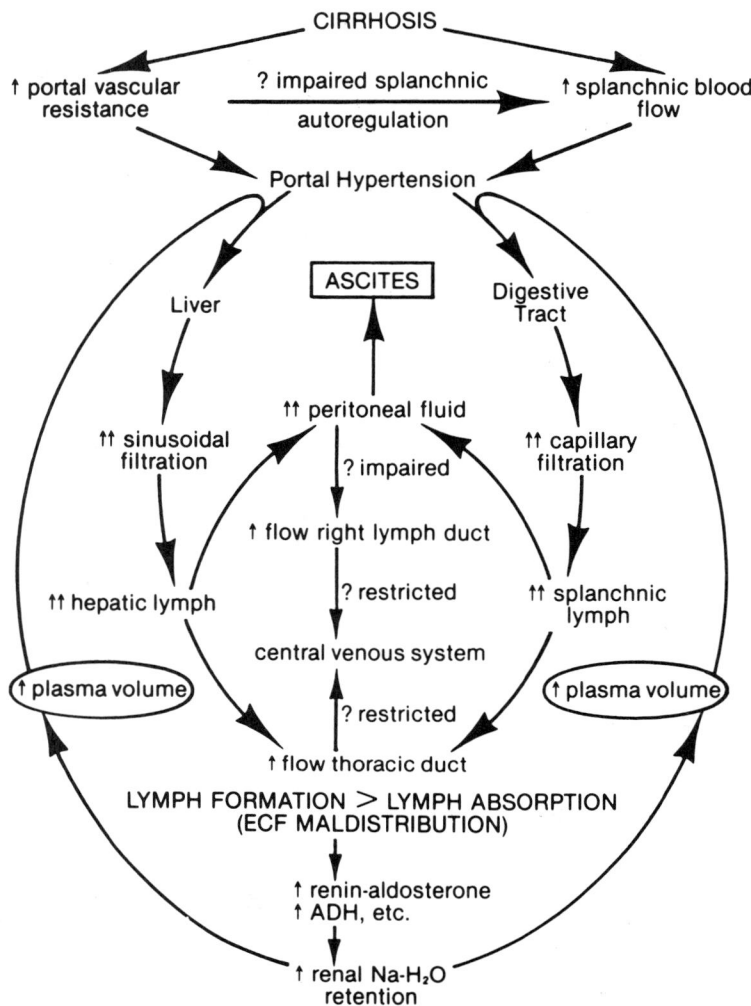

FIG. 2. "Lymph imbalance" theory of ascites. Ascites in hepatic cirrhosis primarily derives from a maldistribution of extracellular fluid volume. Driven by elevated portal pressure, edema fluid extravasates into the liver, digestive tract, and peritoneal cavity. When lymph formation exceeds lymph return, homeostatic renal-endocrine responses are activated. Further expansion of the plasma compartment increases fluid extravasation in the liver and extrahepatic portal bed aggravating the lymph imbalance and leading to progressive ascites. (From Witte et al., ref. 17, with permission.)

cirrhotic liver, similar elevations of hepatic wedge and splenic pulp pressure in alcoholic cirrhosis, and enlarged hepatic lymphatics adjacent to the portal vein further substantiate the existence of perisinusoidal obstruction in patients with cirrhosis and the likelihood of hepatic origin of ascitic fluid (17,19).

Other findings question whether the cirrhotic liver is the sole or even major source of ascites in most patients. Anatomically the multinodular fibrotic liver bears only a superficial resemblance to a congested liver (14), and the dense thickened capsule seems a distinct mechanical barrier to free passage and "weepage" of hepatic tissue fluid. On the other hand, in portal hypertension from cirrhosis, weeping of excessive fluid from the parietal peritoneum and serosal surfaces of the bowel is often striking at operation along with widely dilated lymphatics on the surface of the small intestine, mesentery, and within the retroperitoneal space. Ascites also accumulates at an accelerated rate when portal vein occlusion from thrombosis or invasion by hepatoma is superimposed upon hepatic cirrhosis. Finally, ascites often subsides after an end-to-side portacaval shunt, an operation much more effective in decompressing the splanchnic bed than the liver (17,19).

To understand these apparent contradictions, it is worthwhile to reexamine tissue fluid composition in the liver and extrahepatic portal bed in light of the underlying microcirculatory dynamics. In the liver, experimental and clinical conditions exhibiting congestion from posthepatic venous obstruction are characterized by an outpouring of hepatic and thoracic duct lymph as well as ascitic fluid rich in protein (17). Prehepatic restriction to portal flow, in contrast, produces an outpouring of splanchnic and thoracic duct lymph of progressively lower protein content ("protein washdown" effect) (17).

A wide range of protein content is found in the visceral fluids of patients with cirrhosis, but the usual pattern is ascitic fluid, splanchnic lymph, and thoracic duct lymph of low protein content, signifying a major contribution from extrahepatic portal capillaries (17,19). After portacaval shunt, thoracic duct lymph flow falls while protein content rises. In some patients with cirrhosis, however, protein content of hepatic lymph is low, indicating again that a cirrhotic liver is not simply a congested liver. Development of a continuous endothelial lining in the sinusoid (so-called capillarization) and collagen accumulation in the spaces of Disse probably restrict free movement of macromolecules (17,19).

Two disorders contributing to confusion over the origin of ascites in portal hypertension are extrahepatic portal block and hepatic vein block or Budd-Chiari syndrome (Table 2). In the former, ascites is rare *(vide supra)*, whereas in the latter, ascitic fluid is common but sometimes low rather than high in protein. These findings have called into question the value of "protein data" in visceral fluids and refocused attention on the liver as the chief source of ascitic fluid. Nonetheless, ascitic fluid that occasionally develops in the course of isolated portal block is uniformly low in protein *(personal observations)* reflecting protein washdown in the digestive tract, its site of origin. On the other hand, patients with Budd-Chiari syndrome who demonstrate low protein ascitic fluid invariably exhibit severe coexistent extrahepatic portal hypertension, often with overtly bleeding esophagogastric varices. Alternatively, hepatic vein block may develop fortuitously with preexistent cirrhosis, or cirrhosis may evolve from long-standing Budd-Chiari syndrome. In these latter two situations, extrahepatic rather than intrahepatic portal hypertension is the predominant hemodynamic derangement, and ascitic fluid is low in protein. When extrahepatic portal block develops in conjunction with hepatic disease, the burden of excess intestinal lymph added to the excess lymph produced by the liver apparently overwhelms regional and central lymph trunks, often producing massive ascites. Furthermore, whether occurring as an isolated phenomenon or in conjunction with cirrhosis, intraabdominal tumors, or peritonitis, ascitic fluid associated with portal block is characteristically low in protein (18). Thus, rather than violating pathophysiologic principles, interpretation of ascitic fluid protein measurements in the clinical context confirms the dual origin of ascites in portal hypertension and the likelihood in liver disease that the major source of ascitic fluid is the digestive tract.

PERITONEO- AND LYMPHATIC-VENOUS SHUNTS

Two major lymphatic pathways are involved in ascitic fluid formation. First, visceral lymph trunks merge into the thoracic duct and transport excess tissue fluid emanating from the liver and digestive tract. Second, the diaphragmatic, retrosternal, and right lymph duct system drain the peritoneal cavity. While lymph spills into the peritoneal cavity when tissue "safety factors" including visceral lymph drainage capacity are overwhelmed, palpable ascites signifies that absorptive capacity of the diaphragmatic system is also exceeded.

Ascites diminishes after lymph formation is slowed *(vide supra)* and should do likewise after lymph return is accelerated. Unfortunately, factors limiting flow and propulsion in the lymphatic system are still speculative but probably include impaired intrinsic pumping action, overdistention, and functional narrowing of the thoracic duct-venous junction. Amelioration of ascites after either construction of a thoracic duct-azygos vein shunt in dogs with hepatic venous outflow block or widening of the central lymph-venous junction by thoracic duct-jugular vein anastomosis in a small number of patients with "cirrhotic" ascites support the lymph imbalance theory. Although technical difficulties in constructing lymphatic shunts preclude wider use, a recent simplified method for recirculating ascitic fluid (spilled lymph) from the peritoneal cavity to the systemic circulation is a practical application of the lymph balance principle. Insertion of a prosthetic peritoneovenous bypass shunt acts as a "megalymphatic" to speed up lymph return to the bloodstream. Although this maneuver, like a portacaval shunt or diuretic drugs with dietary salt restriction, does not directly improve hepatocellular function, conversion of high output failure of lymph flow to a high output compensated state not only reduces even massive ascites (Fig. 3) but may also promptly reverse profound disturbances in salt and water homeostasis, including the hepatorenal syndrome (17). Hazardous complications of local and systemic infections, superior vena cava thrombosis, and disseminated intravascular coagulopathy, however, preclude frivolous implantation of the device (4).

ONCOTIC PRESSURE

Because portal pressure does not reliably predict the presence of ascites, a concomitant derangement in colloid osmotic pressure has frequently been invoked as an important contributory factor. Patients with liver ailments often have low plasma albumin and, accordingly, decreased plasma oncotic pressure. This disturbance is usually attributed to defective protein synthesis by the diseased liver. Although such an explanation for hypoalbuminemia is open

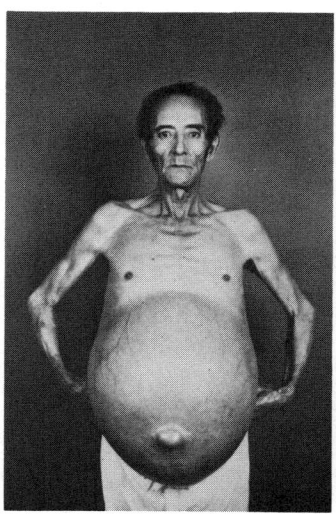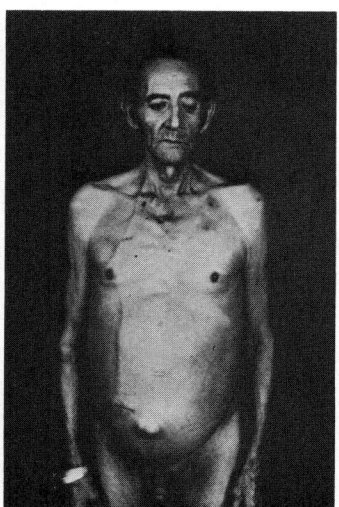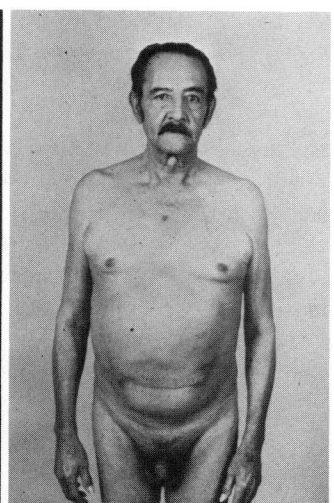

FIG. 3. Marked improvement in a 60-year-old man with massive ascites from hepatic cirrhosis before **(left)**, 10 days after **(middle)**, and 2 years after **(right)** insertion of peritoneovenous shunt, following which a prompt diuresis and natriuresis ensued, and high plasma renin activity and aldosterone level fell to normal.

to question in view of normal or increased albumin synthesis in many cirrhotic patients (9), it is nonetheless the gradient in oncotic pressure between plasma and tissues rather than the absolute level of plasma oncotic pressure that tends to counterbalance the elevated transcapillary gradient in hydrostatic pressure. Although Starling's "Law" defines the direction and magnitude of net transcapillary fluid flux, ultimately the balance between the amount of lymph removed and net filtration determines whether excess tissue fluid accumulates. When the issue of oncotic pressure is reexamined in this light, it appears unlikely that hypoalbuminemia contributes significantly to ascites formation. In the hepatic sinusoid with its large endothelial gaps, plasma oncotic pressure plays little or no role in regulating transsinusoidal fluid fluxes and, therefore, hepatic lymph formation. [In the cirrhotic liver a slight or greater restriction to movement of macromolecules apparently develops, but the overall effect is to raise, not lower, the oncotic gradient and thereby oppose, not aggravate, formation of excess hepatic lymph from elevated hydrostatic pressure (16).] In the splanchnic bed, the protein washdown effect lowering tissue oncotic pressure either parallels or exceeds the fall in plasma oncotic pressure, maintaining or even widening the oncotic gradient, thereby minimally aggravating or even opposing excess capillary filtration (17) (Fig. 4).

Thus, it is not surprising that the plasma albumin level correlates poorly with the presence of ascites. Low plasma albumin may simply signify "dilution" of the albumin pool from an extracellular fluid expansion set into motion by the cycle of ascites formation. Exogenous administration of albumin is also of little practical use in treatment of ascites. Portal hypertension may worsen during plasma volume expansion, and any slight rise in plasma albumin is dissipated through equilibration with tissue albumin levels (17).

SUMMARY

Although bleeding esophagogastric varices and ascites are the major complications of portal hypertension, the pathogenesis of these phe-

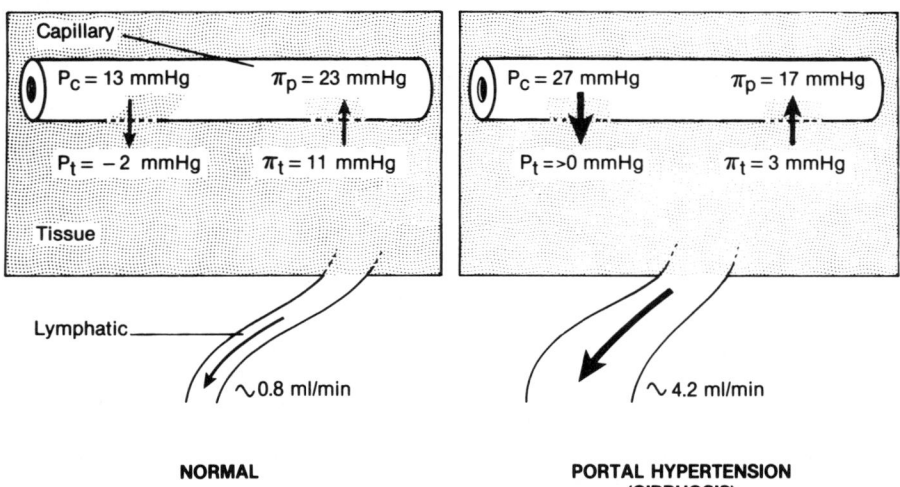

FIG. 4. Estimated capillary (Starling) forces in the normal and portal hypertensive digestive tract. Note that in cirrhosis marked elevation in capillary hydrostatic pressure (P_c) promotes increased intestinal capillary filtration and lymph flow as well as "protein washdown" of the interstitium (π_t). Thus, despite a substantial reduction in plasma oncotic pressure (π_p) from hypoalbuminemia, effective oncotic pressure gradient ($\pi_p - \pi_t$) remains high. P_t, tissue hydrostatic pressure.

nomena involves much more than mere elevation of portal pressure.

Spontaneous rupture of esophagogastric varices develops when increased splanchnic blood flow encounters heightened and relatively fixed portal venous resistance. The greater the restriction to transhepatic portal venous flow, the less the increment in splanchnic blood flow required to generate portal pressure ultimately exceeding the bursting tensile strength of thin-walled varices. Operative treatment includes interrupting varices directly, lowering resistance to esophagogastric venous flow (generalized or segmental portasystemic shunt), or, in selected patients, restricting hyperdynamic arterial inflow. Drug therapy generally aims to curtail splanchnic inflow either by constricting splanchnic arterioles or by reducing cardiac output and, secondarily, splanchnic inflow.

Elevated hydrostatic pressure within both the diseased liver and the digestive tract is the primary driving force for intraabdominal fluid accumulation. Despite a variety of compensatory factors tending to minimize edema, some patients develop an imbalance between the rates of formation and absorption of visceral lymph. Visceral edema (i.e., lymph imbalance) and translocation of blood volume to the splanchnic bed, not ascites per se, precede retention of salt and water by the kidney. Subsequent reexpansion or overexpansion of the extracellular fluid volume with further stepwise increase in visceral lymph formation eventually exceeds central lymph return ("overflow") leading to palpable ascites. As fluid partition in the extracellular space becomes progressively more abnormal, renal-endocrine adjustments further aggravate lymph imbalance, leading to progressive ascites and, in some instances, functional renal failure. Maneuvers that effectively restore lymph dynamics either by reducing lymph formation (e.g., diuretic drugs, dietary salt restriction, portacaval shunt) or by accelerating lymph return (e.g., peritoneovenous shunt) interrupt this vicious cycle and ameliorate ascites. Conversely, approaches that aggravate lymph imbalance by intensifying portal hypertension (e.g., salt ingestion and salt-retaining hormones) worsen ascites.

REFERENCES

1. Bengmark, S., Borjesson, B., Hoevels, J., Joelsson, B., Lunderquist, A., and Owman, T. (1979): Obliteration of esophageal varices by PTP. *Ann. Surg.*, 190:549–554.
2. Blanchet, L., and Lebrec, D. (1982): Changes in splanchnic blood flow in portal hypertensive rats. *Eur. J. Clin. Invest.*, 12:327–330.
3. Burchell, A. R., Moreno, A. H., Panke, W. F., and Nealon, T. (1976) Hepatic artery flow improvement after portacaval shunt: a single hemodynamic correlate. *Ann. Surg.*, 184:289–302.
4. Grieg, P. D., Langer, B., Blendis, L. M., Taylor, B. R., and Glynn, M. F. (1980): Complications after peritoneovenous shunting for ascites. *Am. J. Surg.*, 139:125–131.
5. Hastbacka, J., and Turunen, M. I. (1979): Intrathoracic and splenic transposition for portal hypertension. *Zentralbl. Chir.*, 104:105–112.
6. Johnson, G., Dart, C. H., Peters, R. M., and Macfie, J. A. (1966): Hemodynamic changes with cirrhosis of the liver: Control of arteriovenous shunts during operation for esophageal varices. *Ann. Surg.*, 163:692–703.
7. Kaplan, A., Davies, J. I., and Field, M. (1969): The hemodynamic bisection of the liver. *Surgery*, 66:357–367.
8. Lebrec, D., Poynard, T., Hillon, P., and Benhamou, J. P. (1981): Propranolol for prevention of recurrent gastrointestinal bleeding in patients with cirrhosis. *N. Engl. J. Med.*, 305:1371–1374.
9. Rothschild, M. A., Oratz, M., Zimmon, D., Schrieber, S. S., Weiner, I., and Caneghen, A. V. (1969): Albumin synthesis in cirrhotic subjects with ascites studied with carbonate-^{14}C. *J. Clin. Invest.*, 48:344–350.
10. Sarfeh, I. J., Juler, G. L., Stemmer, E. M., and Mason, G. R. (1982): Results of surgical management of hemorrhagic gastritis in patients with gastroesophageal varices. *Surg. Gynecol. Obstet.*, 144:167–170.
11. Sigiura, M., and Futagawa, S. (1977): Further evaluation of the Sigiura procedure in the treatment of esophageal varices. *Arch. Surg.*, 112:1317–1321.
12. Vorobioff, J., Bredfeldt, J. E., and Groszmann, R. J. (1983): Hyperdynamic circulation in portal-hypertensive rat model: A primary factor for maintenance of chronic portal hypertension. *Am. J. Physiol.*, 244:G52–G57.
13. Warren, W. D. (1983): Control of variceal bleeding: Reassessment of rationale. *Am. J. Surg.*, 145:8–16.
14. Witte, C. L., and Witte, M. H. (1981): The congested liver. In: *Hepatic Circulation in Health and Disease*, edited by W. Wayne Lautt, pp. 307–328, Raven Press, New York.

15. Witte, C. L., and Witte, M. H. (1983): Splanchnic circulatory and tissue fluid dynamics in portal hypertension. *Fed. Proc.*, 42:1685–1689.
16. Witte, C. L., Witte, M. H., and Dumont, A. E. (1978): The portal triad in hepatic cirrhosis. *Surg. Gynecol. Obstet.*, 146:965–974.
17. Witte, C. L., Witte, M. H., and Dumont, A. E. (1980): Lymph imbalance in the genesis and perpetuation of the ascites syndrome in hepatic cirrhosis. *Gastroenterology*, 78:1059–1068.
18. Witte, M. H., Witte, C. L., Davis, W. M., Cole, W. R., and Dumont, A. E. (1972): Peritoneal transudate. A diagnostic clue to portal system obstruction in patients with intraabdominal neoplasms or peritonitis. *JAMA*, 221:1380–1383.
19. Witte, M. H., Witte, C. L., and Dumont, A. E. (1971): Progress in liver disease: Physiological factors involved in the causation of cirrhotic ascites. *Gastroenterology*, 61:742–750.

Intestinal Circulation During Arterial Hypertension

Henry W. Overbeck

Department of Medicine, Cardiovascular Research and Training Center, The University of Alabama in Birmingham, Birmingham, Alabama 35294

Systemic arterial hypertension is a hemodynamic disorder in which mean arterial pressure is elevated because of increased total peripheral vascular resistance (PVR), increased cardiac output, or both (46). This chapter reviews our as yet meager knowledge of the status of the intestinal circulation in this disease. The reader is also referred to a recent review of the splanchnic circulation in hypertension (38).

The paucity of studies of the intestinal circulation in hypertension may be ascribed, at least in part, to its relative inaccessibility and its anatomic and physiologic complexity. Thus, measurement of its hemodynamics is difficult, expecially in man. Nevertheless, the status of this circulation in hypertension should receive considerably more attention, because 20% to 30% of the cardiac output perfuses the splanchnic organs, and the splanchnic veins contain 20% of the total blood volume. Furthermore, splanchnic vascular function changes rapidly and greatly in response to stresses, including posture, exercise, and shock, as is described in Chapters 5, 6, and 13. Thus, this circulation contributes importantly and variably to the PVR and to venous return and cardiac output. Finally, the hepatic portion of the splanchnic circulation has metabolic buffering functions involving substances implicated in hypertension, such as aldosterone and other steroids (36).

In studies of the intestinal circulation during arterial hypertension, measurement of blood flow presents the greatest source of difficulties. These difficulties, as well as variations in the stage and severity of the hypertension, differences among models of hypertension, and species variation, probably account for the discrepancies in splanchnic flows and resistances reported in hypertension. Direct methods of splanchnic blood flow measurement in experimental animals involve considerable surgical and anesthetic trauma that likely alter the hemodynamic state. Microsphere technology, although bringing increasingly recognized problems of its own in validation and interpretation, has the advantage of being applicable to conscious animals and to small animals such as the rat. Chronically implanted electromagnetic or ultrasound flowmetry in conscious unrestrained animals is only beginning to be applied to the study of the splanchnic circulation in hypertension.

In hypertensive man, measurement of splanchnic blood flow presents even more formidable problems, with techniques restricted to indirect methods based on hepatic dye clearance. These methods do not allow us to measure separately hepatic portal venous flow and hepatic arterial flow. Furthermore, flow must be measured in resting, reclining subjects, so the hemodynamic state differs from that of normal activity. Accordingly, most information about the status of splanchnic and intestinal circulation has come from studies of animal models of hypertension. We must always bear in mind that these findings may not be applicable to hypertension in man, especially essential hypertension, which accounts for 90% of human hypertension.

With these many caveats, I shall review measurements of blood flow in the splanchnic vascular bed in hypertension. I will then briefly discuss evidence for certain abnormalities in cell membrane function that have been observed in intestinal vessels in hypertensives. These abnormalities may underlie the altered hemodynamic state.

INTESTINAL HEMODYNAMICS IN HYPERTENSION

Flow, Pressure, and Resistance

Man

The earlier studies (8,10,61) of the splanchnic circulation in hypertensive man may be criticized because of inadequate definition of the type and severity of hypertension. However, in general, the results of these earlier studies have been confirmed by a later more acceptable study (36), indicating that, in resting, supine, postabsorptive patients in the established uncomplicated stages of essential hypertension, total splanchnic blood flow remains unchanged and resistance is elevated to the same extent as PVR. One study of patients with presumptive renovascular hypertension (35) indicated decreased splanchnic blood flow with disproportionately high splanchnic resistance. The investigators suggested that decreased hepatic blood flow in these patients with renal hypertension may impair steroid metabolism and thus contribute to the hypertension.

Experimental Hypertension

Spontaneously hypertensive rats (SHR) of the Aoki-Okamoto strain have been considered a reasonable model of essential hypertension in man (58). However, this view is challenged by many investigators (35). Furthermore, it is generally felt that the parent Wistar-Kyoto strain (WKY) is an insufficient normotensive control for hemodynamic studies of SHR because body and organ weights differ among SHR, WKY, and unrelated Wistar strains, and blood flow is expressed in terms of weight (37). Additionally, several metabolic and endocrine anomalies have been identified in WKY (35). Thus, the simultaneous use of both WKY and an unrelated Wistar strain is preferred; increased credibility is given to findings in SHR that differ from those in both control strains.

Several studies (17,29,37,55,56,62) suggest that SHR with hypertension of 2 to 8 months duration may have normal to decreased splanchnic flow and elevated resistance. Some of these studies were conducted in unanesthetized rats (17,37,56,62). In three studies (17,29,55), cardiac output was measured, allowing calculation of splanchnic blood flow and resistance. In the other studies, only fractional distribution of cardiac output could be assessed. In four studies (17,37,56,62), the intestinal component of the splanchnic circulation was distinguished, with hemodynamics similar to that of the total splanchnic circulation. In only one study (37) were hemodynamics in SHR compared to both WKY and an unrelated Wistar strain (NR). Unfortunately, fractional flow to the intestinal circulation was elevated in both SHR and WKY, as compared with NR, so interpretation was difficult.

The splanchnic circulation has not been studied in other forms of genetic hypertension, in which more adequate control normotensive strains are available, for instance, Dahl salt-sensitive and salt-resistant rats (50), Lyon hypertensive, normotensive, and hypotensive rats (13).

Findings are confusing in rats with experimental renal hypertension. In the chronic stages (more than 4 weeks duration) of Goldblatt hypertension in rats, splanchnic (11) or intestinal (7,17,18,62) percentage of cardiac output (7,11,18,62), or blood flow (17) is reported as decreased (11,62), normal (7,17,18), or elevated (11,18). One group (11,18) suggests that the one-kidney, one-clip model (unilateral nephrectomy with the contralateral renal artery partially constricted), which may be a volume-dependent hypertension, is characterized by elevated intestinal blood flow. In contrast, according to this group, the two-kidney, one-clip model (both kidneys intact with one renal artery partially constricted), which may be a renin-dependent model, is characterized by unchanged intestinal blood flow and elevated resistance. However, other investigators do not confirm these findings (7,62). Certain of these studies in rats with renal hypertension were performed with invalid techniques or techniques considered questionable, such as the use of Rb distribution or distribution of macroaggregated albumin to measure regional blood flow (7,11,18). Furthermore, little information is supplied in these papers to allow the reader to assess the severity of the hypertension. In the hands of many investigators, Goldblatt hypertension in rats, especially the one-kidney, one-clip variety, fairly rapidly enters a severe, complicated stage in which hemodynamics are altered by secondary factors, such as volume depletion, anemia, or uremia, and likely do not resemble those of the uncomplicated stages. Clearly, the stage and severity of hypertension in renal hypertensive rats must be better described to aid interpretation of future studies.

In chronic stages of DOCA-salt hypertension (subcutaneous implantation of DOCA with unilateral nephrectomy and high salt intake) in conscious rats, the results of one study (62) indicated that the proportion of cardiac output perfusing the gastrointestinal tract (hepatic arterial circulation excluded) was normal. Unfortunately, in the only reported studies of animals with neurogenic hypertension (sinoaortic denervation), the tissue uptake of Rb was used to measure regional blood flow (1,2).

In none of the above studies were longitudinal observations of splanchnic hemodynamics made over the course of development of the hypertension. Such longitudinal studies have been made in dogs. In conscious dogs in the very early stages (less than 1 week) of one-kidney, one-clip Goldblatt hypertension (3) or salt-induced hypertension with reduced renal mass (32,33), microsphere injections were used to assess flow in the various vascular beds, including the intestine. Both forms of hypertension are probably volume-dependent. The investigators reported significant increases in small intestinal blood flow and decreased or unchanged intestinal vascular resistance in these animals. In contrast, skeletal muscle blood flow by day 5 was unchanged or reduced, with significant increases in resistance in that vascular bed. We have found similar hemodynamics in the ileum and limb, respectively, of dogs with one-kidney, one-wrapped (perinephritic) hypertension, also likely a volume-dependent form of renal hypertension. Our experiments will be described in further detail below.

Canine perinephritic hypertension

For several years we have been studying the circulation in various vascular beds of dogs with perinephritic hypertension. We designed these studies to trace the hemodynamic development of the hypertension from the early until the chronic, established phases. Our interest in the longitudinal development of the hemodynamic state in hypertension arose as the result of studies of systemic hemodynamics by Guyton and his colleagues (20) and Ferrario and his co-investigators (15,16). From experimental data and computer modeling, Guyton and Coleman (20) had explained the elevated total peripheral vascular resistance of established hypertension, at least volume-dependent forms of hypertension, as a "long-term, whole body" autoregulatory response of the peripheral vasculature to early increases in cardiac output and resulting tissue hyperperfusion (Fig. 1). Ferrario et al. (15,16) measured cardiac output and calculated PVR in dogs with renovascular hypertension (both one-kidney, one-wrapped perinephritic, and one-kidney, one-clipped Goldblatt). In both forms of hypertension, they found cardiac output increased early (up to 4 weeks) and returned to normal levels after that time. Accompanying the early increases in cardiac output was a decreased to unchanged PVR. The return of cardiac output to normal levels as the hypertension entered the chronic phase (after 4–6 weeks) was accompanied by a rise in PVR, which then solely sustained the hypertension. These findings added support to the hypothesis developed by Guyton and his colleagues. Because they found elevated mean systemic filling pressure (equilibrated intravascular pressure following abrupt cessation of cardiac output) and unchanged blood volume, Ferrario and his co-investigators suggested that decreases in venous compliance in their dogs might underlie the primary increases in cardiac output.

We felt that such observations of total body hemodynamics and hypotheses derived therefrom must be supported by parallel observations

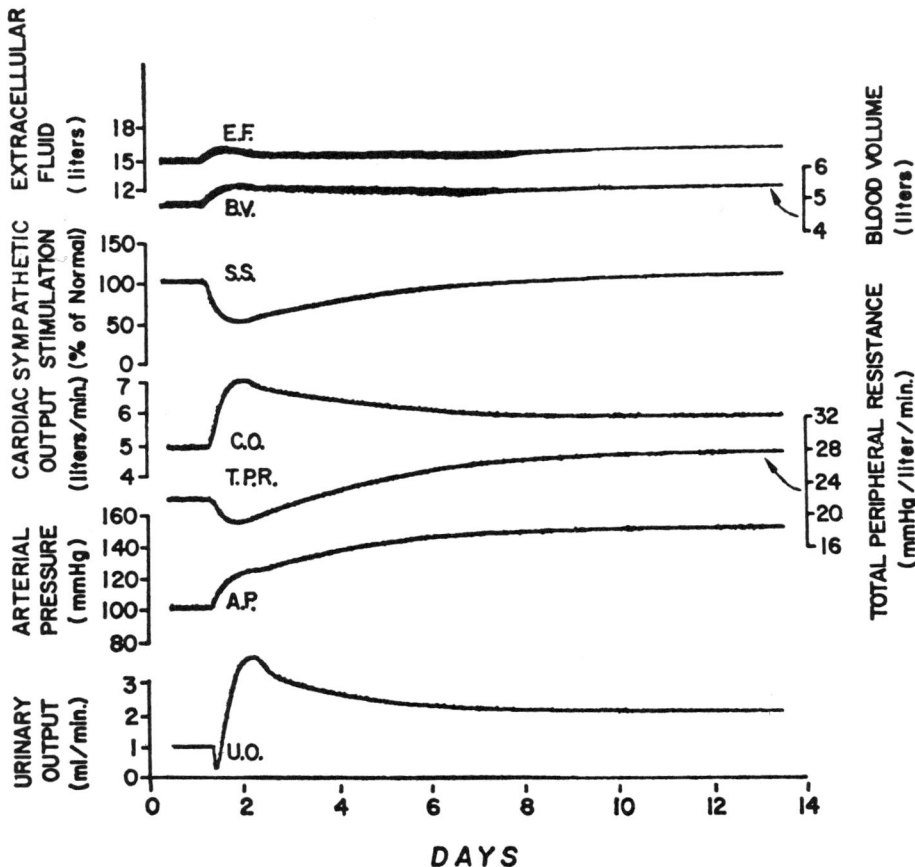

FIG. 1. Computer simulation of changes in body fluid volumes, cardiac sympathetic stimulation, urinary output, and systemic hemodynamics following reduction of renal mass by two-thirds and five times increase in salt intake at point where curves break. (From Guyton et al., ref. 21, with permission.)

in the individual vascular beds. We first studied the hemodynamics of the vascularly isolated, pump-perfused (blood), *in situ* forelimb in pentobarbital-anesthetized dogs in the early and then chronic, uncomplicated stages of one-kidney perinephritic hypertension (39,47). This is a vascular bed composed primarily of skeletal muscle and skin. In both the very early (less than 2 weeks) and the later-established stages (greater than 4 weeks) of hypertension, we found forelimb blood flow to be normal and resistance to be elevated (Fig. 2). Thus, our results indicated that the hemodynamics of the forelimb vascular beds may not parallel whole-body hemodynamics during the development of the hypertension.

We then turned our attention to the hemodynamics of the gut. In anesthetized dogs similarly prepared, we studied the naturally perfused, innervated but vascularly isolated *in situ* ileal preparation developed by Texter et al. (54) (see Fig. 3). We measured venous outflow from the ileal segment (by graduated cylinder and stopwatch) and intravascular pressures in the segment and calculated resistances. Our findings in the ileum were in striking contrast to those in the forelimb. In the ileum in the early stages of canine perinephritic hypertension, we found elevated blood flow and unchanged vascular resistance (51). Most interestingly to us (49), this hemodynamic situation persisted unchanged into the chronic stages

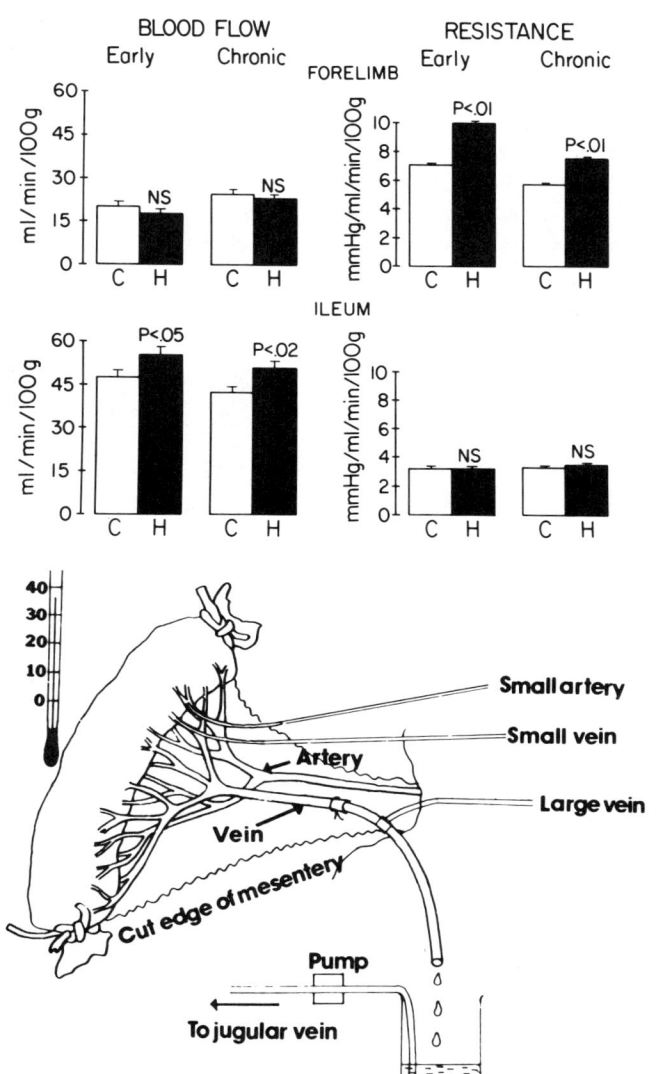

FIG. 2. Forelimb **(top)** and ileal **(bottom)** blood flows and vascular resistances (M ± SEM) in early (<2 weeks) and chronic (>4 weeks) stages of perinephritic hypertension in pentobarbital-anesthetized dogs. Control normotensive *(open bars labeled C)* and hypertensive *(closed bars labeled H)* values compared by Student's *t*-test.

FIG. 3. Diagram of the innervated, collateral-free, naturally perfused *in situ* ileal segment preparation. Venous outflow collected and returned by pump to jugular vein. Intravascular pressures sampled as indicated. (From Simon et al., ref. 51, with permission.)

of the hypertension (Fig. 2). Again, hemodynamics of this individual vascular bed appeared not to parallel whole-body hemodynamics.

It is necessary to point out here that the unchanged ileal arterial resistance in the hypertensive dogs actually represented a degree of increased arterial constriction. This is because the elevated intraarterial pressure would otherwise have passively dilated these vessels and reduced their resistance. This, of course, would also be true for whole-body hemodynamics; an unchanged PVR in face of elevated arterial pressure (15,16) would represent a degree of arterial constriction (9). Finally, we believe it is unlikely that the results of our observations in the ileum were artefactual, due, for example, to the surgical trauma or anesthesia, because, as noted above and presented in Fig. 2, we had found the opposite hemodynamic situation in the forelimb vascular beds in dogs prepared identically (39,47). Furthermore, independent investigators had also documented similar hemodynamics in the small intestine of conscious dogs in the early stages of similar forms of renal hypertension (3,32,33), as noted above.

Data from our two studies of ileal hemodynamics, one in the early- and one in the later-established phases of hypertension, appeared, on the surface, not to support the concept of long-term, whole-body autoregulation in hypertension. The increases in ileal blood flow that occurred in early hypertension persisted, apparently unchanged, for at least 2 to 3 weeks into the chronic stages. These prolonged increases in ileal blood flow were unaccompanied by evidence for the increases in mesenteric vascular resistance that would be predicted by the hypothesis (Fig. 1).

On the other hand, our experiments certainly did not exclude the possibility that the increased ileal blood flow we observed may be entirely appropriate for this vascular bed, serving to maintain normal relations between blood flow and tissue demands. It is possible, for example, that underlying increases in metabolic rate of these ileal tissues exist in hypertension requiring excess flow. Alternatively, diffusion barriers, due, for example, to the tissue "waterlogging" known to occur in hypertension (57), might impair movement of respiratory gases, nutrients, and metabolites between blood and tissue. Thus, more blood flow would be appropriate to maintain normal levels of exchange. Also, it is certainly possible that the increased ileal blood flow merely represents that proportion of flow shunted through arteriovenous anastomotic connections in the ileum, perhaps in passive response to the elevated arterial pressure (34). (We recognize that the existence of anatomically well-defined A-V shunts in the ileum is controversial, at least at normal intravascular pressures.) Finally, it is also possible that long-term autoregulation occurs more slowly in the ileum than in most other vascular beds or that local regulation of ileal blood flow is modified in hypertension.

To investigate these possible explanations for the persistent elevations of ileal blood flow in canine renal hypertension, we recently studied the ileal segment preparation in pentobarbital-anesthesized dogs with chronic, one-kidney, one-wrapped perinephritic hypertension (4). In these experiments, we measured ileal pressures, blood flows, blood gas contents, and oxygen consumption in the naturally perfused segments.

We then interposed a blood pump between the dog's femoral artery and the mesenteric artery serving the vascularly isolated ileal segment, so that segmental blood flow could be controlled and resistance monitored from changes in perfusion pressure. We measured pressure-flow relationships, reactive hyperemia, nonentrapment of 9-μm microspheres (34), and maximal vasodilation in response to nitroprusside injected into the pump tubing. On autopsy, we assessed the dogs' state of health, measured serum creatinine, sodium, and potassium, and sampled small mesenteric arteries for wall water content.

In dogs with hypertension, as compared to normotensive control dogs (unilaterally nephrectomized with the remaining kidney sham wrapped), we observed the following. Body weights and ileal segment weights were similar. Ileal segment blood flow was elevated by an average of 35% ($p<0.001$), and ileal total, arterial, small vessel, and venous segmental vascular resistances were unchanged ($p>0.9$). These results confirmed our previous findings (49) shown in Fig. 2. Oxygen consumption of the ileal segment was unchanged, but ileal segment venous PO_2 was significantly elevated ($p<0.05$). Pressure-flow relationships over a wide range of perfusion pressures (50–180 mm Hg) were unchanged, as was the magnitude and duration of reactive hyperemia in response to a flow cessation of 60 sec.

Nonentrapment of 9-μm microspheres, as assessed by collecting ileal segment venous effluent following injection of well-mixed microspheres upstream from the pump with flow set at the same rate in each dog, was directly related to pump perfusion pressure ($r = 0.69$; $p<0.05$) as has previously been reported (34). When perfusion pressure and flow were adjusted to levels similar to those of the resting hemodynamic state of anesthetized hypertensive dogs ("high pressure"), nonentrapment exceeded that at normotensive perfusion pressures ("low pressure"). This was true in both hypertensive and normotensive control dogs, which did not perceptibly differ in this regard (Table 1). Values in this table are similar to those

TABLE 1. *Percent nonentrapment of 9-μm microspheres by ileal circulation as a function of perfusion pressure (M ± SEM)*

Low pressure (144–148 mm Hg)		High pressure (155–193 mm Hg)	
Normotensive dogs ($N = 11$)	Hypertensive dogs ($N = 8$)	Normotensive dogs ($N = 11$)	Hypertensive dogs ($N = 8$)
20.4 ± 2.0%	18.4 ± 1.8%	28.4 ± 3.7%[a]	26.8 ± 2.6%[b]

[a] $p < 0.05$, high pressure vs low pressure, paired t-test.
[b] $p < 0.02$, high pressure vs low pressure, paired t-test.

previously observed in normal dogs (34). Finally, maximal vasodilation of the ileal segment was similar in hypertensive and normotensive dogs, as was arterial wall water content, serum creatinine, sodium, and potassium. Except for expected increases in heart-weight/body-weight ratios in the hypertensives and encapsulation of their remaining kidney, the general health of the hypertensive dogs at time of experiment was equivalent to that of the normotensive controls.

We interpret these observations as indicating that the increased ileal blood flow in the hypertensive dogs is not attributable to increased metabolic rate or oxygen demands of the tissues. The findings are unlikely to be related to diffusion barriers (there was no evidence for arterial wall waterlogging in this particular bed), and they are not attributable to anomalies in local blood-flow regulatory phenomena. The elevated flows seem best explained on the basis of increased arteriovenous shunting of blood. Apparently, physiologically normal bypass channels in the hypertensive dogs were opened passively by the increased arterial pressure.

It is interesting to speculate about the hemodynamic, structural and functional consequences of the postulated opening of bypass channels in response to increases in ileal arterial pressures in hypertension. Modeling indicates that such shunts would reduce pressures in the precapillary and capillary portion of the ileal circulation toward normal levels. The resulting near-normal pressures at the level of the precapillary resistance vessels may protect these vessels from the wall-thickening that occurs in hypertensives in response to elevated intravascular pressures (19). Thus, we found normal levels of ileal vascular resistance at maximal vasodilation. Increases in minimal resistance (resistance at maximal vasodilation) have been seen in most other vascular beds studied in hypertension (19), including the forelimb vascular bed in our previous studies (47) and have been interpreted as reflecting increases in wall-to-lumen ratio of resistance vessels (vascular-wall-thickening). One may also speculate that the increased A-V shunting serves to maintain near-normal capillary hydrostatic pressures in the ileal vascular bed in face of elevated arterial pressures, reducing loss of fluid into the gut lumen, and perhaps attenuating the increases that have recently been observed in intestinal lymph flow in chronic one-kidney, one-clip canine hypertension (30). These increases in lymph flow, which were accompanied by evidence of reduced sieving of large molecular weight proteins by capillary endothelium, were interpreted as indicating increased intestinal microvascular permeability, perhaps secondary to elevated capillary hydrostatic pressure.

Venous Compliance

It is also interesting to speculate that the increased A-V shunting in hypertensive dogs, by elevating venous return to the heart, may play a role in the increases in cardiac output seen in the early stages of hypertension. Alterations in venous compliance, as suggested by Ferrario et al. (16), might also be involved. In our earlier studies of limb hemodynamics in dogs with perinephritic hypertension, we had found direct evidence for decreased compliance of limb veins (39). Complete pressure-volume curves in temporarily isolated limb venous segments *in situ* were shifted toward the pressure axis. Because the mesenteric veins are considerably more important than those of the limbs in volume homeostasis and control of cardiac filling, we also studied pressure-volume relations in temporarily isolated mesenteric venous segments *in situ*. Our findings (Fig. 4) were similar to those in the limb veins; pressure-volume curves of veins of hypertensive dogs were shifted toward the pressure axis, indicating significant decreases in venous compliance (51). These changes persisted into the chronic stages of the hypertension (2). Decreases in peripheral venous compliance have also been reported in patients with essential hypertension, even in the very early stages (53,60).

Although it is certainly likely that these decreases in mesenteric venous compliance are mediated in part by increased contractile state of the venous smooth muscle, perhaps secondary to elevated sympathetic neural discharge (19), structural changes in the veins, not related to smooth muscle tone, also appear to play a role. Venous compliance was decreased in hypertensives (51) even after cyanide treatment. Greenberg and Bohr (22) found decreased distensibility in SHR venous segments treated with EDTA to deplete Ca^{2+} stores, thereby preventing smooth muscle contraction. Greenberg et al. (23) propose that the decreased venous compliance in hypertension may be related to the venous smooth muscle hypertrophy, but we have suggested (39) a relationship to venous wall waterlogging (48).

MEMBRANE ABNORMALITIES IN ILEAL VASCULAR SMOOTH MUSCLE IN HYPERTENSION

It is unlikely that the venous wall waterlogging that occurs in hypertension is the direct effect of elevated intravascular pressure (48). In hypertension at least some of the excess water and salt appears to be located intracellularly (14,59). Furthermore, such vascular wall waterlogging occurs in dogs and rats treated chronically with digitalis (41,46). These observations support the suggestion made a number of years ago by Tobian (57) that vascular waterlogging in hypertension may reflect primary abnormalities in ion metabolism of the vascular smooth muscle cells.

We studied the effects of digitalis on vascular wall water and salt content, because (26,40, 44,45) certain forms of hypertension might be characterized by widespread decreases in activity of cell membrane Na,K-ATPase, perhaps genetically induced (44,45), perhaps in response to circulating ouabain-like inhibitor (26, 45). A major portion of the evidence leading to this hypothesis had come from our studies of mesenteric vessels in perinephritic hypertensive dogs (45). In these dogs, prepared in a manner identical to those in the studies of ileal hemodynamics, we found evidence (Fig. 5) for significant decreases in *in vitro* ouabain-sensitive ^{86}Rb uptake by small mesenteric arteries and veins. Ouabain-sensitive uptake of Rb^+ paral-

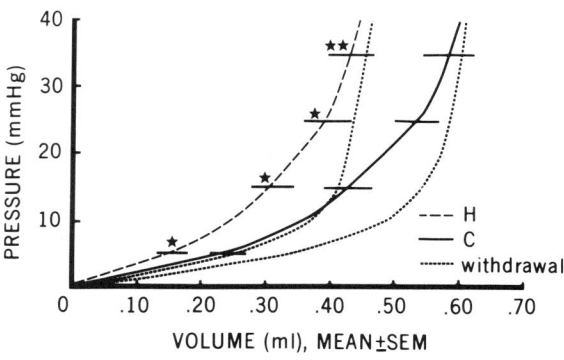

FIG. 4. Mesenteric vein pressure-volume curves. Shown are the injection phase curves of control normotensive dogs *(solid line)* and dogs with chronic 1-kidney, 1-wrapped hypertension *(dashed line)*. Withdrawal curves *(dotted lines)* are also shown. Data are mean values ± SEM. *(Asterisk)* $p<0.05$; *(double asterisk)* $p<0.01$. (From Simon et al., ref. 51, with permission.)

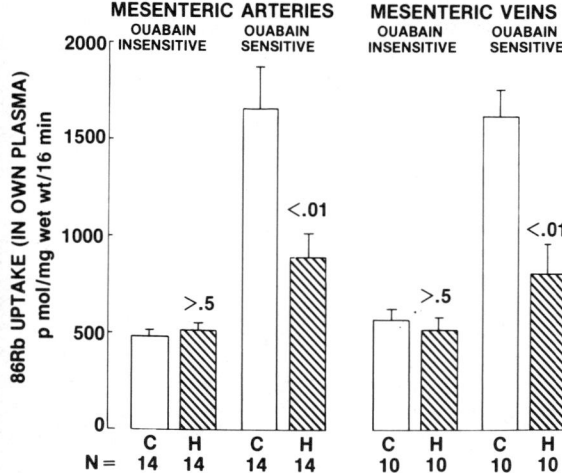

FIG. 5. Decreased ouabain-sensitive ^{86}Rb uptake *in vitro* by mesenteric arteries and veins from dogs with chronic perinephritic hypertension. *(Open bars)* values in control normotensive dogs; *(cross-hatched bars)* values in hypertensive dogs. Values are mean ± SEM. *p* values for comparison calculated by Student's *t*-test. (From Overbeck, ref. 42, with permission.)

lels that of K^+ (5) and is an indicator of the activity of the sarcolemmal sodium-potassium pump (and Na,K-ATPase) in the vascular smooth muscle cells. Because the sodium pump of the cell membrane plays an important role in cell volume homeostasis, we suggested (45) that decreased pump activity might account for the vessel waterlogging characteristic of most forms of hypertension, including essential hypertension in man (57). More importantly, pump function contributes to cell membrane potential (28), cell sodium and, hence, sarcoplasmic levels of activator Ca^{2+} in vascular smooth muscle (6,45). Thus, such decreased pump activity might underlie the arterial and venous vasoconstriction characteristic of hypertension (40,45). Recently, considerable evidence has appeared to support this hypothesis and to suggest that there are indeed circulating substances in certain forms and stages of hypertension that have ouabain-like actions on cardiovascular muscle (12,24, 25,27). In other forms of hypertension, there is evidence for genetically induced reductions in numbers of sodium pump sites in cardiovascular tissue (31). Clearly, such inhibitor substances, reduced pump numbers, and the resulting decreases in active sodium pumping by the vascular smooth muscle cells could mediate the alterations in the intestinal circulation, as well as other circulations, during arterial hypertension.

SUMMARY

The intestinal circulation is significantly involved in the altered hemodynamic state in hypertension. In forms of hypertension considered volume-dependent, often characterized by early increases in cardiac output, decreases in the compliance of mesenteric and other veins may play a primary role. Furthermore, these forms of hypertension may be characterized by increases in nonnutritional blood flow in the intestinal circulation. This flow, by elevating venous return, may also contribute to the increased cardiac output. Pressure-activated opening of these bypass channels may serve to maintain near-normal levels of pressures at the arterioles and in the capillary bed, thus reducing vascular wall hypertrophy and the increases in transcapillary fluid transport.

In other forms of hypertension, including human essential hypertension and possibly spontaneous hypertension in rats, forms felt not to be volume-dependent, intestinal blood flow appears to be unchanged, with resistance elevated to the same extent as total peripheral resistance. Thus, the intestinal arterioles appear to participate in the generalized vasoconstriction that elevates arterial pressure in these forms of hypertension. However, there are methodological problems in most published studies. Thus, further study of the intestinal circulation in these forms of hypertension will be necessary, with special attention to the time course of the hemodynamic changes.

Underlying these changes in function of intestinal arteries and veins, at least in part, appear to be alterations in the sarcolemmal sodium-potassium pump in the vascular smooth muscle cells. These alterations may be produced, in some cases, by circulating ouabain-like inhibitor substances, and, in other cases, by genetically induced anomalies in membrane Na,K-ATPase molecules.

ACKNOWLEDGMENT

Special thanks is due to David R. Bell, M.S., who conducted our most recent investigations of intestinal hemodynamics in perinephritic hypertensive dogs and supplied data for Table 1 and who also provided helpful comments during the writing of this chapter. This research was supported in part by a Public Health Service Research Grant, HL-23312 (NHLBI).

REFERENCES

1. Alexander, N., and DeQuattro, V. (1974): Regional and systemic hemodynamic patterns in rabbits with neurogenic hypertension. *Circ. Res.*, 35:636–645.
2. Alexander, N., and DeQuattro, V. (1974): Gastrointestinal and mesenteric hemodynamic patterns in neurogenic hypertensive rabbits. *Circ. Res.*, 35:646–651.
3. Allotey, J. B. K. (1978): Distribution of regional blood flow and vascular resistance in experimental renal hypertension. *Diss. Abstr.*, 38:3061-B.
4. Bell, D. R., and Overbeck, H. W. (1982): Intestinal hemodynamics in perinephritic hypertensive dogs. *Physiologist*, 25:280 (abstract).
5. Bernstein, J. C., and Israel, Y. (1970): Active transport of ^{86}Rb in human red cells and rat brain slices. *J. Pharmacol. Exp. Ther.*, 174:323–329.
6. Blaustein, M. P. (1977): Sodium ions, calcium ions, blood pressure regulation and hypertension: A reassessment and a hypothesis. *Am. J. Physiol.*, 232:C165–C173.
7. Bralet, A. M., Wepierre, J., and Bralet, J. (1973): Distribution of cardiac output and nutritional blood flow in the unanesthetized rat: Alterations during experimental renal hypertension. *Pflüegers Arch.*, 343:257–266.
8. Brod, J. (1963): Hemodynamic basis of acute pressor reactions and hypertension. *Br. Med. J.*, 25:227–245.
9. Conway, J. (1968): Blood flow and peripheral resistance in normotensive and hypertensive dogs. *Proc. Soc. Exp. Biol. Med.*, 128:272–274.
10. Culbertson, J. W., Wilkins, R. W., Ingelfinger, F. J., and Bradley, S. E. (1951): The effect of the upright posture upon hepatic blood flow in normotensive and hypertensive subjects. *J. Clin. Invest.*, 30:305–311.
11. Dahners, H., Breull, W., Kikis, D., Redel, D., Schotte, J., Stoepel, K., and Flohr, H. (1972): Regional peripheral resistance in experimental hypertension. In: *Vascular Smooth Muscle*, edited by E. Betz, pp. 143–145. Springer-Verlag, Berlin, Heidelberg, New York.
12. deWardener, H. E., and MacGregor, G. A. (1980): Dahl's hypothesis that a saluretic substance may be responsible for the sustained rise in arterial pressure: Its possible role in essential hypertension. *Kidney Int.*, 18:1–9.
13. Dupont, J., Dupont, J. C., Froment, A., Milon, H., and Vincent, M. (1973): Selection of three strains with spontaneously different levels of blood pressure. *Biomedicine*, 19:36–41.
14. Edmondson, R. P. S., Thomas, R. D., Hilton, P. J., Patrick, J., and Jones, N. F. (1975): Abnormal leucocyte composition and sodium transport in essential hypertension. *Lancet*, 1:1003–1009.
15. Ferrario, C. M. (1974): Contribution of cardiac output and peripheral resistance to experimental renal hypertension. *Am. J. Physiol.*, 226:711–717.
16. Ferrario, C. M., Page, I. H., and McCubbin, J. W. (1970): Increased cardiac output as a contributory factor in experimental renal hypertension in dogs. *Circ. Res.*, 27:799–810.
17. Ferrone, R. A., Walsh, G. M., Tsuchiya, M., and Frohlich, E. D. (1979): Comparison of hemodynamics in conscious spontaneous and renal hypertensive rats. *Am. J. Physiol.*, 236:H403–H408.
18. Flohr, H., Breull, W., Dahners, H. W., Redel, D., Conradi, H., and Stoepel, K. (1976): Regional distribution of vascular resistance in two models of experimental renovascular hypertension. *Pflüegers Arch.*, 362:157–164.
19. Folkow, B. (1982): Physiological aspects of primary hypertension. *Physiol. Rev.*, 62:347–504.
20. Guyton, A. C., and Coleman, T. G. (1969): Quantitative analysis of the pathophysiology of hypertension. *Circ. Res. (Suppl.)*, 24/25(I):I-1–I-19.
21. Guyton, A. C., Coleman, T. G., and Granger, H. J. (1972): Circulation: Overall regulation. *Annu. Rev. Physiol.*, 34:13–46.
22. Greenberg, S., and Bohr, D. F. (1975): Venous smooth muscle in hypertension. Enhanced contractility of portal veins from spontaneously hypertensive rats. *Circ. Res. (Suppl.)*, 36/37(I):I-208–I-215.
23. Greenberg, S., Palmer, E. C., and Wilborn, W. M. (1978): Pressure-independent hypertrophy of veins and pulmonary arteries of spontaneously hypertensive rats. Characterization of function, structural and histochemical changes. *Clin. Sci. Mol. Med.*, 55:31s–36s.
24. Gruber, K. A., Rudel, L. L., and Bullock, B. C. (1982): Increased circulating levels of an endogenous digoxin-like factor in hypertensive monkeys. *Hypertension*, 4:348–354.
25. Haddy, F. J. (1980): Mechanism, prevention and therapy of sodium-dependent hypertension. *Am. J. Med.*, 69:746–758.
26. Haddy, F. J., and Overbeck, H. W. (1976): The role of humoral agents in volume expanded hypertension. *Life Sci.*, 19:935–948.
27. Hamlyn, J. M., Ringel, R., Schaeffer, J., Levinson,

27. P. D., Hamilton, B. P., Kowarski, A. A., and Blaustein, M. P. (1982): A circulating inhibitor of (Na⁺ + K⁺) ATPase associated with essential hypertension. *Nature*, 300:650–652.
28. Hendrickx, H., and Casteels, R. (1974): Electrogenic sodium pump in arterial smooth muscle cells. *Pflüegers Arch.*, 346:299–306.
29. Hiley, C. R., and Yates, M. S. (1978): The distribution of cardiac output in the anesthetized spontaneously hypertensive rat. *Clin. Sci. Mol. Med.*, 55:317–320.
30. Laine, G. A., and Granger, H. J. (1983): Permeability of intestinal microvessels in chronic arterial hypertension. *Hypertension*, 5:722–727.
31. Lee, S. W., Whitmer, K., Wallick, E. T., Adams, R. J., and Schwartz, A. (1982): Decrease in Na,K-ATPase activity and (³H)ouabain binding sites in hearts of spontaneously hypertensive rats. *Fed. Proc.*, 41:1645 (abstract).
32. Liard, J. F. (1981): Regional blood flows in salt loading hypertension in the dog. *Am. J. Physiol.*, 240:H361–H367.
33. Liard, J. F., and Silenzio, R. (1982): Baroreceptor reflex influence on peripheral circulations in salt-loading hypertension in dogs. *Hypertension*, 4:597–603.
34. Maxwell, L. C., Shepherd, A. P., and Riedel, G. L. (1982): Vasodilation or altered perfusion pressure moves 15-μm spheres trapped in the gut wall. *Am. J. Physiol.*, 243:H123–H127.
35. McGiff, J. C., and Quilley, C. P. (1981): The rat with spontaneous genetic hypertension is not a suitable model of human essential hypertension. *Circ. Res.*, 48:455–463.
36. Messerli, F. H., Genest, J., Nowaczynski, W., Kuchel, O., Honda, M., Latour, Y., and Dumont, G. (1975): Splanchnic blood flow in essential hypertension and in hypertensive patients with renal artery stenosis. *Circulation*, 51:1114–1119.
37. Nishiyama, K., Nishiyama, A., and Frohlich, E. D. (1976): Regional blood flow in normotensive and spontaneously hypertensive rats. *Am. J. Physiol.*, 230:691–698.
38. Nyhof, R. A., Laine, G. A., Meininger, G. A., and Granger, H. J. (1983): Splanchnic circulation in hypertension. *Fed. Proc.*, 42:1690–1693.
39. Overbeck, H. W. (1972): Hemodynamics of early experimental renal hypertension in dogs: Normal limb blood flow, elevated limb vascular resistance, and decreased venous compliance. *Circ. Res.*, 31:653–663.
40. Overbeck, H. W. (1972): Vascular responses to cations, osmolality and angiotensin in renal hypertensive dogs. *Am. J. Physiol.*, 223:1358–1364.
41. Overbeck, H. W. (1981): Elevated arterial pressure, vascular wall "waterlogging", and impaired cardiac growth in rats chronically receiving digoxin. *Proc. Soc. Exp. Biol. Med.*, 167:506–513.
42. Overbeck, H. W. (1984): Function of the sodium pump in vascular smooth muscle in hypertension. In: *Pathophysiological Mechanisms of Hypertension*, edited by H. Villareal and M. P. Sambhi, pp. 196–209. Martinus Nijhoff, The Hague.
43. Overbeck, H. W., Berne, R. M., Chien, S., Cowley, A. W., Jr., Haddy, F. J., Heistad, D. D., Honig, C. R., Kirkendall, W., Rapela, C. E., Wells, R., Abboud, F. M., Lindheimer, M. D., and Yipintsoi, T. (1980): Report of the Hypertension Task Force of the National Heart, Lung, and Blood Institute. Current research and recommendations from the Subgroup on Local Hemodynamics. *Hypertension*, 2:342–369.
44. Overbeck, H. W., Derifield, R. S., Pamnani, M. B., and Sözen, T. (1974): Attenuated vasodilator responses to K⁺ in essential hypertensive men. *J. Clin. Invest.*, 53:678–686.
45. Overbeck, H. W., Pamnani, M. B., Akera, T., Brody, T. M., and Haddy, F. J. (1976): Depressed function of a ouabain-sensitive sodium-potassium pump in blood vessels from renal hypertensive dogs. *Circ. Res., (Suppl.)*, 38(II): II-48–II-52.
46. Overbeck, H. W., Pamnani, M. B., and Ku, D. D. (1980): Arterial wall "waterlogging" accompanying chronic digoxin treatment in dogs. *Proc. Soc. Exp. Biol. Med.*, 164:401–404.
47. Overbeck, H. W., Swindall, B. T., Cowan, D. F., and Fleck, M. C. (1971): Experimental renal hypertension in dogs. Forelimb hemodynamics. *Circ. Res.*, 29:51–62.
48. Pamnani, M. B., and Overbeck, H. W. (1976): Abnormal ion and water composition of veins and normotensive arteries in coarctation hypertension in rats. *Circ. Res.*, 38:375–378.
49. Pamnani, M. B., Simon, G., and Overbeck, H. W. (1979): Increased mesenteric blood flow and decreased mesenteric venous compliance in dogs with chronic perinephritic hypertension. *Proc. Soc. Exp. Biol. Med.*, 161:397–401.
50. Rapp, J. P. (1982): Dahl salt-susceptible and salt-resistant rats, a review. *Hypertension*, 4:753–763.
51. Simon, G., Pamnani, M. B., Dunkel, J. F., and Overbeck, H. W. (1975): Mesenteric hemodynamics in early experimental renal hypertension in dogs. *Circ. Res.*, 36:791–798.
52. Simon, G., Pamnani, M. B., and Overbeck, H. W. (1976): Decreased venous compliance in dogs with chronic renal hypertension. *Proc. Soc. Exp. Biol. Med.*, 152:122–125.
53. Takeshita, A., and Mark, A. L. (1979): Decreased venous distensibility in borderline hypertension. *Hypertension*, 1:202–206.
54. Texter, E. C., Chou, C. C., Merrill, S. L., Laureta, H. C., and Frohlich, E. D. (1964): Direct effects of vasoactive agents on segmental resistance of the mesenteric and portal circulation. *J. Lab. Clin. Med.*, 64:624–633.
55. Tobia, A. J., Lee, J. Y., and Walsh, G. M. (1974): Regional blood flow and vascular resistance in the spontaneously hypertensive rat. *Cardiovasc. Res.*, 8:758–762.
56. Tobia, A. J., Walsh, G. M., Tadepalli, A. S., and Lee, J. Y. (1974): Unaltered distribution of cardiac output in the conscious young spontaneously hypertensive rat: Evidence for uniform elevation of regional vascular resistances. *Blood Vessels*, 11:287–294.
57. Tobian, L. (1960): Interrelationship of electrolytes, juxtaglomerular cells and hypertension. *Physiol. Rev.*, 40:280–312.
58. Trippodo, N. C., and Frohlich, E. D. (1981): Simi-

larities of genetic (spontaneous) hypertension, man and rat. *Circ. Res.*, 48:309–319.
59. Villamil, M. F. (1972): Angiotensin, hypertension and vascular ionic composition. *Medicina (Suppl.)*, 32(1):57–62.
60. Walsh, J. A., Hyman, C., and Maronde, R. F. (1969): Venous distensibility in essential hypertension. *Cardiovasc. Res.*, 3:338–349.
61. Wilkins, R. W., Culbertson, J. W., and Rymut, A. A. (1952): The hepatic blood flow in resting hypertensive patients before and after splanchnicectomy. *J. Clin. Invest.*, 31:529–531.
62. Yates, M. S., and Hiley, C. R. (1979): Distribution of cardiac output in different models of hypertension in the conscious rat. *Pflüegers Arch.*, 379:219–222.

Diabetes Mellitus and the Splanchnic Vasculature

H. Glenn Bohlen

Department of Physiology, Indiana University School of Medicine, Indianapolis, Indiana 46223

The microvascular consequences of diabetes mellitus have been studied in great detail in virtually all organ systems except the gastrointestinal tract. Although a variety of gastrointestinal complications accompany diabetes, the relationship of these symptoms to microvascular disease is, at best, speculative. This chapter reviews the microvascular changes observed in splanchnic organs and relates these changes to the general pattern of microvascular disease throughout the cardiovascular system. In addition, the suspected causes of microvascular derangements in diabetes is considered, in particular, those that have been shown to affect the splanchnic vasculature.

In animal models of diabetes mellitus (11,35), the intestinal glucose and fatty acid absorption rates both *in vivo* and *in vitro* are as much as twice the normal rate, at least in the uncontrolled diabetic state. This difference in transport rates has been tentatively attributed to mucosal conditions such as a reduction in diffusion distances through unstirred layers (35), increased passive permeability of the mucosal layer (35), and increased numbers of transport sites (11,35). Recently, Madara et al. (26) have shown the density of microvillus membrane proteins did not change after severe short-term (5 days) hyperglycemia. Therefore, if more glucose carriers exist in diabetic animals, the increased number of carrier molecules is probably due to a greater total mucosal surface area (35). The shape of the villus changes during diabetes and, therefore, surface area for transport apparently increases. The most frequently observed change is an increase in villus height (12,29) in diabetic experimental animals. The increase in height and surface area could also reduce the resistance to diffusion through unstirred layers according to Thomson (35). In diabetic humans, Costrini et al. (10) have not found increased intestinal glucose absorption, although others have (20,36). Whether or not data obtained in man and animals can be compared is questionable because, as Costrini et al. (10) point out, diabetic humans usually receive some form of insulin or diet therapy so that they are nearly normoglycemic whereas laboratory animals usually have severe uncontrolled hyperglycemia. Therefore, the metabolic status may have an effect on absorption. For example, Csáky and Fischer (11) using normal rats found that systemic hyperglycemia for about 4 hr induced an increase in glucose transport equivalent to that in diabetic animals.

A recent review by Falchuk (18) points out that a large portion (20–30%) of the human diabetic population has demonstrable impairment of gastrointestinal motor activity. Although the motor impairment generally is readily tolerated or even unnoticed, motility-related dysfunction such as prolonged gastric emptying, constipation, and diarrhea is a significant clinical problem, particularly diabetic diarrhea (18,27,37). I have routinely found that virtually all diabetic rats and mice develop diarrhea if severe hyperglycemia is allowed to persist for 4 to 6 weeks. The incidence of gastrointestinal motor dysfunction in diabetic humans is often correlated with the presence of autonomic neuropathy (21,27,37). However, other factors such as bacterial overgrowth, exocrine pancreatic function, and generalized pathology should be routinely considered as possible contributors at this time (18,21,27,37).

The degeneration of the macro- and microvasculature during diabetes mellitus is perhaps the best-known physical characteristic of the disease. In general, diabetic microangiopathy in advanced cases is best described as an occlusive disease; small vessels are lost due to atrophy, and large vessels are gradually impaired by a form of atherosclerotic plaque formation. The neovascularization of the retina, an anomalous growth of retinal capillaries, is a major risk to vision but neovascularization in other tissues has not been described. An illustrative example of the microvascular occlusive process was presented by Ditzel et al. (15,16,17). The conjunctival vasculature of human diabetics was observed, and two major disease patterns were encountered. The first pattern is vasodilation with little or no loss of microvessels. The second pattern is vasoconstriction and a loss of small microvessels. The second vascular pattern is frequently seen in diabetics who have experienced a rapid progression of microangiopathy; the severity of hyperglycemia or duration of hyperglycemia had little effect on the pattern of vascular disease. Fenton et al. (19) have shown that the primary site of vessel loss in the human conjunctiva is vessels smaller than 30 μm at ages from 10 to 55 years; vessels larger than 30 μm are apparently spared from the occlusive process. The loss of small vessels, particularly capillaries, has also been suggested by Katz and Janjan (23) for the skeletal muscle vasculature of man. In well-controlled diabetics, they (23) found that the capillary filtration coefficient (K_f) of the forearm tissue was as little as half normal. This indicated a major loss of microvessels because capillary permeability usually increases in diabetes (32). Thus, the decreased K_f reflects a loss of exchange surface area, that is, a loss of capillaries. Whether the loss of capillaries is primarily related to the generalized decrease in the number of small vessels or a specific degeneration of the capillary wall is unknown. However, there is no question that both diabetic man and experimental animals experience capillary basement membrane thickening (1,9,13,33,34), which is a hallmark of diabetic microangiopathy.

There are undoubtedly many factors that contribute to the development of diabetic microangiopathy as reviewed by Little (24) and Christensen (9). However, I am taking an intentionally biased point of view for the circumstances that have a bearing on the intestinal vasculature, biased in the sense that the role of elevated glucose per se will be emphasized. In observations of the skeletal muscle and skin vasculatures of diabetic animals, my co-workers and I (4–8) have shown that atrophy of the arteriolar wall and loss of arterioles and capillaries occurred whether the hyperglycemic animal had a hyper- or hypoinsulinemic form of diabetes. It also did not matter whether the diabetes began in juvenile or adult life. Therefore, hyperglycemia per se may be a direct or indirect causative factor in diabetic microangiopathy. Papachristodoulou, Heath, and Kang (22,30,31) have shown that excessive glucose intake in normal rats is associated with a retinopathy very similar to that in diabetic animals. Furthermore, the umbilical arteries from normoglycemic infants born to diabetic human mothers, who were occasionally hyperglycemic, demonstrated thickening of the basement membrane (2). These observations (2,22,30,31) indicate that there is a relationship between excess glucose and vascular anomalies.

In a recent study by Bohlen and Hankins (4), normal rats were subjected for 4 to 5 weeks to twice-daily intraperitoneal injections of either isotonic physiological salt solution or an isotonic mixture that contained 300 mg% glucose. The intent of this protocol was to increase the glucose concentration to which the intestinal microvasculature was exposed without causing systemic hyperglycemia. The abdominal cavity did maintain a glucose concentration equal to or greater than 200 mg% for 2 to 2.5 hr, and the systemic plasma glucose concentration was increased less than 20 mg%. When compared to equal age rats made hyperglycemic (>400 mg%) with streptozotocin or to normal rats, the rats that only received physiological saline had normal microvascular characteristics in the submucosal and muscle layers of the gut. However, as shown in Table 1, the majority of arterioles

TABLE 1. *Arteriolar diameter and vessel wall characteristics in normal (N), streptozotocin diabetic (STZ), and intraperitoneal glucose injected (G) rats*[a,b]

Arteriolar order	Animal type	Control diameter (μm)	Vessel wall thickness (μm)	Vessel wall area (μm)	Wall-to-lumen ratio	No. of vessels	No. of animals
1A	N	71.0 ± 5.1[c]	16.1 ± 0.7	4477 ± 80	0.24 ± 0.03	9	12
	STZ	68.5 ± 3.9	11.2 ± 0.4[d]	2887 ± 219[d]	0.17 ± 0.01[d]	31	9
	G	70.1 ± 4.4	12.6 ± 1.1[d]	3474 ± 337[d]	0.20 ± 0.02[d]	25	9
2A	N	17.7 ± 0.9	6.9 ± 0.4	817 ± 101	0.42 ± 0.01	14	12
	STZ	21.3 ± 1.5[d]	6.0 ± 0.4[d]	540 ± 62[d]	0.29 ± 0.02[d]	26	9
	G	22.1 ± 2.5	6.7 ± 0.5	695 ± 74	0.35 ± 0.03[d]	34	9
3A	N	9.3 ± 0.7	6.0 ± 0.3	357 ± 57	0.67 ± 0.02	14	12
	STZ	11.1 ± 0.8[d]	5.3 ± 0.3[d]	272 ± 25[d]	0.49 ± 0.03[d]	24	9
	G	10.2 ± 0.3[d]	5.8 ± 0.2	311 ± 24	0.58 ± 0.03[d]	26	9

[a] Diabetic and glucose-treated rats had been exposed to hyperglycemia for 4–5 weeks.
[b] Reproduced from *Diabetologia* 22: 344-348, 1982.
[c] All data are mean ± SEM.
[d] $p < 0.05$ for control value different from experimental value.

in diabetic and glucose-treated animals were diluted at rest. Their vessel wall thickness, wall area and wall-to-lumen ratio were decreased. The normal animals that received glucose showed both intestinal vessel wall atrophy and the vasodilation that accompanied the early stages of diabetes. The atrophy of the vessel wall is assumed to be a consequence of vascular smooth muscle degeneration. Angervall and Säve-Söderbergh (1) found that human diabetics have a very atrophied or absent smooth muscle coat around intestinal vessels. This condition also applies to other splanchnic tissues, the kidney, and reproductive organs (1). The vasodilation observed by Bohlen and Hankins (4) is consistent with Lucas and Foy's (25) finding that intestinal blood flow increases 40% to 50% in rats made diabetic with streptozotocin.

The distances between capillaries of the intestinal muscle layer during maximum dilation (topical 10^{-4} M adenosine) are shown in Fig. 1 for normal, diabetic, and glucose-treated rats in (4). The distributions of distances in glucose-treated rats and diabetic rats are similar; both experienced 7- to 10-μm increase in the mean and median capillary separation. The loss of capillaries in the diabetic intestine was consistent with similar findings in the skeletal muscle vasculature of diabetic rodents (6,7,8). In addition, Diani et al. (12), Meyer et al. (28), and Angervall and Säve-Söderbergh (1) have shown that the splanchnic capillaries of diabetic chinese hamsters and man experience the same basement membrane thickening that occurs in other organs. Therefore, the intestinal muscle layer capillaries are apparently as damaged by diabetes as capillaries in other organ systems, and the loss of capillaries is similar to that of the vasculature in general. Capillaries in the intestine are lost rapidly after diabetes begins, but then the capillarity apparently becomes stable. For example, after 4 to 5 weeks of diabetic hyperglycemia, the average distance between capillaries is 44.6 ± 1.1 μm (4) and only increases to 46.8 ± 2.9 μm (3) after 12 to 15 weeks of hyperglycemia; the normal control animals had a spacing of 33.8 ± 1.4 μm (4) and 37.6 ± 2 μm (3), respectively. The observation (4) that localized hyperglycemia in otherwise normal animals can precipitate capillary analomalies qualitatively and quantitatively similar to those in diabetic rats raises the possibility that glucose when present in excess triggers the development of diabetic microangiopathy.

One of the most controversial hypotheses to explain the development of diabetic angiopathy is that microangiopathy is caused by acute episodes of hypoxia. In formulating this hypothesis, Ditzel (14) proposed that the downward shift of the P_{50} for the oxygen disassociation

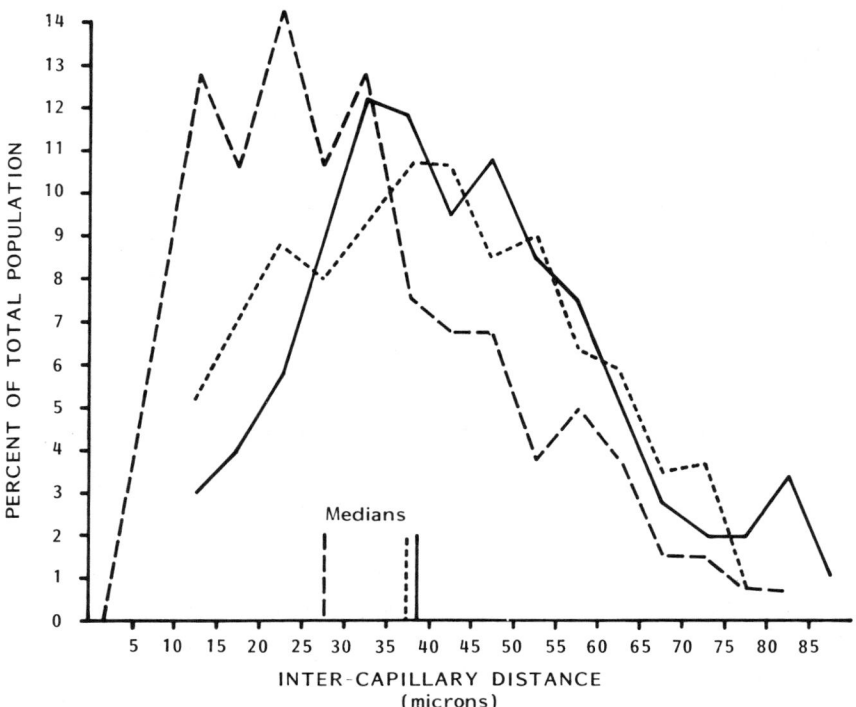

FIG. 1. Intercapillary distance distribution in the intestinal muscle layer of normal *(dashed line)* glucose-treated *(solid line)*, and streptozotocin (STZ) diabetic *(dotted line)* rats. The medians are shown. Mean ± SEM distances were 33.8 ± 1.4 μm in normal, 44.6 ± 1.1 μm for glucose-treated and 41.3 ± 0.9 μm for STZ rats. The number of distance measurements were 132, normal; 296, glucose-treated; and 375, diabetic rats. (From Bohlen and Hankins, ref. 4, with permission.)

curve caused by glycolsylation of hemoglobin (HbAlc) and by the decrease in 2,3-diphosphoglycerate produces intermittent tissue hypoxia. The tissue hypoxia component of this hypothesis is very difficult to test because only brief transient periods of hypoxia may cause tissue damage. Thus, the hypoxic periods may not occur during measurements of tissue Po_2. However, I recently measured tissue Po_2 along capillaries in the intestinal muscularis in normal and severely diabetic rats and found no significant differences at rest or during maximum dilation (3). These data are presented in Fig. 2. The red blood cell velocity, which is analogous to red blood cell flow, was about one-half normal in diabetic animals both at rest and during maximum vasodilation as shown in the upper panel of Fig. 3. The red cell transit time, shown in the lower panel of Fig. 3, was much greater in diabetic than normal animals. This occurred because the velocity of flow is slower in diabetic than normal rats, while the capillary lengths in the two groups are not significantly different (3). It is not known whether the similar tissue Po_2 values in normal and diabetic rats are related to the longer red cell transit time in diabetic animals (this would improve gas exchange), or whether the diabetic animals have a lower than normal oxygen usage. This study (3) does not conclusively rule out the possibility of intermittent hypoxia. However, the data do indicate that both resting and maximum tissue Po_2 values can be normal in diabetic animals despite the loss of capillaries and reduced capillary flow. In addition, tissue Po_2 values measured in the apical half of villi in both the normal

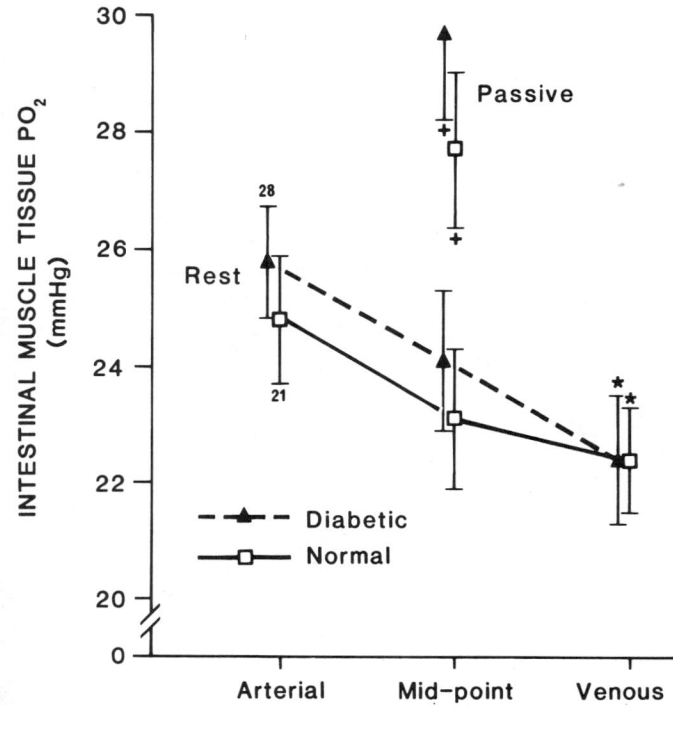

FIG. 2. Tissue Po_2 15 μm from the arterial, midpoint, and venous ends of intestinal muscle layer capillaries. The arterial and venous end Po_2 are significantly (*asterisk*; $p<0.05$) different from each other in both normal and diabetic rats. During maximum passive flow, induced with adenosine (10^{-4}), the midpoint Po_2 increased in both normal and diabetic rats. The N values with arterial end Po_2 are the number of observations for that and all other points. (From Bohlen, ref. 3, with permission.)

($Po_2 = 19.8 \pm 0.8$ mm Hg) and diabetic ($Po_2 = 21.3 \pm 1.0$ mm Hg) animals were not significantly different (3).

Intermittent hypoxia could conceivably cause a loss of capillaries, but it is less likely that arterial damage could be directly related to hypoxia. Measurements of the blood and vessel wall Po_2 in intestinal arterioles and venules of normal and diabetic animals (3) reveal that for comparable locations in the vasculature, the recorded Po_2 values are essentially identical in the two groups of animals (3). Blood flow in vessels larger than 20 μm (i.d.) rarely stops without external stimulation or compression. Therefore, the walls of the vast majority of microvessels have access to the abundant oxygen in the blood. Consequently, a direct deleterious effect of hypoxia on the arteriolar or venular wall is unlikely, although noxious chemicals released as a result of parenchymal tissue hypoxia cannot be excluded as a cause of microangiopathy.

SUMMARY

The single concept that is reasonably well established regarding diabetic microangiopathy is that the vasculatures of virtually all organs experience approximately the same type of microvascular pathology. The typical format of the disease is a gradual atrophy of the vessel wall and a loss of small microvessels. The proposed mechanisms of vascular degeneration are speculative at this time. Furthermore, it is simply unknown to what extent the various gastrointestinal pathologies described in this chapter are related to vascular or parenchymal tissue damage.

ACKNOWLEDGMENTS

The author wishes to thank Miss Marsha Hunt for typing the manuscript. Studies cited for Dr. Bohlen were supported by the Indiana University School of Medicine Diabetes Research and Training Center (PHSP60 AM 20542-SRC) and PHS Grant HL 25824. Dr. Bohlen is a recipient of an NIH Research Career Development Award HLO1089.

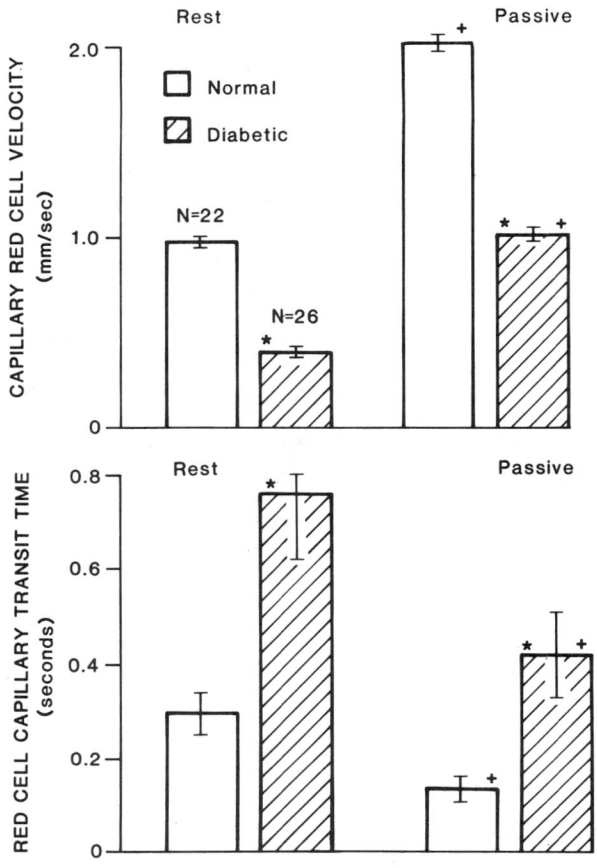

FIG. 3. Red cell velocity and transit times at rest in the capillaries of rat intestinal muscle. Rest refers to conditions of resting vascular tone. Passive conditions of maximum vasodilation were caused by topical application of adenosine (10^{-4} M). *(Asterisks)* A significant difference ($p<0.05$) between normal and diabetic rats at rest or in the passive state. *(Crosses)* Significant difference ($p<0.05$) between rest and passive conditions in a given animal type. The numbers of measurements of flow velocity and transit times are equal. (From Bohlen, ref. 3, with permission.)

REFERENCES

1. Angervall, L., and Säve-Södenbergh, J. (1966): Microangiopathy in the digestive tract in subjects with diabetes of early onset and long duration. *Diabetologia*, 2:117–122.
2. Asmussen, I. (1980): Ultrastructure of human umbilical arteries: Studies of arteries from newborn children delivered by nonsmoking, white group D, diabetic mothers. *Circ. Res.*, 47:620–626.
3. Bohlen, H. G. (1983): Tissue PO_2 in the intestinal muscle layer of rats during chronic diabetes. *Circ. Res.*, 57:677–682.
4. Bohlen, H. G., and Hankins, K. D. (1982): Early arteriolar and capillary changes in streptozotocin-induced diabetic rats and intraperitoneal hyperglycaemic rats. *Diabetologia*, 22:344–348.
5. Bohlen, H. G., and Hankins, K. D. (1983): Early microvascular pathology during hyperglycemia in bats. *Blood Vessels*, 20:213–220.
6. Bohlen, H. G., and Niggl, B. A. (1979): Adult microvascular disturbances as a result of juvenile onset diabetes in Db/Db mice. *Blood Vessels*, 16:269–276.
7. Bohlen, H. G., and Niggl, B. A. (1979): Arteriolar anatomical and functional abnormalities in juvenile mice with genetic or streptozotocin-induced diabetes mellitus. *Circ. Res.*, 45:390–396.
8. Bohlen, H. G., and Niggl, B. A. (1980): Early arteriolar disturbances following streptozocin-induced diabetes mellitus in adult mice. *Microvasc. Res.*, 20:19–29.
9. Christensen, N. J. (1972): Diabetic angiopathy and neuropathy. *Acta Med. Scand. Suppl.*, 541:3–60.
10. Costrini, N. V., Ganeshappa, K. P., Wu, W., Whalen, G. E., and Soergel, K. H. (1977): Effect of insulin, glucose and controlled diabetes mellitus on human jejunal function. *Am. J. Physiol.*, 233:E181–E187.
11. Csáky, T. Z., and Fischer, E. (1981): Intestinal sugar transport in experimental diabetes. *Diabetes*, 30:568–574.
12. Diani, A. R., Gerritsen, G. C., Stromsta, S., and Murray, P. (1976): Study of the morphological changes in the small intestine of the spontaneously diabetic chinese hamster. *Diabetologia*, 12:101–109.
13. Diani, A. R., Weaver, E. A., and Gerritsen, G. C. (1981): Capillary basement membrane thickening associated with the small intestine of ketonuric diabetic chinese hamster. *Lab. Invest.*, 44:388–391.
14. Ditzel, J. (1976): Oxygen transport impairment in diabetics. *Diabetes (Suppl.)*, 25(2):832–838.
15. Ditzel, J., and Duckers, J. (1957): The bulbar conjunctival vascular bed in diabetic children. *Acta Paediatr.*, 46:535–552.

16. Ditzel, J., and Saglid, U. (1954): Morphological and hemodynamic changes in the smaller blood vessels in diabetes mellitus. *N. Engl. J. Med.*, 250:587–594.
17. Ditzel, J., Sargeant, L., and Hadley, W. B. (1958): The relationship of abnormal vascular responses to retinopathy and rephopathy in diabetics. *A.M.A. Arch. Int. Med.*, 101:912–920.
18. Falchuk, K. R. (1982): Motor and absorptive abnormalities of the gastrointestinal tract. *NY State J. Med.*, 82:914–917.
19. Fenton, B. M., Zweifach, B. W., and Worthen, D. M. (1979): Quantitative morphometry of conjunctival microcirculation in diabetic mellitus. *Microvasc. Res.*, 18:153–166.
20. Gottesbüren, H., Schmitt, E., Menge, H., Block, R., Lorenz-Moyer, H., and Riechen, E. O. (1973): The effect of insulin on the intestinal absorption in man. II. The effect of endogenous and intravenously injected insulin on absorption. *Res. Exp. Med.*, 161:262–271.
21. Hosking, D. J., Bennet, T., and Hampton, J. R. (1978): Diabetic autonomic neuropathy. *Diabetes*, 27:1043–1055.
22. Kang, S. S., Price, R. G., and Bruckdorfer, K. R. (1977): Retinal damage in rats caused by dietary sucrose. *Biochem. Soc. Trans.*, 5:235–236.
23. Katz, M. A., and Janjan, D. (1978): Forearm hemodynamics and responses to exercise in middle aged adult-onset diabetic patients. *Diabetes*, 27:726–731.
24. Little, H. L. (1976): The role of abnormal hemorrhemodynamics in the pathogenesis of diabetic retinopathy. *Trans. Am. Ophthamol. Soc.*, 74:573–636.
25. Lucas, P. D., and Foy, J. M. (1977): Effects of experimental diabetes and genetic obesity on regional blood flow in the rat. *Diabetes*, 26:786–792.
26. Madara, J. L., Wolf, J. L., and Trier, J. S. (1982): Structural features of the rat small intestinal microvillus membrane in acute experimental diabetes. *Dig. Dis. Sci.*, 27:801–806.
27 Malins, J. M., and French, J. M. (1957): Diabetic diarrhea. *Q. J. Med.*, 26:467–480.
28. Meyer, H. W., Missmahl, H. P., and Siebner, H. (1973): Basement membrane thickness of rectal capillaries in diabetes. *Lancet*, 1:1317–1318.
29. Miller, D. L., Hanson, W., Schedl, H. P., and Osborne, J. W. (1977): Proliferation rate and transit time of mucosal cells in small intestine of the diabetic rat. *Gastroenterology*, 73:1326–1332.
30. Papachristodoulou, D., Heath, H., and Kang, S. S. (1976): The development of retinopathy in sucrose-fed and streptozotocin-diabetic rats. *Diabetologia*, 12:367–374.
31. Papachristodoulou, D., and Heath, H. (1977): Ultrastructural alterations during the development of retinopathy in sucrose-fed and streptozotocin-diabetic rats. *Exp. Eye Res.*, 25:371–384.
32. Parving, H. H. (1976): Increased microvascular permeability to plasma proteins in short- and long-term juvenile diabetics. *Diabetes (Suppl.)*, 25(2):884–889.
33. Siperstein, M. D. (1972): Capillary basement membranes and diabetic microangiopathy. *Adv. Intern. Med.*, 18:325–344.
34. Tchobrontsky, G. (1978): Relation of diabetic control to development of microvascular complications. *Diabetologia*, 15:143–152.
35. Thomson, A. B. R. (1983): Experimental diabetes and intestinal barriers to absorption. *Am. J. Physiol.*, 244:G151–G159.
36. Vinnik, I. E., Kern, F., and Sussman, K. E. (1965): The effect of diabetes mellitus and insulin on glucose absorption by the small intestine of man. *J. Lab. Clin. Med.*, 66:131–136.
37. Whalen, G. E., Soergel, K. H., and Grenen, J. E. (1969): Diabetic diarrhea: A clinical and pathophysiological study. *Gastroenterology*, 56:1021–1032.

The Pathophysiology of Nonocclusive Intestinal Ischemia

*T. E. Bynum, **Robert H. Gallavan, Jr., and **Eugene D. Jacobson

*Division of Gastroenterology, Department of Internal Medicine, Brigham Women's Medical Center, Harvard Medical School, Boston, Massachusetts 02115; and **Department of Physiology, College of Medicine, University of Cincinnati, Cincinnati, Ohio 45267

Several decades ago Wilson and Qualheim provided the first careful description of nonocclusive intestinal ischemia (12). This entity is a significant disease in the U.S. for three reasons. First, although it was considered a rarity when first described, the disorder has considerable frequency; an analysis of autopsy material indicated that 3% of deaths in one series were attributable to nonocclusive intestinal ischemia (9). Second, this disorder is difficult to diagnose in the living; most published cases involving the full-blown disease were diagnosed post-mortem. Third, until recently, medical science had little to offer in the treatment of nonocclusive intestinal ischemia, and mortality rates for this condition hovered close to 100% (8).

Given a clinical condition that is common, confusing, and catastrophic, the first step in improving its prognosis is to reach a clearer comprehension of the pathophysiology of the disease. Through such understanding it is possible to identify the steps in the sequence of pathophysiological events at which medical intervention may benefit the patient.

There is a strong anatomical emphasis to the education of a physician. His usual inference, when considering the cause of a severe decrease in blood flow to an organ, is that there must be some obstruction or stricture in the main artery carrying blood to the organ. This is not necessarily the case. As seen in Fig. 1, the initial superior mesenteric arteriogram in a subject demonstrated a marked narrowing of the artery near the origin of the middle colic artery. An atherosclerotic plaque in the inner lining of the vessel had reduced the internal diameter by half. The anatomical bias of the physician would cause two predictions to be made, both of which could be tested. First, blood flow through the artery to the intestine should be significantly decreased. Second, it should not be possible to restore blood flow to normal using a vasodilator drug because the stricture is not going to be responsive to drugs, since it is a structural defect.

Both predictions were tested in this patient (4). Reflux angiography showed that blood flow in this subject's superior mesenteric artery was only 180 ml/min, a value that is about one-third of that predicted for a healthy individual of his weight. Thus, the first prediction, that the artery had a low blood flow (presumably on anatomical grounds because of the stricture in the vessel), was confirmed. The second prediction was also tested in this patient by injecting a small dose of the vasodilator, prostaglandin E_1, directly into the artery and measuring blood flow again with reflux angiography. The result was a marked increase in blood flow from the control value.

This case is illustrative of vasospastic or functional ischemia, which can be overcome with a dilator drug. This type of vasospastic disease leading to ischemia in the gut is comparable to Prinzmetal's angina of the heart or transient ischemic attacks of the cerebral circulation. Nonocclusive intestinal ischemia is due to excessive tension in the smooth muscle of the

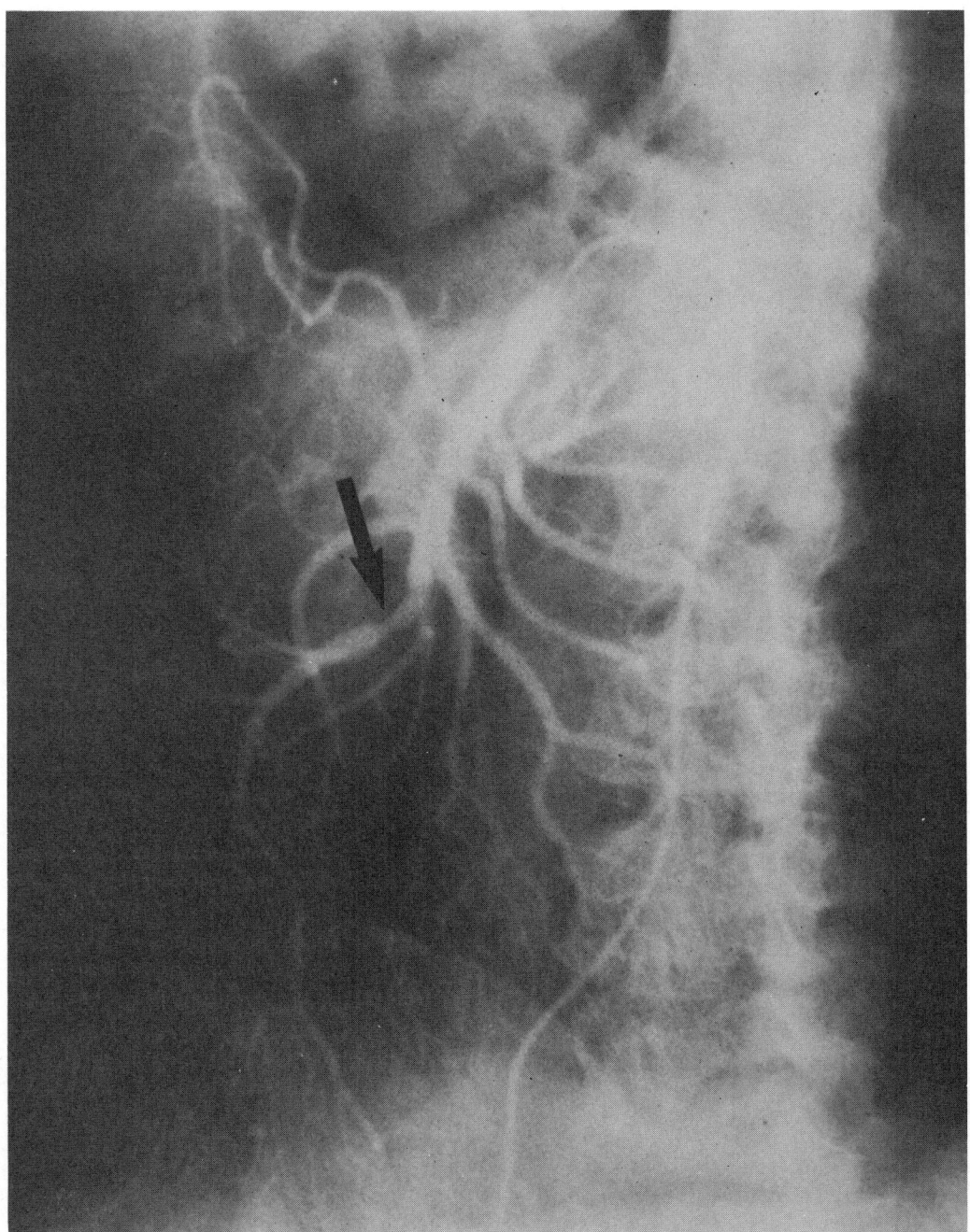

FIG. 1. Superior mesenteric arteriogram showing partial occlusion of the vessel near the origin of the middle colic artery. Blood flow determined by reflux angiography was 180 ml/min, which was about one-third the predicted value for the patient.

arterioles, the major site of control of blood flow to the gut. In the aforementioned case, the stricture of the superior mesenteric artery was a "red herring." By analogy, in experimental animals, mechanical constriction of the superior mesenteric artery causing a reduction of one-half in vessel diameter will cause only a transient decrease in blood flow because the arterioles dilate and restore flow to normal. Between one-fourth and one-half of all patients with a compromised intestinal circulation are suffering from nonocclusive intestinal ischemia, that is, a disease in which the ischemia is not due to an occlusion of the main artery or of its first, second, and third-order branches.

The descriptions of the normal regulation of mesenteric blood flow that provides the context in which the pathophysiology of acute nonocclusive mesenteric ischemia may be understood are given in Chapters 3–5, 7, and 25. The typical patient with this usually fatal disorder is elderly and is a victim of a chronic coexistent cardiovascular disease, such as congestive cardiac failure being treated with digitalis. Heart failure compromises the cardiac output and paradoxically forces the heart to reduce its output in the face of even ordinary stresses such as exercise. In heart failure there is excessive alpha-adrenergic activity and increased production of angiotensin II, the latter substance being both a mesenteric vasoconstrictor and an amplifier of sympathetic vasoconstriction because it interferes with norepinephrine uptake at sympathetic terminals. Furthermore, cardiac glycosides, which are standard therapy in congestive cardiac failure, are also mesenteric vasoconstrictors, because of their direct binding to the Na^+, K^+-ATPase of vascular smooth muscle and their stimulation of local catecholamine release (1).

Prolonged vasoconstriction leads to ischemic hypoxia of the villus tip, which is aggravated by the oxygen countercurrent mechanism (Chapter 7). The ensuing hypoxic necrosis of the lining of the gut destroys a key function of that epithelium, namely, containment of the luminal contents in the lumen. Absorption of bacterial exotoxins and endotoxins, luminal proteins, and digestive enzymes, and the products of necrotic tissue, including lysosomal cathepsins and hydrolases, ensues. The addition of these toxins to a dying circulation contributes to irreversible shock. Within the gut the stagnant circulation manifests disseminated thrombi, further slowing the blood flow. The process of necrosis consumes the villi and advances into the deeper mucosa. Figure 2 is a schematic illustration of this sequence.

It is hardly surprising that most elderly people with heart failure, shock, a necrotic bowel, and a profound toxemia die. Until recently, only rarely did the patient with nonocclusive ischemia of the small bowel survive an encounter with this disorder (8).

CLINICAL CONSIDERATIONS

Intestinal ischemia literally means an insufficient blood supply to adequately perfuse intestinal tissues. Of course, if the ischemia persists there will be pathologic changes in the bowel. When these appear, the condition is termed ischemic bowel disease, mesenteric vascular disease or, simply, intestinal ischemia. When

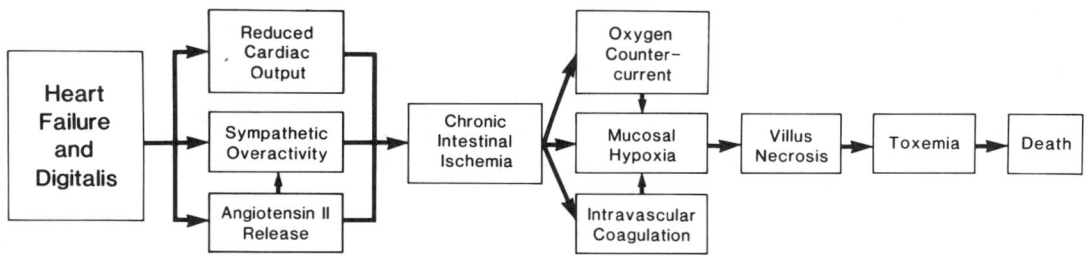

FIG. 2. Sequence of pathophysiological events in fatal nonocclusive intestinal ischemia.

the ischemia is very severe, *intestinal infarction* is the term used to describe the necrotic gut. The various forms of intestinal ischemia can be classified in several ways, each of which affords useful perspectives on clinical aspects of the disease (Fig. 3).

Site of Ischemia

Intestinal ischemia usually involves only the small bowel or the colon. Ischemia of the small bowel is usually much more severe, progresses more often to infarction, is more often associated with an acute abdomen and peritonitis, and has a high mortality rate (90% in one collected series of patients). Chronic occlusive ischemia of the small bowel may present as abdominal angina (the small meal syndrome). Under these circumstances the patient eats only small and infrequent meals because the ingestion of food induces significant abdominal pain. Other patients with chronic ischemia of the gut may present with a malabsorption syndrome, in which there is such extensive malfunction of small bowel mucosa due to ischemia that normal absorption cannot occur.

Ischemia of the colon (Fig. 4), often called ischemic colitis, is relatively less severe and certainly less catastrophic (2). It is often transient and self-limiting. Only rarely does it progress to late scarring with obstruction or become associated with an acute abdomen, perforation, or peritonitis. The initial clinical presentation frequently mimics inflammatory bowel disease (especially ulcerative colitis) or lower gastrointestinal bleeding from a diverticulum of the colon or angiodysplasia. Because of the extensive microbial population in the normal colon, bacteria, endotoxin, and other bacterial products may gain access to the general circulation owing to disruption of the normal barrier when ischemia occurs. Hence, it is somewhat surprising that ischemia of the colon is less severe than small bowel ischemia. The reason small bowel ischemia is more severe than colonic ischemia is not known. Among the speculations are that a greater length or total mass of bowel is usually involved in small bowel ischemia or that the small intestine may release a variety of peptide substances into the circulation, which cause marked vasodilation, myocardial depression, or capillary leakage. Much of the small bowel is also at a distance from the vessels which are collateral to the superior mesenteric artery.

Occlusive Versus Nonocclusive Disease

The small bowel or the colon can be affected by either occlusive or nonocclusive ischemia. In

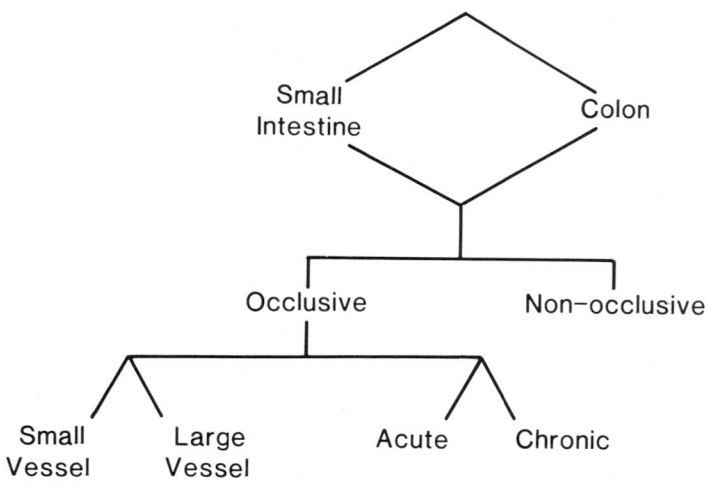

FIG. 3. Forms of intestinal ischemia.

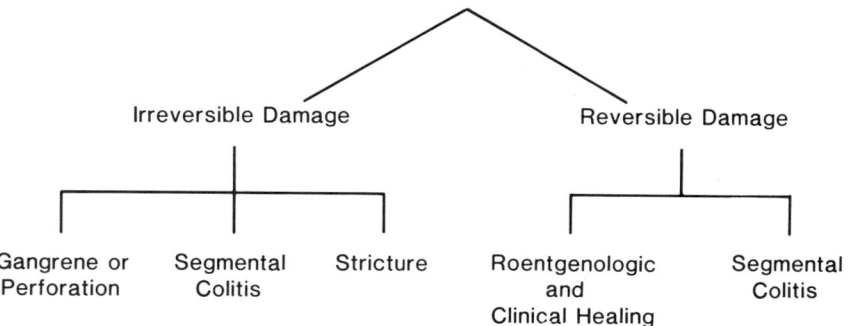

FIG. 4. Results of colonic ischemia.

occlusive disease, ischemia of the gut results from some type of mechanical obstruction to the flow of blood through the supplying vessel. Occlusion of large vessels may be due to an embolus, a thrombus on (or hemorrhage into) an atherosclerotic plaque, a tumor surrounding or invading the vessel, surgical ligation, or a dissecting aneurysm. Small vessel occlusion is associated with vasculitis (systemic lupus erythematosis, polyarteritis nodosum, allergic reactions, Henoch-Schoenlein purpura), radiation injury (radiotherapy with subsequent radiation enteritis), and thrombotic thrombocytopenic purpura. Occlusive disease is most often acute (embolus) or subacute (vasculitis, thrombotic thrombocytopenic purpura), but it may be chronic (gradual occlusion to ultimate total obstruction of major mesenteric arteries by atherosclerosis). The symptoms of acute occlusive intestinal ischemia can appear early in the illness as the bowel undergoes infarction. Chronic mesenteric vascular occlusion allows the development of an extensive collateral circulation so that intestinal ischemia occurs late, and symptoms do not occur unless two of the three major mesenteric arteries are completely occluded.

Nonocclusive intestinal ischemia (Fig. 5) is a low flow state in which there is no vascular occlusion or in which the degree of vascular narrowing, owing to atherosclerosis, for example, is not enough by itself to account for the failure of intestinal perfusion (Fig. 1). Normal mesenteric vessels constrict when there is a contraction in volume (hypovolemia) in the general circulation, thereby providing more blood for presumably more essential organs and tissues, such as the myocardium, brain, and kidneys. Therefore, in hypovolemic circumstances (e.g., following a massive gastrointestinal hemorrhage), mesenteric vasoconstriction can be combined with systemic hypotension and decreased cardiac output secondary to a decreased venous return. These deficits will make the bowel ischemic. Even without hypovolemia, low flow occurs in septic shock and a variety of cardiovascular diseases (severe valvular disease, especially aortic stenosis, arrhythmias, severe cardiomyopathies). Nonocclusive intestinal ischemia often occurs with the hypervolemia of congestive cardiac failure. Nonocclusive intestinal ischemia is usually acute in onset, but may occur against a background of chronic cardiovascular disease. Vasoconstrictive drugs, such as norepinephrine and digitalis (3,6,7), can further compromise mesenteric blood flow. Commonly, such drugs have been administered to patients who subsequently developed intestinal ischemia.

The final result of either occlusive or nonocclusive intestinal ischemia is the same: if the deficit in perfusion is sustained and is severe enough, with sufficient deprivation of oxygen and other nutrients, intestinal epithelial cells begin to die. In the small bowel, necrosis occurs first at the tips of the intestinal villi, because the enterocytes are more active metabolically (being most active in absorption) and are already relatively hypoxic because of countercurrent oxygen shunting along the length of the villus (see Chapters 7 and 26). As the vascular

1. Failure of Blood Flow

2. Vascular disease often present but no total occlusion, and vascular abnormalities are themselves not sufficient to significantly impair blood flow

3. Vasoconstriction of mesenteric arteries is often present

4. Analogies:
    A. Coronary Artery Spasm
    B. Acute Renal Failure (Pre-renal Azotemia, "Acute Tubular Necrosis")

FIG. 5. Features of nonocclusive mesenteric ischemia.

deficiency grows over time, necrosis burrows deeper and deeper into the mucosa, then into the submucosa, and finally infarction extends through the entire bowel wall.

Clinical Evaluation

When the small bowel or colon infarcts, the clinical manifestations of the patient are characteristic of the acute abdomen. The patient has severe abdominal pain, fever, tachycardia, leukocytosis, often a distended abdomen with absent bowel sounds, blood in the stools, and so-called peritoneal signs—rigidity of the abdominal wall and diffuse abdominal tenderness with severe rebound tenderness. Even without knowing specifically what caused these symptoms and signs, the physician knows that the patient must have surgery. At the time of operation, the surgeon finds a variable length of ischemically necrotic bowel, often with one or more perforations, accompanied by extensive peritonitis. The dead bowel must be resected in an effort to save the patient's life. Most of the few patients who survive the drastic resection of so much bowel become severe digestive cripples. Many patients die in shock post-operatively or at the time of surgery.

Intestinal ischemia, particularly of the small bowel, with its pathologic consequences, may represent the point of irreversibility in hemorrhagic, septic, or cardiogenic shock. Hence, for the patient requiring surgical correction of intestinal ischemia, the outlook is nearly hopeless. By the time the patient manifests symptoms requiring surgery, it is always too late to save his intestine, and it is usually too late to save his life. Therefore, when possible, a physician must suspect intestinal ischemia before it progresses to infarction. In early, mild intestinal ischemia, diffuse abdominal pain or periumbilical pain is the important symptom. The pain is usually sudden in onset and often quite severe. Early in the course of intestinal ischemia, pain is totally out of proportion to physical findings. In some patients examined quite early, the abdomen is unremarkable, with normal bowel sounds, no significant tenderness or any rebound tenderness, and no abdominal distention. Occult blood may not yet be present in the stool. Suspicion is increased if the patient is elderly or, at any age, if the patient has been hypotensive for any reason, or has underlying cardiovascular or circulatory disease and is receiving digitalis.

When intestinal ischemia is suspected, there should be little hesitation in performing mesenteric arteriography. Too often, to confirm their suspicion, and to "justify" doing what is often felt to be a hazardous, invasive procedure, namely, mesenteric angiography, clinicians have waited until more definite physical findings have developed. This intervention has become a remarkably safe procedure with extremely low mortality and an acceptable morbidity. Conversely, if one waits for the development of abnormal physical findings, or an abnormal plain X-ray film of the abdomen, it is usually too late to save the patient. Therefore, the first ingredients in making the timely diagnosis of intestinal ischemia are an alert suspicion combined with readiness to perform early mesenteric arteriography based solely on that suspicion (Fig. 6).

In acute intestinal ischemia, mesenteric arteriography would be expected to demonstrate one of three findings: (a) an embolus or thrombus occluding (usually) a first- or second-order branch of one of the principal mesenteric arteries, most commonly a branch of the superior mesenteric artery; (b) arteriographic evidence for vasoconstriction, without high-grade or total occlusion; or (c) normal mesenteric vessels, or atherosclerotic vessels without sufficient occlusion to significantly alter blood flow and without vasoconstriction. The first finding would indicate occlusive intestinal ischemia. The second and third findings are highly compatible with nonocclusive intestinal ischemia. The importance of arteriographic evidence for vasoconstriction has been inappropriately and often erroneously emphasized. Angiographic contrast medium is a vasodilator. Therefore, the vasoconstriction may be temporarily relieved by injection of the dye. More important, the major resistance vessels in the mesenteric circulation are the precapillary arterioles, the size of which is far too small to be seen on even the best arteriogram. An arteriogram cannot determine whether these vessels are constricted.

If arteriography shows occlusion and the patient is in any condition to tolerate an operation, surgery should be undertaken immediately for the purpose of either removing the embolus or performing vascular bypass around the obstructed segment of artery. If arteriography is compatible with nonocclusive intestinal ischemia, efforts should be made to provide general circulatory support as well as specific pharmacologic therapy to increase mesenteric blood flow. This will frequently be successful in reversing intestinal ischemia and preventing infarction of the bowel. If there is clinical evidence, by physical examination, plain X-ray films, or laboratory tests, suggesting that infarction has occurred, surgery must be done to remove dead bowel, but supportive efforts must be undertaken prior to and during surgery to limit the extent of infarction, rescue as much bowel as possible, and improve the patient's chances of surviving surgery.

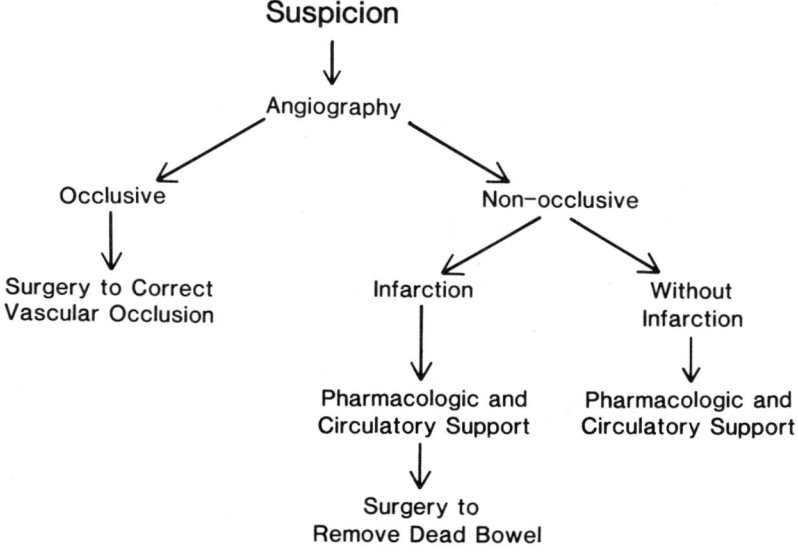

FIG. 6. Steps in the evaluation and management of severe ischemic bowel disease.

There are two contributions that can be provided by general circulatory support. The first is restoration of the effective circulating blood volume if the patient is actually hypovolemic or is functionally hypovolemic (e.g., due to sepsis). The second benefit of this support is improvement of cardiac output without utilizing vasoconstrictor medications. In this latter regard, digitalis and other cardiac glycosides do not cause vasoconstriction in humans when administered orally, unless digitalis toxicity occurs; however, digitalis is a potent mesenteric vasoconstrictor if administered intravenously, even when given in a dose that is far short of toxicity (3,7).

Vasodilator Therapy

Specific pharmacologic therapy to increase mesenteric blood flow involves the administration of vasodilator agents. This is best accomplished by direct intraarterial infusion of these agents by way of the arteriographic catheter following mesenteric arteriography. The agent that has been most often used for this purpose is papaverine, as it is the medication that is most readily available to the vascular radiologist (10). Another agent that has been used and is readily available is glucagon. The E group of prostaglandins are effective vasodilators of mesenteric arteries (11). B group prostaglandins are vasodilators if given in low doses by constant infusion (5).

Vasodilator therapy should be used only if general circulatory support has been accomplished or is being done concomitantly. It is particularly important to correct hypovolemia. If there is reduction in effective circulating blood volume, dilation of mesenteric vessels threatens to pull blood away from the general circulation, thereby further reducing effective blood volume in the general circulation and potentially jeopardizing blood flow to the brain, kidneys, and heart.

SUMMARY

Intestinal ischemia is occlusive or nonocclusive, acute or chronic, and tends to involve either the small bowel or the colon. Nonocclusive disease represents failure of blood flow to a variety of events, without a significant obstruction of the vascular lumen, and is at least as common as occlusive disease. For uncertain reasons, small bowel ischemia is a far worse disease than ischemia of the colon and is usually fatal if appropriate therapy is not instituted promptly. Modern techniques in vascular surgery contribute favorably to the management of occlusive intestinal ischemia, and vasodilator drugs such as papaverine, glucagon, and prostaglandins may save a patient's bowel and life in nonocclusive ischemia.

REFERENCES

1. Adams, R. J., Wallick, E. T., Asano, G., DiSalvo, J., Fondacaro, J. D., and Jacobson, E. D. (1983): Canine mesenteric artery Na^+, K^+-ATPase: Vasopressor receptor for digitalis. *J. Cardiovasc. Pharm. (In press)*
2. Boley, S. J., Schwartz, S. S., and Williams, L. F. (1971): *Vascular Disorders of the Intestine.* Appleton Century Crofts, New York.
3. Bynum, T. E., and Hanley, H. G. (1982): Effect of digitalis on estimated splanchnic blood flood. *J. Lab. Clin. Med.*, 99:84–90.
4. Clark, R. A., Colley, D. P., Jacobson, E. D., Herman, R., Tyler, G., and Stahl, D. (1980): Superior mesenteric angiography and blood flow measurement following intra-arterial injection of prostaglandin E_1. *Radiology*, 134:327–333.
5. Fara, J. W., Barth, K. H., and Bynum, T. E. (1979): Mesenteric vascular effects of prostaglandins F_2 alpha and B_2. *Radiology*, 133:317–321.
6. Gazes, P. C., Holmes, C. R., Mosly, V., and Pratt-Thomas, R. R. (1961): Acute hemorrhage and necrosis of the intestines associated with digitalization. *Circulation*, 23:358–367.
7. Levinsky, R. A., Lewis, R. M., Bynum, T. E., and Hanley, H. G. (1975): Digoxin induced intestinal vasoconstriction. *Circulation*, 52:130–137.
8. Pierce, G. E., and Brockenbrough, E. C. (1970): The spectrum of mesenteric infarction. *Am. J. Surg.*, 119:233–239.
9. Price, W. E., Rohrer, G. V., and Jacobson, E. D. (1969): Mesenteric vascular diseases. *Gastroenterology*, 57:599–604.
10. Siegelman, S. S., Sprayragen, S. S., and Boley, S. J. (1974): Angiographic diagnosis of mesenteric arterial vasoconstriction. *Radiology*, 112:533–540.
11. Tyler, G., Clark, R. A., and Jacobson, E. D. (1982): Nonocclusive intestinal ischemia treated with intraarterial infusion of prostaglandin E_1. *Cardiovasc. Interv. Radiol.*, 5:16–19.
12. Wilson, R., and Qualheim, R. E. (1954): A form of acute hemorrhagic enterocolitis afflicting chronically ill individuals. *Gastroenterology*, 27:431–444.

Vasopressin and Vasoconstrictor Therapy

*Andres T. Blei and **Roberto J. Groszmann

*Gastroenterology Section, Department of Medicine, Lakeside VA Medical Center, Northwestern University, Chicago, Illinois 60611; and **Liver Disease Unit, Department of Medicine, West Haven VA Medical Center, Yale University, West Haven, Connecticut 06516

Our goal in this chapter is to assess the therapeutic role of intestinal vasoconstrictors in man. Although a large number of drugs have been shown to cause splanchnic vasoconstriction, few have been used clinically to treat gastrointestinal hemorrhage. This is probably due to a less than optimal experience with these agents and a fear of serious side effects. Few studies have been performed in animal models of hemorrhage, and randomized clinical trials in humans are difficult to perform, as these patients are seriously ill with life-threatening conditions. In spite of these limitations, some diseases of the digestive tract associated with gastrointestinal bleeding have been treated with these agents. In addition, newer applications have been suggested, such as their use during radiotherapy.

Vasopressin is the most commonly used splanchnic vasoconstrictor and typifies the problems of research in this area. We will therefore concentrate our discussion on this agent. It is also clear that the use of newer agents, such as somatostatin and propranolol, has accelerated in the last 10 years. Other intestinal vasoconstrictors that have not undergone clinical testing are listed on Table 1.

VASOPRESSIN

This naturally occurring nonapeptide, when infused at pharmacological doses, causes splanchnic vasoconstriction in the rat (34), cat (45), dog (33), monkey (25), and man (65). The intracellular mechanism of this effect has not been elucidated. However, vasopressin's antidiuretic effect involves binding to a specific receptor followed by cyclic AMP activation (78). It is unknown whether its action on vascular smooth muscle is similar.

Two different forms of vasopressin, differing by only one amino acid, are available for clinical use: lysine vasopressin and arginine vasopressin. Lysine^8-vasopressin is a peptide extracted from the hypophysis of the pig; some of the European data were obtained with this form. Almost all other mammals (including man) secrete arginine^8-vasopressin, the drug available in the United States. These two vasopressin molecules differ in their antidiuretic potency (47), but their pressor activities appear to be similar. In this discussion, we express the infusion rate of both molecules in biological units of their pressor activity. Pitressin was originally made as a mixture of arginine^8- and lysine^8-vasopressin. Recently, only arginine^8-vasopressin has been used (Parke-Davis, *personal communication*).

Route of Administration

In the initial studies in man, posterior pituitary extracts were administered as intravenous boluses over 10 to 20 min. Davis et al. (18), using an indicator-dilution technique with splenic injection of ^{131}I-labeled serum albumin and hepatic vein sampling, demonstrated that both cardiac output and splanchnic blood flow were decreased by vasopressin in normal and cirrhotic individuals. Intrasplenic pressure, a reflection of portal venous pressure, was also reduced. However, the obvious disadvantages of the short duration of action and the substantial side effects caused this route of administration to be abandoned.

TABLE 1. *Splanchnic vasoconstrictors*

A. Splanchnic vasoconstrictors used therapeutically in man:
   Vasopressin
   Triglycyl-vasopressin
   Somatostatin
   Propranolol
B. Drugs with splanchnic vasoconstrictive effects used for other therapeutic indications in man:
   Norepinephrine
   Epinephrine
   Dopamine
   Ouabain
   Digoxin
C. Splanchnic vasoconstriction in experimental animals, not tested for therapeutic use in man:
   Angiotensin II
   Calcium chloride
   Prostaglandin F_2

In 1968, it was postulated that intraarterial (i.a.) administration of vasopressin into the splanchnic vasculature would cause local vasoconstriction with few systemic hemodynamic repercussions (49). However, this hypothesis has been disproven in experimental animals (2,73) and in man (12,37). Intraarterial vasopressin produced changes in splanchnic blood flow (2), intestinal oxygen consumption (31,73), portal pressure (2,31), arterial pressure and cardiac output (2,31) similar to those seen with continuous intravenous (i.v.) administration. This may be explained in part by data (4) that indicate the liver is not the main site of elimination of the hormone. Intraarterial infusions require an expertise not always available and are fraught with higher risks. Thus, constant i.v. infusions are the route of choice at this time.

Effects on Splanchnic Blood Flow

In experimental animals, the effects of vasopressin on splanchnic blood flow have been studied mainly with two techniques: electromagnetic flow probes and radioactive microspheres. In man, available techniques preclude the measurements in individual splanchnic blood vessels. Most determinations have utilized hepatic venous sampling to estimate total splanchnic blood flow.

Vasopressin has generalized vasoconstrictive effects, but it exerts a more pronounced vasoconstrictive action in the splanchnic bed (63). In the dog, renal blood flow is not affected by bolus doses of lysine^8-vasopressin that clearly decrease gastrointestinal blood flow (64). The dose that results in 50% of maximal flow reduction (D_{50}) was 3 mU/kg in the superior mesenteric artery, but was 30 mU/kg in the renal, coronary and carotid arteries (64). Similar differences between the mesenteric and renal beds in the dog are seen after doses of 0.75 and 6.7 mU/kg of lysine^8-vasopressin, although muscle and carcass blood flow appear even more sensitive than the splanchnic area (20). These differences may depend not only on direct effects of the drug but also on autoregulatory mechanisms within each organ.

The mechanism of action of vasopressin on the resistance vessels is mediated by neither alpha- nor beta-adrenergic receptors (67). It is controversial whether or not escape from the constrictor effects occurs (see Chapter 5). No such escape is seen in the intestinal circulation of the cat (59). In the dog, however, some escape from vasoconstriction occurs at a dose of 2.5 mU/ml (67). In addition, administering vasopressin for several hours can result in tachyphylaxis in man (22).

Vasopressin reduces blood flow and increases vascular resistance in all gastrointestinal organs. In a dog study, the *stomach* appeared to exhibit greater reductions in flow than the intestine (73% and 45%, respectively) with both i.a. and i.v. infusions of 3 mU/kg/min (17). Similar differences occur after bolus injections of lysine^8-vasopressin in the dog (64). No regional differences in gastric perfusion are seen; flows are similar in the area perfused by the left gastric artery and in the remainder of the stomach (17). Additional studies are needed to confirm the preferential effect of vasopressin on gastric perfusion.

Dose-response studies in the *small bowel* of the cat reveal a plateau of mesenteric arterial response at a dose of 10 mU/kg/min (13). Post-infusion hyperemia is absent (59). The distribution of microspheres in the muscular and submucosal-mucosal layers is not altered by the infusion of vasopressin (29). However, the microsphere technique for fractionating intramural flow has limitations, as reviewed recently by Shepherd (68).

The effects of vasopressin on *colonic* blood flow appear to be similar to those on the small bowel. In the monkey, inferior mesenteric blood flow is reduced by 50% with an infusion of 10 mU/kg/min and autoregulatory escape is not evident (40). In denervated segments of dog colon, vascular resistance rises during drug infusion (58). Microsphere studies reveal simultaneous changes of similar magnitude in the small and large bowels (17,20).

The response of the *hepatic artery* to vasopressin is more complex, and its effect on hepatic oxygenation is controversial. An initial decrease in hepatic arterial flow is seen in experiments with either bolus injections or continuous infusions. In a preparation in which portal venous flow is kept constant (9), a biphasic response is seen with an initial reduction in flow followed by a sustained increase. An increase in hepatic arterial blood flow is also seen with constant pressure perfusion (3). These experiments suggest that the hepatic artery vasodilatory response is unique, is not dependent on the portal venous flow, and is not affected by sympathetic or parasympathetic blockade (9). Other investigators, using a vasopressin bolus in a denervated preparation (56) or perfusing the hepatic artery and portal vein simultaneously (57), do not demonstrate this vasodilatory phase. Differences in the systemic hemodynamic response may also influence the results; in a free-flow preparation in the dog, we have shown that the hepatic artery values are dependent on the effect of vasopressin on cardiac output (Fig. 1) (5).

Portal venous flow is also reduced in a dose-dependent fashion (2). In the dog, a linear re-

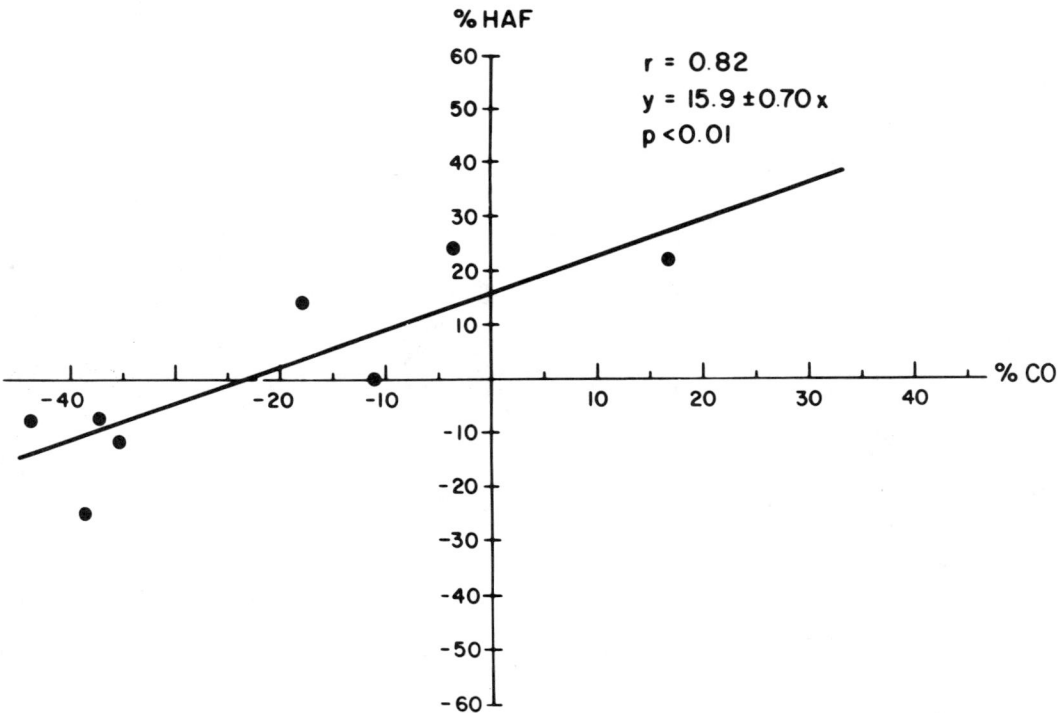

FIG. 1. Correlation between changes in hepatic arterial blood flow (HAF) and cardiac output (CO) during vasopressin infusion in the dog. A positive correlation is noted over a wide range of changes in CO. (From Blei et al., ref. 5, with permission.)

lation between superior mesenteric venous flow and portal venous pressure is seen with either vasopressin or mechanical obstruction of the superior mesenteric artery (31). This relation supports the rationale of using intestinal vasoconstrictors in the treatment of portal hypertension.

Finally, few studies have examined the effects of vasopressin during hemorrhage. In dogs with decreased splanchnic perfusion induced by hemorrhage, Ericsson (20) shows *increased* visceral flow during vasopressin infusion. He relates the increased flow to an increase in perfusion pressure and cardiac output. This issue deserves further attention because of the obvious implications in bleeding patients. In an experiment in which the clinical situation is more closely simulated, vasopressin is infused into dogs hypotensive from induced hemorrhage in which intravascular volume is being replaced (70). In this model, vasopressin prevents portal venous pressure and portal flow from returning to prehemorrhage levels.

Effect on Intestinal Oxygen Consumption

In our studies in which intestinal blood flow is reduced by inflating a balloon catheter placed in the superior mesenteric artery, increased oxygen extraction occurs (Fig. 2). Thus, oxygen

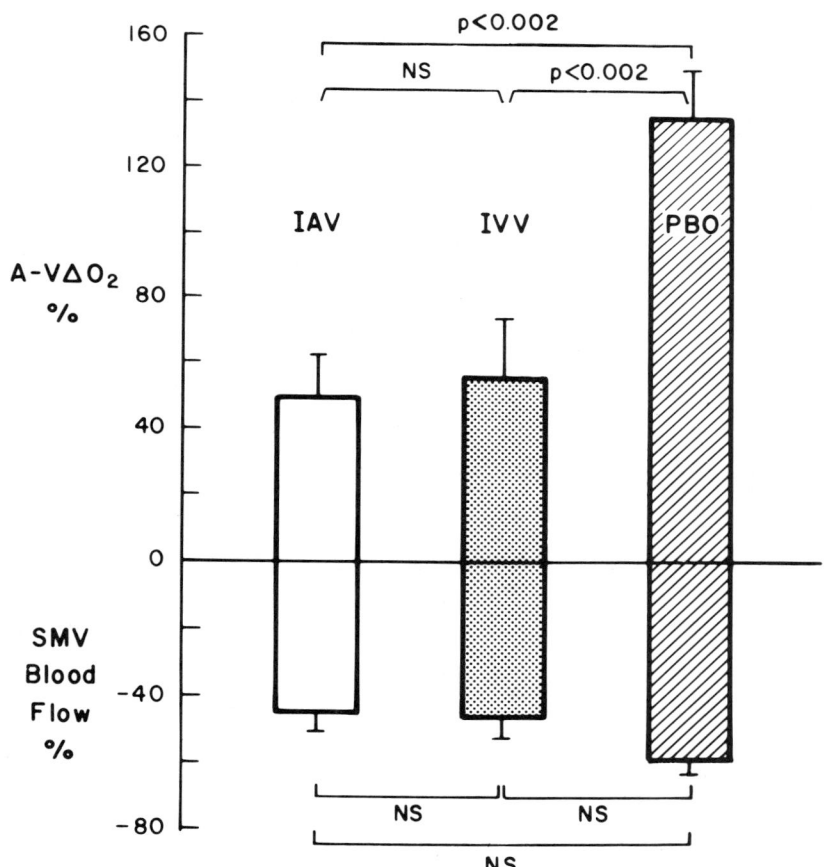

FIG. 2. Effect of vasopressin infusion and partial balloon obstruction (PBO) on superior mesenteric venous (SMV) flow and arteriovenous O_2 difference (A-Vo_2) in the dog. The compensatory response of A-Vo_2 is significantly decreased during intraarterial (IAV) or intravenous (IVV) vasopressin. All values are mean ± SE. (From Groszmann et al., ref. 31, with permission.)

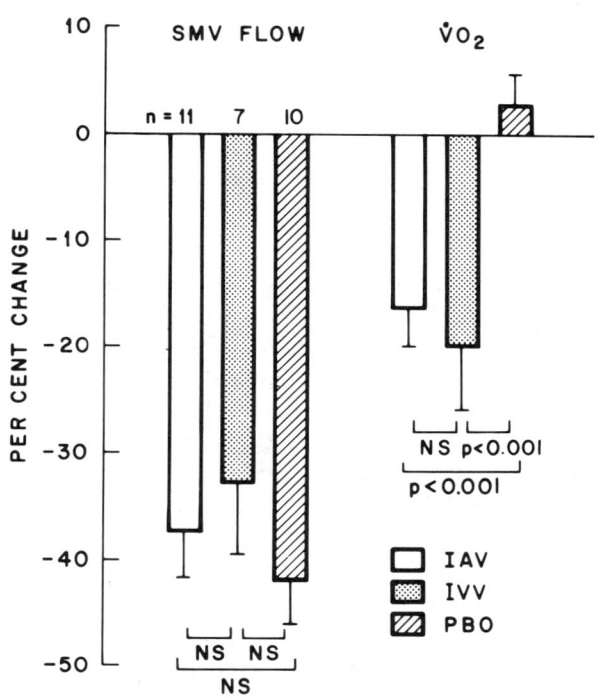

FIG. 3. Intestinal oxygen consumption ($\dot{V}O_2$) during superior mesenteric venous (SMV) flow reductions in the dog. Mechanical obstruction of the superior mesenteric artery flow (PBO) by 40% does not depress $\dot{V}O_2$; a significant decrease is observed with both intraarterial (IAV) and intravenous (IVV) vasopressin. All values are mean ± SE. (From Groszmann et al., ref. 31, with permission.)

consumption, as shown in Fig. 3, remains constant (30,31). A normal oxygen consumption occurs until blood flow is reduced to 40% of base-line values (31). A compensatory increase in oxygen extraction also occurs when vasopressin is infused, but the increased O_2 extraction is insufficient to correct for the reduced blood flow. Thus, oxygen consumption falls (Figs. 2 and 3). Furthermore, reductions in oxygen consumption occur at vasopressin doses that do not affect blood flow (51).

Neither a reduction in oxidative metabolism of the intestine nor villus countercurrent shunting of oxygen explains this phenomenon. However, vasopressin may reduce the number of perfused capillaries and the surface area for oxygen exchange (67). Although precapillary sphincter constriction cannot be directly measured, capillary filtration in the cat ileum is reduced (54). Estimates of capillary transport, using $^{86}RbCl$, are also reduced in constant-flow preparations (67). As with blood flow, the effect of vasopressin on capillary perfusion is not affected by alpha or beta blockade (67).

Is vasopressin contraindicated for clinical use owing to its effect on intestinal oxygen consumption? We do not think so. The majority of intestinal vasoconstrictors reduce bowel oxygenation (42), and the relation between flow and oxygen uptake suggests that it is difficult to have the desired effect on blood flow without some compromise on oxygenation (42). Doing so would require either mechanical reduction in blood flow (30), a maneuver that preserves bowel oxygenation, or the use of a drug that constricts the arteriole and not the precapillary sphincter. Only epinephrine at certain doses appears to possess such a property (42,51). Furthermore, clinical experience with vasopressin indicates that bowel necrosis occurs infrequently. Finally, mechanical reduction of intestinal blood flow in cirrhotic patients does not decrease portal venous pressure (wedge pressure) in a significant and predictable manner (R. J. Groszmann, *unpublished data*), making this a less satisfactory alternative.

Dose-Response

Studies in experimental animals suggest that the responses of both intestinal blood flow and oxygen extraction are dose-dependent (Table 2). Mesenteric blood flow reaches a plateau with an infusion of 10 mU/kg/min in the dog (13).

It is difficult to extrapolate from the dose-response relations in normal anaesthesized animals to patients. Doses between 0.1 and 4.0 U/min have been used therapeutically, but it is difficult to perform dose-response studies in man with a drug that has substantial side effects. The optimal dose for clinical use is discussed under Clinical Efficacy (also see Table 3).

Systemic Effects

Vasopressin causes generalized vasoconstriction and elevates systemic vascular resistance and mean arterial pressure (15). Vasopressin also lowers cardiac output in experimental animals (2,5) and in man (18,32). In addition to peripheral vasoconstriction, baroreceptor-mediated bradycardia (75) and decreased coronary blood flow (79) may contribute to the reduction in cardiac output. An increased sensitivity to the pressor action of vasopressin can be seen in barodenervated preparations (48), suggesting that baroreceptors normally attenuate the pressure response. Direct injections of vasopressin into the cerebral ventricles of the dog causes no changes in blood pressure, but marked bradycardia ensues (75), suggesting a centrally mediated action. Detailed studies of cardiac performance in the dog have shown a reduction in indices of myocardial contractility and coronary blood flow (79). Arrhythmias and myocardial infarction have been reported with the use of vasopressin in man (14).

Studies of other regional circulations have been performed mostly in experimental animals. We have discussed the response of the renal bed where autoregulatory mechanisms appear to be in effect. A similar preservation of blood flow is seen in the cerebral circulation (20,64). Vasoconstriction in muscle and skin appears to be significant (20,63). Clinically, blanching and mottling of the skin are conspicuous in humans given vasopressin.

Antidiuresis occurs with the previously mentioned doses but is rarely a major side effect

TABLE 2. *Selected dose-response studies in the experimental animal*

Ref.	Exp. condition	Organ and animal	Vasopressin dose (mU/kg/min)	Effect on blood flow	Effect on intest. oxygen consumpt.
13[a]	Constant pressure SMA	Small bowel, cat	0.5	−10%	NS
			1.0	−20%	NS
			2.5	−40%	NS
			5.0	−50%	NS
			10.0	−70%	NS
			50.0	−70%	NS
51	Free flow, isolated Ileal loop	Small bowel, dog	0.3	0	−7%
			0.7	−28%	−23%
			4.0	−60%	−54%
58	Free flow, isolated colonic segment	Large bowel, dog	0.5	−2%[b]	−1%[b]
			1.0	−15%	−12%
			2.0	−20%	−20%
			5.0	−33%	−31%
40	Free flow IMA	Large bowel, monkey	0.01[c]	−11%	NS
			0.1	−17%	NS
			1.0	−28%	NS
			10.0	−52%	NS

SMA, measurements in the superior mesenteric artery trunk; IMA, measurements in the inferior mesenteric artery trunk; NS, not studied.
[a]Blood flow changes expressed as conductance.
[b]Adapted from the authors' data.
[c]Bolus injections.

TABLE 3. Randomized clinical trials of vasopressin treatment

Ref.	Bleeding episodes[a] Vasopressin	Bleeding episodes[a] Control	Vasopressin dose	Cessation of hemorrhage Vasopressin	Cessation of hemorrhage Control	Survival in hospital Vasopressin	Survival in hospital Control	Comments
14	17 (V), 11 (NV)	16 (V), 16 (NV)	0.05–0.40 U/min	71% (V)[b], 73% (NV)[c]	25% (V), 31% (NV)	46%	44%	Control group treated with antacids, gastric hypothermia, Sengstaken-Blakemore tube, transfusions
46	5 (V), 13 (NV)	6 (V), 14 (NV)	0.2–0.4 U/min	44%[c]	15%	56%	55%	Control groups received nasogastric lavage and Sengstaken-Blakemore tube, transfusions
24	14 (V), 15 (NV)	19 (V), 12 (NV)	0.60/min	29% (V), 86% (NV)	36% (V), 62% (NV)	72%	65%	Control group received placebo (double-blind) and blood transfusions

Ref.	I.V. vasopressin	I.A. vasopressin	Vasopressin dose	I.V. vasopressin	I.A. vasopressin	I.V. vasopressin	I.A. vasopressin	Comments
12	10	12	I.V. = 0.3–1.5 U/min. I.A. = 0.1–0.5 U/min	50%	50%	30%	25%	No significant differences between groups. Only variceal bleeders
37	11	14	I.V. = 0.4 U/min I.A. = 0.4 U/min	64%	50%	64%		Survival not described for each group

[a] V, variceal; NV, nonvariceal.
[b] $p \leq 0.01$ vs control.
[c] $p \leq 0.05$ vs control.

when the drug is infused over a 24- to 48-hr period. Activation of fibrinolysis, however, is a potentially important effect. Vasopressin releases plasminogen activator from endothelial cells and therefore activates the fibrinolytic cascade (19). It is not known whether this counteracts the therapeutic goal of vasoconstriction and clot formation in the bleeding area. This problem is difficult to study, as these individuals are both losing intravascular volume and receiving blood products, making plasminogen/plasmin determinations difficult to interpret.

Clinical Efficacy

The rationale for the therapeutic use of vasopressin in gastrointestinal bleeding is based on the effects of splanchnic vasoconstriction, but other mechanisms may be operative. In the dog, a claim has been made that blood flow through esophageal varices (measured with ^{85}Kr injections in the portal vein) is decreased during a vasopressin bolus, suggesting a constriction of the esophageal musculature with resultant compression of the submucosal varices (1). This observation needs further confirmation.

In spite of extensive clinical experience, only three randomized clinical trials of continuous vasopressin infusions have been reported (14,24,46), and only one (24) is double-blind (Table 3). In two additional trials, intraarterial vasopressin is compared to intravenous infusions (12,37). Most of the patients in these five studies had bleeding esophageal varices and portal hypertension, but non-variceal hemorrhages were also included.

These trials have not yielded uniform results. Furthermore, the same institution (14) reporting a 75% to 80% success in controlling hemorrhage with intraarterial infusion in 1975 reports only 50% reduction 4 years later (12). Comparison of these trials is further complicated by different vasopressin dosages, differences in the clinical status of the patients, varied definitions of therapeutic success, and the tendency of gastrointestinal bleeding to cease spontaneously.

The Stanford study (24) deserves special attention because its conclusions challenge current thought. The trial reports a double-blind design that is difficult to accomplish with a drug that has obvious side effects (mottling of the skin, abdominal cramps). Variceal bleeding was less responsive to vasopressin (29%) than non-variceal hemorrhage (87%). Similar differences in the placebo response were seen (Table 3). Previous studies had shown that 44% to 71% of variceal bleeders respond to vasopressin (Table 3). As in the other studies, no beneficial effect on survival was seen; the total number of transfusions was similar in both groups. The authors postulated that the lack of beneficial effects of vasopressin in controlling hemorrhage provide little support for the use of this drug in upper gastrointestinal bleeding.

In the study from Stanford (24), the need for surgery in the first 24 hr was decreased with vasopressin administration, although not significantly by chi-square testing (10/31 placebo patients vs. 3/29 drug). In addition, the infusion was terminated in 17 placebo and 9 drug recipients because of persistent bleeding ($p = 0.10$). These differences, not fully discussed by the authors, indicate at least one therapeutic role of vasopressin: a treatment that allows time to be gained while other, more definitive therapeutic measures are planned. We therefore disagree with the conclusions of this study.

We still recommend vasopressin infusions as an initial treatment at a dose of 0.4 U/min. Because a dosage of 0.9 U/min (12) may be effective, dosage increases after an initial failure could be tried, but we are skeptical about their efficacy. Tapering the dose before discontinuing therapy appears unnecessary.

These trials illustrate the need for more-effective and less-toxic therapy, problems addressed in recent investigations.

Vasopressin Analogs

Altering the amino acid structure of the vasopressin molecule profoundly changes its activity. Thus, the presence of D-arginine instead of the L-isomer in position 8 (dDVAP) results in a loss of the pressor activity with maintenance of the antidiuretic effect (16). Addition of a (glycyl)$_3$ residue to the N-terminal of lysine^8-vasopressin yields a hormonogen, triglycylysine-vasopressin (tGLVP), which has undergone clinical testing in the treatment of gastrointestinal bleeding (26,76). Three advantages have been described for the use of this analog. First, enzymatic cleavage of the residue by endothelial endopeptidases may release lysine^8-vasopressin over a prolonged period (52). Consequently, a bolus injection may provide an "endogenous" infusion. Only 5% to 10% of the hormonogen administered is actually released as lysine-vasopressin (55). Second, the levels of the plasminogen activator, which activates the fibrinolytic cascade, rise with lysine^8-vasopressin, whereas the levels are unchanged with tGLVP (19). Finally, the drug may not depress cardiac output (76).

In a portal vein constriction model in the dog, the mean duration of portal venous pressure reduction is 104 min with a tGLVP bolus (5). tGLVP and a continuous vasopressin infusion cause similar reduction in cardiac output. In cirrhotic men, tGLVP decreases portal venous pressure without altering the cardiac output (76). The latter results are suspect, as the method to measure cardiac output was questionable and mean arterial pressure increased during tGLVP.

Two clinical trials in patients with bleeding esophageal varices have been reported with tGLVP. In a nonrandomized comparison with conventional treatment (Sengstaken-Blakemore tube and blood transfusion), tGLVP has controlled variceal bleeding in 80% of individuals (76). The second study, in which VP and tGLVP were compared in a randomized trial, shows 9% and 70% efficacy in controlling hemorrhage, respectively (26). The extremely low response in the vasopressin group casts doubt on the validity of these results. Clearly, more information is needed to substantiate the claims raised by these two trials, but tGLVP unfortunately is unavailable for widespread clinical testing.

Toxicity

The complications of vasopressin therapy can be grouped into several categories (Table 4). Most are due to generalized vasoconstriction.

TABLE 4. *Complications of vasopressin therapy*

A. Related to vasoconstriction
  1. Systemic effects
     Arrhythmias
     Myocardial infarction
     Heart failure
     Cardiorespiratory arrest
     Intracerebral bleeding
     Peripheral gangrene
  2. Splanchnic effects
     Bowel infarction
     Mesenteric thrombosis
     Ischemic colitis
B. Related to route of administration
  1. Intraarterial infusion
     Dissection of superior mesenteric artery
     Femoral pseudoaneurysm
     Sepsis
  2. Intravenous infusion
     Extravasation with gangrene

Hypertension, bradycardia, and abdominal cramping are considered side effects not complications.

The critical toxic dose is difficult to estimate, as it is also related to the previous cardiovascular status of the individual. However, initial bolus injections suggest that doses above 1 U/min are associated with unacceptable cardiotoxicity.

The problem of prior myocardial status is well illustrated in alcoholic cirrhotics, in whom subclinical cardiomyopathy may be present and who are prone to develop complications with vasopressin. The drug is contraindicated in patients with known coronary artery disease, and the infusion should be stopped if ventricular arrhythmia or chest pain develops. In addition, the drug has been associated with respiratory arrest (14) and death due to intracerebral hemorrhage (24). We believe strongly that vasopressin should only be administered in a closely monitored setting with frequent hemodynamic measurements and careful evaluation of side effects.

Attempts have been made to preserve the desired splanchnic vasoconstriction while minimizing the deleterious systemic hemodynamic effects. In the dog, the addition of isoproterenol may decrease the hazards of vasopressin by improving cardiac performance (69); however, the increase in myocardial oxygen consumption seen with both drugs may result in a higher rate of myocardial complications. Experimental evidence suggests that nitroglycerin (32,79) and nitroprusside (28,79) correct the changes in cardiac output, arterial pressure, and myocardial contractility. However, only nitroglycerin corrects the deleterious effects of vasopressin on coronary blood flow (79). Studies in portal hypertensive patients (32) confirm the beneficial effects of sublingual nitroglycerin (Fig. 4).

In addition, studies in dogs with experimental cirrhosis (32) demonstrate that vasopressin increases portal venous resistance, reducing, in part, the beneficial effects of vasopressin on portal pressure. Nitroglycerin, by diminishing portal venous resistance, enhances the benefi-

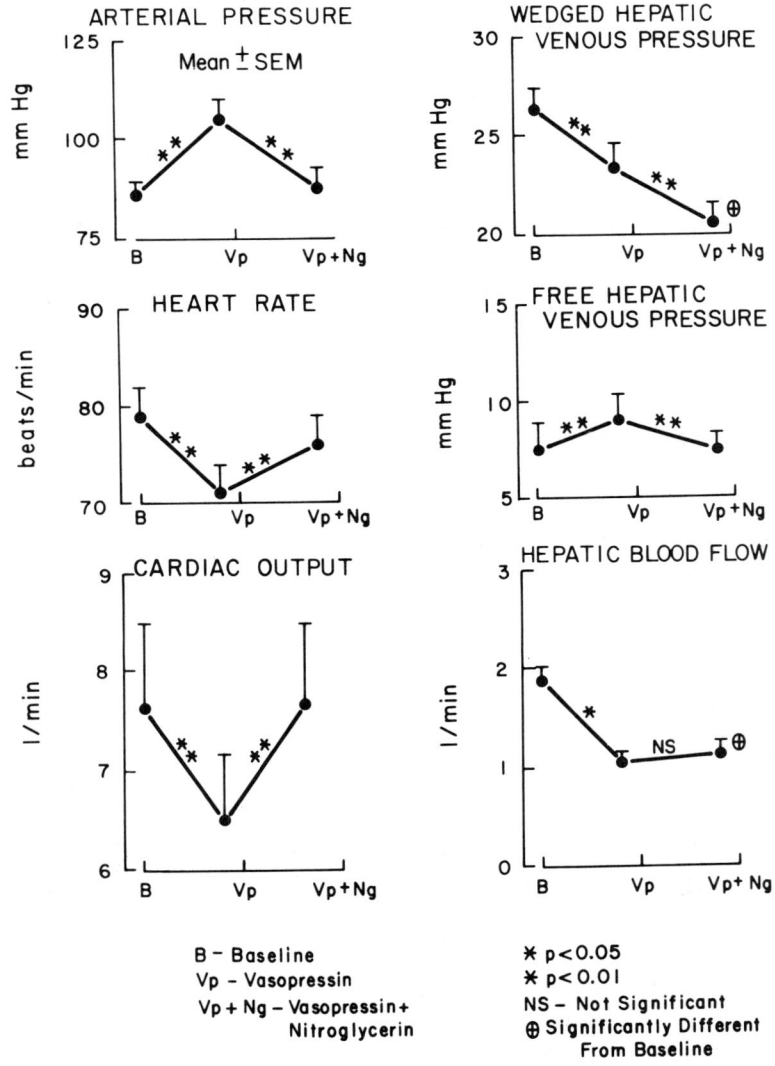

FIG. 4. Nitroglycerin (0.4 mg sublingually) reverses all the detrimental effects of vasopressin on systemic hemodynamics ($n = 15$). A further reduction of wedged hepatic venous pressure was seen with nitroglycerin without a return of hepatic blood flow to baseline levels. The hepatic venous pressure gradient (wedge-free pressures) decreased significantly with vasopressin (19.0 ± 1.4 to 14.6 ± 1.4 mm Hg, $p<0.01$). Addition of nitroglycerin resulted in an additional but not significant decrease in HVPG from 14.6 ± 1.4 to 13.6 ± 1 mm Hg. (From Groszmann et al., ref. 32, with permission.)

cial effects of vasopressin (32). Nitroglycerin, unfortunately, does not correct the decrease in intestinal oxygen consumption seen with vasopressin (R. J. Groszmann et al., *unpublished results*). When infused 1 hr after a digoxin bolus, nitroglycerin does not improve bowel oxygenation (6). Cardiac glycosides exert effects on intestinal oxygen uptake similar to vasopressin (50). In another study, nitroprusside decreased arterial pressure and systemic vascular resistance to values seen prior to the administration of vasopressin (11). The efficacy and safety of these combinations need to be tested in clinical trials.

Other Potential Applications of Vasopressin

The small intestine is vulnerable to radiation damage during radiotherapy of abdominal and pelvic malignancies. This damage by ionizing radiation from photons and electrons is dependent on both the radiation dose and the oxygen tension of the tissue. The ability of vasopressin to induce intestinal hypoxia and ischemia (and hence radiation protection) was studied in normal dogs (72) and mice (55) with results that suggest a radioprotective effect on the normal tissue. The critical hypoxic level that protects the intestine, however, is unknown. Furthermore, the response of tumor vessels to vasopressin is also unknown; a reduction in tumor blood flow may render the therapeutic effect of radiation ineffectual. Further studies are needed to substantiate a possible use of vasopressin during radiotherapy.

SOMATOSTATIN

This hypothalamic tetradecapeptide was isolated in 1972, and only a few years later it became clear that it exerted numerous extrahypophyseal effects. Thus, in 1976, estimated total splanchnic blood flow in man was shown to decrease with infusions of this hormone (77). Several studies in experimental animals (36,41,60) and in man (61,74) confirm these observations.

The *mechanisms* by which somatostatin decreases splanchnic blood flow are unclear. Gastric mucosal blood flow in the dog, estimated by the clearance of aminopyrine, is reduced in parallel to gastric secretion and aminopyrine concentrations are similar in gastric juice and plasma (41). Konturek et al. (41) claim that the reduction in blood flow is the result rather than the cause of secretory inhibition.

Somatostatin decreases the response to and inhibits the secretion of several pancreatic hormones, including gastrin, insulin, and glucagon. Since glucagon can increase splanchnic blood flow when infused at pharmacological doses, the suppressive effect of somatostatin on glucagon release has been studied in normal individuals (71). No correlation was seen between estimated hepatic blood flow and glucagon release. Alternatively, there is evidence to suggest a direct effect of somatostatin on smooth muscle. In isolated canine ileal loops, somatostatin decreases mesenteric flow, oxygen extraction, and oxygen consumption (41). The prompt onset of action and the simultaneous changes in different regional flows of experimental animals (60) and man (74) support a direct effect on vascular smooth muscle mediated through yet unspecified receptors.

In addition, *responses in other circulatory beds* appear to be different. In the human external iliac artery, flow measured with electromagnetic flowmeters at surgery increases 43% during a 1-min i.v. infusion of somatostatin (1 μg/kg/min). At the same time, arterial inflow to the splanchnic vascular bed decreases (74), but internal carotid flow is unaffected. The clinical observation that systemic vascular resistance is unchanged when the splanchnic blood flow is reduced (7) indicates there are regional differences in this agent's effects.

Bolus injections in the dog show *dose-dependent* effects. A plateau in the hemodynamic response is seen at 2 and 15 μg/kg/min during a 1-min infusion. Flow decreases by 20% in the mesenteric and gastric circulations (60). However, at a dose of 0.2 μg/kg/min maintained for 9 min, blood flow in the splanchnic area returns to normal after an initial decrease, suggesting autoregulatory escape (60). The decrease in portal venous blood flow plateaus at a dose ranging between 1 and 2 μg/kg/min (36).

In cirrhotic individuals, estimates of *hepatic blood flow* progressively decrease with infusion

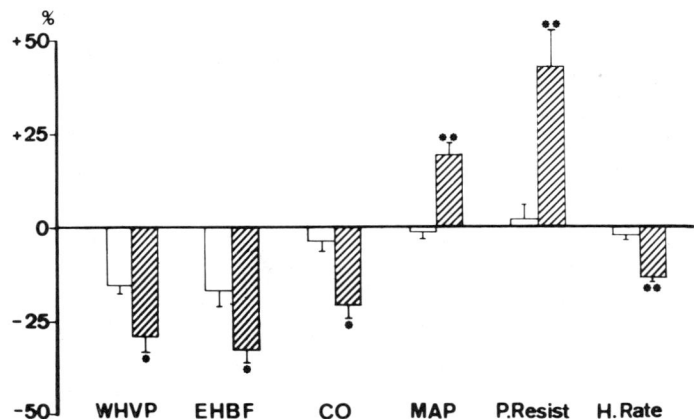

FIG. 5. Comparison of the effects of somatostatin (SMT) and vasopressin (VP) on the wedge hepatic vein pressure (WHVP), hepatic blood flow (EHBF), cardiac output (CO), mean arterial pressure (MAP), peripheral resistance, and heart rate in 6 patients with cirrhosis. Data represents mean ± SE of the present change from control periods. Both drugs reduce splanchnic blood flow, but the effect of vasopressin is more marked, as are the changes in systemic hemodynamics. *(Open bars)* SMT; *(hatched bars)* VP; *(asterisk)* $p<0.02$; *(two asterisks)* $p<0.01$. (From Bosch et al., ref. 7, with permission.)

rates of 2.5, 7.5, and 30 µg/min (7); no significant differences are seen between the last two doses. The effects of somatostatin in normal man are surprisingly more marked with an infusion of 4.2 µg/min than with 8.4 µg/min (71). Near the end of 1-hr infusions, hepatic blood flow returns toward normal, suggesting the possibility of tachyphylaxis (71). The optimal dose for clinical use is still controversial.

Systemic hemodynamic effects of somatostatin appear to be minimal. In experimental animals, doses between 0.2 and 15 µg/kg/min do not produce changes in cardiac output, arterial pressure, or heart rate (60). Infusion rates between 2.5 and 30 µg/min in man are also devoid of systemic hemodynamic effects (7,71). However, a 20% increase in arterial pressure is seen in anesthetized individuals with 1 µg/kg/min (74).

These hemodynamic properties are different from those of vasopressin. These hormones have been compared in stable cirrhotic individuals (7). The reductions in estimated hepatic blood flow and wedge hepatic pressure are more marked with vasopressin. Also, prominent systemic hemodynamic effects are seen that are not observed with somatostatin (Fig. 5).

Preliminary results in a randomized trial of somatostatin infusion (250–500 µg/hr) versus vasopressin (0.4 U/min) show they have equal effectiveness in controlling hemorrhage (53% and 58%, respectively) (8). A striking difference is seen in the rate of complications; somatostatin has a much lower morbidity, but the mortality of the bleeding episode was similar in both groups. Somatostatin also appears more effective in controlling persistent bleeding due to peptic ulcer disease when compared to cimetidine (38). In addition to its effects on gastric blood flow, somatostatin inhibits gastric acid secretion. Confirmation of its efficacy in ulcer bleeding is awaited with interest.

PROPRANOLOL

The use of propranolol in the treatment of patients with portal hypertension highlights the role of the adrenergic system in the regulation of intestinal blood flow (see Chapter 5). Therefore, we will discuss the evidence supporting the use of propranolol as a splanchnic vasoconstrictor.

In the dog, when intraarterial propranolol (0.1–0.3 mg) is added to a vasoconstrictive infusion of epinephrine (50 µg/kg/min), a further reduction in mesenteric flow ensues (51). In addition, propranolol diminishes the extent of autoregulatory escape seen with norepinephrine infusions (59). However, no effects are seen when propranolol is added to a norepinephrine infusion (66). Therefore, the decrease in splanchnic blood flow seen with propranolol could be explained by an alpha-adrenergic constriction enhanced by the blockade of silent beta-receptors.

At a dose of 0.13 mg/kg, propranolol decreases estimated splanchnic blood flow in man by 29%. Splanchnic vascular resistance rises significantly whereas total peripheral resistance is unchanged (53). Furthermore, preadministration of phenoxybenzamine (an alpha-adrenergic blocker) decreases but does not abolish the effect of propranolol on the splanchnic bed, a finding that suggests a direct effect of the drug on the splanchnic circulation.

Propranolol has been shown to decrease wedged hepatic vein pressure in cirrhotic individuals. In a randomized double-blind controlled trial, propranolol was administered to cirrhotic individuals who had had an episode of upper gastrointestinal hemorrhage. The drug successfully prevented the recurrence of bleeding within 1 year when compared to placebo (43). These results have opened a new dimension for the use of intestinal vasoconstrictors not only in the treatment but also in the prevention of bleeding. The need for better and safer vasoconstrictors is now clear.

OTHER VASOCONSTRICTOR AGENTS

Intravenous administration of *ouabain* or *digoxin* consistently decreases mesenteric blood flow in experimental animals (44,50). Pawlik et al. (50) have shown that splanchnic vascular resistance increases and that intestinal oxygen extraction falls. The reduction in intestinal oxygen consumption parallels the effects of other vasoconstrictors (except epinephrine). Digitalis preparations vasoconstrict other circulatory beds (27), raise mean arterial pressure independently of its effects on cardiac performance, and increase peripheral vascular resistance when administered to normal man. The mechanisms responsible for this effect are unclear. Inhibition of Na-K ATPase could be responsible for the direct effect on vascular smooth muscle, but central nervous system pathways may also be involved (27).

In man, the effects of digitalis on intestinal hemodynamics are more controversial. Cardiac glycosides have been implicated in the pathogenesis of nonocclusive mesenteric ischemia (35), a disease in which vasospasm is present in small mesenteric arteries. Ferrer et al. (23) report a decrease in splanchnic blood flow and a rise in splanchnic vascular resistance with i.v. digoxin. However, Bynum and Hanley (10) have shown that the effects of digitalis are dependent on the route of administration and on prior myocardial status. Ouabain and digoxin, administered intravenously, decrease splanchnic blood flow in normal volunteers, but oral digoxin has no effect. These differences might be related to different peak blood levels (higher when digoxin was infused intravenously). In 3 of 6 patients with heart failure, the rise in cardiac output seen with i.v. digoxin was associated with an increase in splanchnic blood flow. It appears, therefore, that the effects of digitalis on splanchnic blood flow were not consistent in the few data available.

Other Agents

The effects of epinephrine, norepinephrine, and other sympathomimetic drugs are discussed in Chapters 5 and 33. Angiotensin, calcium chloride, and prostaglandin F are all intestinal vasoconstrictors when infused intraarterially; they cause concomitant reductions in intestinal oxygen consumption. The effects of prostaglandin F are opposite to those of prostaglandin E, which increases mesenteric blood flow and oxygen consumption (51). The role of prostaglandins in the intestinal circulation is discussed in Chapter 8.

ACKNOWLEDGMENTS

This work was supported by the Veterans Administration Research Service. The authors thank Dr. Robert M. Craig for his careful review of the manuscript.

REFERENCES

1. Aronsen, K. F., Bjorkman, L., Lindstrom, K., Nylander, G., and Mulder, J. (1979): The mechanism of

lysine-vasopressin hemostasis in bleeding esophageal varices. *Acta Chir. Scand.*, 145:231–234.
2. Barr, J. W., Lakin, R. C., and Rosch, J. (1975): Similarity of arterial and intravenous vasopressin on portal and systemic hemodynamics. *Gastroenterology*, 69:13–19.
3. Barr, J. W., Lakin, R. C., and Rosch, J. (1975): Vasopressin and hepatic artery: Effect of selective celiac infusion of vasopressin on the hepatic artery flow. *Invest. Radiol.*, 10:200–205.
4. Baumann, G., and Dingman, J. F. (1976): Distribution, blood transport and degradation of anti-diuretic hormone in man. *J. Clin. Invest.*, 57:1109–1116.
5. Blei, A. T., Groszmann, R. J., Gusberg, R., and Conn, H. O. (1980): Comparison of vasopressin and triglycyl-lysine vasopressin on splanchnic and systemic hemodynamics in dogs. *Dig. Dis. Sci.*, 25:688–694.
6. Blei, A. T., Stern, R., and Yao, J. (1981): Digoxin and nitroglycerin: Its potential for the medical treatment of portal hypertension. *Hepatology*, 1:A6 (abstr).
7. Bosch, J., Kravetz, D., and Rodes, J. (1981): Effects of somatostatin on hepatic and systemic hemodynamics in patients with cirrhosis of the liver. *Gastroenterology*, 80:518–525.
8. Bosch, J., Kravetz, D., Teres, J., Bruix, A., Rimola, A., and Rodes, J. (1982): A controlled comparison of continuous somatostatin and vasopressin infusions in the treatment of acute variceal hemorrhage. *Hepatology*, 2:707 (abstr).
9. Bynum, T. E., and Fara, J. W. (1980): Hepatic artery response to vasopressin. *Am. J. Physiol.*, 239:G378–G381.
10. Bynum, T. E., and Hanley, H. G. (1982): Effect of digitalis on estimated splanchnic blood flow. *J. Lab. Clin. Med.*, 99:84–91.
11. Chandler, J. G. (1982): Vasopressin and splanchnic shunting. *Ann. Surg.*, 295:543–553.
12. Chojkier, M., Groszmann, R. J., Atterbury, C. E., Bar-Meir, S., Blei, A. T., Frankel, J., Glickman, M. G., Kniaz, J. L., Schade, R., Taggart, G. J., and Conn, H. O. (1979): A controlled comparison of continuous intraarterial and intravenous infusions of vasopressin in hemorrhage from esophageal varices. *Gastroenterology*, 77:540–546.
13. Cohen, M. M., Sitar, D. S., McNeill, J. R., and Greenway, C. V. (1970): Vasopressin and angiotensin on resistance vessels of spleen, intestine and liver. *Am. J. Physiol.*, 218:1704–1706.
14. Conn, H. O., Ramsby, G. R., Storer, E. H., Mutchnik, M. G., Joshi, P. H., Phillips, M. M., Cohen, G. A., Fields, G. N., and Petroski, D. (1975): Intraarterial vasopressin in the treatment of upper gastrointestinal hemorrhage: A prospective, controlled trial. *Gastroenterology*, 68:211–221.
15. Corliss, R. J., McKenna, D. H., Sialer, S., O'Brien, G. S., and Rowe, G. G. (1968): Systemic and coronary hemodynamic effects of vasopressin. *Am. J. Med. Sci.*, 256:293–299.
16. Cort, J., Albrecht, I., Novakova, J., Mulder, J., and Jost, K. (1975): Regional and systemic hemodynamic effects of some vasopressins: Structural features of the hormone which prolong activity. *Eur. J. Clin. Invest.*, 5:165–175.
17. Davis, G. B., Bookstein, J., and Hagan, P. L. (1976): The relative effects of selective intraarterial and intravenous vasopressin infusion. *Radiology*, 120:537–538.
18. Davis, W. D., Jr., Gorlin, R., Reichman, S., and Storaasli, J. P. (1957): Effect of pituitrin in reducing portal pressure in the human being: Preliminary report. *N. Engl. J. Med.*, 256:108–111.
19. Douglas, J. G., Forrest, J. A. H., Prowse, C. V., Cash, J. D., and Finlayson, N. D. C. (1979): Effects of lysine-vasopressin and glypressin on the first fibrinolytic system in cirrhosis. *Gut*, 20:565–567.
20. Ericsson, B. F. (1971): Hemodynamic effects of vasopressin. *Acta Chir. Scand. (Suppl.)*, 414:1–29.
21. Erwald, R., Wiechel, K. L., and Strandell, T. (1976): Effect of vasopressin on regional splanchnic blood flows in conscious man. *Acta Chir. Scand.*, 142:36–42.
22. Erwald, R. (1976): Vasopressin tachyphylaxis. *Acta Chir. Scand.*, 143:30–33.
23. Ferrer, M. I., Bradley, H. O., Wheeler, H. O., Enson, Y., Preisig, R., and Harvey, R. M. (1965): The effect of digoxin in the splanchnic circulation in ventricular failure. *Circulation*, 32:524–537.
24. Fogel, M. R., Knauer, C. M., Andres, L. L., Mahal, A. S., Stein, D. E. T., Kemeny, J., Rinki, M. M., Walker, J. E., Siegmund, D., and Gregory, P. (1982): Continuous intravenous vasopressin in active upper gastrointestinal bleeding. *Ann. Intern. Med.*, 96:565–569.
25. Freedman, A. R., Kerr, J. C., Swan, K. G., and Hobson, R. W., II (1978): Primate mesenteric blood flow: Effects of vasopressin and its route of delivery. *Gastroenterology*, 74:875–878.
26. Freeman, J. G., Lishman, A. H., Cobden, I., and Record, C. O. (1982): Controlled trial of terlipressin (glypressin) versus vasopressin in the early treatment of oesophageal varices. *Lancet*, 2:66–68.
27. Garan, H., Smith, T., and Powell, W. J., Jr (1974): The central nervous system as a site of action for the coronary vasoconstrictor effect of digoxin. *J. Clin. Invest.*, 54:1365–1372.
28. Gelman, S., and Ernst, E. A. (1980): Nitroprusside prevents adverse hemodynamic effects of vasopressin. *Arch. Surg.*, 113:1465–1471.
29. Greenway, C. V., and Murthy, V. S. (1972): Effects of vasopressin and isoprenaline infusions on the distribution of blood flow in the intestine: Criteria for the validity of microsphere studies. *Br. J. Pharmacol.*, 46:177–188.
30. Groszmann, R. J., Blei, A. T., Kniaz, J. L., Storer, E. H., and Conn, H. O. (1978): Portal pressure reduction induced by balloon obstruction of the superior mesenteric artery. *Gastroenterology*, 75:187–192.
31. Groszmann, R. J., Blei, A. T., Storer, E. H., and Conn, H. O. (1980): Intestinal O_2 consumption during mechanical and pharmacological reduction in portal pressure. *Am. J. Physiol.*, 238:G502–G508.
32. Groszmann, R. J., Kravetz, D., Bosch, J., Glickman, M., Bruix, J., Bredfeld, T., Conn, H. O., Rodes, J., and Storer, E. H. (1982): Nitroglycerin improves the hemodynamic response to vasopressin in portal hypertension. *Hepatology*, 2:757–762.
33. Hanson, K. M. (1970): Vascular response of intestine and liver to intravenous infusion of vasopressin. *Am. J. Physiol.*, 219:779–784.
34. Holliger, C., Radzyner, M., Villiger, A., Anliker, M., and Knoblauch, M. (1979): Effects of glucagon,

vasoactive intestinal peptide (VIP) and lysine-vasopressin on villous microcirculation and superior mesentery artery blood flow of the rat. *Bibl. Anat.*, 18:129–131.
35. Jacobson, E. D., and Lanciault, G. (1976): The gastrointestinal circulation. *Gastroenterology*, 71:851–873.
36. Jaspan, J., Polonsky, J., Lewis, M., and Moosa, A. R. (1979): Reduction of portal vein blood flow by somatostatin. *Diabetes*, 28:888–892.
37. Johnson, W. C., Widrich, W. C., Ansell, J. E., Robbins, A. H., and Nasbeth, D. C. (1977): Control of bleeding varices by vasopressin: A prospective randomized study. *Ann. Surg.*, 186:369–376.
38. Kayasseh, L., Gyr, K., Keller, V., Stalder, G. A., and Wall, M. (1980): Somatostatin and cimetidine in peptic ulcer hemorrhage. *Lancet*, 1:844–846.
39. Kehne, J. H., Hughes, F. A., and Gompertz, M. L. (1956): The use of surgical pituitrin in the control of esophageal varix bleeding: An experimental study and report of two cases. *Surgery*, 39:917–925.
40. Kerr, J. C., Hobson, R. W., II, Seelig, R. F., and Swan, K. G. (1977): Influence of vasopressin on colon blood flow in monkeys. *Gastroenterology*, 72:474–478.
41. Konturek, S. J., Tasler, J., Jaworek, J., Pawlik, W., Walus, K. M., Schusdziarra, V., Meyers, C. A., Coy, D. H., and Schally, A. W. (1981): Gastrointestinal, secretory, motor, circulatory and metabolic effects of prosomatostatin. *Proc. Natl. Acad. Sci.*, 78:1967–1971.
42. Kvietys, P. R., and Granger, N. (1982): Vasoactive agents and splanchnic oxygen uptake. *Am. J. Physiol.*, 243:G1–G9.
43. Lebrec, D., Poynard, T., Hillon, P., and Benhamou, J. P. (1981): Propranolol for prevention of recurrent gastrointestinal bleeding in patients with cirrhosis: A controlled study. *N. Engl. J. Med.*, 305:1371–1374.
44. Levinsky, R. A., Lewis, R. M., Bynum, T. E., and Hanley, H. G. (1975): Digoxin-induced intestinal vasoconstriction: The effects of proximal arterial stenosis and glucagon administration. *Circulation*, 52:130–136.
45. Lote, K., Folling, M., Levken, J., and Rosengren, B. (1981): Mesenteric arterial vasopressin in cats: Local and systemic effects. *Am. J. Roentg.*, 136:969–975.
46. Mallory, A., Schaefer, J. W., Cohen, J. R., Holt, S. A., and Norton, L. W. (1980): Selective intraarterial vasopressin infusion for upper gastrointestinal tract hemorrhage. *Arch. Surg.*, 115:30–32.
47. Miller, L., Fisch, L., and Kleeman, C. R. (1967): Relative potency of arginine[8]-vasopressin and lysine[8]-vasopressin in humans. *J. Lab. Clin. Med.*, 69:270–291.
48. Montani, J. P., Liard, J. F., Schoun, J., and Mohring, J. (1980): Hemodynamic effects of exogenous and endogenous vasopressin at low plasma concentrations in conscious dogs. *Circ. Res.*, 47:346–355.
49. Nusbaum, M., Baum, S., Kuroda, K., and Blakemore, W. S. (1968): Control of portal hypertension by selective mesenteric arterial infusions. *Arch. Surg.*, 97:1005–1013.
50. Pawlik, W., Shepherd, A. P., Mailman, D., and Jacobson, E. D. (1974): Effects of ouabain on intestinal oxygen consumption. *Gastroenterology*, 67:100–106.
51. Pawlik, W., Shepherd, A. P., and Jacobson, E. D. (1975): Effects of vasoactive agents on intestinal oxygen consumption and blood flow in dogs. *J. Clin. Invest.*, 56:484–490.
52. Pliska, V., Chard, T., Rudinger, J., and Forsling, M. L. (1976): In vivo activation of synthetic homonogenens in the cat. *Acta Endocrinol.*, 61:474–481.
53. Price, H. L., Cooperman, L. H., and Warden, J. C. (1967): Control of the splanchnic circulation in man: Role of beta-adrenergic receptors. *Circ. Res.*, 21:333–340.
54. Quillen, E. W., Granger, D. N., and Taylor, A. E. (1977): Effects of arginine vasopressin on capillary filtration in the cat ileum. *Gastroenterology*, 73:1290–1295.
55. Rapplaye, A. T., Johnson, G. H., Olsen, J. D., and Lagasse, L. D. (1975): The radioprotective effects of vasopressin on the gastrointestinal tract of mice. *Radiology*, 117:199–203.
56. Richardson, P. D. I., and Withrington, P. G. (1977): The effects of intraportal injections of noradrenaline, adrenaline, vasopressin and angiotensin on the hepatic portal vascular bed of the dog: Marked tachyphylaxis to angiotensin. *Br. J. Pharmacol.*, 59:293–301.
57. Richardson, P. D. I., and Withrington, P. G. (1978): The effects of intraarterial and intraportal injections of vasopressin on the simultaneously perfused hepatic arterial and portal venous vascular beds of the dog. *Circ. Res.*, 43:496–503.
58. Richardson, P. D. I., Granger, D. N., and Kvietys, P. R. (1980): Effects of norepinephrine, vasopressin, isoproterenol and histamine on blood flow, oxygen uptake and capillary filtration coefficient in the colon of the anesthetized dog. *Gastroenterology*, 78:1537–1544.
59. Ross, G. (1971): Escape of mesenteric blood vessels from adrenergic and non-adrenergic vasoconstriction. *Am. J. Physiol.*, 221:1217–1222.
60. Samnegard, H., Thulin, L., Andreen, M., Tyden, G., Hallberg, D., and Efendic, S. (1979): Circulatory effects of somatostatin in anaesthesized dogs. *Acta Chir. Scand.*, 145:209–212.
61. Samnegard, H., Tyden, G., Thulin, L., Friman, L., and Uden, R. (1980): Effect of somatostatin on regional splanchnic blood flows in man: Angiographic studies. *Acta Chir. Scand. (Suppl.)*, 500:71–73.
62. Schapiro, H., and Britt, G. L. (1972): The action of vasopressin on the gastrointestinal tract: A review of the literature. *Am. J. Dig. Dis.*, 17:649–667.
63. Schmid, P. G., Abboud, F. M., Wendling, M. G., Ramberg, E. S., Mark, A. L., Heistad, D. D., and Eckstein, J. W. (1974): Regional vascular effects of vasopressin: Plasma levels and circulatory responses. *Am. J. Physiol.*, 227:998–1004.
64. Schuurkes, J. A. J., Brouwers, H. A. A., Beijer, H. J. M., Charbon, G. A., and Schapiro, H. C. (1976): Lysine-vasopressin: Hemodynamic effects in the anesthesized dog. *Am. J. Dig. Dis.*, 21:1012–1019.
65. Shaldon, S., Dolle, W., Guevara, L., Iber, F. L., and Sherlock, S. (1961): Effect of pitressin on the splanchnic circulation in man. *Circulation*, 24:797–807.
66. Shepherd, A. P., Mailman, D., Burks, T. F., and Granger, H. J. (1973): Effects of norepinephrine and sympathetic stimulation on extraction of oxygen and ^{86}Rb in perfused canine small bowel. *Circ. Res.*, 39:166–174.
67. Shepherd, A. P., Pawlik, W., Mailman, D., Burks,

T. F., and Jacobson, E. D. (1976): Effects of vasoconstrictors on intestinal vascular resistance and oxygen extraction. *Am. J. Physiol.*, 230:298–305.
68. Shepherd, A. P., Maxwell, L. C., and Jacobson, E. D. (1981): Limitations of the microsphere technique to fractionate intestinal blood flows. In: *Measurement of Blood Flow*, edited by D. N. Granger and G. B. Bulkley, pp. 195–200. Williams and Wilkins, Baltimore.
69. Sirinek, K. R., Martin, E. W., Jr., and Thomford, N. R. (1976): Simultaneous isoproterenol affords cardiodynamic advantages during vasopressin administration. *J. Surg. Res.*, 20:229–308.
70. Skivolocki, W. P., Sirinek, K. R., and Pace, W. G. (1979): Effect of vasopressin on portal pressure during volume replacement after acute hemorrhage. *World J. Surg.*, 3:241–247.
71. Sonnenberg, G. E., Keller, J., Perruchoud, A., Burckhardt, D., and Gyr, K. (1981): Effects of somatostatin on splanchnic hemodynamics in patients with cirrhosis of the liver and in normal subjects. *Gastroenterology*, 80:526–532.
72. Steckel, R. J., Snow, H. D., Collins, J. D., Barenfus, M., and Patin, T. (1974): Successful radiation protection of the normal intestinal tract in the dog. *Radiology*, 111:451–455.
73. Steckel, R. J., Kolin, A. K., MacAlpin, R. N., Snow, H. D., Juillard, G. F., Tesler, A. S., and Metzger, J. (1978): Differential effects of pitressin on blood flow and oxygen extraction in canine vascular beds. *Am. J. Roentgenol.*, 130:1025–1032.
74. Tyden, G., Samnegard, H., Thulin, L., Muhrbreck, D., and Efendic, S. (1979): Circulatory effects of somatostatin in anaesthesized man. *Acta Chir. Scand.*, 145:443–446.
75. Varma, S., Jaju, B. P., and Bhargava, K. P. (1969): Mechanisms of vasopressin induced bradycardia in dogs. *Circ. Res.*, 24:787–792.
76. Vosmik, J., Jedlicka, K., Mulder, J. L., and Cort, J. H. (1977): Action of glypressin in patients with liver cirrhosis and bleeding esophageal varices. *Gastroenterology*, 72:605–609.
77. Wahren, J., and Felig, P. (1976): Influence of somatostatin on carbohydrate disposal and adsorption in diabetes mellitus. *Lancet*, 2:1213–1216.
78. Weitzman, R. E., and Fisher, D. A. (1978): Arginine vasopressin metabolism in dogs. I: Evidence for a receptor mediated mechanism. *Am. J. Physiol.*, 235:E591–E597.
79. Zito, R. A., Diez, A., and Groszmann, R. J. (1984): Comparative effects of nitroglycerin and nitroprusside on vasopressin-induced cardiac dysfunction in the dog. *J. Cardiovasc. Pharmacol.* (In press)

Pharmacology of Intestinal Blood Flow and Oxygen Uptake

P. D. I. Richardson

Astra Pharmaceuticals Limited, Home Park Estate, Kings Langley, Hertfordshire, WD4 8DH, England

A wide range of drugs alters intestinal blood flow and oxygen uptake. Of these drugs, some have been used to investigate physiological control of the intestinal circulation and others have more direct therapeutic applications. Drugs used clinically may enhance or compromise intestinal perfusion, and any chronic reduction in intestinal blood flow is at least potentially a source of adverse drug reactions.

Interpretation of drug-induced changes in intestinal perfusion may be complicated by technical and physiological differences between an experimental preparation and the intact conscious animal or patient. A drug effect observed in an experimental study, for example, that intraarterial vasopressin reduces intestinal blood flow and oxygen uptake (13,17,41), may be directly applicable to man and be of therapeutic importance, in this case, in controlling portal venous hypertension and esophageal varix bleeding by reducing mesenteric blood flow.

However, such direct, uncomplicated extrapolations from an experimental observation to a therapeutic role are rare. Problems include the following:

1. Direct vascular effects may be overridden *in vivo* by reflex responses, for example, a baroreceptor-mediated vasoconstriction in response to a hypotensive effect of a dilator drug. Experimental preparations in anesthetized animals or with sectioned sympathetic nerves may well give a misleading impression of the responses of the normal human circulation to a drug.
2. The concentration of a drug in the bloodstream during an experiment may far exceed that attained therapeutically, especially if comparing an intraarterial infusion with plasma concentrations attained after oral administration of a drug or after physiological release of a hormone.
3. Drugs may release or inhibit release of catecholamines from intraneuronal or adrenal medullary stores (e.g., histamine, guanethidine) thereby altering intestinal perfusion.
4. The intestine is properly regarded as an endocrine organ, but it is still uncertain what role, if any, hormones such as secretin and cholecystokinin-pancreozymin (CCK-PZ) have in controlling intestinal perfusion (19). The intestinal vasoregulatory significance of hormones such as enteroglucagon or vasoactive intestinal peptide (VIP) remains unestablished.
5. Species or "circumstantial" differences may exist in drug-receptor types or density. Not only may an observation in an experimental animal be misleading when one considers man, but also there may be interindividual differences. For example, changes in beta-adrenergic receptor function may result from long-term beta blockade.

Even if we assume that ultimately our interest lies in the control and modification of human intestinal oxygenation, what is an "ideal" experiment? Leaving aside species differences, a demonstrable effect in an autoperfused innervated preparation with plasma concentrations of drug comparable to those occurring clinically would be valuable evidence of a probable effect in man. However, such experiments may not be compatible with an analytical approach to circulatory studies or with the generation of detailed, accurate data. In this review, a pragmatic view of drug effects on the intestinal circulation is taken with the aims of summarizing the present position and of proposing areas requiring further study. Recent reviews (8,19,30,31) have given details of the effects of many drugs on intestinal blood flow and oxygen uptake, and it is not the purpose of this chapter to repeat these detailed data presentations, some of which are summarized in Table 1.

Kvietys and Granger (31) have reviewed the effects of a wide range of drugs on oxygen uptake by the intestine *in vivo*. The general rule is clearly that vasodilators increase and vasoconstrictors decrease intestinal oxygen uptake. Most of the exceptions to this very simple rule are apparently easily explained. For instance, a complex effect would be expected for epinephrine depending on the relative degree of alpha- (vasoconstrictor; reduced oxygen uptake) and beta- (vasodilator; increased oxygen uptake) adrenoceptor stimulation by a mixed agonist. There is no reason to suppose that dose-response relationships for two effects such as blood flow and oxygen uptake should lie in exactly the same part of the dose range, so fortuitous selection of epinephrine doses would potentially result in varied combinations of changes in blood flow and oxygen uptake. Similarly, there are attractive explanations for the lack of apparent effect on oxygen uptake of some drugs. For example, angiotensin, where tachyphylaxis is often a major feature of responses, or in some cases the doses may simply be inadequate to ensure demonstrable effects.

That there is a clear relationship between drug-induced changes in blood flow or vascular resistance and oxygen uptake in the intestine is well established (30,46) and it appears to hold true for a wide range of drugs. Two important questions remain—What are the explanations for this relationship? Is it of biological significance or an artefact of the experiments that established it?

DRUG EFFECTS ON INTESTINAL BLOOD FLOW

The effects of drugs on intestinal blood flow depend on the segment of gut and vary among the tissue layers of any particular gut segment. For example, total blood flow could increase, yet regional blood flow in the mucosa or muscularis could decrease or remain unaltered.

Many studies of intestinal pharmacology have been published, but because of methodological differences, many are not directly comparable. In this section, an overview of the pharmacological effects of a range of drugs is given, and an attempt is made to assess the physiological and clinical relevance of these observations.

Alpha-Receptor Stimulants and Blockers

The pure alpha-receptor stimulants, methoxamine and phenylephrine, cause intestinal vasoconstriction in the cat (44) and dog (1), as does the naturally occurring catecholamine, norepinephrine, which is predominantly an alpha-receptor stimulant (9,22,26,33,43,52). The vasoconstrictor effects of norepinephrine are blocked by phentolamine (9,43), which itself causes vasodilation in the innervated gut (9,10, 43,44).

Beta-Receptor Stimulants and Blockers

Intestinal vasodilation occurs in response to intraarterial or intravenous isoproterenol (23, 26,41,44,54), and this response is blocked by propranolol (23,26,41,44,54). In most preparations, beta-blockade alone does not produce any consistent change in intestinal blood flow, suggesting the absence of a "tonic" stimulation of intestinal vascular beta-receptors. In the dog and cat at least, the receptors mediating intestinal vasodilation are predominantly of the beta$_2$ type (44,55).

Epinephrine

Early reports of the intestinal vascular responses to epinephrine were variable, and with the benefit of hindsight, the reasons are clear. Epinephrine, by stimulating both alpha- and beta-

TABLE 1. *Drug effects on intestinal oxygenation*

	Resistance vessels (19)	Capillary density (47)	Oxygen uptake	
			In vitro	In vivo
Adrenergics				
Phenylephrine	Constriction	Reduction		
Methoxamine	Constriction			
Norepinephrine	Constriction	Reduction		Reduction
Epinephrine	Variable[a]		Increase	Variable
Isoproterenol	Dilation	Increase	No change	Variable
Salbutamol	Dilation			
Dopamine	Variable[b]			Reduction
Phentolamine	Dilation	Reduction		
Propranolol	(Constriction)	(Reduction)		
Cholinergics				
Acetylcholine	Dilation[c]		Increase	Increase
Atropine	No effect			
Peptide hormones				
Vasopressin	Constriction	Reduction	Reduction	Reduction
Angiotensin	Constriction	Reduction		Reduction
Pentagastrin	Dilation[d]	Reduction		Increase
Secretin	Dilation	Increase		Increase
CCK-PZ	Dilation	Increase		Increase
VIP	Dilation			Increase
Glucagon	Dilation	Reduction[e]		Increase
"Dilators"				
Sodium nitrite	Dilation	Increase		
Papaverine	Dilation			No change
Aminophylline	Dilation	Increase		
Nitroprusside	Dilation	Increase		
Prostaglandins[f]				
PGE_1	Dilation		Increase	Increase
PGE_2	Dilation			
$PGF_{2\alpha}$	Constriction			Variable
Adenine group				
Adenosine	Dilation	Reduction	Reduction	Variable
ATP	Dilation			
AMP	Dilation			
Autacoids				
Histamine	Dilation	Increase[e]	Increase	Increase
Dimaprit	Dilation	—		
5-HT	Variable	Variable		
Bradykinin	Dilation	Increase		

[a] Alpha-mediated constriction, beta-mediated dilation.
[b] Alpha-mediated constriction, DA-receptor mediated dilation.
[c] Intestinal contraction reduces blood flow at high doses.
[d] Pentagastrin.
[e] An alpha-mediated reduction.
[f] Species variations.

receptors, can cause either alpha-mediated constriction or beta-mediated dilation (5,27,34). Changes in blood flow depend on the concentration of epinephrine and the concomitant alterations in systemic arterial pressure. Vasoconstrictor responses to epinephrine (high doses) are potentiated by beta-blockade (41) and vasodilator responses (low doses) by alpha-blockade (54).

Experimentally, vascular responses to epinephrine depend on the existing level of vasoconstrictor tone, since no dilation will be apparent in an atonic vasculature, although even in atonic, denervated preparations the vasoconstrictor response to epinephrine may be enhanced by beta$_2$-receptor blockade.

Dopamine

The intestinal vasculature, like other splanchnic beds, contains specific dopamine receptors that when stimulated cause vasodilation (59). At higher concentrations, dopamine stimulates alpha-adrenoceptors, causing vasoconstriction (42, 59). Neither effect is likely to be of physiological interest, as elevated dopamine levels only occur concomitant with overwhelming elevated epinephrine concentrations. However, dopamine is commonly used clinically.

Cholinergics

There are conflicting reports of the vascular effects of acetylcholine, but it seems most likely that acetylcholine causes intestinal vasodilation (2,52,56), particularly at low doses and by intraarterial administration. Higher doses may actually reduce intestinal blood flow due to systemic hypotension, the baroreflex response of splanchnic vasoconstriction, and vascular compression due to intestinal smooth muscle contraction. These vascular effects of acetylcholine can be blocked by atropine (2), although possibly higher doses are needed than are required to block the nonvascular (intestinal smooth muscle) effects of acetylcholine.

Histamine

Histamine causes intestinal vasodilation predominantly by stimulating vascular H$_1$ receptors (16,44). Although the role of vascular H$_1$ receptors in the dilator response to histamine is clear, it seems that H$_2$ receptors also mediate vasodilation (16,39), but the importance of intestinal vascular H$_2$ receptors is not established.

Serotonin

Intestinal vascular responses to serotonin (5-HT) are variable and occur only at high doses. The responses depend on dose, route of administration, and the tone of the vasculature. Moderate doses evoke vasodilation that is reversed to constriction by dihydroergotamine (19). On balance, a physiologic role for 5-HT in gut vasoregulation seems improbable, despite the large amounts localized in the intestinal wall (19).

Bradykinin

Intestinal vasodilation is the sole response to bradykinin (15,43,52), though pulmonary deactivation ensures that responses to intravenous administration are minor compared with intraarterial doses.

Vasopressin

Vasopressin is a pure intestinal vasoconstrictor that has been used for this purpose in the clinical control of bleeding from esophageal varices secondary to portal hypertension (28, 37,43,54; see also Chapter 31). It is conceivable that vasopressin has a pathophysiologic role following hemorrhage: release of ADH would tend to maintain intravascular volume by causing arteriolar constriction in the gut and thus mobilize fluid from pericapillary spaces.

Angiotensin

Angiotensin is a less-potent intestinal vasoconstrictor than vasopressin or methoxamine (44,56), but it may have a pathophysiologic role in hemorrhagic shock (35).

Gastrointestinal Hormones

Intestinal vasodilation has been demonstrated in response to secretin (7,45,49), CCK-PZ (7), VIP (12), and pentagastrin (51), but a number of problems remain in the establishment of a physiological vasoregulatory role for these hormones. Classical perfusion experiments often use higher concentrations of hormones than occur physiologically, or impure preparations. If difficulty exists in assessing whether or not a hormone has a physiological role in increasing gut blood flow postprandially, a greater difficulty exists in knowing whether the concomitant release of two or more hormones (e.g., secretin + CCK-PZ) evokes physiological dilation (19).

Glucagon

Glucagon causes intestinal vasodilation (14, 50,57) at concentrations well in excess of those occurring naturally. Unlike other polypeptide hormones, glucagon also inhibits intestinal vasoconstriction (29,58), an effect similar to that in the hepatic arterial bed (48), which has been proposed as of potential pathophysiologic importance in stress and hypoglycemia (48).

"Nonspecific Vasodilators"

Smooth muscle relaxant drugs that evoke intestinal dilation include sodium nitroprusside (40), sodium nitrate (43), aminophylline (44), papaverine (24), adenosine, ATP and AMP (36).

Prostaglandins

PGE_2 is an intestinal vasodilator (25), as is PGE_1 (11), whereas $PGF_{2\alpha}$ causes vasoconstriction, at least in the dog (52).

EXPLANATIONS OF A POSITIVE RELATIONSHIP BETWEEN BLOOD FLOW AND OXYGEN UPTAKE

In the absence of drugs, there is a curvilinear relationship between blood flow and oxygen uptake in most splanchnic organs (30,31). At blood flows in and above the normal physiological flow, oxygen uptake remains constant; as blood flow decreases below normal, the oxygen uptake becomes flow-limited as both variables approach zero (Fig. 1). This reduced oxygen

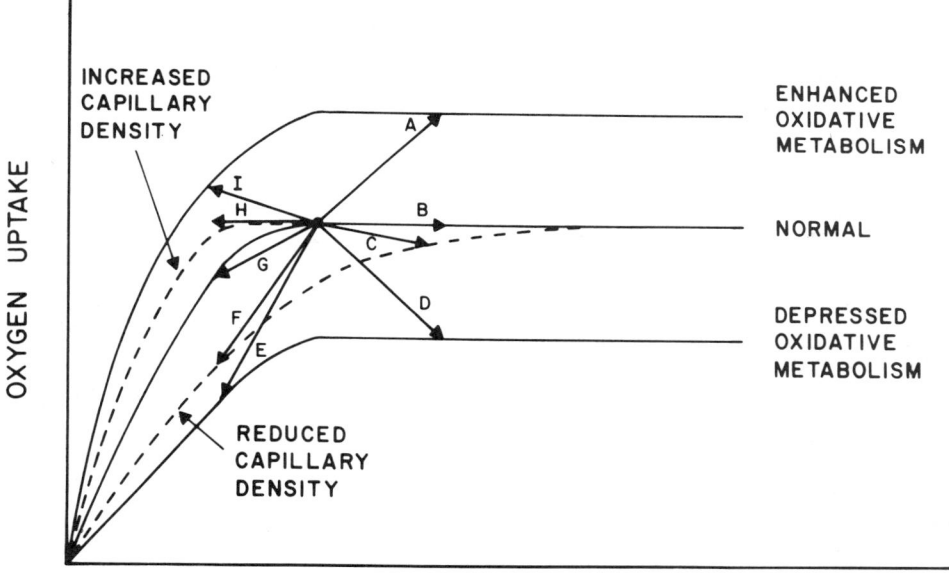

FIG. 1. Diagrammatic representation of relation between blood flow and oxygen uptake and factors that alter this relationship. Note that alterations in tissue oxidative metabolism shift curves vertically, whereas alterations in capillary density shift curves horizontally. *(Dot)* Control blood flow under normal conditions. *Pathway A* is taken by vasodilator that increases oxidative metabolism. *Pathway B* is taken by vasodilator that either does not affect metabolism or increase capillary density. *Pathway C* is taken by vasodilator that decreases capillary density. *Pathway D* is taken by vasodilator that decreases metabolism. *Pathway E* is taken by vasoconstrictor that decreases metabolism. *Pathway F* is taken by vasoconstrictor that decreases capillary density. *Pathway G* is taken by vasoconstrictor that does not affect metabolism or capillary density. *Pathway H* is taken by vasoconstrictor that increases capillary density. *Pathway I* is taken by vasoconstrictor that increases metabolism. (From Kvietys and Granger, ref. 31, with permission.)

uptake at low blood flows probably reflects a reduction in intracellular P_{O_2} due to reduced oxygen diffusion from blood to cells, so that normal intracellular metabolism cannot be sustained.

Drugs Altering Metabolism

Theoretically, any combination of drug effects in intracellular metabolism and blood flow is possible: vasoconstriction with increased or decreased metabolism, vasodilation with increased or decreased metabolism. To profile a drug accurately requires that these two sets of data are acquired independently, that is, that vasoconstriction or dilation are assessed *in vivo* (while measuring oxygen uptake) and that changes in oxidative metabolism are assessed using comparable drug concentrations *in vitro*.

This is necessary to ensure that only direct effects on metabolism and not indirect effects such as flow limitation of oxygen supply are studied. Figure 1 illustrates that vasoactive agents that do not directly alter oxidative metabolism merely move oxygen uptake along the normal blood flow–oxygen uptake curve *(pathways B and G)*. Agents that directly alter oxidative metabolism shift the blood flow–oxygen uptake relationship either up (increased metabolism) or down (decreased metabolism). The more common drug profiles are of vasodilation with increased oxygen uptake *in vitro* [histamine (4,20), acetylcholine (4), and PGE_2 (20)] and vasoconstriction with reduced oxygen uptake [vasopressin (20) and ouabain (18)]. Additional studies are required to extend these important observations to a wider range of drugs and a substantial dose range. Complex effects are to be expected from drugs such as epinephrine (18), which have actions resulting from multiple receptor interaction.

Drugs Altering Capillary Density

One would expect a relationship between drug-induced changes in capillary density and oxygen uptake. If capillary density is increased, a lower blood flow will be capable of maintaining normal oxygen uptake because there will be a reduced distance for oxygen to diffuse from blood to tissue. Put crudely, the cells have better access to the available oxygenated blood supply. Conversely, if capillary density is reduced, a higher blood flow will be required to serve the tissue's oxygen needs, but once that higher than normal blood flow has been attained, the reduction in capillary density is irrelevant, and oxygen uptake will be maintained constant at the normal level (see Fig. 1).

Capillary density can be readily assessed from measurements of intestinal capillary filtration coefficient ($K_{f,c}$ 44,47). In general, vasodilator drugs increase $K_{f,c}$ and vasoconstrictors decrease it. The effects on $K_{f,c}$ often occur at drug concentrations lower than are required to alter blood flow (44). Of the exceptions, epinephrine is expected to have dose-dependent effects due to beta- and alpha-receptor simulation, whereas some of the dilators that reduce $K_{f,c}$ (histamine, glucagon, 5-HT, pentagastrin) may do so indirectly through catecholamine release, or have an effect only at near-toxic concentrations (47). Adenosine is an established exception to the rule and dilates while reducing $K_{f,c}$ (21). However, adenosine also reduces oxygen uptake *in vitro*, so adenosine's effects on tissue oxygen uptake *in vivo* may be due to a reduced capillary density, depressed oxidative metabolism, or both.

Drug Effects on Countercurrent Exchange

A theoretical contribution to drug effects on tissue oxygen uptake could arise from an alteration in the gradient of tissue P_{O_2} from villus tip (low) to base (high) (3). This gradient would be expected to be reduced by an increased villus blood flow (vasodilation) and vice versa. With vasodilation to increase blood flow above normal, no increase in oxygen uptake occurs (30,32), a finding that suggests that this contribution from a dilator-induced change in countercurrent exchange is of little practical significance. A vasoconstrictor would be expected to exaggerate the tip-to-base P_{O_2} gradient with an increase in the relative hypoxia of the villus tip as blood flow is compromised, and the contribution that this effect makes to the general reduction in tissue oxygen uptake associated with constrictor drugs is hard to assess, though probably it is rather small.

Blood Flow Distribution

It is inaccurate to regard the intestine as a homogeneous structure: some vasoactive drugs may alter tissue oxygen uptake by redistributing blood flow among the mucosa, submucosa, and muscularis (8).

At present there are insufficient data to permit more than speculation on the contribution this might make to total tissue oxygen uptake, but it is an attractive hypothesis that a drug might redistribute blood flow from a metabolically active to a less-active area and so reduce total tissue oxygen uptake (21). This is an area that requires considerable additional experimentation so that its importance can be assessed (see Chapter 3).

EXPERIMENTAL PROBLEMS

As well as the five pharmacological variables discussed above, several features of an experimental preparation can influence the results of an investigation of drug effects on oxygen uptake. Luminal distension (38) causes intestinal oxygen uptake to become flow-dependent. Thus, if the lumen were to become distended during an investigation, in which, for example, secretagogs were infused, aberrant results dependent not on the vascular effects of the drug under investigation but on the luminal distension would be obtained.

Changes in the oxygen-carrying capacity of the blood, by a reduced hematocrit or hemoglobin concentration, would alter the relationship between oxygen uptake and blood flow (53). This factor can be monitored easily during an investigation.

Partial perfusion of a tissue is perhaps a more difficult technical problem to solve. It has been shown (6) that gastric oxygen uptake is flow-independent in stomachs perfused via the celiac artery but flow-dependent in stomachs perfused solely via the left gastroepiploic artery, suggesting that under- or partial perfusion results in oxygen uptake becoming flow-dependent. This may be a result of changes during the experiment in the proportion of the total tissue mass that is actually perfused. A similar phenomenon may occur if discrete regions of an organ are not perfused (e.g., due to thrombotic occlusion or vasospasm).

Many of these "technical" problems are difficult to monitor in experimental preparations, and it is almost impossible to assess the contribution that they may have made to the pharmacological observations discussed earlier.

CONCLUSIONS

Drug Profiles

With increasing technical sophistication, it becomes more apparent that to establish a profile of a drug's effects on the intestinal circulation, several complimentary studies are necessary. It should go without saying that, in all these studies, the same concentrations of drug must be used to ensure comparability, and where possible a range of concentrations encompassing the pathophysiological or therapeutic range should be tested.

It is not long since accurate measurements of blood flow and intravascular pressures would have been regarded as major advances. Now we should add to these an assessment of capillary exchange, probably measuring drug-induced changes in capillary filtration coefficient or permeability–surface area product. In separate experiments, drug-induced changes in osmotic reflection coefficients can be assessed (see Chapter 20), and consequently "pure" effects on microvessel permeability established. Comparisons of the effects of a drug on filtration coefficients and reflection coefficients can determine whether that drug alters perfused capillary surface area or microvessel permeability. It is critical in such studies that the same drug concentrations be used in both types of experiments, and that a range of concentrations is studied, since at low concentrations a drug may alter capillary surface area, and at high concentrations there may be alterations in microvessel permeability.

Additional vascular studies should include assessments of drug effects on countercurrent exchange and on blood flow distribution within the gut wall and oxygen uptake. Clearly *in vivo* studies in which oxygen uptake, blood flow, and possibly $K_{f,c}$ are measured form the basis of these determinations, but they need complimenting by *in vitro* studies in which metabolism cannot be "substrate-limited" by impaired blood flow.

By putting results of all of these types of studies together, the mechanism of a drug's effects on intestinal blood flow and oxygen uptake can be delineated.

Precautions must be observed to ensure that the tissue does not become edematous, that luminal distension does not occur, and that the hematocrit is constant. Arterial PO_2 and oxygen capacity should remain within normal limits as should pH and PCO_2. Finally, an assessment of the completeness of the perfusion of a gut loop should be made, for example, by injecting a fluorescent dye at the end of each experiment.

Although fragmentary data for many drugs exist in the literature, further physiological and pharmacological studies are needed. In particular, the role of gastrointestinal hormones in the control of intestinal blood flow and oxygen uptake is of potential importance. Postprandial vascular changes could be mediated not only by GI hormones but also by modulations in plasma osmolality, another area requiring detailed examination.

Pathological changes, although a more challenging experimental problem than pharmacological changes, represent an area requiring study. The effects of portal hypertension, brief intestinal ischemia, and toxins would all be of interest.

Finally, the chronic effects of drugs may need separate study from the acute effects. Many drugs, antihypertensives and centrally active drugs are obvious examples, may be administered for many years. Whether or not chronic drug administration affects peripheral vascular function is at present poorly understood.

REFERENCES

1. Aviado, D. M. (1959): Cardiovascular effects of some commonly-used pressor amines. *Anesthesiology*, 20:71–97.
2. Boatman, D. L., and Brody, M. J. (1963): Effects of acetylcholine on the intestinal vasculature of the dog. *J. Pharmacol. Exp. Ther.*, 7:185–191.
3. Bohlen, H. G. (1980): Intestinal tissue PO2 and microvascular responses during glucose exposure. *Am. J. Physiol. (Heart Circ. Physiol. 7)* H164–H174.
4. Bulbring, E. (1953): Measurements of oxygen consumption in smooth muscle. *J. Physiol. (Lond.)*, 122:111–134.
5. Bulbring, E., and Burn, J. H. (1936): Sympathetic vasodilation in the skin and intestine of the dog. *J. Physiol. (Lond.)*, 87:254–274.
6. Bulkley, G. M. A., Kvietys, P. R., and Granger, D. N. (1981): Interrelationship between gastric oxygen uptake and blood flow (Abstract). *Physiologist*, 24:50.
7. Chou, C. C., Hsieh, C. P., and Dabney, J. M. (1977): Comparison of vascular effects of gastrointestinal hormones on various organs. *Am. J. Physiol.*, 232:H103–H109.
8. Chou, C. C., and Kvietys, P. R. (1981): Physiological and pharmacological alterations in gastrointestinal blood flow. In: *Measurement of Blood Flow: Applications to the Splanchnic Circulation*, edited by D. N. Granger and G. B. Bulkley, pp. 475–509. Williams & Williams, Baltimore.
9. Collis, M. G., and Alps, B. J. (1973): The evaluation of the -adrenoreceptor blocking action of indoramin, phentolamine, thymoxamime on rat and guinea-pig isolated mesenteric vascular and aortic spiral preparations. *J. Pharm. Pharmacol.*, 25:621–628.
10. Collis, M. G., and Alps, B. J. (1975): Vascular reactivity to noradrenaline, potassium chloride and angiotensin-II in the rat perfused mesenteric vasculature preparation, during the development of renal hypertension. *Cardiovasc. Res.*, 9:118–126.
11. Davis, L. J., Anderson, J., and Wallace, S. (1975): Experimental use of prostaglandin E in nonocclusive mesenteric ischemia. *Am. J. Roentgenol.*, 125:99–110.
12. Eklund, S., Jodal, M., Lundgren, O., and Sjoquist, A. (1979): Effects of vasoactive intestinal polypeptide on blood flow, motility and fluid transport in the gastrointestinal tract of the cat. *Acta Physiol. Scand.*, 105:461–468.
13. Fara, J. W., Borth, J. H., White, R. I., and Bynum, T. E. (1979): Mesenteric vascular effects of prostaglandins F_2 alpha and B_2: Possible advantages over vasopressin in control of gastrointestinal bleeding. *Radiology*, 13:317–320.
14. Fasth, S., and Hulten, L. (1971): The effect of glucagon on intestinal motility and blood flow. *Acta Physiol. Scand.*, 83:169–173.
15. Feruglio, F. S., Greco, F., Cesano, L., and Enson, Y. (1964): Effect of drug infusion on the systemic and splanchnic circulation. I. Bradykinin infusion in normal subjects. *Clin. Sci.*, 26:487–491.
16. Flynn, S. B., and Owen, D. A. A. (1975): Histamine

receptors in peripheral vascular beds in the cat. *Br. J. Pharmacol.*, 55:181–188.
17. Freedman, A. R., Kerr, J. C., and Swan, K. G. (1978): Primate mesenteric blood flow, effects of caopressin and its route of delivery. *Gastroenterology*, 74:875–878.
18. Frizzell, R. A., Markscheid-Kaspi, L., and Schultz, S. G. (1974): Oxidative metabolism of rabbit ileal mucosa. *Am. J. Physiol.*, 226:1142–1148.
19. Granger, D. N., Richardson, P. D. I., Kvietys, P. R., and Mortillaro, N. A. (1980): Intestinal blood flow. *Gastroenterology*, 78:837–863.
20. Granger, D. N., and Taylor, A. E. (1979): Intestinal secretagogues: Effects on in vivo and in vitro oxygen consumption (Abstract). *Fed. Proc.*, 38:952.
21. Granger, D. N., Valleau, J. D., Parker, R. E., Lane, R. E., and Taylor, A. E. (1978): Effects of adenosine on intestinal hemodynamics, oxygen delivery and capillary fluid exchange. *Am. J. Physiol.*, 235 *(Heart. Circ. Physiol.*, 4):H707–H719.
22. Greenway, C. V., and Lawson, A. (1966): The effects of adrenaline and noradrenaline on venous return and regional blood flow in the anesthetized cat with special reference to intestinal blood flow. *J. Physiol. (Lond.)*, 187:579–595.
23. Greenway, C. V., and Murthy, V. S. (1972): Effects of vasopressin and isoprenaline infusions of the distribution of blood flow in the intestine: Criteria for the validity of microsphere studies. *Br. J. Pharmacol.*, 46:177–188.
24. Hamilton, T. C. (1972): The effects of some phosphodiesterase inhibitors on the conductance of the perfused vascular beds of the chloralosed cat. *Br. J. Pharmacol.*, 46:386–394.
25. Houvenaghel, A., and Wechsung, E. (1977): Influence of prostaglandins on blood flow through the superior mesenteric artery in the pig. *Arch. Int. Pharmacodyn.*, 230:332–334.
26. Immink, W. F. G. A., Beijer, H. J. M., and Charbon, G. A. (1976): Hemodynamic effects of norepinephrine, and isoprenaline in various regions of the canine splanchnic area. *Pfluegers Arch.*, 365:107–118.
27. Innes, I. R., and Nicherson, M. (1975): Norepinephrine, epinephrine and the sympathomimetic amines. In: *The Pharmacological Basis of Therapeutics*, edited by L. S. Goodman and A. Gilman, Chapter 24, pp. 447–513. Macmillan, New York.
28. Kerr, J. C., Hobson, R. W., Seelig, R. F., and Swan, K. G. (1977): Influence of vasopressin on colon blood flow in monkeys. *Gastroenterology*, 72:474–478.
29. Kock, N. G., Tibblin, S., and Schenk, W. G. (1971): Modification by glucagon of the splanchnic vascular responses to activation of the sympathicoadrenal system. *J. Surg. Res.*, 11:12–17.
30. Kvietys, P. R., and Granger, D. N. (1982): Relation between intestinal blood flow and oxygen uptake. *Am. J. Physiol.*, 242 *(Gastrointest. Liver Physiol.*, 5):G202–G208.
31. Kvietys, P. R., and Granger, D. N. (1982): Vasoactive agents and splanchnic oxygen exchange. *Am. J. Physiol.*, 243 *(Gastrointest. Liver Physiol.*, 6):G1–G9.
32. Lutz, J., Henrick, H., and Bauereisen, E. (1975): Oxygen supply and uptake in the liver and the intestine. *Pfluegers Arch.*, 360:7–15.
33. McGregor, D. D. (1965): The effect of sympathetic nerve stimulation on vasoconstrictor responses in perfused mesenteric blood vessels of the rat. *J. Physiol. (Lond.)*, 177:21–30.
34. McMichael, J. (1932): The portal circulation. I. The action of adrenaline and posterior pituitary pressor extract. *J. Physiol. (Lond.)*, 75:241–263.
35. McNeill, J. R., Stark, R. D., and Greenway, C. V. (1970): Intestinal vasoconstriction after hemorrhage: Roles of vasopressin and angiotensin. *Am. J. Physiol.*, 219:1342–1347.
36. Mailman, D., Pawlik, W., Shepherd, A. P., Tague, L. L., and Jacobson, E. D. (1977): Cyclic nucleotide metabolism and vasodilation in canine mesenteric artery. *Am. J. Physiol.*, 232:H191–H196.
37. Nusbaum, M., Baum, S., Sakiyalak, P., and Blakemore, W. S. (1967): Pharmacologic control of portal hypertension. *Surgery*, 62:299–310.
38. Ohman, U. (1976): Blood flow and oxygen consumption in the feline small intestine; responses to artificial distention and intestinal obstruction. *Acta Chir. Scand.*, 142:329–333.
39. Owen, D. A. A., Flynn, S. B., Harvey, C. A., and Levy, R. (1979): The evidence for histamine receptors in the gastro-mesenteric circulation. In: *Cimetidine Symposium at the Westminster Hospital*, edited by C. Wastell and P. Lance, pp. 207–219. Churchill-Livingstone, Edinburgh, London, New York.
40. Page, I. H., Corcoran, A. C., Dustan, H. P., and Oparil, S. (1955): Cardiovascular actions of sodium nitroprusside in animals and hypertensive patients. *Circulation*, 11:118–198.
41. Pawlik, W., Shepherd, A. P., and Jacobson, E. D. (1975): Effects of vasoactive agents on intestinal oxygen consumption and blood flow in dogs. *J. Clin. Invest.*, 56:484–490.
42. Pawlik, W. W., Shepherd, A. P., Mailman, D., and Jacobson, E. D. (1976): Effects of dopamine and epinephrine on intestinal blood flow and oxygen uptake. *Adv. Exp. Med. Biol.*, 75:511–516.
43. Richardson, P. D. I. (1973): *Pharmacological responses of the vasculature of the mammalian small intestine, with particular regard to the responses of the microcirculation*. Ph.D. Thesis, University of London.
44. Richardson, P. D. I. (1974): Drug-induced changes in capillary filtration coefficient and blood flow in the innervated small intestine of the anaesthetized cat. *Br. J. Pharmacol.*, 52:491–498.
45. Richardson, P. D. I. (1976): The actions of natural secretin on the small intestinal vasculature of the anaesthetized cat. *Br. J. Pharmacol.*, 58:127–135.
46. Richardson, P. D. I., Granger, D. N., and Kvietys, P. R. (1980): Effects of norepinephrine, vasopressin, isoproterenol, and histamine on blood flow, oxygen uptake, and capillary filtration coefficient in the colon of the anaesthetized dog. *Gastroenterology*, 78:1537–1544.
47. Richardson, P. D. I., Granger, D. N., and Taylor, A. E. (1979): Capillary filtration coefficient: The technique and its application to the small intestine. *Cardiovasc. Res.*, 13:547–561.
48. Richardson, P. D. I., and Withrington, P. G. (1978): The effects of intraportal infusions of glucagon on

the hepatic arterial and portal venous vascular beds of the dog: Inhibition of hepatic arterial vasoconstrictor responses to noradrenaline. *Pfluegers Arch.*, 378:135–140.
49. Ross, G. (1970): Cardiovascular effects of secretin. *Am. J. Physiol.*, 218:1166–1170.
50. Ross, G. (1970): Regional circulatory effects of pancreatic glucagon. *Br. J. Pharmacol.*, 38:735–742.
51. Rudick, J., Werther, J. L., and Chapman, M. L. (1972): Effects of physiologic and supramaximal doses of pentagastrin on mucosal blood flow in antral and fundic pouches. *Surgery*, 71:405–411.
52. Schehadeh, Z., Price, W. E., and Jacobson, E. D. (1969): Effects of vasoactive agents on intestinal blood flow and motility in the dog. *Am. J. Physiol.*, 216:386–392.
53. Shepherd, A. P., and Riedel, G. L. (1982): Optimal hematocrit for oxygenation of canine intestine. *Circ. Res.*, 51:233–243.
54. Swan, K. G., and Reynolds, D. G. (1971): Effects of intra-arterial catecholamine infusions on blood flow in the canine gut. *Gastroenterology*, 61:863–871.
55. Tairi, N., Yabuuchi, Y., and Yamashita, S. (1977): Profile of B-adrenoceptors in femoral, superior mesenteric and renal vascular beds of dogs. *Br. J. Pharmacol.*, 59:557–583.
56. Texter, E. C., Chou, C. C., and Merrill, S. L. (1964): Direct effects of vasoactive agents on the segmental resistance of the mesenteric and portal circulations. Studies with L-epinephrine, levarterenol, angiotensin, vasopressin, acetylcholine, methacholine, histamine, and 5-hydroxytryptamine. *J. Lab. Clin. Med.*, 64:624–633.
57. Tibblin, S., Kock, N. G., and Schenk, W. G. (1970): Splanchnic haemodynamic responses to glucagon. *Arch. Surg.*, 100:84–89.
58. Tibblin, S., Kock, N. G., and Schenk, W. G. (1971): Response of mesenteric blood flow to glucagon. *Arch. Surg.*, 102:65–70.
59. Yeh, B. K., McNay, J. L., and Goldberg, L. I. (1969): Attenuation of dopamine renal and mesenteric vasodilation by haloperidol: Evidence for a specific receptor. *J. Pharmacol. Exp. Ther.*, 168:303–309.

Pharmacology of Intestinal Transcapillary Fluid Exchange

James J. Szwed

Nephrology Section, Community Hospital, Indianapolis, Indiana 46219

Only recently have the pharmacological characteristics of the gastrointestinal tract's microcirculation been explored. The effects produced by many naturally occurring as well as synthetic compounds must be ascertained to more effectively understand health and disease in the gastrointestinal tract. A large number of drugs have been studied. The drugs that affect transcapillary fluid and protein movement have been studied in a number of different ways. Essentially two different techniques have been used to study pharmacological effects on capillary function: determinations of the capillary filtration coefficient (K_f) and determinations of osmotic reflection coefficients.

We can divide the drugs that affect intestinal capillary function into two major lists: the drugs that increase K_f and those that decrease K_f (Table 1). Some agents are felt to have a direct effect on the capillary endothelial barrier and hence enhance or restrict the fluid filtration rate (J_v) and in some cases alter the solute flux (J_s). Table 2 contains reported values for osmotic reflection coefficients; however, before discussing particular pharmacological agents, it must be pointed out that the determination of capillary filtration coefficients in the intestine is controversial. The K_f has often been used as an index of functional exchange capacity of an organ (7,21,23). However, when measured by the gravimetric technique, K_f is a measure of hydraulic conductance, that is, it relates net fluid filtration (or absorption) to a pressure gradient across a membrane. K_f is influenced by several factors, such as the size and number of pores and the number of filtering capillaries. These factors probably account for the wide range of K_f values reported for different tissues. Values of the order of 0.025 (3,23), 0.325 (5,30), 0.055 to 0.25 (8,19,26,33), 2.26 (17), and 1.10 (4) ml·min^{-1}·mm Hg^{-1}·100 g^{-1} have been reported for skeletal muscle, lung, intestine, liver, and spleen, respectively.

Richardson et al. (29) reviewed the methods for determining K_f. The first technique was the volumetric or gravimetric technique. With this technique the tissue is placed in a plethysmograph or on a weighing pan to continuously record changes in either tissue volume or weight. When the tissue is isovolumetric, that is, neither losing nor gaining volume, the venous pressure (P_v) is elevated. The resulting volume or weight recordings in all tissues examined so far are biphasic. The first, sharp phase (phase 1) is usually attributed to passive vascular distension and increased local blood volume; the second, slow and more continuous response (phase 2) is usually attributed to the filtration of fluid from the vasculature into the perivascular space, a result of the elevated capillary hydrostatic pressure (P_c) and the consequent disturbance of the Starling equilibrium. The rate of volume or weight gain during phase 2 (30-sec slope, zero-time extrapolation) is divided by the increase in capillary hydrostatic pressure. Thus, K_f is expressed in cm^3 of fluid gained/min/kPa rise in pressure/100 g of tissue, that is, in ml·min^{-1}·mm Hg^{-1}·100 g^{-1}.

The volumetric methods of determining capillary filtration coefficient suffer from two fundamental problems (8). First, the endpoint of the passive increase in vascular volume (phase

TABLE 1. *Effects of physiologic, pathologic, and pharmacologic conditions on the capillary filtration coefficient (K_f) in the small intestine*

Conditions or agents that increase k_f	
Glucose absorption	Histamine
Arterial hypotension	Secretin
Hyperthermia	Aminophylline
Denervation	Glucagon
Hemorrhagic shock	Acetylcholine
Nitroglycerin	Serotonin
Isoproterenol	Cholecystokinin
Phentolamine	Prostaglandin E_1
Neostigmine	Propranolol
Bradykinin	Epinephrine
Sodium nitroprusside	Cholera toxin
Sodium nitrite	
Conditions or agents that decrease K_f	
Sympathetic nerve stimulation	Pentagastrin
Lumenal distention	Adenosine
Portal hypertension	Norepinephrine
Acute arterial hypertension	Phenylephrine
Hypothermia	Angiotensin II
Serotonin	Ergotamine

1 of the volume response) is difficult to determine. Second, following elevation of the venous pressure, tissue forces continuously readjust to compensate for transcapillary filtration. The vascular (venous) distension and the readjustment of tissue forces have markedly different time courses: the former occurs within seconds and the latter within 2 to 3 min of venous pressure elevation (11). Ideally, therefore, the rate of increase in tissue volume used to estimate the capillary filtration coefficient should lie between the end of the vascular distension and the onset of the tissue forces readjustment.

Wallentin (33), using radioactively labeled red blood cells, showed that the bulk of the blood volume shift on elevating the superior mesenteric venous pressure of the cat by 15 mm Hg is complete within about 30 sec. This indicates that measuring the rate of volume increase from a point 30 sec after the venous pressure elevation gives an acceptable basis for capillary filtration measurements. These conclusions are supported by the data of Johnson and Hanson (19), which show a separation of the phase 1 and phase 2 responses in dog intestine at a point well under 30 sec on a semilogarithmic plot of the change in intestinal weight against time following venous pressure elevation from 0 to 10 mm Hg. In contrast, studies in the cat ileum (12) suggest a separation in the two phases at approximately 60 sec when the rate of ileal volume change is plotted semilogarithmically against time. Friedman et al. (10) utilized a method similar to Wallentin's ^{51}Cr-labeled red blood cells to monitor changes in vascular volume following venous pressure elevations of 10 and 20 mm Hg. The vascular transient was not complete for at least 1 to 1.5 min.

An alternative approach to the use of radioactively labeled red blood cells in assessing the end of the blood volume shift has been described by Granger (13). On elevation of the superior mesenteric venous pressure, venous outflow from the intestine falls initially to a low value and subsequently attains a plateau lower than the control level. The point of attainment of this plateau ("flow equilibrium") represents the end of the blood volume shift. Thus, measuring the rate of intestinal volume increase from that point gives K_f values in agreement with those determined from the end of the blood

TABLE 2. *Effects of physiologic and pharmacologic interventions on the osmotic reflection coefficient of intestinal capillaries to total plasma proteins*

Experimental condition	Reflection coeff.
Controls	0.92
Isoproterenol	0.92
Bradykinin	0.65
Secretin	0.91
Cholecystokinin	0.89
Fat absorption	0.70
Glucagon	0.81
EDTA	0.73
E. coli endotoxin	0.78
Arterial hyperglycemia (20 mM)	0.64
Ischemia	0.59
Ischemia + superoxide dismutase	0.86
Histamine	0.56
Cimetidine + histamine	0.90
Benadryl + histamine	0.56
Compound 48/80	0.76
Goldblatt hypertension	0.55
Angiotensin II	0.91

volume shift assessed using radioactively labeled red blood cells, or K_f values obtained by the zero-time extrapolation technique. The time required for phase 1 to end should theoretically be influenced by alterations in vascular tone due to drug infusions, provided vascular compliance is sufficiently altered. Johns and Rothe (18) have shown that norepinephrine decreases whereas papaverine increases intestinal vascular compliance. The data of Granger et al. (16) suggest that local intraarterial infusions of adenosine nearly double the time at which there is separation of the phase-1 and phase-2 components of ileal volume change following venous pressure elevations, presumably owing to an adenosine-induced increase in vascular compliance.

In terms of the transcapillary protein leakage that occurs during venous pressure elevation, it must be pointed out that a large source of transcapillary fluid movement results from protein leakage. This tends to overestimate K_f to some degree (9,10,18). Whereas Granger et al. (12) estimate the increased transcapillary fluid flux associated with protein leakage to be 1% of the total volume being filtered in a range of venous pressure elevation of 10 to 30 mm Hg, Friedman et al. (10) have estimated that 40% to 60% of the total filtered volume of fluid is due to protein leakage. When one considers the theoretical bases for both estimates, one still must conclude that the Granger estimate is much too low considering the nature of the capillaries involved and the methods involved. In the first place, the intestine has fenestrated capillaries that should be much more permeable than muscle capillaries in which the small protein leakage is explainable in terms of the continuous endothelium. Friedman reported a 3% increase in transcapillary fluid movement associated with increased transcapillary protein leakage at 20 mm Hg. This 3% figure compares favorably with Granger's value for muscle capillaries.

Friedman loaded his perfusion system with albumin-labeled ^{125}I, was careful to assay for the presence of free ^{125}I-albumin, and measured transcapillary protein leakage from the rate of accumulation of radioactivity in the tissue. Using this technique, transcapillary protein leakage rate was measured (32) by counting the radioactivity in whole feline jejunum entirely removed from its donor. A support cat was used as an oxygenator-deoxifier. The disadvantage of this technique is that the support animal may affect the organ studied. Therefore, control periods must be carried out carefully before any pertubation. With venous pressure elevations of 10 and 20 mm Hg, fluid filtration increased by 0.156 and 0.274 ml·min^{-1}·100 g^{-1}, respectively; the protein flux rose to 4.09 mg·min^{-1}·100 g^{-1} and 7.88 mg·mm^{-1}·100 g^{-1}, respectively. Mortillaro and Taylor (22) reported values of 0.9 and 5.0 mg·min^{-1}·100 g^{-1}, whereas Granger et al. (12) reported values of 1.6 and 5.5 mg·min^{-1}·100 g^{-1}, respectively. The Friedman estimates were conducted on tissue accumulation data, whereas the others were obtained from lymph recovery data. The discrepancy between the values obtained at a venous pressure of 10 mm Hg could represent undetected protein accumulation in the interstitial space in their study even though the lymph flow had achieved an apparent steady state. The K_f of the Friedman study averaged 0.09 ml·min^{-1}·100 g^{-1} mm Hg compared with the reported intestinal range of K_f of 0.03 to 0.56 (29). The high values of this range undoubtedly represent overestimations because they were obtained at 30 sec following venous pressure elevation, although approximately 1 to 2 min are required for the vascular volume transient to be completed, as mentioned earlier. Thus, elevations of K_f by drugs can be deceiving. Furthermore, since drugs can affect microvascular hemodynamics, agents such as *papaverine* can increase the fluid flux by 250% and the protein leakage by 14%, thus dramatically increasing K_f.

Histamine has variable effects on K_f. Low doses (0.1–1.0 µg·kg^{-1}·min^{-1}) of histamine infused intravenously reduce K_f with variable changes in blood pressure and blood flow; higher doses (up to 40 µg·kg^{-1}·min^{-1}) or smaller doses after histaminase inhibition increase K_f. Richardson (27) suggested that the increases in K_f could be due either to precapillary sphincter dilatation or to increases in microvessel premeability to protein or both. The latter concept fits well with the proposal of Friedman (9) relating enhanced K_f to enhanced transcapillary protein leakage rate and its positive effect for filtration on the transcapillary oncotic pressure gradient.

A more sophisticated study of histamine was reported by Mortillaro and Taylor (22). Using an isolated ileum preparation in cat, they found that histamine selectively increases the ileal vascular permeability to plasma proteins of a molecular radius up to 96 Å. Diphenhydramine, an H_1-receptor antagonist, did not block the permeability changes seen with histamine alone. However, cimetidine, the H_2-receptor antagonist, significantly reduced the permeability changes associated with histamine while having only a slight effect on the initial vasodilation.

Mortillaro and Taylor concluded that H_1 receptors mediated the initial vasodilation and H_2 receptors mediated permeability changes.

We (32) studied the effects of large doses (100 $\mu g \cdot kg^{-1} \cdot min^{-1}$) of histamine administered intraarterially both in total isolated small bowel and in isolated jejunum from cats (Fig. 1). The increase in transcapillary protein and fluid movement was enormous. Transcapillary protein leakage was enhanced by a factor of 6 (1.4–8.0 mg·min^{-1}·100 g^{-1}). Transcapillary fluid movement increased by a factor of 3, and lymph flow was greatly enhanced (100%) with marked increases in protein concentration (Fig. 2). The preparations were perfused at constant flow, and the blood pressure of the isolated organs declined significantly in both studies. K_f declined slightly. One can postulate that precap-

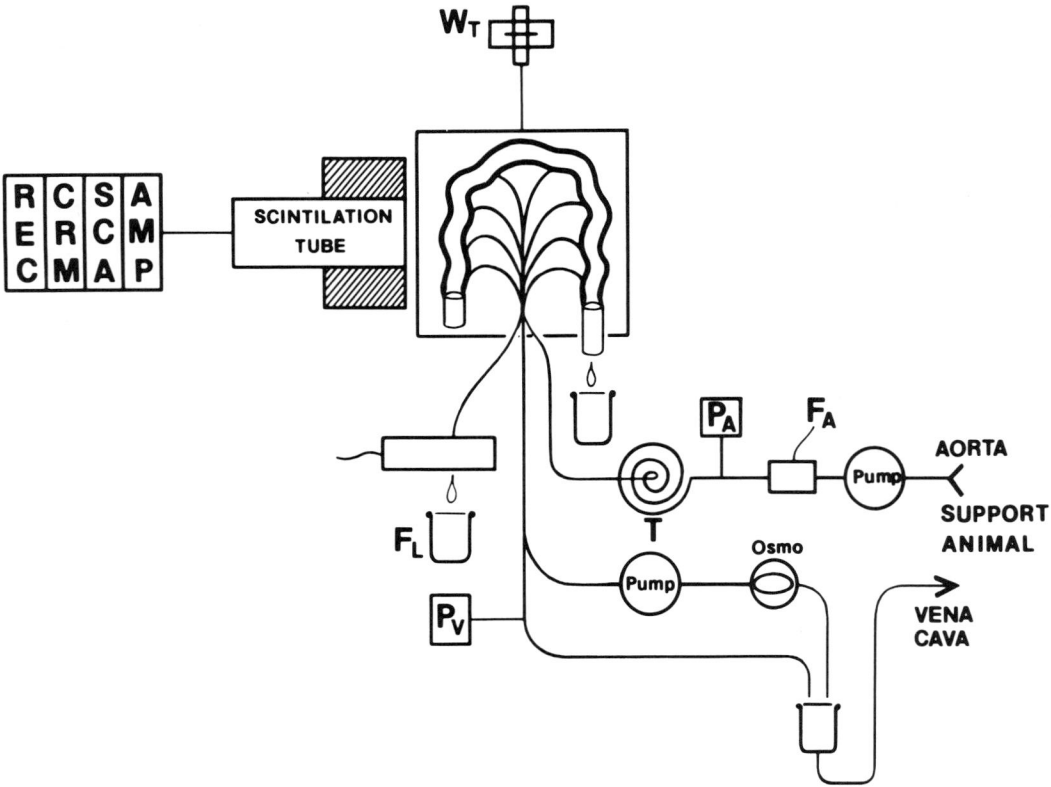

FIG. 1. Experimental small bowel cat set-up. Aorta and vena cava belong to "support" animal. F_a, arterial flow probe; P_a, arterial blood pressure; Wt, weight of tissue; scintillation tube-radioisotope detector (counting entire tissue); F_l, lymph flow; P_v, venous pressure measurement; Osmo-colloidal osmotic transducer (Prather with Friedman modification).

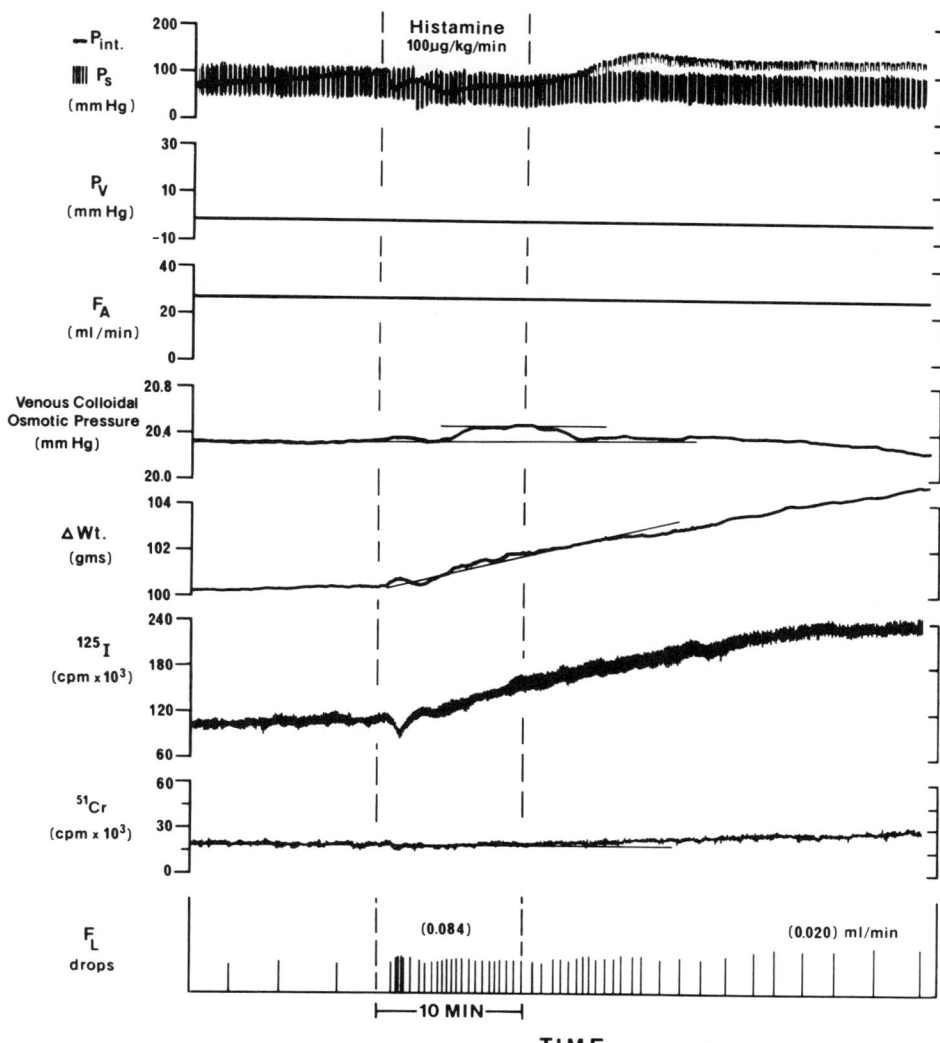

FIG. 2. Record of small bowel of cat during histamine infusion as well as control state. P_{int}, arterial pressure in intestine; P_s, arterial pressure of support cat; P_v, venous pressure; F_a, arterial blood flow; Δ Wt, change in weight of tissue; ^{125}I, accumulation of protein-labeled ^{125}I in intestine; ^{51}Cr, accumulation of chromium labeled red blood cells in gut; F_1, lymph flow.

illary resistance increased and that circulating capillary surface area fell because, although perfusion pressure dropped during the first few minutes of infusion, it subsequently rose and even surpassed the control level. This secondary vasoconstriction may have been due to histamine reaching the support animal and stimulating the adrenal medulla to release catecholamines. Catecholamines would definitely have a profound effect on precapillary resistance. Unfortunately, levels of circulating catecholamines were not measured.

Glucagon and *pentagastrin* have been studied by Richardson (25). Glucagon was infused intravenously into cats to assess its influence on K_f. In a dose of 0.25 μg·kg^{-1}·min^{-1}, glucagon produced a significant decline in K_f of 55 ± 14% (0.023 ± 0.004–0.009 ± 0.003 ml·min^{-1}·mm Hg^{-1}·100 g^{-1}. The effect of glucagon before and after phentolamine was highly significant.

Glucagon releases catecholamines from the adrenal glands, so phentolamine's ability to block this endogenous source of catecholamines revealed an entirely different effect of glucagon than previously seen.

Granger et al. (14) studied *isoproterenol* and found that it did not increase vascular permeability. This indicates that the rise in K_f observed by Folkow et al. (7) and Richardson (28), using isoproterenol, results from capillary recruitment. A low dose of *bradykinin* (36 ng/ml), which is known to increase K_f, does not alter intestinal vascular permeability. However, higher doses of bradykinin (about 680 ng/ml) increased both K_f and capillary permeability.

Fasth and Hulten (6) found an interesting nuance to Granger's work employing isoproterenol and bradykinin. The K_f increase due to bradykinin was considerably enhanced by concomitant isoproterenol infusions. The authors suggested that bradykinin increases the permeability of the intestinal exchange vessels. One would imagine that the rate of transcapillary protein leakage increased, but unfortunately the authors did not measure protein flux. Atropine was used in the Fasth study (6) to "reduce intestinal secretion." This maneuver raises some concern about the results because interstitial tissue pressure may have been raised and interstitial oncotic pressure could have been diminished owing to blockage of secretion with atropine. These changes could significantly impede the fluid flux and hence decrease K_f. Fasth infused intraarterial bradykinin (1–20 ng·ml^{-1} of whole blood.) The dose selected was too low to produce significant changes in blood flow or motility, but K_f did increase. The Friedman hypothesis may be germane to this study. The increase in K_f could have been due, in part at least, to enhanced transcapillary protein leakage from intravascular to extravascular compartments. This would decrease the transmural oncotic pressure difference and favor capillary filtration.

Richardson (27) infused large doses of bradykinin intravenously with a resultant increase in K_f. The large dose employed, 8 to 10 μg·kg^{-1}·min^{-1}, was needed because of the rapid deactivation of bradykinin in the blood and pulmonary vasculature.

Biber et al. (2) found administration of 20 to 50 μg/ml of *5-hydroxytryptamine* (5-HT) increased intestinal blood flow and capillary filtration coefficients. At infusion rates of 10 to 15 μg/min, 5-HT increased K_f without increasing intestinal blood flow. Since 5-HT is a compound released from the gastrointestinal tract by neoplasms such as argentaffinoma as well as pancreatic neoplasms, careful study must be carried out with these agents for a more thorough understanding of symptomatology in human disease processes.

Prostaglandin E$_1$ (PGE$_1$) was studied by Weiner et al. (34) in the rat mesoappendix. Locally applied PGE$_1$ dilated all muscular microvessels. PGE$_1$ antagonized the constrictor action of angiotensin, epinephrine, norepinephrine, and vasopressin after PGE$_1$'s vasodilator activity had vanished. On the other hand, PGE$_1$ did not interfere with the vasoconstrictor activity of serotonin, nor did it alter vascular responsiveness to the dilators, bradykinin, and histamine. The study was performed using direct *in vivo* microscopic observation, and all applications of drug were local. Therefore, no quantitative data are available.

The effect of arginine *vasopressin* (intraarterial infusion) were studied by Quillen et al. (24) in the cat ileum. The drug decreased the post- to precapillary resistance ratio and hence capillary hydrostatic pressure. K_f, lymph flow, and lymphatic protein clearance all declined with vasopressin infusion. The dose of drug employed in these studies was 17.5 mU·kg^{-1}·mm^{-1} ADH.

Altura (1) published data on a new analog of vasopressin, (2-phenylalanine, 8-ornithine) vasopressin. The administration of this vasopressin analog systemically to rats subjected either to lethal hemorrhage or bowel ischemia shock increased survival significantly over Ringer's solution, produced a "plateau-like" effect on arterial blood pressure while returning arterial hematocrits toward normal after hemorrhage, regenerated vasomotion and venular tone, decreased the microvascular hyperreactivity characteristic of shock syndrome, restored constricted arterial lumen sizes toward normal, prevented stasis and petechiae, and restored capillary perfusion and outflow to near normal. The optimum dose (100% survival) was 5 mU/min for 60 min after hemorrhage. In intestinal ischemic shock, Altura found a dose of 10 mU/min for 60 min produced a survival of 61% of the animals as compared with 7.5% for the control.

A number of investigators have examined the effect of drugs such as *norepinephrine* on transcapillary fluid exchange. Norepinephrine reduced K_f 19% to 24% (15). Shepherd et al. (31) found a decrease in ^{86}Rb extraction in a constant-flow perfused canine small bowel. They concluded that norepinephrine caused a sustained reduction in the density of the perfused capillary bed and that the decline in K_f as well as ^{86}Rb extraction are a consequence (31). Richardson found that *phenylephrine* and *angiotensin* depressed K_f, but that isoproterenol, propanolol, aminophylline, and 5-HT increased K_f. Histamine in a dose of up to 10 $\mu g \cdot kg^{-1} \cdot mm^{-1}$ intravenously caused a fall in K_f, but the higher doses or smaller doses after histaminase inhibition increased in K_f. Alpha-adrenoceptor blockade reversed the fall in K_f caused by small doses of histamine (26).

Finally, *acetylcholine* infusions have been studied in the jejunum of the cat. Kewenter (20) found an enormous progressive increase in intestinal motility with marked rhythmicity. His intraluminal pressure measurements ranged from 30 to 200 mm Hg. Although K_f was not measured, these severe changes with acetylcholine resulted in enhanced intestinal volume, which was probably due to enhanced transcapillary fluid movement from intra- to extravascular spaces.

Many of the studies in this chapter mention only transcapillary fluid flux; they did not measure transcapillary protein flux. Often this was due to the nature of the study, but the fact that fluid and protein leave the vascular compartment together, and that the transcapillary fluid balance is affected by both fluid and protein fluxes, underscores the need for more study of pharmacological agents affecting the gut. The intestine is a fragile organ. If obstruction occurs due to a neoplasm or internal adhesion, strangulation of the bowel with necrosis of normal bowel can follow within hours. This occurs clinically because small bowel obstruction is often surprisingly difficult to diagnose. Only when severe leukocytosis, hyperkalemia, and life-threatening systemic acidosis occur, is the diagnosis often made. Therefore, a renewed vigor in the study of the bowel is extremely important. Some drugs can produce profound therapeutic effects in patients, as in the case of vasopressin infusion with gastrointestinal bleeding, that is, decrease or stoppage of the bleeding. More studies are needed to determine which drugs are potentially helpful and which are potentially harmful. The microcirculatory study of the gut is difficult because the intestinal tract is delicate and surgical manipulation or extensive surgery in the animal may alter the results dramatically. Hence, great care must be taken in the study of pharmacological agents' effects on microcirculatory dynamics.

REFERENCES

1. Altura, B. M. (1976): Microcirculatory approach to the treatment of circulatory shock with a new analog of vasopressin, (2-phenylalanine, 8-orinthine) vasopressin. *J. Pharmacol. Exp. Ther.*, 198:187–196.
2. Biber, B., Fara, J., and Lundgren, O. (1973): Intestinal vascular responses to 5-hydroxytryptamine. *Acta Physiol. Scand.*, 87:525–534.
3. Chen, H. I., Granger, H. J., and Taylor, A. E. (1976): Interaction of capillary, interstitial and lymphatic forces in the canine hindpaw. *Circ. Res.*, 39:245–254.
4. Davies, B. N., Richardson, P. D. I., and Withrington, P. G. (1974): The effects of post-ganglionic sympathetic nerve stimulation on the "capillary filtration coefficient" of the isolated, blood-perfused dog spleen. *J. Physiol.*, 241:46–47P.
5. Drake, R., Garr, K. A., and Taylor, A. E. (1978): Estimation of the filtration coefficient of pulmonary exchange vessels. *Am. J. Physiol.*, 234:H266–H274.
6. Fasth, S., and Hulten, L. (1973): The effect of bradykinin on the consecutive vascular sections of the small and large intestine. *Acta Chir. Scand.*, 139:707–715.
7. Folkow, B., Lundgren, O., and Wallentin, I. (1963): Studies on the relationship between flow and resistance, capillary filtration coefficient and regional blood volume in the intestine of the cat. *Acta Physiol. Scand.*, 57:270–283.
8. Folkow, B., and Mellander, S. (1970): Measurements of capillary filtration coefficient and its use in studies of the control of capillary exchange. In: *Capillary*

Permeability, edited by Alfred Benzon Symposium II, Munksgaard, Copenhagen.
9. Friedman, J. J. (1976): Transcapillary protein leakage and fluid movement: Effect of venous pressure. *Microvasc. Res.*, 12:275–290.
10. Friedman, J. J., Szwed, J. J., and Johns, B. (1982): The mass balance approach for estimating transcapillary protein transport. *Am. J. Physiol.*, 242:H227–H237.
11. Granger, D. N. (1977): *Interstitial fluid volume regulation in the feline small intestine: An analysis of the interactions between transmucosal flows and lymph flow.* Ph.D. Thesis, University Medical Center, Jackson, Mississippi.
12. Granger, D. N., Brace, R. A., Parker, R. E., and Taylor, A. E. (1979): Analysis of the permeability characteristic of intestinal capillaries. *Circ. Res.*, 44:335–343.
13. Granger, D. N., Richardson, P. D. I., and Taylor, A. E. (1979): Volumetric assessment of the capillary filtration coefficient in the cat small intestine. *Eur. J. Physiol.*, 381:25–33.
14. Granger, D. N., Richardson, P. D. I., and Taylor, A. E. (1979): The effects of isoprenaline and bradykinin on capillary filtration in the cat small intestine. *Br. J. Pharmacol.*, 67:361–366.
15. Granger, D. N., Richardson, P. D. I., and Taylor, A. E. (1979): Volumetric assessment of the capillary filtration coefficient in the cat small intestine. *Pfluegers Arch.*, 381:25–33.
16. Granger, D. N., Valleau, J. D., Parker, R. E., Lane, R. S., and Taylor, A. E. (1979): Effects of adenosine on intestinal vascular hemodynamics, oxygen delivery, and capillary fluid exchange. *Am. J. Physiol.*, 235:H707–H719.
17. Greenway, C. V., and Lautt, W. W. (1972): Effects of adrenaline, isoprenaline and histamine on transsinusodal fluid filtration in the cat liver. *Br. J. Pharmacol.*, 44:185–191.
18. Johns, B. L., and Rothe, C. F. (1978): Delayed vascular compliance and fluid exchange in the canine intestine. *Am. J. Physiol.*, 234:H660–H669.
19. Johnson, P. C., and Hanson, K. M. (1966): Capillary filtration in the small intestine of the dog. *Circ. Res.*, 19:766–773.
20. Kewenter, J. (1971): Effects of graded acetylcholine infusions on intestinal motility, volume, and blood flow. *Scand. J. Gastroenterol.*, 67:435–440.
21. Landis, E. M., and Gibbon, J. H. (1933): The effects of temperature and of tissue pressure on the movement of fluid through the human capillary wall. *J. Clin. Invest.*, 12:105–138.
22. Mortillaro, N. A., and Taylor, A. E. (1976): Interaction of capillary and tissue forces in the cat small intestine. *Circ. Res.*, 39:348–358.
23. Pappenheimer, J. R., and Soto-Rivera, A. (1948): Effective osmotic pressure of the plasma proteins and other quantities associated with the capillary circulation in the hindlimbs of cats and dogs. *Am. J. Physiol.*, 152:471–491.
24. Quillen, E. W., Granger, D. N., and Taylor, A. E. (1977): Effects of arginine vasopressin on capillary filtration in the cat ileum. *Gastroenterology*, 73:1290–1295.
25. Richardson, P. D. I. (1975): The effects of glucagon and pentagastrin on capillary filtration coefficient in the innervated jejunum of the anesthetized cat. *Proc. Br. Pharmacol. Soc.*, 225 p.
26. Richardson, P. D. I. (1974): Drug-induced changes in capillary filtration coefficient and blood flow in the innervated small intestine of the anesthetized cat. *Br. J. Pharmacol.*, 52:481–498.
27. Richardson, P. D. I. (1973): *Pharmacological responses of the vasculature of the mammalian small intestine with particular regard to the responses of the microcirculation.* PhD Thesis, University of London.
28. Richardson, P. D. I. (1974): The actions of natural secretin on the small intestinal vasculature of the anesthetized cat. *Br. J. Pharmacol.*, 52:481–498.
29. Richardson, P. D. I., Granger, D. N., and Taylor, A. E. (1979): Capillary filtration coefficient: The technique and its application to the small intestine. *Cardiovasc. Res.*, 13:547–561.
30. Staub, N. C. (1974): Pulmonary edema. *Physiol. Rev.*, 54:678–811.
31. Shepherd, A. P., Mailman, D., Burks, R. F., and Granger, H. J. (1973): Effects of norepinephrine and sympathetic stimulation on extraction of oxygen and ^{86}Rb in perfused canine small bowel. *Circ. Res.*, 33:166–174.
32. Szwed, J. J., Johns, B. J., and Friedman, J. J. (1981): Effect of histamine on transcapillary protein and fluid movements in the cat small intestine. In: *Proc. VIIIth International Congress of Lymphology, Florence, Italy, 1979*, edited by H. Weissleder, V. Bartos, L. Clodius, and P. Malek, pp. 44–47. Avicenum, Czechoslovak Medical Press, Prague.
33. Wallentin, I. (1966): Importance of tissue pressure for the fluid equilibrium between the vascular and interstitial compartments in the small intestine. *Acta Physiol. Scand.*, 68:304–315.
34. Weiner, R., and Kaley, G. (1969): Influence of prostaglandin E_1 on the terminal vascular bed. *Am. J. Physiol.*, 217:563–566.

Subject Index

Abdominal visceral cardiovascular reflexes
significance of
under normal conditions, 172–173
under pathological conditions, 173–174
stimulation of
by acetylcholine, 170–171
by bradykinin, 170–171
by other naturally occurring chemical substances or solutions, 171–172
Absorption, *see* Intestinal absorption
tissue oxygenation during, 145–148
Absorptive hyperemia, as response to changes in availability of oxygen, 146–148,149
Acetylcholine, effects of
on intestinal blood flow, 111–113
on lymphatic contractility, 204
on stimulation of reflex cardiovascular response, 170–171
on transcapillary fluid exchange, 409
Active intestinal secretion
discussion of, 227
effects of drugs and hormones on, 228–230
evidence for neural component in, 227
Active secretory responses, in capillary exchange and secretion, 227–230
Active vasoconstriction, effects of, 74
Adenosine
as candidate vasodilator metabolite, 43
role as a potential feedback signal, 43
Adrenergic receptor mechanisms, in neural responses, 66–68
Afferent fibers, from abdominal viscera, classification of, 165,166
Alimentary tract, role of microcirculation of, 9
Anesthetics, effects on lymphatic contractility, 204
Angiotensin, effects on intestinal blood flow, 396
Angiotensin II, effects of infusion of, on intestinal blood flow, motility, and oxygen consumption, 113,115
Appearance rate, determination of, 293–295
Arterial hypertension
description of, 349
intestinal circulation during, 349–360
Arterial hypotension, small bowel in, 305–319
Arterial hypoxia, effects of
on intestinal oxygenation, 34–36
on intestinal vasculature, 36
Arterial pressure
diameter changes in mesenteric arterioles during stepwise changes in, with free flow and no flow, 53–54
diameter and pressure changes in mesenteric arterioles during single step change in, 54,55
and flow, relationship of, 53,54
step rises in, blood flow and vascular resistance in dog intestine during, 49
Arteriolar constriction, with venous pressure elevation, 54

Arteriolar diameter, and vessel wall characteristics in normal, STZ, and glucose-injected rats, 362–363
Artificial distension, of bowel, effects of, 321–325
Ascites
causes and origins of, 341–343
lymph imbalance theory of, 341,342
treatment of, 339–341
diuretic drugs in, 341
salt reduction in, 341
shunt operations in, 341–344
Atropine, effects on intestinal secretions, 228
Autonomic neural control, effects of, on general fetal and neonatal circulation, 187
Autoregulation, of intestinal blood flow, 37–39,269–271
effect of metabolic rate, 38–39
gain of autoregulatory control, 40
pressure-flow relationship, 38
role of passive factors in, 270,271
Autoregulatory escape
description of, 61,63–64
during norepinephrine infusion, 64–65
in intestinal bed perfused at constant inflow pressure, 63
mechanism of, 61,65–66
and neural control, 61–71
role of flow redistribution in, 65,66
role of vasodilator antagonist in, 66
and sympathetic nerve stimulation, 64

Blood circulation, of small and large bowel, differences between, 131,132
Blood exchange vessels, fine structure of, 19–25
Blood flow
and bowel distension, effects of, 321–325
and capillary density, 40,42
changes in
during digestion in general, 99–100
in jejunal segments containing polyethylene glycol or food, 102
dependence of appearance rate on
from intestinal venous blood, 293
from rat jejunal blood, 294
dependence of disappearance rate on, from intestinal lumen, 293
drug effects on, 102–104,399
and motility, relationship of, 323–324
overshoot of, mechanisms that contribute to, 36
and oxygen uptake, 40,41,102–104,397–399
effects of drugs on, 102–104,399
explanation of positive relationship between, 397–399
Blood volume compensation, mechanisms in, 74
Blood volume shift, methods for assessing, 404–405
Bradykinin
effects of

Bradykinin, effects of *(contd.)*
  on abdominal organs and cardiovascular system, 170–171
  on intestinal blood flow, 396
  on spinal afferent fibers, 165–166
  on transcapillary fluid exchange, 408
Brunner's glands, *see* Duodenal glands
Budd-Chiari syndrome, in ascites, 343
Bulk exchange of oxygen, determination of, 144–145

Candidate vasodilator metabolites, in intestinal circulation, 42–44
Canine perinephritic hypertension, 351–355
  blood flow and vascular resistances in acute and chronic stages of, 352–353
  computer simulation of changes in, 351,352
  ileal hemodynamics in, 353–355
  ileal preparations for representation of, 352,353
  venous compliance in, 355–356
Capacitance vessels
  control of, 73–81
  response to ischemia and shock by, 307–308
Capillaries, parameters of, 19
Capillary density
  drug effects on, 398
  local control of, 39–42
Capillary exchange processes, discussion of, 223
Capillary filtration coefficient
  and artificial bowel distension, effects with and without obstruction, 322–323,327,328,329
  changes in, during capillary exchange and filtration, 225
  factors that alter, 134–135
  and fluid absorption, 217
  in the small intestine
    effects of physiologic, pathologic, and pharmacologic conditions on, 403–404,405–409
    effects of protein leakage on, 405
    problems in determination of, 403–404
  reduction in, in response to arteriolar constriction due to venous pressure elevation, 56–57
Capillary filtration rate, and lymph-to-plasma protein concentration ratio, 281–283
Capillary fluid exchange
  capillary and interstitial forces in, 137–138
    interaction of, 138–139
    mathematical relationship of factors in, 137–138
  and intestinal secretion, 223–232
Capillary fluid fluxes, in nonabsorbing and absorbing small bowel, summary of, 219
Capillary forces
  in nonabsorbing and absorbing small bowel, summary of, 219
  in normal and portal hypertensive digestive tract, 345
Capillary perfusion, effects of bowel distension on, 321–322
  comparison with effects on blood flow, 322–323
Capillary pressure changes, during fluid absorption, 216–217
Capillary recruitment, role in oxygen uptake, 42
Cardiopulmonary receptors, and reflex control of splanchnic blood volume reservoir, 76
Cardiovascular changes, during digestion
  general, 99–100
  in mesenteric organs, 100–102

Cardiovascular effects, of intestinal ischemia, 314–316
  in cats, 315
Cardiovascular reflexes
  of gastrointestinal origin, 165–177
  thresholds of, in stomach and small intestine of cats, 174
Carotid sinus pressure, effects of changes in, 75–76
Catecholamines, response of gastrointestinal tract to, 188
Chemical agents, effect on intestinal motility and blood flow, 111–113
Chemohumeral control, of intestinal circulation, during development, 188
Chemosensitive receptors, reflexes from, 170–172
Cholecystokinin (CCK)
  effect on intestinal blood flow, 102–103,104,121–124
  vasodilator effects of, comparison with effects of gastrin and secretin, 125
Cholera toxin, effect on active intestinal secretion, 227
Cholinergics, effects on intestinal blood flow, 396
Chylomicra, in endothelium of initial lymphatics, 28
Circulation agents, effect on colonic circulation, capillary filtration, and oxygen uptake, 134–135,137,138
Clinical efficacy, of vasopressin, 384
Colonic blood flow, factors that alter, 134–135
Colonic circulation
  capillary fluid and solute exchange in, 137–139
  extrinsic regulation of, 136–137
  and functional hyperemia, 136
  hemodynamics of, 131–133
  intrinsic regulation of, 133–136
  nervous influences on, 137
  parasympathetic nerve stimulation effects on, 137
  physiology, pharmacology, and pathology of, 131–142
  and pressure-flow autoregulation, 133–136
  sympathetic control of, 137
  and venous pressure elevation, 136
Colonic ischemia, results of, 373
Colonic microcirculation, discussion of, 16–17
Compliance
  calculation of, 73
  effect of vasoconstriction on, 74
Countercurrent exchange
  drug effects on, 398–399
  in intestinal absorption and blood flow, description of models and derivation of equations for, 298–302
  mechanisms in the small intestine for, 83–97
    anatomical considerations for, 83–84
    demonstration of and evidence for, 85,89–90
    experimental observations and functional implications for, 85–95
    general theoretical considerations for, 84–85
Crypts, mucosal microvascular architecture of, 14

Decompression, of obstructed bowel, effects of, 328
Denervation, effect on intestinal microvascular pressures, 254–257
Diabetes mellitus, and the splanchnic vasculature, 361–367
Diabetic microangiopathy, factors contributing to the development of, 362
Diffusible solute, amount left in circulation relative to a vascular tracer, 234–237
Diffusion
  from capillaries to central arterial vessel, 85–90
  from central arterial vessel to capillaries, 90–91

of substances in capillary exchange, 223–224
theoretically calculated times for, 88
Diffusive oxygen flux, determination of, 263
Digestion
cardiovascular changes in mesenteric organs during, 100–102
effects of
on blood flow to neonatal stomach, small intestine and colon, 185–186
on neonatal gastrointestinal oxygen delivery, 185–186,187
general cardiovascular changes during, 99–100
Disappearance rate, determination of, 293–295
Distal splenorenal shunt, for portal hypertension, 340
Distended bowel, intestinal circulation in, 321–334
when combined with obstruction, 327–328
Diuretic drugs, for treatment of ascites, 341
Dopamine, effects on intestinal blood flow, 396
Drug effects
on blood flow metabolism, 398
on intestinal circulation, 188
Drug profiles, utility of establishment of, 399–400
Duodenal glands, microvascular architecture of, 16

Electrical activity, of lymphatic muscles, 208
Electrical stimulation, of splanchnic nerves of cat, effects of, 75
Epinephrine
discovery of, 4
effects of
on intestinal blood flow, 394–396
on lymphatic contractility, 203
Exchange vessels, response to ischemia and shock, 306–307
Exclusion phenomenon, discussion of, 212–213
Exercise
circulatory response to
in dogs, 159
in humans, 160
regional oxygen transport during, 156–157
Experimental hypertension, in rats, intestinal hemodynamics of, 350–351
Extracellular space (ECS), determination of, 211
Extramural vessels of intestine, microcirculatory structure and organization of, 9–10
Extrinsic innervation, in intestinal vascular responses, 68

Fasting, lipid transport during, 195–196
Fat absorption, and intestinal lymph flow, 197
Fenestrae, of capillaries
description of, 19–23
fine structure and distribution of, 22
permeability of, 22–23
Fluid absorption
capillaries in, 216–218
and changes in capillary filtration coefficient, 216,217
and excluded volume fraction of albumin, 212
hydrostatic pressure during, 213,214
interaction of interstitium, lymphatics, and capillaries during, 218–220
and intestinal interstitial volume expansion
illustration of, 212
physiologic consequences of, 212–213
lymphatics in, 215–216

role of plasma oncotic pressure in, 217
and vascular permeability, 217–218
Fluid flux, determination of, 276
Food, mesenteric vascular response to, mechanisms in the, 102–104
Functional hyperemia
countercurrent multiplier in, 95
effect on colonic circulation, 136
and intestinal circulation, 37
regional effects, 44–45

Gastric inhibitory polypeptide, effects on gastrointestinal blood flow, 129
Gastrin, effects on intestinal blood flow, 124–126
comparison with CCK and secretin effects, 125
Gastrointestinal hormones
and intestinal blood flow, 121–130,396
vascular effects of, in small intestine, 122–123
Glucagon, effects of
on intestinal blood flow, 126,397
on intestinal secretion and absorption, 228–229
on transcapillary fluid exchange, 407–408
Glucose, PS product in small intestine and other organs, 237
Glucose-electrolyte absorption, events in, 218–219
implications for absorption of other substances, 219–220
Glucose-stimulated oxygen demand, metabolic response to, 37

Heat stress, regulatory problems with, 157
Heat transport
blood volume shifts with, 157–158
splanchnic and renal vasoconstriction associated with, 158
Hemodynamics, of colonic blood flow, 131–133
Hemorrhage, in humans
blood volume effects of, 75
splanchnic response to, 154
stimulation of, 154
Histamine
effects of
on intestinal blood flow, 396
on intestinal secretion, 230
on lymphatic contractility, 204
on transcapillary fluid exchange, 405–407
5-Hydroxytryptamine, role in mesenteric hyperemia, 104
Hypercapnia, as candidate vasodilator metabolite, 43
Hyperosmolar compartment, of intestinal villi, 94–95
Hypertension
ileal vascular smooth muscle membrane abnormalities in, 356–357
intestinal hemodynamics in
in dogs, 351–355,357
in man, 350,357
in rats, 350–351,357
and intestinal microvascular pressures, 258–259
Hypoxia
as candidate vasodilator metabolite, 43–44
regional oxygen transport during, 157
Hypoxic hypoxemia, response of fetal and neonatal intestine to, 182,184

Ileal blood flow, in hypertensive dogs, 353–355
Ileal vascular smooth muscle, membrane abnormalities in, in hypertension, 356–357

Indicator dilution studies, for determining intestinal capillary permeability
  factors influencing, 238–239
  results in other splanchnic organs, 236–238
  results in small intestine of, 235–236
  theory behind, 233
Inflammatory bowel disease
  and colonic circulation, 141
  factors in, 140–141
Initial lymphatics, intestinal
  endothelial intercellular junctions of, 27,28
  general fine structure of, 26–27
  illustration of, 17,26
  permeability of, 27–28
  role in absorption, 26
Insulin
  extraction pattern in rat small intestine for, 238
  PS product in small intestine and other organs, 236–238
  factors influencing, 238–239
Interstitial edema, in small intestine, safety factors against, 139
Interstitial forces, in nonabsorbing and absorbing small bowel, summary of, 219
Interstitial hydrostatic pressure, effects of active absorption on, 283–286
Interstitial oncotic pressure changes, induced by net fluid absorption, factors in measurement of, 213–215
Interstitium, in intestinal lymph flow, 191–192
Interstitium, role in transcapillary exchange during intestinal fluid absorption, 211–215
Intestinal absorption
  countercurrent delay of, 88–89
  discussion of, 85–87
  equation for, 85
  and lymph flow, 193–194
  permeability factors affecting, 88
  transcapillary exchange during, role of interstitium in, 211–215
Intestinal absorption and blood flow, models of the relationship of, 289–304
  interrelationships among, 290,292,296,298,300
  predictions of, 293–294,297,301–302
  with countercurrent exchange, 298–302
  with more than one absorptive site and without countercurrent exchange, 294–298
  with one absorptive site and without countercurrent exchange, 289–294
Intestinal arterioles, innervation of, 61–62
Intestinal blood flow
  chemical agent effects on, 111–114
  CNS control of, 61–62
  drug effects on, 394–397
  early studies of, 5
  of the fetus
    calculation of, 180
    methodology in determining, 180
  gastrointestinal hormone effects on, 121–130
  intraarterial acetylcholine effects on, 111,112
  and luminal distension of intestinal wall, effects of, 109–110
  and motility, 107–120
  and nerve stimulation, effects of, 62–63,110–111
  pharmacology of, 393–402
  relationship with oxygen consumption, 149–150
    model of, 150
  rhythmic vs tonic contraction effects on, 107–109
Intestinal blood volume
  effect of flow changes on, equation for, 77
  and intestinal vascular capacitance, 76
Intestinal capacitance
  and blood volume, 76
  effects of drugs and hormones on, 78–79
  future research on, 79
  and hemorrhage, 78
  reflex control of, 78
Intestinal capillaries, permeability characteristics of, 233–248
  indicator dilution studies of, 233–239
  to macromolecules, 239–247
  osmotic transient studies of, 239
  to small solutes, 233–239
  vascular washout studies of, 247
Intestinal capillary exchange
  and active fluid absorption, 283–286
  and active fluid secretion, 283,284
  mathematical model of, 275–287
    computer techniques in development of, 277–278
    flow chart of, 278
    methods in, 275–278
    simulation of, 279–286
    variables used in determination of, 277
  venous pressure elevation or plasma dilution effects on, model predictions for, 279–280
Intestinal circulation
  capillary recruitment in, 33,34,35
  concepts regarding, historical perspective on, 1–8
  during arterial hypertension, 349–360
  effect of arterial hypoxia on, 35–36
  effect of functional or metabolic hyperemia on, 37
  effect of luminal distension and obstruction on, 321–324
  mechanisms that regulate, 33–47
  myogenic and venous-arteriolar responses in, 49–60
  and oxygen uptake, 39
  perinatal, 179–190
    chemical correlations in the study of, 188
    effects of catecholamines on, 188
    effects of changes in oxygen supply and demand on, 181–186
    effects of gastrointestinal peptides on, 188
    growth and development of, 180–181
    methodology in the study of, 179–180
    neural and neurohumoral control of, 186–188
  physiology of
    milestones in research on the, 3
    modern study of, 5–7
  precapillary sphincter in, 33–34
Intestinal compliance, passive effects of, 76–77
Intestinal countercurrent exchanger
  evaluation of, for absorption of various solutes, 85–90
  extravascular short circuiting in, 91
  factors affecting permeability of exchange area, 87–88
  functional implications for, 85,89
  importance of mean transit time for efficacy of, 88
  and lipid absorption, 90
  as a multiplier, 91–95
  substances trapped in, 90

Intestinal countercurrent multiplier
  components of, 91–93
  effect of, on Starling forces across subepithelial villus capillaries, 95
  factors determining efficacy of, 92
  proposed mechanism for, 91–92
  role in functional hyperemia of gut, 95
  substantiation of theory for, 92–94
Intestinal growth, of fetus and neonate, 179
Intestinal hemodynamics, in hypertension
  in dogs, 351–355
  in man, 350
  in rats, 350–351
Intestinal interstitial volume
  effect of active fluid secretion on, 283, 284
  forces governing regulation of, 276
Intestinal ischemia
  forms of, 372
  general cardiovascular effects of, 314–316
  and intestinal secretion, 229
  occlusive vs nonocclusive, 372–374
  site of, 372
Intestinal lymph
  composition of, 192–193
  flow of, 192–195, 197
  formation of, 191–200
  and lipid transport, 195–198
Intestinal microcirculation, spacial organization and fine structure of, 9–31
Intestinal motility
  effects on blood flow, 107–111, 323–324
  and hypoxia or ischemia, 115–116
  and nerve stimulation, effects of, 110–111
  with reduced bowel flow, 115–116
Intestinal mucosal damage, in ischemia and shock, 310–314
Intestinal obstruction, effects of, 325–327
Intestinal oxygenation
  anatomical and physiological bases of, mathematical model of, 262
  balance between oxygen supply and uptake in, 261–267
  drug effects on, 395
  future directions in the study of, 273
  graphic analysis of, 264–267
  local microvascular control of, 267–271
    autoregulation in, 269–271
    general considerations in, 267–268
    mathematical model of, 268–269
    other phenomena in, 272–273
    postprandial hyperemia in, 271–273
    vasopressin effects on, 380–381
  vasoregulation of, 261–273
Intestinal secretion, and lymph flow, 194–195
Intestinal shock, red blood cell flow before, during and after, 308
Intestinal transcapillary fluid exchange
  effects of acetylcholine on, 409
  effects of bradykinin on, 408
  effects of histamine on, 405–407
  effects of glucagon on, 407–408
  effects of isoproterenol on, 408
  effects of pentagastrin on, 407–408
  effects of prostaglandin E_2 on, 408
  effects of vasopressin on, 408
  effects of vasopressin analogs on, 408–409
  pharmacology of, 403–410
Intestinal vascular capacitance, discussion of, 76–79
Intestinal vascular responses, role of extrinsic innervation in, 68
Intestinal vasculature, early portrayal and studies of, 1–4
Intestinal vasoconstrictors, therapy with, 377–392
Intestinal villi, early microscopic examination of, 2
Intestine
  modern study of, 5
  role in pathogenesis of hemorrhagic shock, 5
Intralymphatic pressures
  and lymphatic contractility, relation between, 204–205
  for various regions of intestinal lymphatic system, 204
Ionic composition, of villus, studies of, 92–94
Irreversible shock, possible events explaining the role of small intestine in, 315–316
Ischemia
  effects of colonic circulation, 140
  intestinal hemodynamics in, 305–310
Ischemic bowel disease
  clinical evaluation in, 374–376
  therapy for, 376
Isoproterenol, effects of
  on lymphatic contractility, 203–204
  on transcapillary fluid exchange, 408
Isovolemic anemia, effect on perinatal intestinal circulation, 182

Krogh's model, of control of splanchnic blood flow, 158–159
Krypton absorption, in small intestine mucosa, 88–90

Lactate dehydrogenase (LDH), in study of blood-lymph exchange, 242–243
Lactoglobulin, PS product in small intestine and other organs, 237
  factors influencing, 238–239
Lavteals, see Initial lymphatics
Lipid absorption
  explanation for variability in, 90
  role of intestinal lymphatics in, 195
Lipid transport
  during fasting, 195–196
  by portal venous blood, 196
  role of lymphatics in, 195, 196
Lipids, partition of absorbed, between portal venous blood and intestinal lymph, 196
Local circulatory control
  factors affecting, 35–44
  future directions in studies of, 45–46
  metabolic theory of, 33
  myogenic theory of, 33
  regional differences in, 44–45
  two-component metabolic model of, 33–35
Local reflex, in moderation of microvascular pressures, 257–258
Lower-body negative pressure (LBNP)
  circulatory response to, 154–155
  and simulation of hemorrhage, 154
Luminal distension, of intestinal wall, effect on blood flow, 109–110
Luminal pressure, of bowel
  in obstruction, 325, 329

Luminal pressure, of bowel *(contd.)*
  relationship with blood flow, 324–325
  with distension, 325,329
Lymph studies, in determining intestinal capillary permeability
  effect of solute charge on, 242–245
  factors influencing, 246–247
  results for other splanchnic organs, 242
  results for small intestines, 241–242
  theory in, 239–241
Lymph-to-plasma (LP) concentration ratios
  effect of charge on, 242–245
  filtration-rate-independent, in study of capillary permeability, 242
  for LDH1 to LDH5, at 0 mm Hg pressure, 245
  relationship to solute radius for several organs, 240
  in small intestine of cat and rat, 240–242
Lymph transport, factors affecting, 201
Lymphatic circulation
  of colon, 131
  of small and large intestine, 132
Lymphatic contractility, 201–210
  effects of drugs or chemicals on, 203–204
  effects of vasoactive substances on, 204
  and intralymphatic pressure, relationship between, 204–205
  methods in the study of, 202–203
  nervous regulation of, 205–208
    effect of propranol and phenoxybenzamine on, 206–208
    effect of tetrodotoxin on, 206
  role in fluid absorption from small intestine, 208–209
Lymphatic ducts, perfusion of, 203
Lymphatic fluid fluxes, in nonabsorbing and absorbing small bowel, 219
Lymphatic muscles, electrical activity of, 208
Lymphatic system
  general architecture of, 25–26
  general fine structure of, 26–27
  microcirculatory structure of, 25–28
  permeability of, 27–28
Lymphatic valve, photomicrograph of, 206,207
Lymphatic-venous shunt, in treatment of ascites, 343–344

Major intramural blood vessels, microcirculatory structure and organization of, 10
Mechanoactive receptors
  effect of stimulation on, 169–170
  reflexes from, 167–170
Membrane abnormalities, in ileal vascular smooth muscle, in hypertension, 356–357
Membrane coefficients, in nonabsorbing and absorbing small bowel, 219
Mesenteric hyperemia
  osmotic and metabolic mechanisms in, 103–104
  role of endogenous chemical substances in, 104
Mesenteric lymphatics, histology of, 201
Mesenteric pedicle, contractility of, 209
Mesenteric vascular response
  to food, mechanisms of the, 102–104
  to intraduodenal installation of various agents, 103
Mesenteric vein pressure-volume curves, in normotensive and hypertensive dogs, 356
Mesentery, microcirculatory structure of, 9–10

Metabolic control theory, in regulation of intestinal circulation during hypoxia, support for, 35–36
Metabolic hyperemia, and intestinal circulation, 37
Metabolic vasodilation, and capillary exchange capacity, 38
Methionine enkephalin (met-enkephalin), effect of infusion of, on intestinal blood flow, motility, and oxygen consumption, 112,114
Microcirculatory structure
  of blood exchange vessels, 19–25
  of colon, 16–19
  of crypts, 14
  of duodenal glands, 16
  of extramural vessels, 9–10
  of fenestrae, 22–23
    fine structure and distribution of, 22
    permeability of, 22–23
  of lymphatic system, 25–28
    fine structure of, 26–27
    general architecture of, 25–26
    permeability of, 27–28
  of mesentery, 9–10
  of small intestine, 11–16
  of tissue channels, 23–25
  of villi, 11–15
    of cat, 12,15
    of dog, 12–14,17
    of human, 14,18
    of rabbit, 12,13
    of rat, 12,15
Microfilaments, and vasoconstriction of villous arcade vessels, 21–22
Microvascular architecture, *see* Microcirculatory structure
Microvascular branching, in rat intestine, 251
Microvascular pressure, in the small intestine, 249–260
  control of, 253–256
  effect of intestinal absorption on, 255–256
  effects of reflex activity by sympathetic nervous system at normal and reduced arterial pressures, 253–255,256,257
  and hypertension, 258–259
  local reflex or myogenic mechanisms in, 257–258
  of rat, 250–253
Minimum flow, use of term, 149
Mitochondrial oxygen utilization, determination of rate of, 263–264
Morphine, effect on intestinal motility, 113–114,116
Motility, *see* Intestinal motility
Mucosal capillary surface area, alteration of, 149
Mucosal damage, in hypotensive states, 310
  grading of, 311
Mucosal epithelial topology, of small intestine, 11
Mucosal fluid fluxes, in nonabsorbing and absorbing small bowel, 219
Mucosal microvascular architecture, *see* Microcirculatory structure
Muscle layer capillary pressures, in innervated and denervated rat intestine preparations at various systemic arterial pressures, 254,255
Myogenic mechanism, in maintenance of intestinal microvascular pressure, 257–258
Myogenic response, in the intestine, 49–60
  of an arteriolar network, 59
  explanation of, 49

to intravascular pressure elevation, evidence for, 50–51
sustained, 50–59
transient, 49–50,57

Nerve endings (receptors), in abdominal viscera, electrophysiological studies of, 165–167
Nerve stimulation, effects of, on gastrointestinal motility and blood flow, 110–111
Nervous influences, on colonic circulation, 137
Net capillary filtration, equation for, 192–193
Net fluid transfer, across capillaries, forces in, 224
Neural control, and autoregulatory escape, 61–71
Neural reflex control, of intestinal circulation of fetus and neonate, 186–187
Neurohumeral control, of intestinal circulation during development, 188
Neurotensin, effect on gastrointestinal blood flow, 128
Neurotransmitters, effects on intestinal secretion, 228
Nociceptive reflex, thresholds in stomach and small intestine, comparison in cats and man, 174
Nonocclusive intestinal ischemia
 causes and consequences of, 372–374
 clinical considerations in, 372
 development of, 371
 diagnosis of, 369–371
 evaluation and management of, 374–376
 features of, 374
 forms of, 372
 pathophysiology of, 369–376
Nonspecific vasodilators, effects of, on intestinal blood flow, 397
Norepinephrine, effect of, on lymphatic contractility, 203

Obstructed bowel
 effects of decompression on, 328
 effects on hemodynamic variables, 326–327
 intestinal circulation in, 321–334
  when combined with distension, 327–328
Occlusive intestinal ischemia, causes and results of, 372–374
Oncotic pressure, in patients with liver disease, 344–345
Opiate agonists, effect on gastrointestinal blood flow, 127
Orthostatic adjustments, in splanchnic blood flow, 156
Osmolality, of villus
 levels in man and cat of, 94
 studies of, 92–94
Osmotic reflection coefficients
 effects of various physiologic and pharmacologic interventions on, 246,403–404
 of intestinal capillaries
  to total plasma proteins, 403–404
  for various macromolecules, 241–242,243
 use of, 240–241
Osmotic transient studies, for determination of intestinal capillary permeability, 239
Ouabain-sensitive ^{86}Rb uptake, by mesenteric arteries and veins, 356–357
Oxygen consumption, in the bowel
 effect of distension on, 322,323
  in obstructed and nonobstructed specimens, 327–328,329
 relationship with blood flow, 41,150,325,326
Oxygen convection, physiological control of, 261–263
Oxygen extraction, mathematical model for, 143

Oxygen supply-uptake interactions
 graphic analysis of, 264–267
 with blood flow changes, 265
 with changes in capillary density, 266
 with changing oxygen demand, 266–267
Oxygen transport, stages of, 261–264
Oxygen uptake
 and blood flow
  drug effects on, 397–399
  experimental problems in, 399
  relationship of, 40,41,397–399
 factors that alter, 134–135
 and intestinal circulation, 39–42

Pancreatic proteases, effects on mucosal damage, from ischemia and shock, 314
Parallel-coupled vascular sections, in arterial hypotension and shock, 308–310
Passive intestinal secretion, methods for induction of, 226
Passive secretory mechanisms, in capillary exchange and secretion, 223–227
Pentagastrin, effects of
 on absorption and secretion, 230
 on transcapillary fluid exchange, 407–408
Perfusion, organ control of, 33
Perinatal intestinal oxygenation
 with increased oxygen demand, 183–186
 with reduced oxygen supply, 181–183
Peripheral chemoreceptor reflexes, and cardiovascular regulation in fetal and neonatal animals, 186–187
Peritoneo-venous shunt, in treatment of ascites, 343–344
Permeability
 of fenestrae, 22–23
 of intestinal capillaries
  characteristics of, 233–248
  to macromolecules, 239–247
  to small solutes, 233–239
Permeability surface area product (PS), for various solutes
 determination of, 233–234,235
 in small intestine and other organs, 236–238
Permeation rate, of transported substances through capillary wall, determination of, 290–291
Phenoxybenzamine, and propranolol, effect on nervous stimulation of lymphatic contraction, 206–208
Plasma oncotic pressure, effects of changes in
 on fluid absorption, 217
 on interstitial volume and hydrostatic pressure, 279–281
Polyethylene glycol (PEG), effect on blood flow in jejunal segments containing, 102
Pore dimensions, in capillaries of small intestine and other organs, 242,244
Pore stripping analysis, for lymphatic protein flux, data from small intestines under control conditions, 243
Portal hemodynamics, major clinical manifestations of, 336,338
Portal hypertension
 discussion of, 335–347
 factors controlling, 336–337
 possible explanation for, 336,345–346
 treatment of, 339–341
  drugs or hormones in, 338–339
  nonoperative, 337–339
  operative, 339–341

Portal hypertension *(contd.)*
  visceral circulation in, 336
    schematic representation of, 337
Portal venous flow, effect of vasopressin on, 379–380
Portasystemic shunt
  in treatment of ascites, 341–343
    possible contraindications to, 343
  in treatment of portal hypertension, 339–340
Postprandial hyperemia, effects on intestinal oxygenation, 271–272
Postprandial mesenteric hyperemia, discussion of, 96–106
Precapillary sphincters, response to ischemia and shock by, 306
Pressure distribution, within rat small intestine, 250–253
Pressure-flow autoregulation
  and colonic circulation, 133–136
  definition of, 133
  effect on isolated small bowel, 38
  effect of metabolic rate of intestine on, 38–39,40
  and intestinal circulation, 37–39
  regional effects of, 44
Propranolol, effects of
  on nervous stimulation of lymphatic contraction, with and without phenoxybenzamine, 206–208
  on splanchnic blood volume, 388–389
Prostaglandin D_2 (PGD_2), effects of infusion of, on intestinal blood flow, motility, and oxygen consumption, 112,114
Prostaglandin E_2 (PGE_2), effects on transcapillary fluid exchange, 408
Prostaglandin F_2 (PGF_2), effects of infusion of, on intestinal blood flow, motility, and oxygen consumption, 113,115
Prostaglandins, effects of
  on intestinal blood flow, 397
  on intestinal secretion, 229
Protein
  flux, determination of, 276–277
  lymphatic transport of, from the intestine, 197–198

Raffinose
  extraction pattern for, in rat small intestine, 238
  PS product for, in small intestine and other organs, 236–238
Reactive hyperemia, intestinal response to
  metabolic control of, 36–37,133
  myogenic control of, 133
  regional differences in control of, 44
Receptor stimulants and blockers, effects on intestinal blood flow, 394
Red cell transit time, in capillaries of normal and diabetic rats, 364–366
Red cell velocity
  in capillaries of normal and diabetic rats, 364–366
  during change in arterial pressure
    discussion of underlying mechanisms in, 49–50
    recording of, 50
Reduced perfusion pressure, effect on intestines of fetus and neonate, 182–183
Reflex cardiovascular effects, caused by traction on mesentery or distension of hollow organs, 167–168
Reflex studies, of mechanosensitive and chemosensitive receptors, 167–172

Regional hypotension, extent of damage found before, during, and after, 312
Regional oxygen transport
  in exercise, 156–157
  in hypoxia, 157
Renkin's equation, for extraction, 143
Resistance vessels, response to ischemia and shock by, 305–306
Rhythmic contractions, of intestinal mucosa
  comparison with tonic contraction effects on blood flow, 108
  effect on intestinal blood flow, 107–109
  indication of, 108
^{86}Rubidium (^{86}Rb) uptake, ouabain-sensitive, by mesenteric arteries and veins, 356–357

Salt hypertension, findings in rats with, 351
Secretin, effects on intestinal blood flow, 124
  comparison with gastrin and CCK effects, 125
Series-coupled vascular sections
  description of, 305
  response to arterial hypotension and shock, 305–308
Serotonin, effects on intestinal blood flow, 396
Shock
  intestinal hemodynamics in, 305–310
  small bowel in, 305–319
Shunt operations
  for ascites, 341–344
  for portal hypertension
    advantages and disadvantages of, 339–340
    alternatives to, 340–341
Small bowel, in arterial hypotension and shock, 305–319
Small intestine
  countercurrent exchange mechanisms in, 83–97
  microvascular pressure in, 249–260
    physical considerations in measurement of, 249–250
Small intramural blood vessels, microcirculatory structure and organization of, 10–19
Solute diffusion, effects of interstitial matrix on, 212–213
Sodium deoxycholate, effect of, on active intestinal secretion, 227
Sodium pump activity, in hypertension, 357
Solute exchange, in colonic circulation, 139
Somatostatin, effects of
  comparison with other drugs of, 388
  on gastrointestinal blood flow, 127–128
  on splanchnic blood flow, 387–388
Spinal afferent fibers
  innervating chemosensitive receptors, existence of, 167
  myelination of, 165
  response to bradykinin or isoproterenol stimulation, 165,166
  terminal structures of, 165–167
Spinal reflex, in response to venous pressure elevation, 51
Splanchnic blood flow (SBF)
  during exercise, 156–157
  response to orthostatic adjustments, 156
  response to pressure changes, 155–156
  role in systemic blood flow regulation, 156–158
  and tissue oxygenation, 143–151
  vasopressin effects on, 377–378,380
Splanchnic blood volume (SBV), effect of hemorrhage on, 154

SUBJECT INDEX

Splanchnic circulation
  and heart rate during exercise, 160–161
  role of
    in blood volume distribution, 158–160
    in reflex control of cardiovascular system, 153–163
Splanchnic nerves, role of, in control of intestinal blood flow, 61
Splanchnic organ oxygen consumption, regulation of, 148–149
Splanchnic region, role of, in blood pressure regulation, 153–156
Splanchnic vascular capacitance, characteristics of, 73–76
Splanchnic vascular conductance, results of changes in, in humans, 76
Splanchnic vascular resistance (SVR)
  effect of hemorrhage on, 154
  response to other pressure changes, 155
Splanchnic vasculature, in diabetes mellitus, 361–367
Splanchnic vasoconstrictors, substances that act as, 378
Starling forces, across subepithelial villus capillaries, influence of countercurrent multiplier on, 95
Starling's hypothesis, in determining capillary fluid exchange, 137–138
Streptozoticine (STZ) diabetic rats, diabetic microangiopathy in, 363–364
Stress-relaxation, and vascular volume change, 77
Submucous microvessels, intestinal microcirculatory structure of, 10–11
Substance P, effect on gastrointestinal blood flow, 128–129
Superoxide dismutase (SOD), effects of treatment with, 310–311,313,314
Superoxide radicals
  cytotoxic effects of, 311
  effects of pretreatment with, 310–314
Sustained myogenic response, in the intestine, 50–59
  possible mechanism for, 57–58
Sympathectomy, effects of, on intestinal secretion, 228
Sympathetic nerve stimulation, in control of capacitance vessels, 77–78

Tension-related myogenic response, morphological basis for, 58–59
Tetrodotoxin, effect of, on nervous stimulation of lymphatic contraction, 206
Tissue channels, in interstitial tissues, 23–25
  electron micrograph of, 24,25
  methods for observation and quantitation of, 23–25
Tissue colloid osmotic pressure
  changes in, 225–226
  estimation of, 224–225
  and LP ratio, 225
Tissue compliance, stages for increases in, 225
Tissue hypoxia, and mucosal damage, 310
Tissue oxygenation
  during absorption, 145–148
  and splanchnic blood flow, 143–151
Tissue PO_2
  in diabetic and normal rats, 364–365
  in intestinal muscle layer, 144–145
    following glucose exposure, 146,147
  at rest, determination of, 143–145
  in villi of rats, 144–147
    following glucose exposure, 146,147
    variation in, 144
Tonic contractions, of intestinal mucosa, effects on intestinal blood flow, 107–109
  comparison with rhythmic contraction effects, 108
Total resistance, in blood vessels, measurement of, 249
Transcapillary fluid exchange, see Intestinal transcapillary fluid exchange
Transcapillary oxygen flux, role of arteriolar feedback, precapillary sphincter feedback, and passive factors in augmenting, 272
Transient myogenic response, in the intestine, 49–50

Vagotomy, effects of, on mesenteric blood flow, 228
Varix hemorrhage, as cause of portal hypertension, 335–337
Vascular anatomy
  of intestine in general, 250
  of rat intestine, 250,251
Vascular capacitance, role of vascular pressure-volume relationship in, 73,74
Vascular permeability, and fluid absorption, 217–218
Vascular pressure-volume relationship, in vascular capacitance, 73,74
Vascular washout studies, for determination of intestinal capillary permeability, 247
Vasoactive agents
  effects of, on colonic circulation and oxygenation, 137,138
  response of lymphatic strips to, 204
    dose response curves for, 205
Vasoactive intestinal polypeptide (VIP), effects of
  on intestinal blood flow, 126–127
    when combined with atropine or guanethidine, 127
  on intestinal secretion, 229
Vasoconstriction, effect of arterial and venous pressure changes on, 54–56
Vasoconstrictor agents, effects of, on splanchnic blood flow, 389
Vasodilator therapy, for intestinal ischemia, 376
Vasopressin
  administration of, route of, 377–378
  clinical efficacy of, 384
  clinical trials of, results of, 383
  complications of therapy with, 385–387
    reversal of, 386
  dose-response studies on, 381–382
  effects of
    on colonic blood flow, 379
    on hepatic arteries, 379
    on intestinal blood flow, 396
    on intestinal transcapillary fluid exchange, 408–409
    on intestinal oxygen consumption, 380–381
  other potential applications of, 387
  systemic effects of, 382–384
Vasopressin analogs
  action of, 385
  effects of, on transcapillary fluid exchange, 408–409
Venous arteriolar response, influence of blood oxygen levels on, 51–53
Venous compliance, in hypertension, 355–356
Venous drainage, of small and large intestines, 9
Venous hypertension, effect on colonic circulation, 140

Venous pressure elevation
    diameter and pressure changes in mesenteric arterioles during a single step change in, 54,55
    effect of, on colonic circulation, 136
    and plasma dilution, 279–281
Villi
    cat
        electron micrograph of, 15,86,87
        plasma mean transit time in, 85,88
        topographical relationship of, 86
    hemodynamics of, 308–310
    microcirculatory architecture of, 11–15,17,18
        of cat, 12,15,86,87
        of dog, 12–14,17
        of human, 14,18
        of rabbit, 12,13
        of rat, 12,15
    permeability of, 84
    vascular anatomy of, schematic representation of, 83,84
Villous hemodynamics, and circulation, 308–310
Villous tissue PO_2, see Tissue PO_2

Wall stress-related myogenic response, see Tension-related myogenic response
Water, see Intestinal absorption